DIGESTIVE SYSTEM

Dr. Greeshma Sharma

ALLIED HEALTH PRESS

Digestive System

Author: **Dr. Greeshma Sharma**

Allied Health Press
4164 Lakeshore Road
Burlington ON L7L 1A4
Canada
www.alliedhealthpress.com
Email: orders@arclereducation.com

ISBN: 978-1-77956-231-9

ABOUT THE AUTHOR

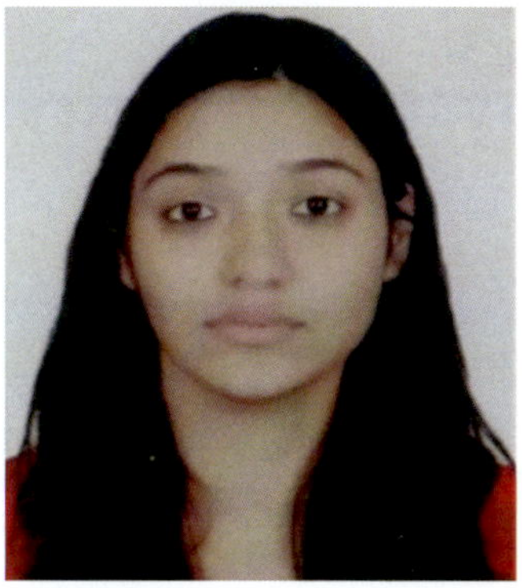

Dr. Greeshma Sharma, a post doctoral Project Scientist, in one of the most reputed research institutes of India. She holds a Ph.D in the field of Maternal and Child health care, with specialization in Neonatalogy, and Molecular Biology. UGC qualified in Forensic Science, with an expertise in Forensic Biotechnology. She has received an international scholarship (Harold Gunson fellowship, International Society of Blood Transfusion) and holds 9+ years of Research experience, which includes reviewing articles, writing research articles as well as proposal for extramural funding. Serving in the field of freelance writing ad research since 2020.

Word Roots, Prefixes, and Suffixes by Chapter

Chapter 1 The Beginning of the Digestive Tract

endo-:within, in
sub-: under, below
dys-: painful, abnormal, difficult, labored
an/o: anus
cec/o: cecum
col/o: colon
-ac: pertaining to
-al: pertaining to
-iasis: condition
-itis: inflammation

Chapter 2 The Stomach: Basic Functions and Control Mechanisms

abdomin/o: abdomen, abdominal
antr/o: antrum
chol/e: gall, bile
choledoch/o: common bile duct
rect/o: rectum
endo-:within, in
sub-:under, below
dys-: painful, abnormal, difficult, labored

Chapter 3 The Pancreas

a/an: Without or none
gram: the image (X-ray)
itis: inflammation
macro: large
micro: small
osis: abnormal condition

Chapter 4 Liver and Biliary System

endo-: within, in
sub-: under, below
dys-: painful, abnormal, difficult, labored
abdomin/o: abdomen, abdominal
cholangi/o: bile duct
col/o: colon
diverticul/o: diverticulum
duoden/o: duodenum
enter/o: intestine

Chapter 5 The Small Intestine

Exo-: Outside
Peri-: Surrounding
Retro-: Backward, back
-ase: Enzyme
-flux: Flow
-ectomy: Surgical removal, cutting out
-iasis: Abnormal condition
-itis: Inflammation
-lithiasis; Calculus or stone

Chapter 6 Digestion and Absorption

endo-:within, in
sub-: under, below
abdomin/o: abdomen, abdominal
chol/e: gall, bile
choledoch/o: common bile duct
colon/o: colon
duoden/o: duodenum
enter/o: intestine
esophag/o: esophagus
gastr/o: stomach
hepat/o: liver

Chapter 7 The Absorptive and Post-Absorptive States

-algia: pain
anti-: attacks, treats condition
-ase: an enzyme
bi-: two of
cardio-: related to the heart
contra-: to go against

-cyst: related to the bladder
-cyt(e,o)-: cell(s)
dys-: abnormal
endo-: inside
erythr(o)-: red cells
extra-: outside
gastr(o)-: stomach

Chapter 8 The Colon

ab-: away
ad-: towards
anti-: against
ante-: before
bi-: two, both
dys-: painful
endo-: inside
epi-: above, upon
hemi-: half
hyper-: excessive, above,
hypo-:decrease, below, less

Chapter 9 The Intestinal Microbiome

Anti-: Against
Auto-: Self
Dys-: Painful or difficult
Endo-: Within
Epi-: Above
Eu-: Normal
Ex-: Outwards
Hypo-: Lower than normal
Hyper-: Higher than normal
Inter-: Between
Intra-: Within
Mal-: Bad
Micro-: Small

Chapter 10 Diseases of the Digestive System

gram: the image (X-ray)
itis: inflammation
mega/ megaly: enlarged
micro: small
osis: bnormal condition
otomy: to cut into
scopy/ scopic: to look, observe
tachy-: fast
trans-: across or through

Table of Contents

3 The Pancreas 57

4 Liver and Biliary System 107

LIST OF FIGURES

LIST OF TABLES

PREFACE

The digestive system is intricately designed to break down the food we consume into its most basic components, such as glucose (a simple sugar), amino acids (the building blocks of proteins), and fatty acids (the primary components of fats). This process of digestion transforms complex food substances into substances that the body can more readily absorb. Once broken down, these nutrients are absorbed through the lining of the small intestine and then enter the bloodstream. From there, they are transported to every cell in the body, where they are utilized for various bodily functions and maintenance of health.

The role of the digestive system is crucial in maintaining overall health because it is responsible for the delivery of essential nutrients to the body. Effective digestion and nutrient absorption are fundamental not only for energy and growth but also for the proper functioning of all bodily systems. Inadequate digestive health can lead to a multitude of uncomfortable and distressing symptoms, including abdominal pain, bloating, indigestion, and other gastrointestinal disturbances. Furthermore, if the digestive system is not functioning optimally, it can lead to insufficient nutrient absorption from the food we eat. This nutritional deficiency can have a profound negative impact on an individual's health and well-being, affecting everything from energy levels to immune response and chronic disease susceptibility. Therefore, maintaining good digestive health is imperative for sustaining overall health and ensuring the body functions at its best.

This textbook "Digestive System" provides a comprehensive and detailed exploration of the human digestive system, tailored specifically for students pursuing studies in the fields of biology, medicine, and health sciences. This textbook aims to equip readers with a thorough understanding of the structure, function, and complex processes of the digestive system, ensuring that they grasp how this critical system contributes to overall health and well-being.

The content of the textbook is for both undergraduate and graduate students who are new to the subject as well as those looking to deepen their existing knowledge. Dealing with the anatomy and physiology of the digestive system, the book covers key topics such as the mechanical and chemical processes of digestion, nutrient absorption, and the intricate management of waste products. It also addresses common disorders and diseases related to the digestive system, providing insights into their diagnosis, treatment, and prevention.

The book employs a multidisciplinary approach, integrating insights from biochemistry, pathology, and nutrition to give a holistic view of how the digestive system interacts with other body systems for optimal health. This approach helps in fostering a deeper understanding and appreciation of the digestive system's role within the human body.

The book also includes a variety of learning tools such as detailed illustrations, and real-life examples that enhance comprehension and facilitate active learning. These features are designed to engage students, stimulate critical thinking, and apply theoretical knowledge to practical scenarios.

This book aims to be an authoritative resource that not only disseminates knowledge but also stimulates curiosity and fosters a profound understanding of the human digestive system, making it an indispensable part of the academic journey for students in the biological and health sciences.

Chapter 1

THE BEGINNING OF THE DIGESTIVE TRACT

Contents

Introduction

The breakdown of all the foods and liquids we ingest, into beneficial nutrients and chemicals is largely dependent on the functioning of the human digestive system. The digestive tract, or the collection of tissues and organs that pass through food and liquids as they are transformed into forms that can be absorbed into the bloodstream and delivered to tissues, makes up the majority of the digestive system. Other important parts of the digestive system include the terminal structures through which solid wastes pass in the process of elimination from the body, as well as the glands that secrete the hormones and juices needed for digestion.

Starting from the lips, the digestive tract terminates at the anus. It is made up of the tongue, which kneads food and combines it with saliva, and the mouth, or oral cavity, with its teeth for grinding food. The pharynx, which is the throat, is followed by the esophagus, the stomach, the duodenum, the jejunum, and the ileum in the small intestine, and the large intestine, which is made up of the sigmoid colon, which ends in the rectum, the ascending colon, the transverse colon, the descending colon, and the cecum, a closed-end sac connected to the ileum. Salivary glands, pancreas, gastric glands in the lining of the stomach, liver, and its adjuncts, the gallbladder and bile ducts, are among the glands that contribute digestive juices. All these glands and organs play a part in the final removal of nondigestible wastes as well as the physical and chemical breakdown of food that has been consumed (Figure 1.1).

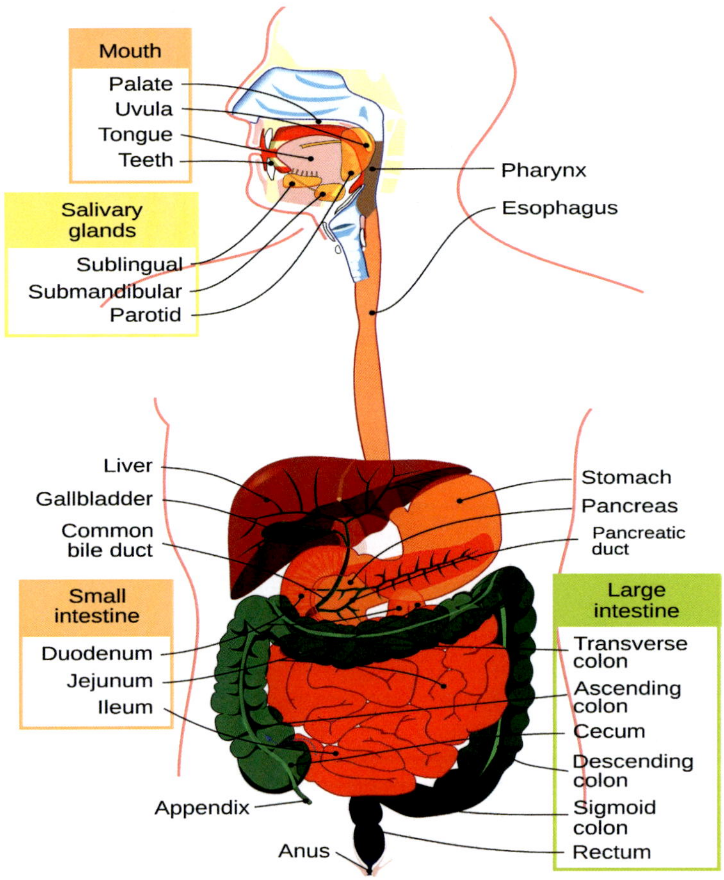

Figure 1.1. *Human digestive system.*

Source: By Mariana Ruiz, Jmarchn – Own work, Public Domain, https://commons.wikimedia.org/w/index.php?curid=2898771.

Orientation and Directional Terms

Term	Definition	Illustration
The vestibule	The space between the soft tissue (lips and cheeks), and the teeth and gums. The vestibule is kept moist by secretions from the parotid salivary glands, which are located in front of the ears and behind the angle of the jaw.	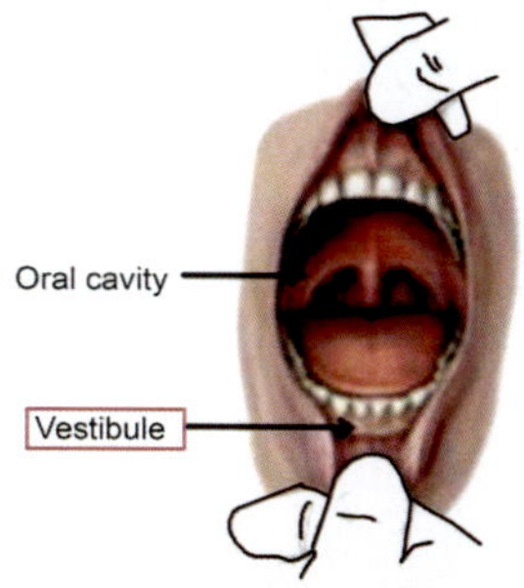
Gums	Gums are made up of the fibrous and dense tissue that lines the alveolar arches and hugs the teeth.	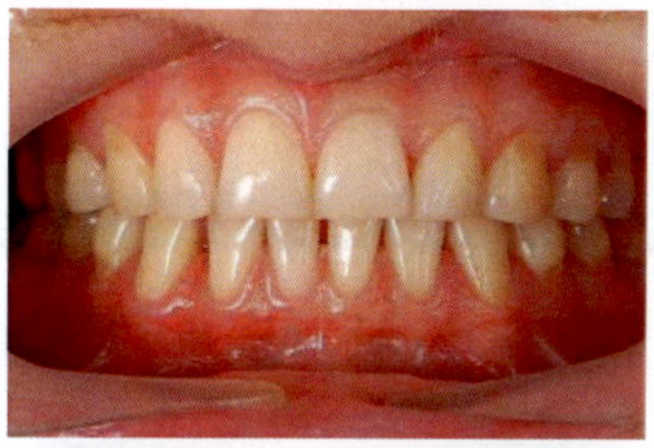
Teeth	A person has two sets of teeth over the course of a lifetime. The average child has their full set of 20 primary (or milk or baby) teeth by the age of three years. The primary teeth start to fall out between the ages of about six and seven years and are gradually replaced by permanent (or secondary or adult) teeth. By about 21 years, the average person has 32 permanent teeth – 16 in the upper jaw and 16 in the bottom jaw.	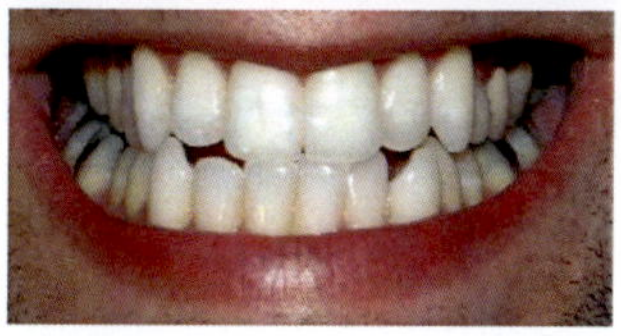
Palate	Consists of the hard and soft palates. The hard palate is the bony roof of the mouth. The soft palate is a fold of membrane that hangs between the mouth cavity and the back of the throat. The little dangling bit you can see when you stick out your tongue and say 'ah' is called the uvula.	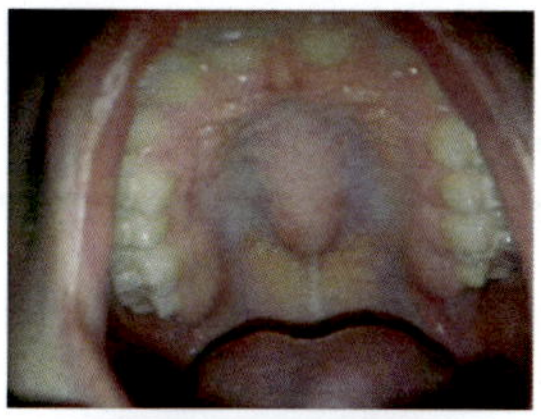
Tongue	The tongue is made up almost entirely of muscle fibers. It is divided into an oral portion (tip, blade, front, center and back) and a pharyngeal (throat) section. The tongue helps us to taste, speak and swallow.	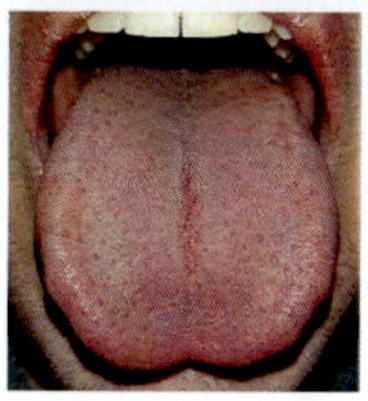

1.1. Mouth and Oral Structures

In reality, very little amount of food is digested in the mouth occurs in the mouth. However, food is prepared in the mouth for its passage through the upper digestive tract and into the stomach and small intestine, where the process of digestion occurs, through the process of mastication, or chewing. The first mechanical process that food goes through is chewing. The masseter, temporal, medial and lateral pterygoids, and buccinator are the masticatory muscles that move the lower jaw while chewing. The force of the bite is not determined by the strength of the masticatory muscles, but rather by the sensitivity of the periodontal membrane that surrounds and supports the teeth.

Adequate digestion does not require mastication. However, by breaking down food into small pieces and combining it with saliva produced by the salivary glands, chewing does help with digestion. While chewing the saliva spreads throughout the food mass, saliva lubricates and moistens dry food. A rounded mass of food, or **bolus**, is formed in part by the movement of the tongue against the cheeks and hard palate.

1.1.1. The Lips and Cheeks

The lips are supple, soft anatomical structures that define the edge of the mouth. They consist of a layer of muscle, connective tissue, and the surface epidermis (skin). The margins of the lips, often referred to as the "vermilion border,"that are rich in delicate nerve endings and have reddish skin all over them. The reddish skin serves as a transitional layer between the inner mucosa, or mucous membrane, and the outer, hair-bearing epidermis. Mucus-secreting glands abound in the mucosa, and they work in tandem with saliva to provide sufficient lubrication for speaking and chewing (Figure 1.2).

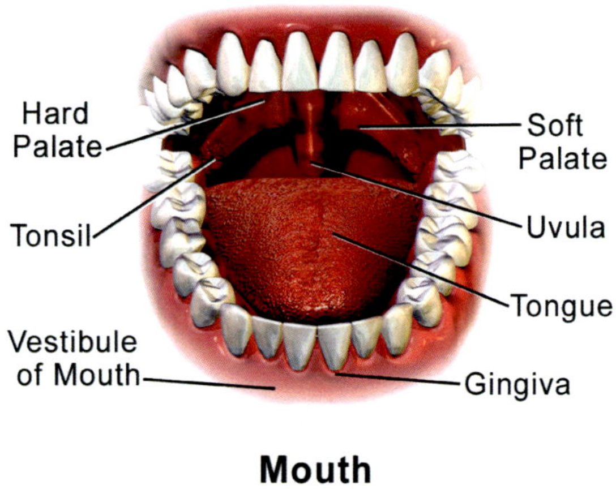

Figure 1.2. *Anatomy of the mouth.*

Source: By BruceBlaus – Own work, CC BY 3.0, https://commons.wikimedia.org/w/index.php?curid=33041243.

The inner surface of newborns has much thicker tissue, sebaceous glands, and tiny projections called papillae. These anatomical modifications appear to facilitate the sucking process. The muscle that surrounds the aperture, the orbicularis oris, supplies the majority of the substance of each lip. The numerous shapes and expressions of the lips are made possible by this muscle and others that extend into the cheeks. The sides of the mouth, or cheeks, share a similar structure and are continuous with the lips. The cheek's subcutaneous tissue, or tissue beneath the skin, contains a noticeable fat pad. This pad, referred to as the sucking pad, is particularly large in newborns. The opening of the parotid duct, which originates from the parotid salivary gland, which is situated in front of the ear, is marked by a small elevation on the inner surface of each cheek, across from the second upper molar tooth. Four to five mucus-secreting glands, the openings of whose ducts face the final molar tooth, are located directly behind this gland.

Diseases like leukoplakia (white patches, which may be precancerous) and herpes simplex (fever blisters, or cold sores) can affect the lips. Ulcers on the lower lip's vermilion border are often malignant in older men. The weather's excessive drying, chemical irritants, inadequate moistening due to infection, or an adverse reaction to antibiotics can also cause the borders to crack and become inflamed.

1.1.2. The Mouth

The opening through which food and air enter the body is the mouth, also referred to as the oral (or buccal) cavity. The mouth empties into the throat at the back after opening to the outside at the lips. The glottis, cheeks, hard and soft palates, and lips all serve as its boundaries. The vestibule, which is the space between the cheeks and the teeth, and the oral cavity proper make up its two sections. The tongue, a sizable muscle that is securely attached to the floor of the mouth by the **frenulum linguae**, occupies the majority of the latter region. The mouth and its structures are crucial for the formation of speech in humans, in addition to its primary function in the intake and initial digestion of food.

The tongue, which positions and mixes food and also carries taste receptors, the palate, which divides the mouth from the nasal cavity to allow separate passages for food and air, and the teeth, which break and grind food into small pieces that are suitable for digestion, are the main components of the mouth. By altering the way air passes through the mouth, all of these structures—along with the lips—assist in producing speech sounds. The mucous membranes that line the oral cavity and vestibule are completely covered in tiny glands. These glands, in addition to the three pairs of salivary glands, produce a fluid that keeps the mouth moist and free of food particles and other debris. Both the surfaces of the tongue and the gums (gingivae), which encircle and support the teeth, are made of specialized membranes. The tongue's surface has a rougher membrane with numerous tiny papillae that house the taste buds. Food is softened by the mouth's moist environment and the enzymes found in its secretions, which makes swallowing easier and kickstarts the digestive process.

The hard and soft palates combine to form the concave roof of the mouth. The palatine portions of the maxillae, or upper jaws, and the horizontal sections of the two palatine bones combine to form the hard palate. A thick, somewhat pale mucous membrane that is continuous with the gums covers the hard palate. Firm fibrous tissue binds the membrane to the upper jaw and palate bones. The hard palate in front and the soft palate in between are continuous. It is continuous with the mucous membrane covering the nasal cavity's floor posteriorly. The palatine aponeurosis, a robust, thin, fibrous sheet, and the glossopalatine and pharyngopalatine muscles make up the soft palate. The uvula is a tiny protrusion that protrudes freely from the back of the soft palate.

Only when the tongue is raised is the floor of the mouth visible. The frenulum linguae, located in the midline, binds each lip to the gums in addition to serving as an anchor for the tongue on the oral cavity floor. The sublingual papilla, a small fold on either side of this, is where the submandibular salivary gland ducts open. The pla sublingual, is, a ridge that extends from each sublingual papilla in both directions, which also indicates the upper border of the sublingual salivary gland, which is located beneath the tongue and is the surface where the majority of the gland ducts open.

1.1.3. The Gums

The mucous membrane covers the connective tissue that makes up the gums, also referred to as the **gingivae**. Thick fibrous tissue connects the mucous membrane to the membrane encircling the jaw bones. Every tooth's exposed portion, or base of the crown, is encircled by a collar made of rising gum tissue. As a result, the gums encircle and are attached to the necks of the teeth as well as the nearby alveolar bone. Healthy gums are tough, pink, and stippled. They also have a low sensitivity to pressure, temperature, and pain. The red alveolar mucosa is divided from the gums by a scalloped line that roughly reflects the shape of the teeth. The free gum margins surrounding the teeth jut outward into the spaces between the teeth (interdental papillae). The gum is firmly held against the teeth by internal periodontal membrane fibers. Early indicators of gum inflammation, or gingivitis, include color changes, loss of stippling, and abnormal sensitivity.

Alveolar arteries branch off into the densely packed blood vessels that make up gum tissue. These vessels, which are also responsible for supplying blood to the teeth and the spongy bone of the upper and lower jaws where the teeth are lodged, are known as alveolar because of their connection to the alveoli dentales, or tooth sockets. Gum pads, which are tiny elevations of the oral mucous membrane above, form prior to the erupting teeth entering the mouth cavity. The neck of each tooth is enveloped by gum tissue upon completion of tooth eruption.

1.1.4. The Teeth

The teeth are the white, hard structures that are part of the mouth. The teeth of various vertebrate species are sometimes specialized and are typically used for mastication. For example, snakes have extremely thin, sharp teeth that typically curve backward. They serve the purpose of capturing prey; however, since snakes swallow their food whole, they cannot chew. Compared to primates, including humans, carnivorous mammals like cats and dogs have sharper teeth than other monkeys. The premolars, which are more suited to cutting and shearing, have long canines and no flat grinding surfaces (often the more posterior molars are lost). However, the canines are frequently completely absent from herbivores like cows and horses, which have very large, flat premolars and molars with intricate ridges and cusps.

Teeth vary in shape because of functional adaptations. Although few animals are able to break down cellulose, herbivores must first break down the cellulose cell walls surrounding the plant cells they consume, for the contents of tcells to be exposed to for the action of the digestive enzymes. In contrast, the animal cells found in meat are directly accessible to the action of digestive enzymes because they are not covered in indigestible material. As a result, unlike herbivores, carnivores do not require as much chewing. Given that they consume both plant and animal tissue, humans are omnivores, meaning that their teeth fall somewhere in between the extremes of specialization that carnivore and herbivore teeth can achieve in terms of function and structure. A crown and one or more roots make up each tooth. The portion of the tooth that can be seen above the gum line is called the crown. The part of the tooth that is not visible but holds it in place in the jawbone is called the root. Animals differ from one another in the forms of their roots and crowns. In essence, the teeth on one side of the jaw are mirror reflections of the teeth on the other. The upper teeth complement the lower teeth and are different from them.

1.1.4.1. Tooth Structure

True teeth are composed of three layers and share the same general structure. Mammals have part or all of their tooth crown covered by an outer layer of enamel, which is the hardest tissue in the body and is completely inorganic. Dentine, which is similar to bone in composition and less hard than enamel, makes up the middle layer of the tooth. Covered by cementum on the roots and enamel on the crown, the dentine, which makes up the majority of a tooth's mass, is practically its whole length. The pulp, which is the tooth's innermost layer, provides nourishment for the dentine.

The pulp, which fills a cavity in the middle of the tooth, is made up of nerves, microscopic blood vessels, and cells. The pulp chamber is an expansion located at the coronal end of the long and narrow pulp canal. Through the apical foramina, or holes, at the end of the roots, the pulp canal, which stretches nearly the entire length of the tooth, connects to the body's nervous and general nutritional systems. The root of the tooth extends below the gum line, at least partially hidden by cementum. Though less hard than dentine, the latter has a structure resembling that of a bone. The cementum provides a thin layer to the root and acts as a medium for the attachment of the fibers (periodontal membrane) that secure the tooth to the surrounding tissue. Fiber bundles connect the gums to both the cementum of each tooth and the nearby alveolar bone.

1.1.4.2. Tooth Form and Function

Throughout their lives, humans have two sets of teeth, just like the majority of other mammals. The term "primary," or deciduous, teeth refers to the first set, and "permanent" teeth to the second. The number of teeth in humans is 32 permanent and 20 primary. Primary teeth are smaller than permanent teeth, with more pointed cusps, a whiter appearance and greater susceptibility to wear, as well as relatively large pulp chambers and small, delicate roots. About six months after birth, the first teeth erupt, and by the time a person is twenty-two and a half, their primary dentition is complete. Shedding starts at age five or six and ends at age thirteen. As the permanent teeth erupt toward the oral cavity during growth, the primary teeth are lost when their roots resorb.

There are 20 teeth in the human primary dentition, with two canines, four molars, and four incisors in each jaw. Premolars, also known as bicuspid teeth, take the place of primary molars in the adult dentition. There are 32 teeth in the permanent dentition overall because the 12 adult molars do not replace any of the primary teeth that erupt (emerge from the gums) behind them. Thus, in each jaw, the permanent dentition consists of four incisors, two canines, four premolars, and six molars. The teeth at the front of the mouth are called incisor teeth, and their functions include holding, tearing, cutting, and plucking. An incisor's biting edge is shaped like a chisel because it is thin and wide. Because of their sensitive tactile sense, the upper incisors can be used to identify objects in the mouth through nibbling. There is a canine, or cuspid, tooth next to the incisor on each side. Like the incisors, it is often pointed and shaped like a peg, and its purpose is to chop and tear food.

Food particles are broken up by the cusps, which are a series of elevations found on premolars and molars. Each canine has two premolars behind it that are capable of grinding and chopping food. Bicuspid refers to the fact that each premolar has two cusps. In contrast, the molars are only utilized for crushing and grinding. These teeth are located at the back of the mouth. Usually, a molar has four or five cusps. In humans, the third molar's size, number of roots, cusp pattern, and eruption are frequently variable. For incisors, canines, and premolars, there is only one root; for molars, there are two or three roots.

1.1.5. The Tongue

In the mouth of a typical tetrapod, the tongue is a muscular organ. It is the main organ of taste and manipulates food for chewing and swallowing during the digestive process. Taste buds contained in multiple lingual papillae cover the dorsum, or upper surface of the tongue. It is sensitive, has a rich blood vessel and nerve supply, and is kept moist by saliva. Additionally, the tongue acts as a natural tooth cleaner. The ability for humans to speak and for other animals to vocalize is one of the tongue's primary roles. The oral and pharyngeal portions of the human tongue are located at the front and rear, respectively. The tongue's lingual septum, a vertical segment of fibrous tissue that creates the median sulcus, a groove on its surface, divides its left and right sides for the majority of its length.

The tongue's muscles are divided into two groups. The tongue's four intrinsic muscles, which are not anchored to the bone, change its shape. The tongue is moved by the four paired extrinsic muscles, which are fixed to the bone.

1.1.5.1. Structure

The tongue is a muscular hydrostat that contributes to the oral cavity's floor. The lingual septum, a vertical segment of fibrous tissue, divides the tongue's left and right sides. This division, which is visible as a groove known as the median sulcus, runs the entire length of the tongue with the exception of the very back of the pharyngeal portion. The terminal sulcus, a V-shaped groove, separates the anterior and posterior regions of the human tongue. A blind foramen called the foramen cecum, a remnant of the median thyroid diverticulum in early embryonic development, marks the apex of the terminal sulcus. The visible portion of the tongue, known as the anterior oral part, is located at the front and accounts for about two-thirds of its length. At about one-third of its length, the posterior part of the throat is the section nearest to the throat. The neural supply and embryological development of these regions vary (Figure 1.3).

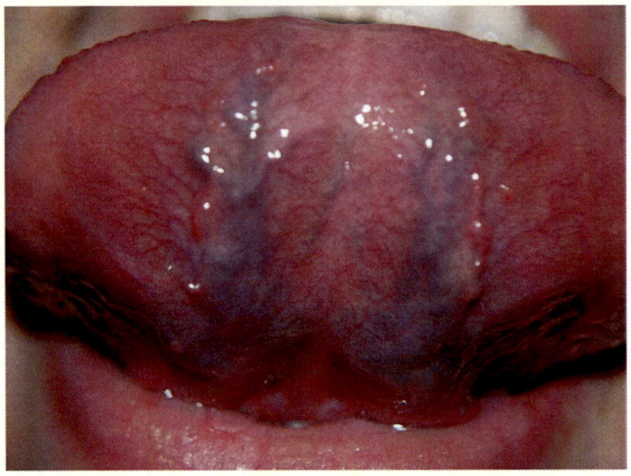

Figure 1.3. *Structure of a tongue.*

Source: By Miserlou at English Wikipedia – Transferred from en.wikipedia to Commons by Faigl.ladislav using CommonsHelper., Public Domain, https://commons.wikimedia.org/w/index.php?curid=7916581.

The anterior tongue is narrow and thin at its tip. It is aimed forward and up against the lower incisor teeth's lingual surfaces. At its root, the posterior part is directed backward. It is connected to the hyoid bone by the hyoglossi and genioglossi muscles and the hyoglossal membrane; to the epiglottis by three mucous membrane folds called the glossoepiglottic folds; to the soft palate by the glossopalatine arches; and to the pharynx by the superior pharyngeal constrictor muscle and the mucous membrane. It also creates the oropharynx's anterior wall.

The human tongue is 10 cm long on average, measuring from the oropharynx to the tip. The average weight of an adult male's tongue is 99g, while that of an adult female tongue is 79g. The tongue tip and the blade (the area directly behind the tip) are distinguished in phonetics and phonology. It is said that sounds produced with the tongue blade are laminal and sounds produced with the tongue tip are apical.

- **Upper Surface**: The tongue's upper surface, known as the dorsum, is split into symmetrical halves by the median sulcus, which forms a groove in it. This division ends at the foramen cecum, which is located approximately 2.5 cm from the tongue root, and the terminal sulcus begins at this point. In addition to serving as the thyroglossal duct's attachment point, the foramen cecum is synthesized when the thyroid diverticulum descends during embryonic development. The terminal sulcus is a shallow groove that extends from the foramen cecum to the borders (margins) of the tongue in a forward-facing V shape. The tongue is divided into an anterior oral part and a posterior throaty part by the terminal sulcus. The glossopharyngeal nerve supplies the pharyngeal part; the chorda tympani, a branch of the facial nerve, supplies the oral part; and the lingual nerve, a branch of the mandibular branch (V3) of the trigeminal nerve, supplies the somatosensory perception. The two tongue segments originate from distinct pharyngeal arches.

- **Undersurface:** The frenulum, a fold of mucous membrane on the underside of the tongue, connects the tongue's midline to the floor of the mouth. The major salivary submandibular glands drain into tiny protrusions called sublingual caruncles on either side of the frenulum.
- **Muscles:** There are two categories for the eight tongue muscles: intrinsic and extrinsic. The tongue's four intrinsic muscles function to alter its shape; they are not affixed to any particular bone. The four extrinsic muscles are attached to the bone and function to move the tongue.
- **Extrinsic:** The tongue is reached by the four extrinsic muscles, which start from the bone. These are the hyoglossus (which frequently includes the chondroglossus), the palatoglossus, the genioglossus, and the styloglossus. Their primary purposes involve; moving the tongue in different directions to facilitate protrusion, retraction, and side-to-side motion. The mandible gives rise to the genioglossus, which extends the tongue. Because it is the only muscle that moves the tongue forward, it is also referred to as the tongue's safety muscle. The tongue is retracted and depressed by the hyoglossus, which emerges from the hyoid bone. This muscle is frequently associated with the chondroglossus. The styloglossus, wh forms a trough for swallowing, is drawn up from the sides of the tongue by the stylooloid process of the temporal bone. The palatoglossus, which develops from the palatine aponeurosis, depresses the soft palate, elevates the back of the tongue during swallowing, and moves the palatoglossal fold toward the midline.
- **Intrinsic:** Along the length of the tongue, four paired intrinsic muscles originate and insert within the tongue. They are the vertical muscle, the transverse muscle, the inferior longitudinal muscle, and the superior longitudinal muscle. These muscles lengthen and shorten the tongue, curl and uncurl its edges

and apex as in tongue rolling, and flatten and round its surface, among other changes to its shape. This gives things shape and makes eating, swallowing, and speaking easier.

The superior longitudinal muscle, which is located beneath the mucous membrane on the tongue's upper surface, shortens and curls the tongue upward. It comes from the median fibrous septum at the hyoid bone, which is close to the epiglottis. The styloglossus muscle is connected to the inferior longitudinal muscle, which runs the length of the tongue. Its purpose is to curl the tongue downward and shorten it. The superior and inferior longitudinal muscles are joined by the vertical muscle, which is situated in the center of the tongue. Its purpose is to make the tongue flatter. The mucous membranes that run along the sides of the tongue are connected to the transverse muscle, which splits it in half. Its purpose is to make the tongue longer and narrower.

- **Blood Supply:** The lingual artery of the external carotid artery is the main source of blood supply for the tongue. The internal jugular vein receives the lingual vein drainage. The lingual artery supplies blood to the floor of the mouth as well. Additionally, the ascending pharyngeal artery and the tonsillar branch of the facial artery provide a secondary blood supply to the root of the tongue. The posterior border of the mylohyoid muscle, the hypoglossal nerve, and the intermediate tendon of the digastric muscle form the area in the neck that is sometimes referred to as the Pirogov triangle. One useful site to stop severe tongue hemorrhage is the lingual artery.
- **Nerve Supply:** The tongue is innervated by motor fibers, general sensory fibers for sensation, and special sensory fibers for taste.
    - Efferent motor nerve fibers from the hypoglossal nerve (CN XII) supply the motor supply for all of the tongue's intrinsic and extrinsic muscles, with the exception of the palatoglossus, which is innervated by the vagus nerve (CN X).

Because the anterior and posterior parts of the tongue are innervated differently and originate from distinct embryological structures (pharyngeal arches 1 and 3, respectively), there are differences in taste and sensation innervation between them.

- Anterior to the vallate papillae, or the anterior two-thirds of the tongue:
    - **Taste:** Through unique visceral afferent fibers, the chorda tympani branch of the facial nerve (CN VII) is connected.
    - **Sensation:** general visceral afferent fibers of the trigeminal nerve (CN V) supply the lingual branch of the mandibular (V3) division.
- Posterior one-third of tongue:
    - **Taste and Sensation:** through a combination of general and special visceral afferent fibers, to the glossopharyngeal nerve (CN IX).
- Base of tongue
    - **Taste and Sensation:** the superior laryngeal nerve's internal branch (which is a branch of the vagus nerve, CN X).

- **Lymphatic Drainage:** The submental nodes receive the tongue's tip drainage. The posterior one-third of the tongue drains to the jugulo-omohyoid nodes, while the left and right halves of the anterior two-thirds drain to the submandibular lymph nodes.
- **Microanatomy:** Masticatory mucosa, a subtype of oral mucosa composed of stratified squamous epithelium that has been keratinized, covers the upper surface of the tongue. Many papillae are embedded in this, some of which contain the taste buds and their receptors. Only the filiform papillae, which are part of the lingual papillae, are not connected to any taste buds. The other papillae types include vallate, foliate, and funiform. The tongue's dorsal and ventral surfaces can be divided. Numerous mucosal projections known as papillae define the stratified squamous keratinized epithelium that makes up the dorsal surface. The dorsal side of the tongue is covered by the lingual papillae in the direction of the terminal groove. Smooth, stratified squamous non-keratinized epithelium covers the ventral surface.

1.1.5.2. Development

The terminal tongue bud (tuberculum impar) of the first pharyngeal arch is the source of the median swelling from which the tongue develops during the fourth week of embryonic development. A pair of lateral lingual swellings form on the first pharyngeal arch in the fifth week, one on the left and one on the right. These lingual swellings cover the median tongue bud and quickly enlarge. They continue to develop during fetal development and comprise the anterior region of the tongue, which accounts for two thirds of its length. The median sulcus indicates the line of their fusion.

The copula, a swelling from the second pharyngeal arch in the midline, manifests itself in the fourth week. The hypoparyngeal eminence, a swelling originating primarily from the third arch and growing into the copula during the fifth and sixth weeks, gives rise to the posterior portion of the tongue (the other third and posterior most portion developing from the fourth pharyngeal arch). The primary process by which the hypopharyngeal eminence develops is the endoderm's growth from the third pharyngeal arch. The terminal sulcus delineates the border between the anterior from the first arch and the posterior from the third arch of the tongue. The terminal sulcus has a V-shaped structure, with the posterior position of the V's tip. The foramen cecum, the point of attachment of the thyroglossal duct where the embryonic thyroid starts to descend, is located at the tip of the terminal sulcus.

1.1.5.3. Function

- **Taste:** Tastants are substances that activate taste receptor cells. Tastants can interact with gustatory hair plasma membranes, which serve as taste transduction sites, once they have been dissolved in saliva. The tongue's dorsal surface is covered in numerous taste buds, each of which has taste receptor cells that are sensitive to specific taste classes. Different kinds of taste receptor cells can distinguish between flavors that are umami, sweet, bitter, salty, sour, and spicy. Since umami receptor cells are the least understood, they are the type that is being studied the most. It's a popular misperception that distinct basic tastes are only produced by specific regions of the tongue. This is untrue; while the tongue map is a common teaching tool in schools, all taste sensations originate from all regions of the tongue, albeit some regions are more sensitive to particular tastes than others.

- **Mastication:** An essential auxiliary organ of the digestive system is the tongue. During mastication, the tongue is used to crush food against the hard palate and manipulate it to make it softer before swallowing. The tongue's dorsal surface, or upper surface, has keratinized epithelium. As a result, the tongue can grate against the hard palate without suffering any harm or discomfort.
- **Speech:** The extrinsic muscles that move the tongue and the intrinsic muscles that change their shape work together to make the tongue one of the main articulators in speech production. More specifically, the articulation of distinct vowels is achieved by modifying the height and retraction of the tongue, which modifies the vocal tract's resonant characteristics. These resonant characteristics attenuate other harmonics while amplifying certain harmonic frequencies (formants), which varies depending on the vowel. For instance, the tongue is lowered and centered when producing [a], and it is raised and fronted when producing [i]. Airflow through the vocal tract is restricted to produce consonants, and many consonants have a constriction between the tongue and another portion of the vocal tract. For instance, the tongue is used to articulate alveolar consonants like [s] and [n] against the alveolar ridge, whereas the tongue is used to articulate velar consonants like [k] and [g] against the soft palate (velum). The shape of the tongue affects how words are pronounced as well. Take retroflex consonants, for instance, where the tongue tip curves backward.

1.1.5.4. Clinical Significance

- **Disease:** Ankyloglossia, commonly referred to as tongue-tie, is a congenital condition of the tongue. A very short and thickened frenulum ties the tongue to the floor of the mouth, which interferes with swallowing, eating, and speaking. The tongue can develop multiple pathologies, such as lingual swellings (bifid tongue), fissured tongue, oral hairy leukoplakia, burning mouth syndrome, bifid tongue (caused by a failure in the fusion of two lingual swellings of the first pharyngeal arch), and generic tongue.

Several forms of oral cancer primarily impact the tongue. These are mostly carcinomas with squamous cells. A visible coating of bacteria, desquamated epithelial cells, and food debris frequently forms on the tongue. This coating has been found to be a significant cause of halitosis, or bad breath, which is treatable with tongue cleaner.

- Medication Delivery: Some drugs are best absorbed into the body through the sublingual area, which is located beneath the front of the tongue. There is a plexus of veins beneath the extremely thin oral mucosa, which covers the tongue. By avoiding the gastrointestinal tract and taking advantage of the oral cavity's high vascularity, the sublingual route expedites the delivery of medication to the cardiovascular system. Other than intravenous therapy, this is the only practical and effective way to give nitroglycerin to a patient with angina pectoris-related chest pain.

1.1.6. The Salivary Glands

The saliva secreted by multiple gland sets is combined with tasted food. The parotid, submandibular, and sublingual glands are the three main pairs of salivary glands, in addition to the numerous tiny glands that also secrete saliva.

The largest pair of the parotid glands are situated in front and below each ear on the side of the face. When the parotid glands become inflamed, as in the case of the mumps, their swelling is constrained by sheaths surrounding them. The rounded submandibular glands are located in front of the sternomastoid muscle, which is the jaw's most noticeable muscle, close to the inner side of the lower jawbone. The mucous membrane that covers the floor of the mouth beneath the tongue directly covers the sublingual glands (Figure 1.4).

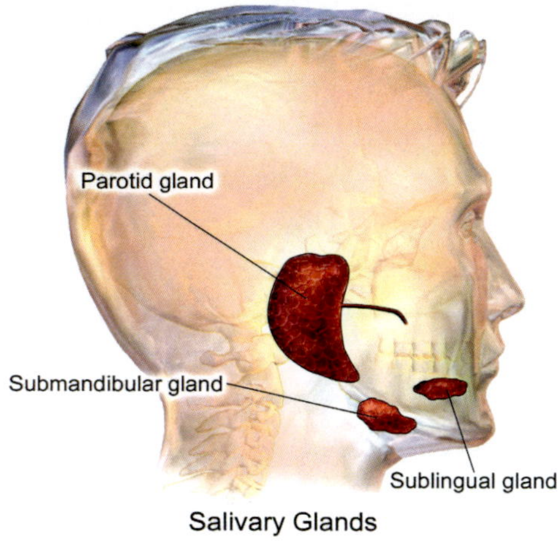

Figure 1.4. *The main salivary glands.*

Source: By BruceBlaus – Own work, CC BY 3.0, https://commons.wikimedia.org/w/index.php?curid=29294590.

The salivary glands are of the type called racemose, from the Latin racemosus ("full of clusters"), because of the cluster like arrangement of their secreting cells in rounded sacs, called acini, attached to freely branching systems of ducts. An alveolus is a small central cavity surrounded by the walls of the acini. Pyramidal secreting cells and flat, star-shaped contractile cells known as myoepithelial, or basket, cells are found in the walls of the acini. It is believed that these cells contract, much like the breast's myoepithelial cells, which contract to release milk from the milk ducts. The cells that secrete can either be mucous or serous in nature. The former secretes a watery fluid that contains the enzyme amylase, while the latter secretes mucin, the main component of mucus. The parotid glands' secreting cells are serous in nature. those of the submandibular glands, both the mucous and serous types, with four times as many serous cells as mucous. The mucous cells that make up the acini of the sublingual glands are the main constituent.

The parasympathetic and sympathetic branches of the autonomic nervous system regulate the salivary glands. The parasympathetic nerve supply dilates blood vessels and controls acinar cell secretion. The sympathetic nervous system controls the secretion of acinar cells, blood vessel constriction, and possibly myoepithelial cell contraction. Saliva is normally secreted continuously, even when food is present in the mouth. Saliva production in a 24-hour period typically reaches a volume of 1–1.5 liters or 0.3–0.4 gallon. Saliva production rises when something touches the gums, tongue, or other parts of the oral cavity, as well as during chewing. Food is not necessary to stimulate salivation; shifting the jaws and tongue when the mouth is empty or even dry sand can do the same thing. The unconditioned salivary reflex is the result of increased salivation following direct stimulation of the oral mucosa. Increased salivary flow may be triggered by a stimulus alone if a person discovers that a specific sight, sound, smell, or other stimuli is consistently linked to food. The conditioned salivary reflex is the name given to this reaction.

1.2. Saliva

The chemical environment that surrounds teeth and soft tissues in the mouth is provided by whole saliva, which is made up of secretions from both major and minor salivary glands as well as gingival crevicular fluid. Both sympathetic and parasympathetic nervous system activation can cause salivation. Saliva plays an essential role in the upkeep and preservation of oral tissue. A complex secretion is saliva. The major salivary glands secrete approximately 93% of the saliva by volume, with the minor glands secreting the remaining 7%. Saliva is 99% water, with the remaining 1% consisting of both organic and inorganic molecules. Saliva contains both fully degraded and partially degraded forms of mRNA, and the partial degradation of salivary RNA may be prevented by its association with macromolecules. Finding significant biomarkers for oral disease will depend on the proteome of the entire saliva, which is relevant to oral health. There is a close relationship between oral and systemic health because sialometry and sialochemistry are used to monitor general health, diagnose systemic illnesses, and serve as risk indicators for diseases. Because saliva regulates and/or modifies oxidative damage in the oral cavity, it may serve as the body's first line of defense against oxidative stress. Saliva is a mirror of overall health. Saliva can be one of the source for DNA, instead of RNA/mRNA; elaborate the role of saliva in different fields of science.

Salivary transcriptome analysis may have positive effects on salivary diagnostics and oral cancer detection. Innate immunity is primarily caused by cationic peptides and other defense proteins such as lysozyme, bactericidal/permeability-increasing protein (BPI), BPI-like proteins, PLUNC (palate lung and nasal epithelial clone) proteins, salivary amylase, cystatins, proline-rich proteins, mucins, peroxidases, and statherin. The protein and ion components transform a 99% water solution into a viscoelastic solution that can serve a variety of purposes, including lubricating, acting as an antimicrobial, preventing tooth dissolution, promoting taste, and assisting in digestion. With the quick progress in saliva omics, saliva may eventually replace blood in the diagnosis and prognosis of diseases because it is a safe, noninvasive source. Through its salivary enzymes, buffering, remineralization, and lubricating properties, saliva plays a significant role in preserving mucosal integrity and indigestion. Saliva is an aqueous fluid that is present in the oral cavity and is essential to the upkeep and preservation of dental health. Taste, mastication, bolus formation, enzymatic digestion, and swallowing are all impacted by saliva. Saliva's protective qualities, such as its ability to preserve mucosal and dental integrity, have an indirect impact on digestion. The review's goal was to go over the various tasks that saliva completes.

1.2.1. Composition of Saliva

Numerous electrolytes, such as sodium, potassium, calcium, magnesium, bicarbonate, and phosphates, are found in saliva. Saliva also contains proteins, enzymes, immunoglobulins, mucins, and nitrogenous products like ammonia and urea. Bicarbonates, phosphates, and urea regulate pH and saliva's buffering ability; (2) mucins and macromolecule proteins clean, agglomerate, and/or attach oral microorganisms and aid in the metabolism of dental plaque; (3) calcium, phosphate, and proteins act as an anti-solubility factor and regulate demineralization and remineralization; and (4) immunoglobulins, proteins, and enzymes have antibacterial action. These constituents interact in related ways in the following general areas. The aforementioned elements typically exist in small quantities and fluctuate according to flow variations, but they consistently perform a variety of crucial tasks. It is crucial to emphasize that saliva must be viewed as a whole that is greater than the sum of its parts because it is a special biological fluid.

Saliva is a very diluted fluid with a water content of over 99%. Saliva is not regarded as an ultrafiltrate of plasma because, while it forms in the acini, it is initially isotonic and then turns hypotonic as it passes through the duct network. Unstimulated saliva's hypotonicity enables taste buds to distinguish between flavors without being obscured by normal plasma sodium levels. Lower levels of glucose, bicarbonate, and urea in unstimulated saliva augment the hypotonic environment to enhance taste. Hypotonicity, especially during low-flow periods, also allows for the expansion and hydration of mucin glycoproteins, which protect the tissues of the mouth.

1.2.2. Organic and Inorganic Constituents of Saliva

Saliva's organic and inorganic compositions can provide insight into changes in enzymatic activity as a result of periodontal inflammation. Alkaline phosphatase (ALP) is an enzyme that hydrolyzes phosphorus and binds to calcium phosphate. ALP is regarded as a phenotypic marker for osteoblast cells and a significant indicator of bone formation. ALP was found in dental plaque bacteria, desquamated epithelial cells, leucocytes, and the parotid, submandibular, and minor salivary glands. The presence of ALP in gingival crevicular fluid and saliva typically indicates periodontal tissue destruction and/or inflammation. Urea is an organic compound present in saliva that is the end result of protein catabolism in humans, among other components.

Ammonia and CO_2 are produced during the hydrolysis of urea by bacterial urease enzymes, which is regarded as a primary mechanism for the oral cavity's production of alkali. Ammonia may also be cytotoxic to the tissues of the periodontal cavity. Ammonia is a major factor in the development of gingivitis because it can make the sulcular epithelium more permeable to other harmful and antigenic substances. Saliva volume in the oral cavity is influenced by many variables, including diet, age, drugs, stimulation, circadian rhythm, and hydrogen (H+) ion concentration. However, pathological conditions like periodontal disease can also change these factors (Table 1.1).

Table 1.1. Components and Functions of Saliva

Salivary Component	Function
Amylase	Digestive
Bicarbonate	Buffering
Calcium	Remineralization
Salivary antibodies	Antimicrobial

Lactoferrin	Antimicrobial
Lysozyme	Hydrolysis of cell membrane
Mucins	Digestion, lubrication, and pellicle formation
Protease	Digestion
Water	Mucosal integrity

Source: Maddu N. Functions of Saliva [Internet]. Saliva and salivary diagnostics. IntechOpen; 2019. Available from: http://dx.doi.org/10.5772/intechopen.84709.

1.2.3. Saliva Functions

Saliva's constituent parts all work together to support daily eating, speaking, and oral hygiene. Saliva serves a variety of purposes, some of which are as follows.

There should be a table depicting every enzyme present in the saliva and the specific function of that enzyme.

1.2.3.1. Immune Functions

Salivary peroxidase, lactoferrin, myeloperoxidase, lysozyme, and thiocyanate concentrations all function as defensive mechanisms for the entire salivary system. The natural defense qualities of salivary secretions through clinical modalities, including the creation of topical vaccines to prevent oral diseases, artificial salivas to treat salivary dysfunction, and diagnostic reagents and tests for local and systemic disease. Salivary mucins are crucial to the processes taking place within the mucosal defense's epithelial perimeter and are widely acknowledged as a crucial component in maintaining the oral cavity's health. Numerous physical, physicochemical, and chemical agents found in human saliva shield oral tissues from harmful substances. It successfully eliminates the continuous presence of immune and nonimmune components in the mouth as well as exogenous and endogenous microorganisms and their byproducts in the gut. The structural foundation of the oral mucosa's local innate immune defense system is the salivary mucosal pellicle.

1.2.3.2. Saliva Proteome Analysis

The rate at which bacterial substrates found in meals and snacks are cleared from the mouth and saliva is significantly influenced by the flow rate of saliva. The self-perceived stress related to work was inversely correlated with salivary IgA and lysozyme levels. The inverse relationship between stress and mucosal immunity is supported by the results, as these salivary biomarkers are indicative of mucosal immunity. Hyaluronidase and hyaluronidase inhibitors were found to be inversely correlated, especially when it came to intraoral wound healing and periodontal disease. Salivary α-amylase (HSA) is a significant secretory protein component that plays a vital biological role in the first stages of starch digestion. Saliva contains the collagen-cleaving enzyme matrix metalloproteinase-8 (MMP-8), which is a quantifiable sign of periodontal disease.

One of the first enzymes identified for the amylolysis of starch and even the physiological function of salivary amylase itself was amylase, which is found in human saliva. Because lactoferrin in saliva can reduce bacterial growth, biofilm formation, iron overload, reactive oxygen formation, and inflammatory processes, it is a valuable defense against bacterial injuries, including those caused by Streptococcus mutans and periodontopathic bacteria. Salivary immune globulins and salivary chaperokine HSP70/HSPAs are examples of defense proteins that are implicated in both innate and acquired immunity. A significant part of physiologically significant mucosal fluids, lactoferrin is necessary for mucosal-mediated immunity.

The salivary proteins lactoferrin and lysozyme have antimicrobial properties in vitro that affect microorganisms, obtaining their minimum inhibitory concentration and minimum bactericidal concentration. It has been suggested that salivary alpha-amylase is a sensitive, noninvasive biomarker for alterations in the body brought on by stress that corresponds with sympathetic nervous system activity. Therefore, salivary α-amylase levels could be a useful marker for the non-invasive evaluation of physical stress. A multifunctional mammalian immunity protein called lactoferrin sequesters the nutrient iron, thereby inhibiting the growth of microorganisms. Saliva contains lysozyme, which has been shown to have antibacterial activity against pathogens. This suggests that lysozyme may have antimicrobial properties in certain medical applications. One potential treatment to stop the effects of radiation on salivary glands could be lactoferrin. LTF is investigated as a molecule essential for regulating oxidative cell function, as well as a first-line mediator in immune defense and response to pathogenic and nonpathogenic injuries. Amylases are involved in the metabolism of starch and adiposity. They hydrolyze starch in the saliva and pancreas. Oral lactoferrin has been shown to reduce psychological stress in people. Lactoferrin is a secretory protein with a variety of physiological functions.

1.2.3.3. Role of Lubrication

An efficient set of mechanisms for lubricating and shielding the hard and soft tissues is provided by the complex mixture of salivary constituents. Saliva has lubricating and antimicrobial properties that are primarily preserved by rest; it flushes the mouth and removes harmful substances and debris. Saliva is a complex fluid with both specific and nonspecific physical and chemical properties that affect oral health. Many antimicrobial proteins found in saliva help shield the oral ecosystem from infectious agents. Via active transportation, passive diffusion, or ultrafiltration, proteins can travel from the blood circulation into the salivary glands. Some of these proteins are then released into the saliva and may therefore function as disease biomarkers. The conditioning film that saliva forms over the oral hard and soft tissues controls the first microbial attachment, an important stage in the development of the oral microflora.

1.2.3.4. Role of Digestion

Saliva of a high caliber is necessary to support digestion and shield the dental components from wear and tear. The main fluid component of the taste receptor cell external environment, saliva is involved in both the transport of taste substances and the taste receptor defense. The part played by human saliva and its constituent parts in the GI processes of swallowing, enzymatic digestion, bolus formation, taste, and mastication. Salivary nonesterified fatty acids (NEFA) may have diagnostic and prognostic value and are thought to contribute to oral health and oral fat detection.

During oral lipolysis, lingual lipase produces nonesterified fatty acids (NEFA) from dietary fats. Rodents' lingual lipase is highly lipolytic and essential for the oral detection of fats. The regulation of basal FFA concentration through salivary lipolytic activity may play a physiological role in the sensitivity to fat taste. Saliva aids in the preparation of the food bolus during chewing by clumping together the formed particles and starting the enzymatic breakdown of food. The sense of taste and the eating process are significantly influenced by saliva. The combination of taste perceptions, aromatics, and chemical feelings that food elicits in the oral cavity is known as flavor.

1.2.3.5. Role of Diagnostic Properties

Saliva analysis has potential applications in the diagnosis of autoimmune diseases, endocrine disorders, cancer, infectious diseases, and hereditary disorders. It can also be used to monitor drug use and determine therapeutic drug levels. The addition of fluids improved dry food chewing and reduced hyposalivation-related feeding problems. Salivary diagnostics have shown enormous promise in clinical applications, and saliva has been shown to be a promising bodily fluid for early disease detection. Because of combinations of biomolecules with clinical relevance and advancements in detection technologies, saliva has the potential to become the preferred first-line diagnostic sample. Saliva is a helpful diagnostic fluid for conditions relating to the mouth. In epidemiological surveys, monitoring salivary biomarkers for systemic and oral diseases may prove to be a valuable adjunct to clinical examinations (Figure 1.5).

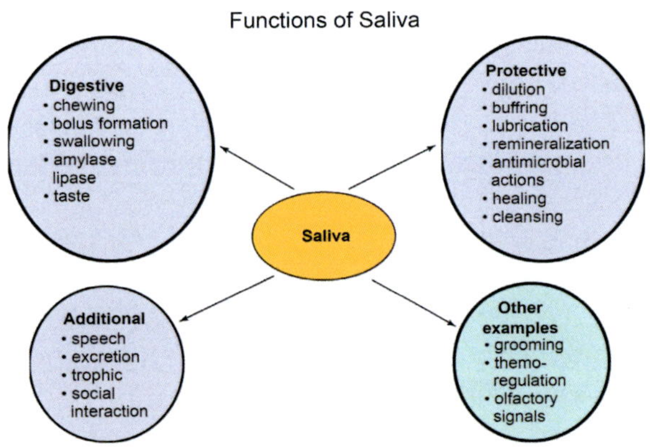

Figure 1.5. *Different functions of the saliva.*

Source: Maddu N. Functions of saliva [Internet]. Saliva and salivary diagnostics. IntechOpen; 2019. Available from: http://dx.doi.org/10.5772/intechopen.84709.

Saliva's high rate of compositional changes makes it useful for tracking different biorhythms and learning more about the physiological features of the human body. The present comprehension of the salivary microbiome in caries is enhanced by the noteworthy impacts of the oral environment noted in this investigation. These findings will help to improve disease diagnosis, prognosis, and treatment options as well as to broaden the scope of research.

1.2.3.6. Role of Maintenance of Health Teeth

The function of saliva, the frequency of dry mouth and the ensuing significance of salivary flow, as well as the connection between xerostomia and hypofunction of the salivary glands, are some of the factors that contribute to dry mouth. When food is consumed, scent and taste molecules are released into saliva, which also coats the taste receptors in the oral cavity. Saliva also contains chemicals and enzymes that have the ability to react with food. Because saliva lubricates the teeth and soft tissues in the mouth, it is a vital fluid. In the process of tooth de-/remineralization and calculus formation, salivary pH, buffer capacity, and mineral content—calcium (Ca), phosphate (P), sodium (Na), and potassium (K)—all play significant roles. The degree of the periodontal disease determines whether the pH will change significantly. The degree of periodontal disease is related to the significant changes in salivary pH. Therefore, salivary pH could be a quick clinical diagnostic biomarker. For an organism to survive, taste perception—which is triggered by food ingredients and made possible by sensory cells in the mouth—is essential. Apart from the quintessential taste modalities of sweet, umami, bitter, sour, and salty, there is a great deal of research done on the orosensory perception of stimuli like fat components.

Teeth have a strong resistance to localized demineralization that is unequaled by bone because they are exposed to food, beverages, and the oral microbiome. Because of demineralization, the pH of saliva and plaque can cause white spot lesions on the tooth surface, which are thought to be the first signs of caries. Reduced salivary flow harms the oral tissues. Saliva is a vital biological fluid that helps mechanically remove food particles and bacteria from the oral cavity and teeth.

1.2.3.7. Antimicrobial, Antiviral, and Antifungal Functions

When salivary proteins like lysozyme, lactoferrin, and lactoperoxidase combine with other salivary constituents, they can directly affect oral bacteria by preventing their growth or eliminating them. By interacting with anions of low charge density chaotropic ions (thiocyanate, perchlorate, iodide, bromide, nitrate, chloride, and fluoride) and bicarbonate, lysozyme can cause bacterial cells, particularly Streptococcus mutans, to lyse. Recent research has demonstrated the bactericidal and growth-inhibitory properties of parotid saliva, a different cationic peptide in saliva that is rich in histidines. The histidine-rich peptides seem to be a potent antifungal agent as well, killing Candida albicans at extremely low concentrations and preventing their growth.

The exocrine gland equivalent of transferrin, lactoferrin, works well against bacteria that need iron for metabolic activities. It has the ability to outcompete the bacteria's iron-chelating molecules and rob them of this vital component. In addition, lactoferrin has bactericidal properties that set it apart from basic iron deficiency. Salivary peroxidase is a component of an antibacterial system that works by oxidizing salivary thiocyanate to hypothiocyanite and hypothiocyanous acids using hydrogen peroxide produced by oral bacteria. These byproducts oxidize the sulfhydryl groups of the enzymes involved in glycolysis and sugar transport, which in turn influences bacterial metabolism (particularly acid production). The antimicrobial activity of salivary peroxidase against S. mutans is greatly increased through contact with secretory IgA. By interacting with mucin, which can serve to concentrate this defense force at the interface of the mucosa and the hostile external environment, all of the protective potential of antibacterial proteins can be increased. The gingival crevice area and its corresponding gingival crevicular fluid will contribute to the oral fluids when teeth are present, particularly if there is some gingivitis. By supplying (a) serum antibodies against oral bacteria, particularly IgG antibodies, (b) phagocytic cells (PMNs), and (c) antibacterial products released from the phagocytic cells, e.g., this fluid can support the oral defense system lysozyme, myeloperoxidase, and lactoferrin.

Saliva from humans contains a significant amount of antiviral and antibacterial proteins. It's interesting to note that the majority of these antibacterial proteins have antiviral activity—usually against particular viral infections. Further, gp340, also known as salivary agglutinin, a protein that interacts with both bacteria and viruses. It is believed that soluble gp340 increases bacterial clearance from the mouth by binding to and aggregating a range of bacteria in the oral cavity. However, gp340 encourages bacterial adherence when it is bound to the tooth surface. The majority of gp340 proteins are soluble in saliva and can specifically inhibit the infectious potential of influenza A and HIV-1 in the oral cavity. On the other hand, the majority of gp340 proteins are attached to the cell surface in the female reproductive tract, where they may facilitate HIV-1 infection.

The antifungal properties of saliva against *Cryptococcus neoformans* and *Candida albicans*. It is therefore imperative to continue searching for novel, low- or non-toxic broad-spectrum antifungals. Histatins are promising antifungal therapeutic agents because of the following characteristics: (1) they are relatively safe or non-toxic; (2) they exhibit strong cidal activity against most tested fungal species as well as azole-resistant ones; and (3) their candidacidal activity is comparable to that of azole-based antifungals. The development of more stable and effective histatin delivery systems, as well as better histatins with increased cidal activity, is the main goal of current research efforts. These and other strategies could aid in overcoming the increasing number of opportunistic and drug-resistant fungi that cause serious, widely spread illnesses. For patients with impaired salivary function, the histatins with enhanced protective qualities may also be utilized as ingredients in artificial saliva.

Saliva contains a variety of proteins and enzymes and is secreted by salivary glands. For the preservation of oral tissues, salivary flow rate and pH are critical factors. Saliva serves a protective role and provides benefits such as immune defense, lubrication, digestion, buffering, remineralization in the healthy oral mucosa, diagnostic purposes, and proteome analysis. Salivary enzymes assist in digestion and help maintain the integrity of the mucosa. Saliva is a crucial component of the pellicle, which shields the tooth from damage following eruption. Regular salivary flow, composition, and function are vital for daily life. It exists in various amounts, regardless of size, and its numerous contributions to the preservation and upkeep of health deserve acknowledgment (Table 1.2).

Table 1.2. Functions of the Digestive Organs

Organ	Major Functions	Other Functions
Mouth	• Ingests food • Chews and mixes food • Begins chemical breakdown of carbohydrates • Moves food into the pharynx • Begins breakdown of lipids via lingual lipase	• Moistens and dissolves food, allowing you to taste it • Cleans and lubricates the teeth and oral cavity • Has some antimicrobial activity
Pharynx	• Propels food from the oral cavity to the esophagus	• Lubricates food and passageways
Esophagus	• Propels food to the stomach	• Lubricates food and passageways
Stomach	• Mixes and churns food with gastric juices to form chyme • Begins chemical breakdown of proteins • Releases food into the duodenum as chyme • Absorbs some fat-soluble substances (for example, alcohol, aspirin) • Possesses antimicrobial functions	• Stimulates protein-digesting enzymes • Secretes intrinsic factor required for vitamin B_{12} absorption in the small intestine
Small intestine	• Mixes chyme with digestive juices • Propels food at a rate slow enough for digestion and absorption • Absorbs breakdown products of carbohydrates, proteins, lipids, and nucleic acids, along with vitamins, minerals, and water • Performs physical digestion via segmentation	• Provides optimal medium for enzymatic activity

Accessory organs	• Liver: produces bile salts, which emulsify lipids, aiding their digestion and absorption • Gallbladder: stores, concentrates, and releases bile • Pancreas: produces digestive enzymes and bicarbonate	• Bicarbonate-rich pancreatic juices help neutralize acidic chyme and provide an optimal environment for enzymatic activity
Large intestine	• Further breaks down food residues • Absorbs most residual water, electrolytes, and vitamins produced by enteric bacteria • Propels feces toward the rectum • Eliminates feces	• Food residue is concentrated and temporarily stored prior to defecation • Mucus eases the passage of feces through the colon

Source: https://courses.lumenlearning.com/suny-ap2/chapter/digestive-system-processes-and-regulation/.

A Closer Look

Dry Mouth

When the salivary glands in the mouth don't produce enough saliva to keep the mouth moist, it's known as xerostomia (Zeer-o-STOE-me-uh). Dry mouth is frequently brought on by aging, drug side effects, or cancer radiation treatment. Dry mouth is less frequently caused by an illness that directly affects the salivary glands. Additionally, you might momentarily experience dry mouth if you're thirsty or nervous. Some people find dry mouth to be just bothersome. For others, the condition of their teeth, gums, and general health may be significantly impacted by dry mouth. It may also have an impact on people's food intake and level of enjoyment. The cause of dry mouth determines how to treat it.

Symptoms: You may experience all or the majority of these symptoms if your salivary flow is inadequate.

- Dryness or a feeling of stickiness in your mouth.
- Saliva that seems thick and stringy.
- Bad breath.
- Having a hard time chewing, speaking and swallowing.
- Dry or sore throat and hoarseness.
- Dry or grooved tongue.
- A changed sense of taste.
- Problems wearing dentures.
- Lipstick stuck to teeth.

By removing sugar and food particles and neutralizing and reducing the harmful effects of bacteria, saliva helps prevent tooth decay. You might have trouble tasting, chewing, and swallowing if you don't have enough saliva. It's possible that you struggle with food digestion.

When to See a Doctor: Schedule a visit with your healthcare provider if you experience persistent symptoms of dry mouth.

Causes: When the mouth's salivary glands don't produce enough saliva to keep the mouth moist, dry mouth results. These glands may occasionally malfunction because of:

Medicines: Numerous over-the-counter and prescription medications are among the hundreds of medications that can induce dry mouth. Medication for anxiety, depression, and high blood pressure, as well as some antihistamines, decongestants, muscle relaxants, and pain relievers, are among the drugs that are more likely to result in issues.

Aging: As they age, dry mouth symptoms are common in older adults. Dry mouth can be brought on by dietary deficiencies, long-term health issues, and modifications in the way the body handles medications.

Cancer Therapy: Chemotherapy, a type of cancer treatment medication, can alter the type and quantity of saliva produced. This might only last temporarily, and once the treatment is over, normal salivary flow will resume. Salivary gland damage from radiation therapy to the head and neck can significantly reduce saliva production. Depending on the area and radiation dose, this could last for a short while or a long time.

Nerve Damage: Dry mouth may be the result of an injury or surgery that damages the nerves in the head and neck region.

Other Health Conditions: Certain medical conditions like diabetes, stroke, oral yeast infections, and Alzheimer's disease can all contribute to dry mouth. Alternatively, autoimmune conditions like Sjogren syndrome or HIV/AIDS may be the cause of dry mouth.

Snoring and Mouth Breathing: Dry mouth can result from breathing with your mouth open and snoring.

Tobacco and alcohol use: More symptoms of dry mouth can result from smoking, chewing tobacco, and alcohol consumption.

- Use of legal or illegal drugs that may be sold on the streets. Using methamphetamine can harm teeth and result in severe dry mouth. The use of marijuana may also result in dry mouth.

Risk Factors: Risk of dry mouth is higher in people who:

- Take medicines that have dry mouth listed as a possible side effect.
- Are being treated for cancer.
- Have nerve damage in the head and neck area.
- Suffer from other medical conditions such as diabetes, stroke, Alzheimer's disease, Sjogren's syndrome, or HIV/AIDS.
- Use tobacco products.
- Drink alcohol.
- Use street drugs.
- Eat sugary or acidic foods or candies.

Complications: Not having enough saliva and getting dry mouth can lead to:

- Increased plaque, tooth decay and gum disease.
- Mouth sores.
- A yeast infection in the mouth, also known as thrush.
- Sores or split skin at the corners of the mouth, or cracked lips.
- Poor nutrition from having problems with chewing and swallowing.

Diagnosis: Your healthcare provider examines your medical history and the medications you take, including over-the-counter medications, to identify the cause of your dry mouth. Your medical practitioner examines your mouth as well. Tests to gage saliva production, blood tests, or imaging scans of your salivary glands may occasionally be necessary. Your dry mouth's cause may be determined with the aid of these scans and tests. Your healthcare provider may send for testing a small sample of cells extracted from the salivary glands in your lip if they believe that Sjogren syndrome is the cause of your dry mouth. We refer to this process as a biopsy.

Treatment: The cause of your dry mouth will determine how you are treated. Your medical practitioner might:

- Modify medications that are causing dry mouth. Your doctor may adjust your dosage if they believe that one of your medications is the problem. Alternatively, you might try a different medication that doesn't make your mouth dry.
- Make suggestions for mouth moisturizers. These goods may consist of over-the-counter or prescription mouthwashes, artificial saliva, mouth moisturizers, or mouthwash dispensers. Mouthwashes with xylitol, in particular, that are intended for dry mouth can be useful. Act Dry Mouth Mouthwash and Biotene Dry Mouth Oral Rinse are two examples.

Your doctor may recommend pilocarpine (Salagen) to help you produce more saliva if you have a highly dry mouth from Sjogren syndrome or radiation therapy for head and neck cancer. If you have Sjogren syndrome, your doctor may prescribe cevimeline (Evoxac) to help you produce more saliva.

Lifestyle and Home Remedies: These suggestions, along with the guidance from your healthcare provider, may help reduce symptoms of dry mouth:

- Drink sugar-free beverages or water, or nibble on ice chips. To keep your mouth moist throughout the day, do this. Moreover, sip water throughout meals to facilitate chewing and swallowing.
- Suck on sugar-free hard candies or chew sugar-free gum. Xylitol-containing products may also aid in the prevention of cavities. However, if taken in excess, xylitol, which is frequently present in sugar-free gum and candies, may give some people gas or diarrhea.
- Consider using over-the-counter xylitol-containing saliva substitutes. These consist of Oasis Moisturizing Mouth Spray and Mouth Kote. Alternatively, try saliva substitutes like Biotene Dry Mouth Oralbalance Gel that contain carboxymethylcellulose or hydroxyethyl cellulose.
- Use your nose to breathe, not your mouth. If your snoring makes you breathe through your mouth at night, you might need to get treated for it.
- At night, add moisture to the air. Put a room humidifier to use.
- Hydrate your lips. This relieves dry, cracked skin.

Products that exacerbate your symptoms should be avoided. These include:

- Caffeine and alcohol. These goods may irritate and dry out the skin. Use of mouthwash containing alcohol is not advised.
- Tobacco. Give up smoking and chewing tobacco. Products made of tobacco can irritate and dry out your mouth.

- Decongestants and antihistamines that are over-the-counter. These medications may make your dry mouth worse.
- Candies and foods high in sugar or acidity. The risk of tooth decay is increased by these foods. Additionally, avoid foods that are salty or spicy as they may irritate your skin.

Maintaining the health of your mouth and teeth depends on saliva. Taking the following preventative measures for your teeth may also help with dry mouth:

- After brushing, floss and use fluoride toothpaste on your teeth. Consult your dentist to see if you would benefit from using a tooth gel to neutralize bacteria acids, betaine-containing toothpaste, or prescription fluoride toothpaste.
- Apply rinses or fluoride. Your dentist may recommend fluoride trays, which you fill with fluoride and place over your teeth at night, to help prevent cavities. Additionally, your dentist might advise you to use a weekly chlorhexidine rinse or brush with fluoride gel before going to bed.
- Make at least two annual visits to your dentist. To help avoid tooth decay, get your teeth examined and have any plaque removed.

Summary

- The lips are soft, pliable anatomical structures that form the mouth margin. They are composed of a surface epidermis(skin), connective tissue, and a muscle layer. The edges of the lips are covered with reddish skin, sometimes called the vermilion border, and abundantly provided with sensitive nerve endings.
- The mouth, which is also known as the oral (or buccal) cavity, is the orifice through which food and air enter the body. The mouth opens to the outside at the lips and empties into the throat at the rear.
- The gums, also known as the gingivae, are made up of connective tissue covered with mucous membrane. The mucous membrane is connected by thick fibrous tissue to the membrane surrounding the bones of the jaw.
- The teeth are hard, white structures found in the mouth. Usually used for mastication, the teeth of different vertebrate species are sometimes specialized. The teeth of snakes, for example, are very thin and sharp and usually curve backward. They function in capturing prey but not in chewing because snakes swallow their food whole.
- The tongue is a muscular organ in the mouth of a typical tetrapod. It manipulates food for chewing and swallowing as part of the digestive process and is the primary organ of taste. The tongue's upper surface (dorsum) is covered by taste buds housed in numerous lingual papillae. It is sensitive and kept moist by saliva and is richly supplied with nerves and blood vessels.
- Food is tasted and mixed with saliva that is secreted by several sets of glands. Besides the many minute glands that secrete saliva, there are three major pairs of salivary glands: the parotid, the submandibular, and the sublingual glands.
- The secretions of the major and minor salivary glands, together with the gingival crevicular fluid, constitute whole saliva which provides the chemical milieu of the teeth and oral soft tissues. Saliva formation can be stimulated by sympathetic and parasympathetic stimulations.
- Saliva is composed of a variety of electrolytes, including sodium, potassium, calcium, magnesium, bicarbonate, and phosphates.
- The organic and inorganic compositions of saliva can supply information about alterations in enzymatic activity in response to periodontal inflammation. Alkaline phosphatase (ALP) is a calcium-phosphate binding protein and a phosphor-hydrolytic enzyme.
- All the components of saliva work together to help you eat, speak and keep your mouth clean every day.

References

1. Balligand, J. L., Feron, O., & Dessy, C. (2009). eNOS activation by physical forces: From short-term regulation of contraction to chronic remodeling of cardiovascular tissues. *Physiological Reviews, 89*(2), 481–534. https://doi.org/10.1152/physrev.00042.2007.

2. Bohlen, H. G., & Nase, G. P. (2000). Dependence of intestinal arteriolar regulation on flow-mediated nitric oxide formation. *American Journal of Physiology-Heart and Circulatory Physiology, 279*(5), H2249–H2258.
3. Busse, R., & Fleming, I. (2006). Vascular endothelium and blood flow. In *Handbook of Experimental Pharmacology,* 2006:(176 Pt 2):43-78.
4. Canagaratnam, M. (2004). *Gastrointestinal System* (R. J. Naftalin, Ed.), Hodder Education Publishers, 2004.
5. Carlson, B. E., & Secomb, T. W. (2005). A theoretical model for the myogenic response based on the length-tension characteristics of vascular smooth muscle. *Microcirculation, 12*(4), 327–338. https://doi.org/10.1080/10739680590934745.
6. Carlson, B. E., Arciero, J. C., & Secomb, T. W. (2008). Theoretical model of blood flow autoregulation: Roles of myogenic, shear-dependent, and metabolic responses. *American Journal of Physiology-Heart and Circulatory Physiology, 295*(4), H1572–H1579. https://doi.org/10.1152/ajpheart.00262.2008.
7. Cheng LK, O'Grady G, Du P, Egbuji JU, Windsor JA, Pullan AJ. Gastrointestinal system. Wiley Interdiscip Rev Syst Biol Med. 2010 Jan-Feb;2(1):65-79.
8. Chan, S. L., & Fiscus, R. R. (2003). Vasorelaxations induced by calcitonin gene-related peptide, vasoactive intestinal peptide, and acetylcholine in aortic rings of endothelial and inducible nitric oxide synthase-knockout mice. *Journal of Cardiovascular Pharmacology, 41*(3), 434–443.
9. Crissinger, K. D., & Granger, D. N. (2003). Gastrointestinal blood flow. In T. Yamada (Ed.), *Textbook of Gastroenterology* (4th ed., pp. 498–520). Philadelphia: William & Wilkins.
10. De Fontgalland, D., Wattchow, D. A., Costa, M., & Brookes, S. J. (2008). Immunohistochemical characterization of the innervation of human colonic mesenteric and submucosal blood vessels. *Neurogastroenterology & Motility, 20*(11), 1212–1226. https://doi.org/10.1111/j.1365-2982.2008.01150.x.
11. Drummond, H. A., Grifoni, S. C., & Jernigan, N. L. (2008). A new trick for an old dogma: ENaC proteins as mechanotransducers in vascular smooth muscle. *Physiology (Bethesda), 23*, 23–31. https://doi.org/10.1152/physiol.00034.2007.
12. Fleming, I., & Busse, R. (2003). Molecular mechanisms involved in the regulation of the endothelial nitric oxide synthase. *American Journal of Physiology-Regulatory, Integrative and Comparative Physiology, 284*(1), R1–R12.
13. Fleming, I., Fisslthaler, B., Dixit, M., & Busse, R. (2005). Role of PECAM-1 in the shear–stress-induced activation of Akt and the endothelial nitric oxide synthase (eNOS) in endothelial cells. *Journal of Cell Science, 118*(Pt 18), 4103–4111. https://doi.org/10.1242/jcs.02541.
14. Gibbins, I. L., Jobling, P., & Morris, J. L. (2003). Functional organization of peripheral vasomotor pathways. *Acta Physiologica Scandinavica, 177*(3), 237–245. https://doi.org/10.1046/j.1365-201X.2003.01079.x.
15. Kachlik, D., & Baca, V. (2006). Macroscopic and microscopic intermesenteric communications. *Biomedical Papers of the Medical Faculty of the University Palacky, Olomouc, Czechoslovakia, 150*(1), 121–124.
16. Koenigsberger, M., Sauser, R., Beny, J. L., & Meister, J. J. (2006). Effects of arterial wall stress on vasomotion. *Biophysical Journal, 91*(5), 1663–1674. https://doi.org/10.1529/biophysj.106.083311.

17. Kuebler, W. M., Uhlig, U., Goldmann, T., Schael, G., Kerem, A., Exner, K., Martin, C., Vollmer, E., & Uhlig, S. (2003). Stretch activates nitric oxide production in pulmonary vascular endothelial cells in situ. *American Journal of Respiratory and Critical Care Medicine, 168*(11), 1391–1398. https://doi.org/10.1164/rccm.200304-562OC.

18. Leung, P. S. (Ed.). (2014). *The Gastrointestinal System*. Dordrecht: Springer Netherlands. ISBN 978-94-017-8770-3 http://dx.doi.org/10.1007/978-94-017-8771-0.

19. Liu, H., Li, Y. Q., Yu, T., Zhao, Y. A., Zhang, J. P., Zhang, J. N., Guo, Y. T., Xie, X. J., Zhang, T. G., & Desmond, P. V. (2008). Confocal endomicroscopy for in vivo detection of microvascular architecture in normal and malignant lesions of upper gastrointestinal tract. *Journal of Gastroenterology and Hepatology, 23*(1), 56–61.

20. Nowicki, P. T., & Granger, D. N. (2008). Gastrointestinal blood flow. In T. Yamada (Ed.), *Textbook of Gastroenterology* (5th ed., pp. 540–556). Wiley-Blackwell. https://doi.org/10.1002/9781444303254.ch22.

21. Rogers, K. (Ed.). (2011). *The Digestive System*. New York, NY: Britannica Educational Publishing in association with Rosen Educational Services 2011. 258 pages, ISBN-13: 978-1615301317

22. Seidel, E. (2006). *Gastrointestinal system, Digestive System,* Philadelphia: Elsevier Mosby.

23. Weinbaum, S., Tarbell, J. M., & Damiano, E. R. (2007). The structure and function of the endothelial glycocalyx layer. *Annual Review of Biomedical Engineering, 9*, 121–167.

24. Xie, H., Ray, P. E., & Short, B. L. (2010). Role of sensory C fibers in hypoxia/reoxygenation-impaired myogenic constriction of cerebral arteries. *Neurological Research, 2010 Jun; 32(5): 487–491.* doi: 10.1179/174313209X408981

25. Xu, Y., Henning, R. H., Sandovici, M., van der Want, J. J., van Gilst, W. H., & Buikema, H. (2009). Enhanced myogenic constriction of mesenteric artery in heart failure relates to decreased smooth muscle cell caveolae numbers and altered AT1- and epidermal growth factor-receptor function. *European Journal of Heart Failure, 11*(3), 246–255. https://doi.org/10.1093/eurjhf/hfn027.

26. Zani, B. G., & Bohlen, H. G. (2005). Sodium channels are required during in vivo sodium chloride hyperosmolarity to stimulate increase in intestinal endothelial nitric oxide production. *American Journal of Physiology-Heart and Circulatory Physiology, 288*(1), H89–H95.

Chapter 2

THE STOMACH: BASIC FUNCTIONS AND CONTROL MECHANISMS

Contents

Introduction

In the gastrointestinal tracts of humans and a wide variety of other animals, including invertebrates, the stomach is a hollow, muscular organ. The stomach is an essential component of the digestive system and has a dilated structure. After chewing, the stomach is involved in the gastric phase of digestion. It uses hydrochloric acid and enzymes to carry out a chemical breakdown. The small intestine and the esophagus are separated by the stomach. To help with food digestion, the stomach secretes gastric acid and digestive enzymes. The duodenum receives partially digested food (chyme) from the stomach, and the pyloric sphincter regulates its passage until peristalsis takes over to move it through the remaining intestines.

Orientation and Directional Terms

Term	Definition	Illustration
Cardia	Part of the stomach surrounding the cardiac orifice (esophageal hiatus).	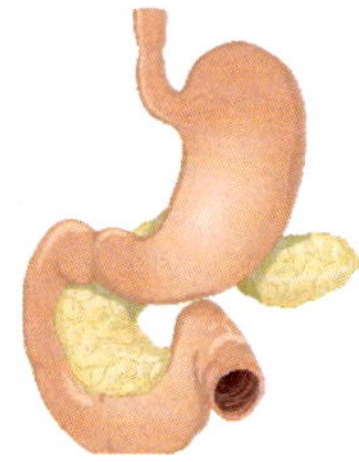
Fundus	Dome-shaped region of the stomach above and to the left of the cardia.	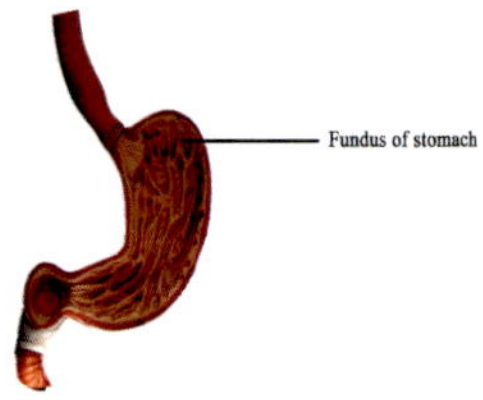
Gastric gland	Gland in the stomach mucosal epithelium that produces gastric juice.	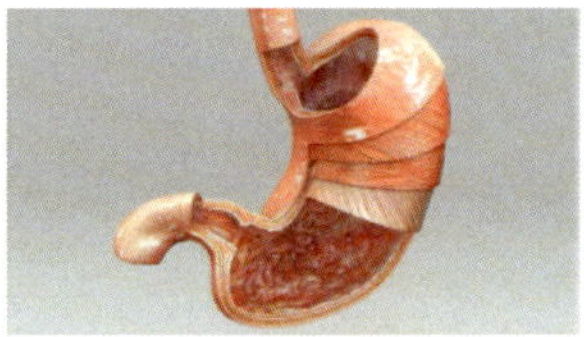
Gastrin	A peptide hormone that stimulates the secretion of hydrochloric acid and gut motility.	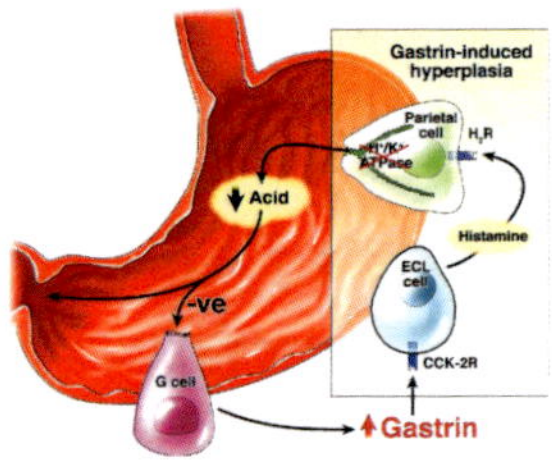
Pylorus	Lower, funnel-shaped part of the stomach that is continuous with the duodenum.	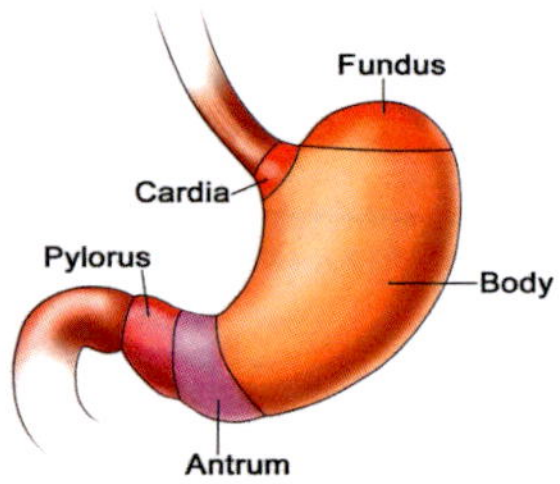

2.1. Anatomy and Morphology of the Stomach

Chemical digestion begins in the stomach, but only a small amount of carbohydrate digestion takes place in the mouth. The stomach is a portion of the alimentary canal that extends immediately below the esophagus. It connects the esophagus to the duodenum, the first segment of the small intestine, and is largely fixed at the esophageal and duodenal ends. In the interim, though, it may exhibit a highly dynamic structure that contracts and varies in size and position continuously. The mechanical support for digestion is given by these contractions. The empty stomach is about the size of your fist, but it can expand to hold up to 4 liters of food and liquid—more than 75 times its empty volume—before contracting back to its resting size. Body weight does not correspond with stomach size, despite the common misconception that an individual's stomach size is a measure of how much food they eat. Instead, eating more food makes your stomach expand more than eating less, as is the case with holiday dinners.

The stomach is frequently described in popular culture as the site of all digestion. Naturally, this is untrue. Being a temporary holding chamber is one of the many important roles of the stomach. Meals can be consumed much faster than they can be broken down and absorbed by the small intestine. As a result, food is stored in the stomach, and only small amounts are passed into the small intestine at a time. Foods are not broken down in the order they are consumed; instead, they are combined with the stomach's digestive juices to form chyme, which is then expelled into the small intestine. The stomach is crucial for the ongoing digestion of carbohydrates as well as the initial digestion of proteins and triglycerides, as you will see in the sections that follow. Apart from the tiny amount of nutrients in alcohol, very little, if any, nutrient absorption happens in the stomach.

2.1.1. Structure

The stomach is divided into four main regions: the cardia, fundus, body, and pylorus. The area where food enters the stomach through the esophagus and joins it is called the cardiac region, or simply the heart. The dome-shaped fundus is situated above and to the left of the cardia, inferior to the diaphragm. The stomach's main portion, the body, is located below the fundus. The duodenum and stomach are connected by the funnel-shaped pylorus. The body of the stomach is connected to the pyloric antrum, the funnel's wider end.

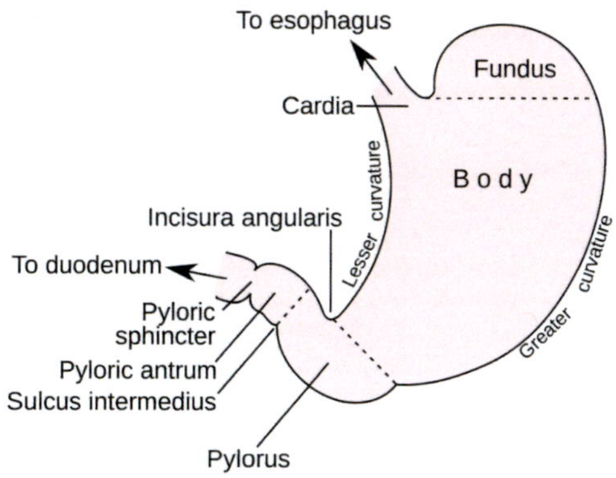

Figure 2.1. *Outline of the stomach, showing its anatomical landmarks.*

Source: By Henry Vandyke Carter, Public Domain, https://commons.wikimedia.org/w/index.php?curid=1420664.

The pyloric canal, which joins the duodenum, is the narrower end. This later point of connection is home to the smooth muscle pyloric sphincter, which regulates stomach emptying. When there is no food present, the stomach contracts inward, causing the mucosa and submucosa to fold into a broad shape known as a ruga (Figure 2.1). The stomach's convex lateral surface is referred to as its greater curvature, while its concave medial border is referred to as its lesser curvature. The lesser omentum, which connects the liver to the lesser curvature, and the greater omentum, which connects the greater curvature to the posterior abdominal wall, keep the stomach in place.

2.1.2. Histology

With modifications to the mucosa and muscularis for the particular purposes of this organ, the stomach wall is composed of the same four layers as the majority of the alimentary canal. The muscularis contains an inner oblique smooth muscle layer in addition to the usual circular and longitudinal smooth muscle layers. As a result, the stomach can churn food vigorously, mechanically breaking it down into smaller particles, in addition to moving food through the canal (Figure 2.2).

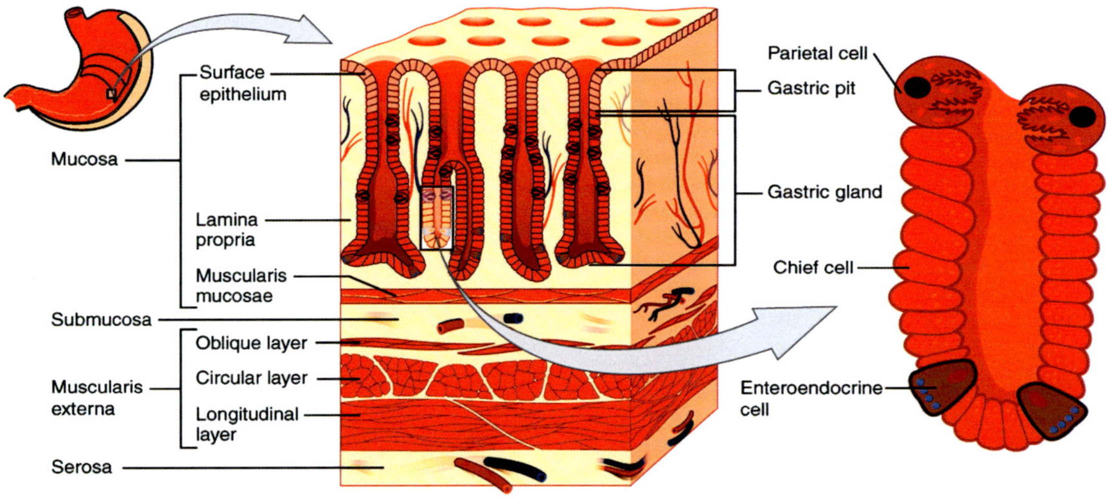

Figure 2.2. *The stomach wall is adapted for the functions of the stomach. In the epithelium, gastric pits lead to gastric glands that secrete gastric juice. The gastric glands (one gland is shown enlarged on the right) contain different types of cells that secrete a variety of enzymes, including hydrochloride acid, which activates the protein-digesting enzyme pepsin.*

Source: https://courses.lumenlearning.com/suny-ap2/chapter/the-stomach/.

Only surface mucus cells, which secrete an alkaline mucus coat for protection, make up the epithelial lining of the stomach mucosa. The surface of the epithelium is covered in a vast number of gastric pits that resemble worn-out pincushion cushions. These pits indicate the entrance to each gastric gland, which secretes gastric juice, a complex digestive fluid. The gastric glands are composed of various cell types, despite the mucus cells that primarily line the walls of the gastric pits. The main component of the cardia and pylorus glands is mucus-secreting cells. Mucus and several hormones, including most of the stimulatory hormone gastrin, are secreted by the cells that comprise the pyloric antrum. The majority of gastric secretions are produced by the much larger glands of the fundus and stomach body, which is where most chemical digestion occurs. These glands consist of different types of secretory cells. These consist of enteroendocrine cells, chief cells, mucous neck cells, and parietal cells.

- **Parietal Cells:** Parietal cells are the most highly differentiated epithelial cells in the body and are mainly found in the middle region of the gastric glands. These comparatively large cells generate both intrinsic factor and hydrochloric acid (HCl). The stomach's contents are highly acidic (pH 1 to 3.5), and the protein-digesting enzyme pepsin needs to be activated. This is caused by hydrochloric acid (HCl). Additionally, the acidity helps to denature proteins, which increases their availability for enzymatic digestion, and kills most of the bacteria that you ingest with food. The small intestine needs intrinsic factor, a glycoprotein, to absorb vitamin B_{12}.

- **Chief Cells:** The chief cells of the stomach glands are mainly found in the basal regions and secrete pepsinogen, which is the inactive proenzyme form of pepsin. For pepsinogen to become pepsin, HCl is required.
- **Mucous Neck Cells:** Mucous neck cells found in the upper portion of the stomach's gastric glands secrete a thin, acidic mucus that is very different from the mucus secreted by the surface epithelium's goblet cells. At present, the function of this mucus remains unclear.
- **Enteroendocrine Cells:** Lastly, different hormones are secreted into the lamina propria's interstitial fluid by enteroendocrine cells, which are located in the stomach glands. Among them is gastrin, which is mostly expelled by enteroendocrine G cells.

The digestive processes of significant hormones secreted by the stomach are outlined in Table 2.1.

Table 2.1. Hormones Secreted by the Stomach

Hormone	Production Site	Production Stimulus	Target Organ	Action
Gastrin	Stomach mucosa, mainly G cells of the pyloric antrum	Presence of peptides and amino acids in the stomach	Stomach	Increases secretion by gastric glands; promotes gastric emptying
Gastrin	Stomach mucosa, mainly G cells of the pyloric antrum	Presence of peptides and amino acids in the stomach	Small intestine	Promotes intestinal muscle contraction
Gastrin	Stomach mucosa, mainly G cells of the pyloric antrum	Presence of peptides and amino acids in the stomach	Ileocecal valve	Relaxes valve
Gastrin	Stomach mucosa, mainly G cells of the pyloric antrum	Presence of peptides and amino acids in the stomach	Large intestine	Triggers mass movements

Ghrelin	Stomach mucosa, mainly fundus	Fasting state (levels increase just prior to meals)	Hypothalamus	Regulates food intake, primarily by stimulating hunger and satiety
Histamine	Stomach mucosa	Presence of food in the stomach	Stomach	Stimulates parietal cells to release HCl
Serotonin	Stomach mucosa	Presence of food in the stomach	Stomach	Contracts stomach muscle
Somatostatin	Mucosa of the stomach, especially pyloric antrum; also the duodenum	Presence of food in the stomach; sympathetic axon stimulation	Stomach	Restricts all gastric secretions, gastric motility, and emptying
Somatostatin	Mucosa of the stomach, especially pyloric antrum; also duodenum	Presence of food in the stomach; sympathetic axon stimulation	Pancreas	Restricts pancreatic secretions
Somatostatin	Mucosa of the stomach, especially pyloric antrum; also the duodenum	Presence of food in the stomach; sympathetic axon stimulation	Small intestine	Reduces intestinal absorption by reducing blood flow

Source: https://courses.lumenlearning.com/suny-ap2/chapter/the-stomach/.

2.1.3. Gastric Secretion

Hormones and nerves work together to control the secretion of stomach juice. The production of gastric juice is either activated or inhibited by stimuli in the brain, stomach, and small intestine. The cephalic, gastric, and intestinal phases are the names given to the three stages of gastric secretion because of this. However, all three stages can happen at once as soon as gastric secretion starts (Figure 2.3).

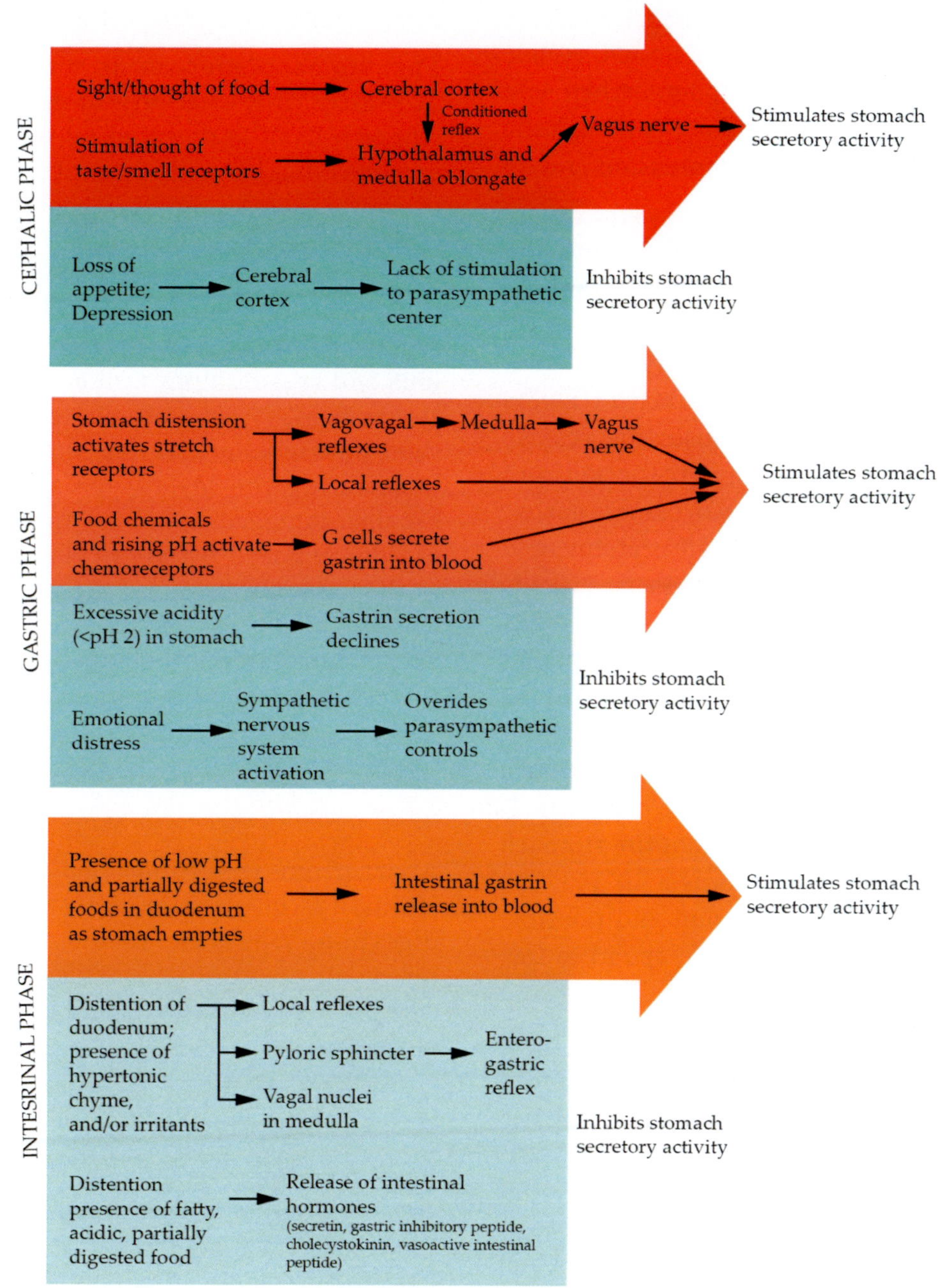

Figure 2.3. *Gastric secretion occurs in three phases: cephalic, gastric, and intestinal. During each phase, the secretion of gastric juice can be stimulated or inhibited.*

Source: https://courses.lumenlearning.com/suny-ap2/chapter/the-stomach/.

Food does not enter the stomach during the relatively short reflex phase (cephalic phase) of gastric secretion. This stage is brought on by the sight, taste, smell, or thought of food. For instance, when a piece of sushi reaches your lips, impulses from your nose or taste buds are transmitted to your brain. Your brain then sends signals back to your stomach, increasing gastric secretion in preparation for digestion. This increased secretion is a conditioned reflex, which means that it only happens when you desire or enjoy a specific food. The cephalic reflex can be suppressed by depression and an appetite decrease.

Triggered by the entry of food into the stomach, local neural and hormonal mechanisms initiate the 3- to 4-hour gastric phase of secretion. For instance, the distention that occurs when sushi enters the stomach triggers the stretch receptors. This causes the release of acetylcholine from parasympathetic neurons, which in turn causes the secretion of more gastric juice. Caffeine, partially digested proteins, and rising pH levels all cause enteroendocrine G cells to release gastrin, which causes parietal cells to produce more HCl. This acidic environment is necessary for the breakdown of proteins and the conversion of pepsinogen to pepsin. Furthermore, strong contractions of smooth muscle are triggered by the release of gastrin. It should be mentioned, though, that the stomach does have a built-in mechanism to prevent overabundance of acid secretion and possible heartburn. The stomach's cells respond to low pH by suspending the secretion of HCl and increasing the secretion of mucous secretions.

Both excitatory and inhibitory factors are present in the intestinal phase of gastric secretion. The duodenum plays a significant part in controlling how the stomach empties. A hormone known as intestinal (enteric) gastrin is released by intestinal mucosal cells when partially digested food fills the duodenum. This hormone then stimulates the secretion of gastric juice. However, this stimulating action is only temporary because the enterogastric reflex suppresses secretion when the intestine spreads due to chyme. The pyloric sphincter closes as a result of this reflex, preventing more chyme from entering the duodenum.

2.1.4. The Mucosal Barrier

The stomach mucosa is subjected to the extremely caustic acidity of gastric juice. The stomach itself is digested by the same gastric enzymes that break down protein. The mucosal barrier prevents the stomach from digesting food on its own. This barrier is made up of multiple parts. First, a thick layer of mucus rich in bicarbonate covers the stomach wall. This mucus neutralizes acid with its bicarbonate ions and creates a physical barrier. Second, the stomach mucosa's epithelial cells converge at tight junctions, preventing stomach juice from penetrating the layers of underlying tissue. Finally, damaged epithelial mucosal cells are rapidly replaced by stem cells at the junction of the gastric glands and the gastric pits when the epithelial cells shed. In actuality, the surface epithelium of the epithelium is entirely replaced every three to six days.

2.1.5. Digestive Functions of the Stomach

Apart from ingestion and defecation, the stomach is involved in almost every aspect of digestion. While the small intestine handles nearly all absorption, the stomach does absorb certain nonpolar substances like aspirin and alcohol.

2.1.5.1. Mechanical Digestion

Mixing waves start to appear at intervals of roughly 20 seconds within a few minutes after food enters your stomach. A special kind of peristalsis called a "mixing wave" combines and softens food with stomach secretions to produce chyme. The first waves of mixing are quite mild, but they are succeeded by waves that are stronger, beginning at the stomach's body and building in strength until they reach the pylorus. It's safe to say that your sushi doesn't look anything like the sushi you ate until well before it passes through the pyloric sphincter.

The pylorus functions as a filter, allowing only liquids and tiny food particles to pass through the mostly, but not completely, closed pyloric sphincter. The pylorus contains about 30 mL (1 fluid ounce) of chyme. Rhythmic mixing waves push around 3 mL of chyme at a time past the pyloric sphincter and into the duodenum during a procedure known as gastric emptying. A larger volume of chyme released all at once would be more than the small intestine could process. The remaining chyme is forced back into the stomach's interior, where it continues to mix. When more chyme is forced into the duodenum by the subsequent mixing waves, this process is repeated. Both the duodenum and the stomach control gastric emptying. Receptors that prevent stomach secretion are activated when chyme is present in the duodenum. By doing this, the stomach is unable to release more chyme before the duodenum is prepared to process it.

2.1.5.2. Chemical Digestion

Due to its ability to hold both undigested food and gases released during chemical digestion, the fundus is crucial to digestion. Food may remain in the stomach's fundus for some time before becoming combined with the chyme. Salivary amylase continues to break down food while it is in the fundus until the food starts to combine with the acidic chyme. In the end, mixing waves combine this food with the chyme, whose acidity causes lingual lipase to be activated and salivary amylase to be inactivated. After that, lingual lipase starts to convert triglycerides into mono- and diglycerides as well as free fatty acids.

Pepsin and hydrochloric acid (HCl) start the breakdown of protein in the stomach. Rennin, an enzyme that aids in the digestion of milk protein, is also produced by the gastric glands during infancy. Despite the stomach's many digestive functions, only one is essential to life: the synthesis of intrinsic factor. Intrinsic factor is required for the intestinal absorption of vitamin B_{12}, which is essential for both the maturation of red blood cells and healthy neurological function. If they receive vitamin B_{12} injections, patients who have total gastrectomy (removal of the stomach)—for example, in cases of life-threatening stomach cancer—can survive with only mild digestive dysfunction.

Within two to four hours of eating a meal, the entire contents of the stomach are emptied into the duodenum. Foods process differently depending on what kind they are. Foods high in protein empty the stomach the fastest, followed by foods high in carbs. The longest-lasting meals are those with a high triglyceride content. When the duodenum is processing fatty chyme, food can remain in the stomach for up to six hours because small intestine enzymes break down fats slowly. But keep in mind that this still only accounts for a portion of the 24 to 72 hours that complete digestion normally requires. With the exception of ingestion and defecation, the stomach is involved in every stage of digestion. The food is churned vigorously. It secretes digestive juices that aid in food digestion and absorbs some medications, such as aspirin and some alcohol. Protein is broken down in the stomach first, followed by the breakdown of carbs and fats. Food is kept in the stomach as an acidic liquid known as chyme, which is subsequently released into the small intestine over time by the pyloric sphincter.

2.2. Important Cell Types Within the Stomach

The gastric pits and glands, which are formed when the epithelium folds into the lamina propria, are home to the specialized cells listed below:

- surface mucous cells (foveolar cells)
- parietal cells
- chief cells
- neuroendocrine cells

2.2.1. Surface Mucous Cells

The stomach is lined by the gastric mucosa, which includes gastric glands that produce various substances. Within the stomach, there is a single layer of columnar epithelial cells on the surface and around the openings of gastric pits, known as surface mucous cells or foveolar cells.

These cells release a thick layer of mucus that coats the stomach lining, shielding it from digestive acids. The mucus also aids in the smooth passage of food through the stomach. Due to the constant regeneration of these surface mucous cells, the stomach lining is always safeguarded.

2.2.2. Parietal Cells

The fundus, or upper portion of the stomach, contains parietal cells in the form of gastric pits. They release hydrochloric acid, which aids in the digestion of food. Moreover, bacteria and other microorganisms that might be present in food are eliminated by hydrochloric acid. These cells secrete a protein called intrinsic factor in addition to hydrochloric acid. In the small intestine, intrinsic factor aids in the body's absorption of vitamin B_{12}.

2.2.3. Chief Cells

The fundus contains the base of the stomach glands, which contain chief cells. Digestive enzymes secreted by them aid in the breakdown of food. Pepsinogen is secreted by the chief cells. If hydrochloric acid is present, it transforms into pepsin. Pepsin aids in the breakdown of proteins into smaller molecules called polypeptides.

2.2.4. Neuroendocrine Cells

There are neuroendocrine cells in the stomach's gastric pits. Different subtypes secrete different hormones:

- **G-Cells:** These produce the hormone gastrin while residing in the pylorus region of the stomach. By inducing the release of histamine from ECL-like cells, glutathione can enhance the production of hydrochloric acid.
- **ECL-Like Cells:** Histamine is secreted by these cells in response to gastrin stimulation. Histamine increases the secretion of hydrochloric acid by binding to receptors on parietal cells. These cells are primarily found in the stomach's fundus.
- **D-Cells:** These cells are located in the stomach's pylorus. Somatostatin is an inhibitory molecule that they secrete. D-cells release somatostatin when the stomach's acidity reaches a particular point, which subsequently reduces the production of gastrin and gastric acid overall.
- **EC-Cells:** Serotonin is secreted by these cells. Serotonin plays a role in controlling fluid secretion and gastrointestinal motility.
- **P/D1 Cells:** The hormone ghrelin is secreted by these cells. The hunger hormone ghrelin stimulates appetite and encourages fat storage.

The stomach's highly specialized cells perform a wide range of tasks. The mucous layer secreted by the surface mucous cells shields the lining of the stomach. Parietal cells release intrinsic factor, which facilitates the absorption of vitamin B_{12}, and hydrochloric acid, which aids in the breakdown of food. Chief cells release digestive-supporting enzymes. Hormones that control hunger, gastrointestinal motility, and stomach acidity are secreted by neuroendocrine cells. Together, the various cell types in the stomach enable efficient food digestion and self-defense against pathogens.

2.3. Composition of Gastric Juice

A digestive fluid produced by the stomach lining is known as stomach acid, gastric juice, or stomach acid. Gastric acid, which has a pH of 1–3, is essential for the breakdown of proteins because it triggers the activity of digestive enzymes, which in turn disassemble the lengthy chains of amino acids found in proteins. In feedback systems, the production of gastric acid is regulated to increase when necessary, such as after a meal. Other stomach cells create the base bicarbonate, which buffers the liquid and maintains a consistent pH. Additionally, these cells create mucus, a viscous barrier that shields the stomach from the damaging effects of gastric acid. To counteract the acidity of the stomach as it enters the digestive tract, the pancreas additionally generates a significant quantity of bicarbonate, which it secretes into the duodenum via the pancreatic duct.

Hydrochloric acid (HCl), which is produced by parietal cells in the stomach's gastric glands, is the main active ingredient in gastric acid. The process of secretion is intricate and comparatively energy-intensive. Parietal cells have a vast network of secretory structures called canaliculi, from which hydrochloric acid is secreted into the stomach's lumen. The pH of gastric acid is 1.5 to 3.5 in the human stomach lumen, a level maintained by the proton pump H^+/K^+ ATPase. In the process, the parietal cell releases bicarbonate into the bloodstream, which results in an alkaline tide—a brief rise in blood pH. The stomach lumen's extremely acidic environment breaks down proteins (e.g., food). Proteins are made up of peptide bonds, which are labeled. The stomach's chief cells, known as the gastric chief cells, secrete pepsinogen and, in infants, renin, which are enzymes used to break down proteins. Because of the low pH, pepsinogen is converted into the enzyme pepsin, which facilitates digestion by proteolyzing amino acid bonds. Additionally, an acidic environment inhibits or destroys a lot of microorganisms, preventing illness or infection.

2.3.1. Secretion

Approximately 1.5 liters of gastric acid are secreted daily by the stomach of an adult human. The production of gastric acid secretion occurs in stages. The cytoplasm of parietal cells secretes hydrogen and chloride ions, which are then combined in the canaliculi. After then, the main stomach lumen is gradually reached by the gastric acid that is secreted into the lumen of the gastric gland. There is debate over the precise route taken by secreted acid to reach the stomach lumen because it must first pass through the mucus layer in the stomach, which has a relatively neutral pH. The parietal cell's cytoplasm actively secretes sodium and chloride ions into the canaliculus lumen. Potassium ions and a trace amount of sodium ions diffuse from the cytoplasm into the parietal cell canaliculi as a result of this creating a negative potential of between -40 and -70 mV across the parietal cell membrane.

The process that creates carbonic acid from carbon dioxide and water is catalyzed by the enzyme carbonic anhydrase. This acid splits into bicarbonate and hydrogen ions right away. H^+/K^+ATPase antiporter pumps allow the hydrogen ions to exit the cell. Sodium ions are actively reabsorbed at the same time. This indicates that most potassium (K+) and sodium

(Na+) ions secreted return to the cytoplasm. Secreted hydrogen and chloride ions combine in the canaliculus before being secreted into the oxygenic gland lumen.

The maximum concentration of gastric acid that can be found in the stomach's canaliculi is 160 mM. This is nearly precisely isotonic with other body fluids, but it is approximately three million times that of arterial blood. The acid secreted has the lowest pH of 0.8, but in the stomach lumen, it is diluted to a pH of one to three. Between meals, there is a tiny, continuous basal secretion of gastric acid that typically occurs at a rate of less than 10 mEq/hour.

To speed up the process of digesting a meal, the gastric acid secretion occurs in three phases:

- **The Cephalic Phase:** The anticipation of food and its aroma or flavor triggers 30% of the total amount of gastric acid secretions to be produced. The vagus nerve (Cranial Nerve X) transmits this signal from higher brain centers. It causes the release of histamine from ECL cells and acid from parietal cells. Gastrin-releasing peptide is also released onto G cells by the vagus nerve (CN X). Lastly, it prevents D cells from releasing somatostatin.
- **The Gastric Phase:** During this phase, about 60% of the total acid for a meal is secreted. The presence of amino acids in food and stomach distension both encourage the secretion of acid.
- **The Intestinal Phase:** The remaining 10% of the acid is secreted when chyme reaches the small intestine and is triggered by amino acids and small intestine distension. Entero-oxyntin is released by the duodenal cells and acts on the parietal cells without interfering with gastrin.

2.3.2. Regulation of Secretion

The production of gastric acid is controlled by multiple hormones and the autonomic nervous system. The hormone gastrin and the parasympathetic nervous system act directly on the parietal cells by stimulating their production of gastric acid through the vagus nerve and the stimulation of the hormone histamine secreted from enterochromaffin-like cells (ECL), respectively. Secretin, cholecystokinin, and vasoactive intestinal peptide all work to suppress production (Figure 2.4).

Positive regulators and negative feedback systems closely control the stomach's production of gastric acid. This process involves four different cell types: enterochromaffine-like cells, G cells, D cells, and parietal cells. In addition, the intramural nervous plexus and the vagus nerve (CN X) endings in the digestive tract have a major impact on secretion.

The stomach's nerve endings release two stimulatory neurotransmitters: acetylcholine and gastrin-releasing peptide. These neurotransmitters act by directly affecting parietal cells, as well as by triggering the secretion of gastrin from G cells and histamine from enterochromaffine-like cells. Gastrin directly and indirectly influences parietal cells by promoting histamine release.

The primary positive regulation mechanism of gastric acid secretion in the stomach is the release of histamine. Somatostatin inhibits its release while gastrin and acetylcholine stimulate it.

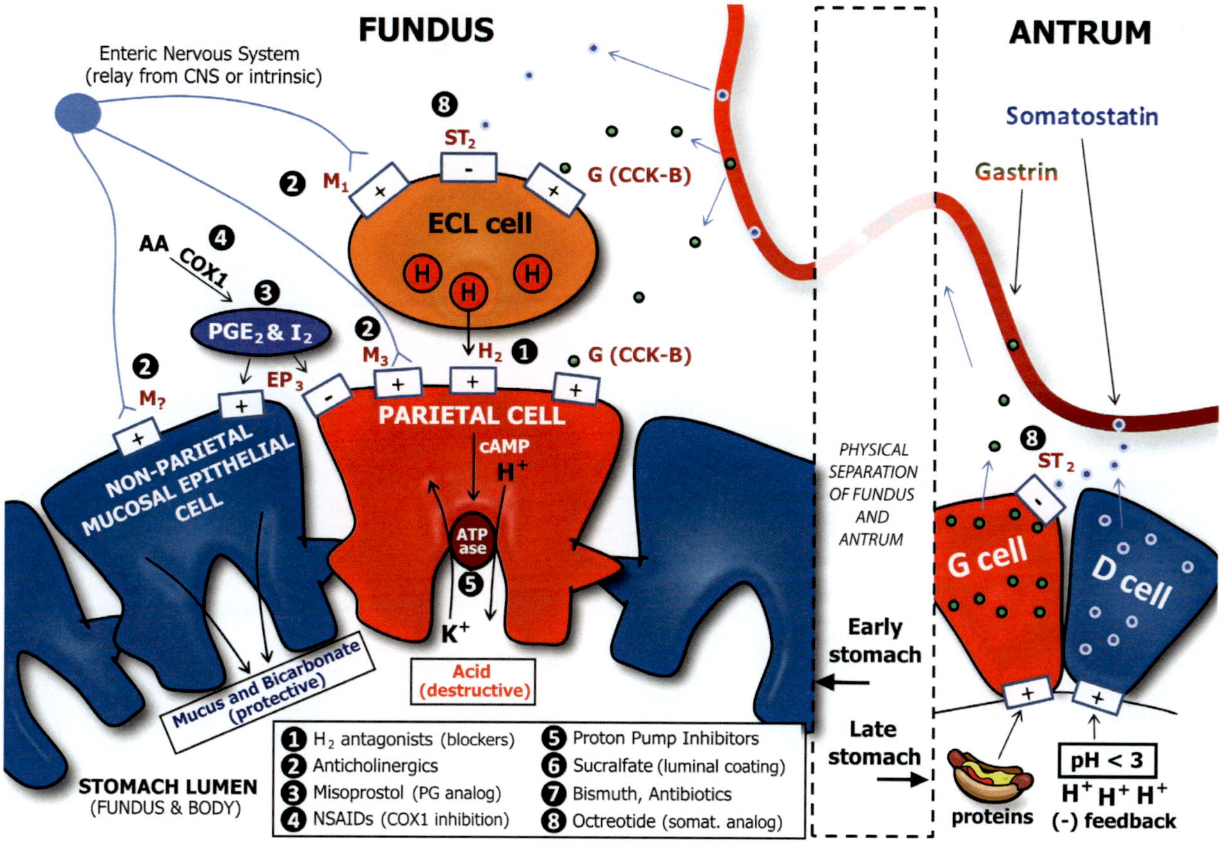

Figure 2.4. *Diagram depicting the major determinants of gastric acid secretion, with inclusion of drug targets for peptic ulcer disease (PUD) and gastroesophageal reflux disease (GERD).*

Source: By Adam L. VanWert, Pharm.D., Ph.D. – Own work, CC BY 3.0, https://commons.wikimedia.org/w/index.php?curid=12677508.

2.3.3. Neutralization

Bicarbonate neutralizes gastric acid in the duodenum. Additionally, this inhibits stomach enzymes whose optimal pH range is in the acidic range. Secretin stimulates the pancreatic production of bicarbonate. When the pH in the duodenum drops below 4.5 to 5.0, the so-called S cells in the mucosa of the duodenum and jejunum activate and secrete this polypeptide hormone. The following equation describes the neutralization:

$$HCl + NaHCO_3 \rightarrow NaCl + H_2CO_3$$

Through the catalysis of carbonic anhydrase enzymes bound to the gut epithelial lining, the carbonic acid quickly equilibrates with carbon dioxide and water, resulting in a net release of carbon dioxide gas within the lumen associated with neutralization. Most of the gas produced during neutralization is exhaled through the lungs because both the dissolved carbon dioxide and carbonic acid will tend to equilibrate with the blood in the absorptive upper intestine, such as the duodenum.

2.3.4. Role in Stomach Disease

The stomach produces little to no gastric acid in hypochlorhydria and amchlorhydria, which can cause issues because the gastric lumen's disinfectant capacity is reduced. Such circumstances increase the risk of developing digestive tract infections, such as those caused by Helicobacter or Vibrio bacteria.

Increased gastrin levels in Zollinger-Ellison syndrome and hypercalcemia result in an excess of gastric acid production, which can cause stomach ulcers. Patients with illnesses that cause excessive vomiting experience hypochloremic metabolic alkalosis, which is characterized by a decrease in blood acidity due to H+ and chlorine depletion. Acid reflux or stomach acid constantly flowing back into the esophagus, can irritate the lining of the esophagus and lead to gastroesophageal reflux disease. Periodically, a lot of people experience acid reflux. On the other hand, acid reflux can result in GERD if it occurs frequently over time. With medication and lifestyle modifications, the majority of people are able to control their GERD discomfort. Although rare, some people may require surgery to relieve their symptoms.

2.3.5. Pharmacology

Proton pump inhibitors, which are used to raise gastric pH and subsequently lower stomach acidity in conditions characterized by excess acid, target the proton pump enzyme. H2 antagonists reduce stomach acid production in an indirect manner. Existing acid is neutralized by antacids.

2.4. Parietal Cells

Parietal cells, also referred to as oxygen cells, are stomach epithelial cells that secrete intrinsic factor and hydrochloric acid (HCl). These cells are found in the gastric glands, which are situated in the stomach's body parts and fundus lining. They have a vast network of secretory canaliculi from which the stomach receives active transport of the HCl. The enzyme known as hydrogen potassium ATPase, or H^+/K^+ ATPase, is exclusive to parietal cells and facilitates the transport of H+ against the steepest ion gradient in the human body, which is a concentration gradient of roughly 3 million to 1. The main modulators of parietal cells are histamine, acetylcholine, and glutamate, which can be obtained from both central and local sources.

2.4.1. Structure

2.4.1.1. Canaliculus

An adaptation present on gastric parietal cells is called a canaliculus. It is a small channel or deep in folding that works to expand the surface area, e.g., to be kept secret. The number of canaliculi varies in response to secretory demand, indicating the dynamic nature of the parietal cell membrane. This is achieved through the membrane fusing with canalicular precursors, or tubulovesicles, to increase surface area, and the canaliculi's reciprocal endocytosis (reforming the tubulovesicles) to decrease surface area.

2.4.2. Function

2.4.2.1. Hydrochloric Acid Secretion

Hydrochloric acid is formed in the following manner:

- Carbonic acid dissociates to produce hydrogen ions. When considering hydrogen ion sources, water pales in comparison to carbonic acid. Carbonic anhydrase converts carbon dioxide and water into carbonic acid.
- An alkaline tide phenomenon results from the bicarbonate ion (HCO_3^-) diffusing into the venous blood and being exchanged for a chloride ion (Cl^-) on the basal side of the cell.
- Chloride (Cl^-) and potassium (K^+) ions permeate into the canaliculi.

- The H^+/K^+-ATPase pumps hydrogen ions from the cell into the canaliculi in exchange for potassium ions. When parietal cells are activated, fusion of tubulovesicles increases the number of these pumps on the luminal side, and during deactivation, they are eliminated. This pump keeps the difference in proton concentration between a million times. The numerous mitochondria produce ATP (Figure 2.5).

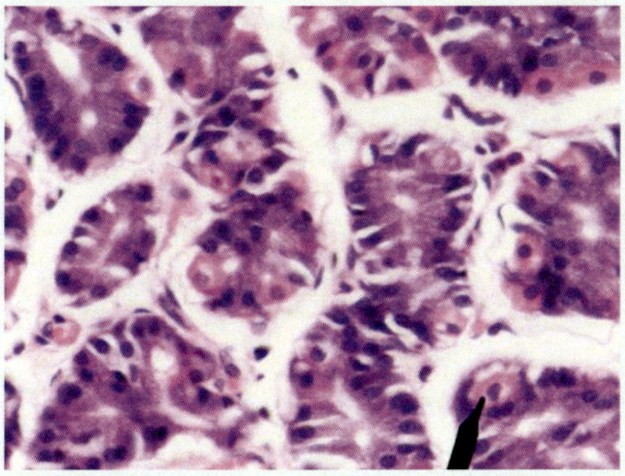

Figure 2.5. *Human parietal cells (pink staining) – stomach.*

Source: By Jpogi at English Wikipedia – Transferred from en.wikipedia to Commons., Public Domain, https://commons.wikimedia.org/w/index.php?curid=3740621.

The highly acidic environment of the gastric lumen is preserved due to the cellular export of hydrogen ions. By encouraging the unfolding (or denaturing) of ingested proteins, the acidity facilitates food digestion. The peptide bonds that hold the amino acids together become visible as proteins unfold. Through a process known as proteolysis, gastric hydrochloric acid simultaneously cleaves the zymogen pepsinogen into active pepsin, an endopeptidase that facilitates the digestive process by rupturing the now-exposed peptide bonds.

2.4.2.2. Regulation

Parietal cells release acid in reaction to three different kinds of stimuli:

- The main contribution of histamine is the stimulation of H_2 histamine receptors.
- Acetylcholine (ACh) stimulates M3 receptors through the vagus nerve and enteric nervous system, resulting from parasympathetic activity.
- Gastrin stimulates CCK2 receptors, which has a minor effect but also causes local ECL cells to secrete histamine.

Intracellular cAMP levels rise in response to histamine activation via the H2 receptor, whereas intracellular calcium levels rise in response to ACh activation through the M3 receptor and gastrin activation through the CCK2 receptor. These receptors are found on the membrane's basolateral side.

Protein kinase A is elevated in response to elevated cAMP levels. Proteins that are involved in moving H^+/K^+-ATPase from the cytoplasm to the cell membrane are phosphorylated by protein kinase A. Further, H^+ ions are secreted and K^+ ions are reabsorbed as a result. The secreted fluid's pH may drop by 0.8. Gastrin mainly causes an indirect increase in histamine synthesis in ECL cells, which then signals parietal cells through the release of histamine and stimulation of H_2. The maximal histamine-stimulated gastric acid secretion is unaffected by gastrin alone. Histamine, acetylcholine, and gastrin have synergistic effects, meaning that their combined effects are greater than the sum of their individual effects. It aids in the physiologically nonlinear increase of secretion in response to stimuli.

2.4.2.3. Intrinsic Factor Secretion

Additionally, parietal cells generate a glycoprotein referred to as intrinsic factor. For vitamin B_{12} to be absorbed from the diet, intrinsic factor is necessary. Long-term vitamin B_{12} deficiency can cause megaloblastic anemia, which is characterized by large, fragile red blood cells. The autoimmune breakdown of stomach parietal cells causes pernicious anemia by preventing the production of intrinsic factor and, consequently, the absorption of vitamin B_{12}. Megaloblastic anemia is also a result of pernicious anemia. Atrophic gastritis can result in deficiencies like decreased DNA synthesis and nucleotide metabolism in the bone marrow, as well as an inability to absorb B_{12}. This is especially true in older patients.

2.4.3. Clinical Significance

Parietal cells (highly magnified) are a component of fundic gland polyps.

- Overacidity in the stomach can lead to peptic ulcers. Antacids can be used to increase the stomach lining's innate tolerance. H2 antihistamines and other antimuscarinic medications, like pirenzepine, can lessen acid secretion. Since the final common pathway of all stimulation of acid production is the stomach, proton pump inhibitors have a greater effect on reducing the production of acid in the stomach.
- Autoantibodies against intrinsic factor or parietal cells reduce the absorption of vitamin B_{12} in pernicious anemia. Vitamin B_{12} replacement shots (methylcobalamin, hydroxocobalamin, or cyanocobalamin) can be used to treat it.
- Another autoimmune condition affecting the parietal cells is achlorhydria. The necessary quantity of gastric acid cannot be produced by the injured parietal cells. This raises the pH of the stomach, impairs food digestion, and raises the risk of gastroenteritis.

2.5. The Mucosal Barrier

The feature of the stomach that permits it to securely hold the gastric acid needed for digestion is called the gastric mucosal barrier. When the barrier is breached, as occurs when acetylsalicylic acid (ASA, aspirin) is dissolved in acid, the acid diffuses back into the mucosa, where it can harm the stomach.

There are three protective parts to the barrier. They give the stomach's mucosal surface an extra layer of resistance. The three elements consist of:

- A dense layer of epithelial cells. Tight junctions between the cells that make up the stomach's epithelium repel harsh liquids that could harm the lining of the stomach.
- a unique mucus layer made of mucus secreted by focal cells and surface epithelial cells. The entire surface of the stomach mucosa is covered in a protective layer of gel-like insoluble mucus. The gastric mucosa is shielded from autodigestion by the mucus e.g., pepsin as well as from deterioration caused by consumed acids and other caustic substances.
- Bicarbonate ions are released by the epithelial cells on the surface. Harsh acids are neutralized by the bicarbonate ions (Figure 2.6).

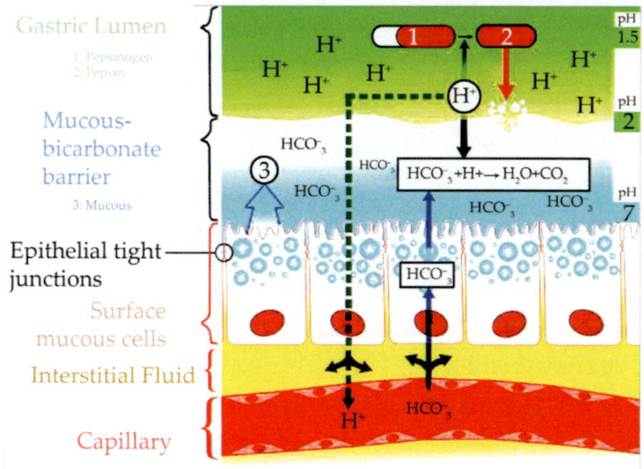

Figure 2.6. *Diagram of the alkaline mucous layer in the stomach with mucosal defense mechanism.*

Source: By Nelson Glyn – Own work, CC BY-SA 4.0, https://commons.wikimedia.org/w/index.php?curid=68205101.

Factors that can damage the barrier:

- Bacterial Infection by *Helicobacter pylori*
- Alcohol
- Aspirin is an example of a non-steroidal anti-inflammatory drug (NSAID).

2.5.1. Tight Junction Composition

Intestinal epithelia create a selective barrier that allows molecules and ions to flow between cells but stops pathogens and commensal bacteria from passing through. The tight junction creates the actual seal between neighboring cells, as was previously mentioned. The strength of the adhesive that holds cells together and inhibits mechanical disruption of the epithelial sheet is provided by adherens junctions and desmosomes. The apical junctional complex, which is made up of these structures, is also the location of the proteins that control epithelial polarization. Proper sorting and delivery of newly synthesized proteins as well as those trafficking through intracellular compartments to the apical or basolateral plasma membrane are integral to epithelial function. This process is known as polarization. This is dependent, in part, on basolateral exocytosis being directed by the exocyst complex binding to the apical junctional complex via cell-adhesion proteins.

The tight junction, when examined using freeze-fracture electron microscopy, appears as a network of interconnected strands believed to be responsible for forming a barrier. The exact makeup of these strands is still being studied, with evidence suggesting an involvement of both lipids and proteins. Lipids, particularly cholesterol-rich microdomains, play a crucial role in regulating the density and composition of tight junction proteins, impacting barrier function. Lowering plasma membrane cholesterol levels can lead to changes in the structure of tight junction strands and barrier integrity. Additionally, caveolar endocytosis, a process dependent on cholesterol, is essential for the internalization of occludin and increased permeability through the leak pathway, such as in response to TNF exposure.

2.5.2. Claudin Proteins Define the Selectivity of Paracellular Permeability

Claudin proteins are an essential part of tight junction strands, as evidenced by the independent observations that some claudin protein expression in tight-junction-deficient fibroblasts leads to the assembly of tight-junction-like strands, while expression of other claudin proteins changes the architecture of epithelial strands. The precise biochemical makeup of tight junction strands is unknown, though. The structure of the tight junction, which forms the barrier, is generally understood to consist of pore-forming claudins that form channels supporting solute flow and barrier-enhancing claudins that occlude the intercellular space. For instance, the pore-forming protein claudin-2 creates gated paracellular channels that allow small uncharged molecules and Na^+ to flow through but not larger solutes. Interestingly, tight junctions have much less relative selectivity for monovalent cations, such as Na^+, K^+, methylamine and ethylamine, and even anions, despite having gating behaviors that are similar to transmembrane ion channels. Water can also pass through a common pore that is enabled by Claudin-2 pores. The first two extracellular loops of claudin-2, which are next to four transmembrane domains with intracellular N- and C-termini, controls the protein's specificity for Na^+. The charge and size selectivity of the high-capacity pore pathway are determined by pore-forming claudins. As a result, transepithelial resistance (TER), a gauge of barrier function, decreases in tandem with the specific increase in Na^+ permeability brought about by claudin-2 expression in cultured epithelial monolayers.

2.5.3. Non-claudin Tight Junction Proteins Regulate the Paracellular Barrier

Other tight junction proteins, such as occludin, tricellulin (also called MarvelD2), and MarvelD3, which all contain the tetra-spanning "myelin and lymphocyte protein and related proteins for vesicle trafficking and membrane link" (MARVEL) domain, can influence the structure and function of claudin-based tight junction strands. TAMPs are targeted to specific tight junction domains; tricellulin is mainly present at tricellular junctions, while occludin and MarvelD3 localize to bicellular and tricellular junctions. These proteins can modify strand architecture and claudin channel function in addition to forming homotypic cis-interactions. Occludin can control the paracellular pore pathway in this way. For instance, in specific circumstances, occludin can interfere with claudin-2 anchoring at the tight junction. Additionally, occludin controls the leak pathway. In MDCK and human intestinal Caco-2 monolayers, occludin knockdown increases the permeability of big monovalent cations and uncharged solutes. Furthermore, cytokine-induced increases in leak pathway permeability are restrained by in vivo overexpression of occludin.

Tricellulin, a constituent of tricellular junctions, controls paracellular flux across them. Overexpression of tubulin causes localization at bicellular and tricellular junctions and enhances epithelial resistance by reducing the paracellular flux of larger molecules and ions. A more restricted level of tricellulin overexpression only improves tricellulin localization at tricellular junctions and reduces permeability to macromolecules ranging in size from 4 to 10 kDa. Furthermore, when tricellulin is eliminated from the tricellular junction, macromolecule permeability rises. These findings suggest that at tricellular junctions, tricellulin regulates the leak pathway.

ZO-family proteins, such as ZO-1, ZO-2 (TJP2), and ZO-3 (TJP3), which are frequently referred to as scaffolding proteins, have direct interactions with TAMPs. The ZO-1 and ZO-2 interactions with claudin proteins through the PDZ1 domain are thought to be necessary for claudin trafficking and tight junction biogenesis. The ZO-family proteins have similar structures and share protein-binding motifs within the N-terminus, including three PDZ domains that mediate binding to claudins, to other ZO-family members, and to signaling proteins like phospholipase C isoforms. After the PDZ domains come the GuK and U5 domains, which mediate binding to occludin, a U6 domain that may control interactions with occludin, and actin-binding regions in the case of ZO-1 and ZO-2. The increased paracellular permeability of large solutes through the leak pathway when ZO-1 is knocked down in MDCK monolayers is evidence that ZO-1 regulates the leak pathway in terms of barrier function. Furthermore, ZO proteins control the organization of cortical actin, as demonstrated by the hypercontraction of cortical actin in cells devoid of ZO-1 and ZO-2. ZO-1 interacts with additional cytoskeletal regulators, according to other data. For instance, TER is decreased upon knockdown of both ZO-1 and afadin, which is in line with the adherens junction's critical function in preserving intercellular adhesion, which is a requirement for tight junction assembly. On the other hand, some information implies that ZO-1 controls adherens junctions as well. Lastly, recent research suggests that in three-dimensional culture, ZO-1 interactions with F-actin and occludin orient epithelial polarization and direct morphogenesis.

2.5.4. Adherens Junctions Contribute to Epithelial Barrier Function by Stabilizing the Tight Junction

Adherens junction components are necessary for tight junction assembly and serve as a basis for cell-cell interactions. E-cadherin, also referred to as CDH1, is a single-spanning transmembrane protein that plays a major role in the epithelial adherens junction. It can interact intracellularly with other adherens junction components as well as homotypic cell-cell adhesion. Studies using in vitro knockdown indicate that while E-cadherin is necessary for tight junction assembly, it may not be necessary for their maintenance.

2.5.5. Activation of the Perijunctional Actomyosin Ring Regulates Tight Junction Barrier Function

The tight junction function is partially regulated by myosin light chain kinase (MLCK), which phosphorylates myosin II regulatory light chain to drive actomyosin contraction and increase tight junction permeability. The perijunctional actomyosin ring is defined as a dense ring of myosin and actin that runs around the circumference of the cell at the region of the adherens and tight junctions. In vitro and in vivo, perijunctional actomyosin can be reorganized and paracellular permeability can be increased by expressing a constitutively active MLCK catalytic domain that lacks regulatory elements. In contrast, inhibition of MLCK blocks the increase in paracellular permeability that occurs after activation of Na^+–glucose cotransport and supports paracellular nutrient absorption. Furthermore, acute cytokine-induced increases in flux through the leak pathway can be prevented in vivo and in vitro by pharmacological or genetic inhibition of MLCK.

2.5.6. Mucin is an Extracellular Component Essential in Barrier Function

The luminal contents and the epithelium layer are shielded by a layer of mucus. In the small intestine, mucus is found in a single detached layer, but in the colon, it is arranged as a mucus bilayer with an adherent inner layer and a loose detached outer layer.

Apart from those that make up the outer layer of the colon, commensal bacteria cannot pass through mucus. The structure, function, and expression sites of mucins, which are highly glycosylated proteins made and secreted by goblet cells, differ. Examples of how transmembrane mucins that are anchored to the epithelium differ from detached gel-forming mucins are through variations in their protein domains. Mucous layer protection is crucial, as demonstrated by diarrhea and mucosal damage when the dominant intestinal mucin gene, *Muc2*, is depleted.

2.5.7. Tight Junction Permeability Pathways in Disease

Disease-related alterations to the barrier parts alter the structure and functionality of tight junctions, which eventually results in barrier dysfunction. The representative cytokines TNF and interleukin (IL)-13 are frequently elevated in inflammatory bowel disease and cause barrier loss by different mechanisms. Research on intestinal epithelia has demonstrated that TNF and IL-13, respectively, impair barrier function by going after claudin-2 and MLCK. More specifically, both in vitro and in vivo, the flux of small cations across the pore pathway is increased by IL-13-dependent claudin-2 expression. On the other hand, TNF causes an increase in the flow of bigger solutes across the leak pathway, which can be specifically stopped by overexpressing occludin or inhibiting MLCK pharmacologically or genetically. There is evidence that the pore and leak pathways converge at the level of intercellular signaling, despite their apparent differences.

It has been demonstrated that intestinal barrier function in Crohn's disease can be restored by anti-TNF antibody (biologic) therapy. It is unclear whether the restoration is solely a result of the general attenuation of the inflammatory activity or if it is partially attributable to the suppression of TNF-induced MLCK activation in intestinal epithelial cells. However, it is noteworthy that MLCK expression and activity are elevated in intestinal epithelial cells during inflammatory bowel diseases, such as ulcerative colitis and Crohn's disease.

2.5.8. The Unrestricted Pathway

Particles of nearly any size can pass through the unrestricted pathway, which opens as a result of epithelial damage and permits the passage of big proteins, viruses, and bacteria, in contrast to the pore and leak pathways. Graft-versus-host disease (GVHD) is a well-researched example of unrestricted pathway flux, where the degree of bacterial flux across the unrestricted pathway is correlated with the disease's severity. A condition known as donor-derived host disease (GVHD) can develop after hematopoietic stem cell or bone marrow transplantation, in which the recipient's body cells are attacked by immune cells derived from the donor. The pathogenesis of GVHD has been found to require epithelial damage, as demonstrated by a clinically relevant mouse model. In line with the critical function of the intestinal barrier in preventing GVHD, intraperitoneal injection of bacterial lipopolysaccharides could avoid the need for epithelial damage. i.e., endotoxin.

2.5.9. Isolated Tight Junction Dysfunction is Insufficient to Cause Disease

Disease-related barrier dysfunction has a variety of causes; modifications to the elements that control and preserve specific permeability pathways as well as mucosal immune stimuli can lead to barrier loss. In fact, many intestinal disorders are believed to be initiated and propagated by barrier loss. From the epithelium to the mucus layer, a complex network of multiple protein and lipid components is required for the mucosal barrier to function. Many proteins, including claudins, that have been classified as either barrier-enhancing or pore-forming make up the tight junction, which is responsible for defining a large portion of the function of the mucosal barrier. However, both this and the overall mechanism of claudin regulation are still poorly understood. To understand how these elements, along with pore and leak pathways, are disturbed during disease, more investigation is required to disentangle the interactions that are crucial to maintaining the integrity of the mucosal barrier. Determining possible therapeutic targets and understanding how cytokines, such as TNF and IL-13, signal to cause barrier loss are significant challenges. Though not sufficient to start a disease, intestinal barrier loss is probably going to be a major factor in how it progresses, and solving the puzzle of barrier loss will probably help treat a lot of diseases.

2.6. The Role of the Stomach in Nutrient Absorption

The cavity of upper small intestine is where ingested food molecules, water, and minerals from the diet are absorbed. The majority of the absorbed materials pass through the mucosa and enter the bloodstream, where they are transported to other bodily regions for storage or additional chemical transformation. The way that various nutrients affect this portion of the digestive system's operation varies.

2.6.1. The Essential Nutrients

According to the Australian Department of Health, carbohydrates, protein, fats, vitamins, water, and even salt are considered essential nutrients because they give the body energy, the components needed for growth and repair, and the materials required to control chemical reactions. The descriptions that follow detail how these nutrients interact with the digestive system and support the body's normal functioning.

2.6.1.1. Carbohydrates

An adult in America typically consumes half a pound of carbohydrates per day. The majority of the calories in some of our most popular foods are carbs.

Bread, potatoes, pastries, candies, rice, spaghetti, fruits, and vegetables are a few examples. Many of these foods have a combination of fiber, which the body cannot digest, and starch, which the body can digest. Enzymes found in saliva, pancreatic juice, and the lining of the small intestine break down the digestible carbohydrates into smaller molecules.

The process of breaking down starch involves two stages: first, an enzyme found in pancreatic juice and saliva converts starch into molecules known as maltose; second, an enzyme called maltase located in the small intestine lining breaks down the maltose into glucose molecules that can be absorbed into the blood. After entering the liver through the bloodstream, glucose is either stored there or used to power the body's operations.

Another carbohydrate that needs to be digested to be useful is table sugar. Table sugar is broken down by an enzyme in the small intestine lining into glucose and fructose, which can then be absorbed into the bloodstream from the intestinal cavity. Another type of sugar found in milk is called lactose, which is converted into molecules that can be absorbed by the intestinal lining by an enzyme called lactase.

2.6.1.2. Protein

Giant protein molecules found in foods like meat, eggs, and beans must be broken down by enzymes for the body to use them for tissue growth and repair. An enzyme in the stomach's juice initiates the breakdown of protein that has been swallowed. In the small intestine, the protein undergoes final digestion. Here, a number of enzymes from the intestinal lining and pancreatic juice break down large protein molecules into smaller ones known as amino acids. These tiny molecules can be taken up by the blood from the small intestine and distributed throughout the body to build cell walls and other components.

2.6.1.3. Fats

The body can get a lot of energy from fat molecules. Dissolving fat, like butter, in the intestinal cavity's water content is the first stage of digestion. The liver secretes bile acids, which serve as natural detergents to dissolve fat in water and enable the breakdown of large fat molecules into smaller ones, some of which are cholesterol and fatty acids, by enzymes. The cholesterol and fatty acids mix with the bile acids to facilitate their entry into the mucosa cells. The small molecules are reassembled into large molecules in these cells, the majority of which enter the lymphatic vessels that are located close to the intestine. These tiny blood vessels transport the reformed fat to the chest veins, while the blood transports the fat to various body storage locations.

2.6.1.4. Vitamins

The walls of the large, hollow organs of the digestive system can move because of the muscles within them. Food and liquid can be propelled by the movement of organ walls, which can also mix the contents within each organ. Peristalsis is the term for the normal movement of the intestine, stomach, and esophagus. Peristalsis appears to be an ocean wave passing through a muscle. The organ's muscle narrows a section, which is then gradually propelled down the organ's length. The food and liquid in front of them are forced through each hollow organ by these waves of narrowing.

2.6.1.5. Water and Salt

The majority of the substance that passes through the small intestine's cavity is water that has dissolved salt in it. The food and liquids we swallow, as well as the secretions from the numerous digestive glands, are the sources of salt and water. Every 24 hours, the intestine absorbs more than a gallon of water containing more than one ounce of salt from a healthy adult.

2.6.2. Digestion Control

The digestive system's ability to regulate itself is an intriguing feature. Several aspects are discussed below:

2.6.2.1. Hormone Regulators

Cells in the stomach and small intestine mucosa produce and release the main hormones that regulate the digestive system functioning. These hormones are discharged into the bloodstream of the digestive tract, return via the arteries and heart, and then enter the digestive system again to stimulate the secretion of digestive juices and induce the movement of organs.

The three hormones that regulate digestion are cholecystokinin (CCK), secretin, and gastrin.

- To dissolve and digest some foods, the stomach produces acid due to the action of gastrin. Furthermore, it is essential for the healthy development of the stomach, small intestine, and colon linings.
- The pancreas secretes a digestive juice that is high in bicarbonate when secretin is present. It also causes the liver to produce bile and the stomach to produce pepsin, an enzyme that breaks down protein.
- Gallbladder emptying and pancreatic growth and production of pancreatic juice enzymes are caused by CCK.

2.6.2.2. Nerve Regulators

The functions are regulated by two different kinds of nerves. The brain's unconscious region and the spinal cord supply extrinsic, or external, nerves to the digestive organs. Acetylcholine and adrenaline are two of the chemicals they release. Acetylcholine increases the force with which the muscles of the digestive organs squeeze, which pushes food and liquids through the digestive tract. The pancreas and stomach both produce more digestive juice when acetylcholine is present. Blood flow to the stomach and intestine is reduced by adrenaline, which also relaxes the muscles present in them.

The intrinsic (inside) nerves, which comprise a dense network embedded in the walls of the esophagus, stomach, small intestine, and colon, are far more significant. When food stretches the walls of the hollow organs, the intrinsic nerves are activated. They release a plethora of substances that either accelerate or decelerate the passage of food through the digestive system and the production of bodily fluids.

A Closer Look

Homeostatic Imbalances: Ulcers

Although the mucosal barrier is highly effective, it is not infallible. Occasionally, gastric juice can damage the superficial lining of the stomach mucosa, leading to erosions that typically heal independently. When the erosions are more severe and extend deeper, they are referred to as ulcers.

Numerous factors can interfere with the mucosal barrier's ability to protect the stomach lining, which is why it breaks down. Most ulcers are brought on by an infection with *Helicobacter pylori* or by overusing non-steroidal anti-inflammatory drugs (NSAIDs), such as aspirin.

Antacids aid in the relief of ulcer symptoms like indigestion and "burning" pain. Transferring to different classes of pain relievers facilitates healing when NSAID use is the cause of ulcers. When brought on by H. antibiotics work well for pylori infection.

One possible side effect of ulcers is perforation, which can lead to peritonitis (peritoneal inflammation) by rupturing the stomach wall. These ulcers need to be surgically repaired.

Summary

- There are four main regions in the stomach: the cardia, fundus, body, and pylorus. The cardia (or cardiac region) is the point where the esophagus connects to the stomach and through which food passes into the stomach. Located inferior to the diaphragm, above and to the left of the cardia, is the dome-shaped fundus. Below the fundus is the body, the main part of the stomach. The funnel-shaped pylorus connects the stomach to the duodenum.
- The wall of the stomach is made of the same four layers as most of the rest of the alimentary canal but with adaptations to the mucosa and muscularis for the unique functions of this organ.
- The secretion of gastric juice is controlled by both nerves and hormones. Stimuli in the brain, stomach, and small intestine activate or inhibit gastric juice production. This is why the three phases of gastric secretion are called the cephalic, gastric, and intestinal phases.
- The mucosa of the stomach is exposed to the highly corrosive acidity of gastric juice. Gastric enzymes that can digest protein can also digest the stomach itself. The stomach is protected from self-digestion by the mucosal barrier.
- The stomach participates in virtually all the digestive activities except for ingestion and defecation. Although almost all absorption takes place in the small intestine, the stomach does absorb some nonpolar substances, such as alcohol and aspirin.
- The epithelium folds into the lamina propria, forming the gastric pits and glands, which contain the specialized cells namely, surface mucous cells (foveolar cells), parietal cells, chief cells, and neuroendocrine cells.
- Gastric acid, gastric juice, or stomach acid is a digestive fluid formed within the stomach lining. With a pH between 1 and 3, gastric acid plays a key role in the digestion of proteins by activating digestive enzymes, which together break down the long chains of amino acids of proteins.
- Gastric acid production is regulated by both the autonomic nervous system and several hormones. The parasympathetic nervous system, via the vagus nerve, and the hormone gastrin stimulate the parietal cell to produce gastric acid, both directly acting on parietal cells and indirectly, through the stimulation of the secretion of the hormone histamine from enterochromaffine-like cells (ECL). Vasoactive intestinal peptide, cholecystokinin, and secretin all inhibit production.
- Parietal cells (also known as oxyntic cells) are epithelial cells in the stomach that secrete hydrochloric acid (HCl) and intrinsic factor. These cells are located in the gastric glands found in the lining of the fundus and body regions of the stomach.
- The gastric mucosal barrier is the property of the stomach that allows it to safely contain the gastric acid required for digestion. If the barrier is broken, as by acetylsalicylic acid (ASA, aspirin) in acid solution, acid diffuses back into the mucosa where it can cause damage to the stomach itself.

- Digested molecules of food, as well as water and minerals from the diet, are absorbed from the cavity of the upper small intestine. The absorbed materials cross the mucosa into the blood, mainly, and are carried off in the bloodstream to other parts of the body for storage or further chemical change.

References

1. Alcaino, C., Knutson, K. R., Treichel, A. J., Yildiz, G., Strege, P. R., Linden, D. R., & Beyder, A. (2018). A population of gut epithelial enterochromaffin cells is mechanosensitive and requires Piezo2 to convert force into serotonin release. *Proceedings of the National Academy of Sciences of the United States of America, 115*(32), E7632–E7641. https://doi.org/10.1073/pnas.1804938115.
2. Bode, C., & Bode, J. C. (2003). Effect of alcohol consumption on the gut. *Clinical Gastroenterology, 17*(4), 575–592. https://doi.org/10.1016/S1521-6918(03)00034-9.
3. Brown, L. M. (2000). Helicobacter pylori: Epidemiology and routes of transmission. *Epidemiologic Reviews, 22*(2), 283–297. https://doi.org/10.1093/oxfordjournals.epirev.a018040.
4. Chaudhari, N., & Roper, S. D. (2010). The cell biology of taste. *Journal of Cell Biology, 191*(2), 429. https://doi.org/10.1083/jcb.20100314420100927c.
5. Chaudhry SR, Nahian A, Chaudhry K. Anatomy, Abdomen and Pelvis, Pelvis. 2023 Jul 25. In: StatPearls [Internet]. Treasure Island (FL): StatPearls Publishing; 2024 Jan–. PMID: 29489173.
6. Engevik, A. C., Feng, R., Yang, L., Nelson, C. E., & Engevik, M. A. (2020). The physiology of the gastric parietal cell. *Frontiers in Physiology, 11*, 737. https://www.ncbi.nlm.nih.gov/pmc/articles/PMC7327232/ (accessed on 23 May 2024).
7. Gropper, S. S., Smith, J. L., & Groff, J. L. (2013). *Advanced Nutrition and Human Metabolism* (6th ed.). Belmont, CA: Wadsworth Publishing Company. 624 pages, ISBN: 0495116572, 9780495116578.
8. Guaraldi, F., & Salvatori, G. (2012). Effect of breast and formula feeding on gut microbiota shaping in newborns. *Frontiers in Cellular and Infection Microbiology, 2*, 94. https://doi.org/10.3389/fcimb.2012.00094.
9. Guyton, A. C., & Hall, J. E. (2006). *Textbook of Medical Physiology* (11th ed.). Philadelphia: Elsevier Saunders. ISBN 0-7216-0240-1
10. Hsu, M., et al. (2022). Physiology, stomach. In *StatPearls*. Retrieved from: https://www.ncbi.nlm.nih.gov/books/NBK535425/ (accessed on 23 May 2024).
11. Hunt, R. H., Camilleri, M., Crowe, S. E., El-Omar, E. M., Fox, J. G., Kuipers, E. J., & Tack, T. (2015). The stomach in health and disease. *Gut, 64*(10), 1650–1668. https://doi.org/10.1136/gutjnl-2014-307595.
12. Johnson, T., Gerson, L., Herschcovici, T., Stave, C., & Fass, R. (2010). Systematic review: The effects of carbonated beverages on gastro-oesophageal reflux disease. *Alimentary Pharmacology & Therapeutics, 31*(6), 607–614. https://doi.org/10.1111/j.1365-2036.2010.04232.x.
13. Marieb, E. N., & Hoehn, K. (2018). *Human Anatomy and Physiology* (11th ed.). Pearson Education. 1272 Pages, ISBN: 9781292260853.

14. Newberry, C., & Lynch, K. (2019). The role of diet in the development and management of gastroesophageal reflux disease: Why we feel the burn. *Journal of Thoracic Disease, 11*(Suppl. 12), S1594–S1601. https://doi.org/10.21037/jtd.2019.06.42.

15. Noel C, Dando R. The effect of emotional state on taste perception. Appetite. 2015 Dec;95:89-95. doi: 10.1016/j.appet.2015.06.003. Epub 2015 Jun 27. PMID: 26122754.

16. Pradhan, G., Samson, S. L., & Sun, Y. (2013). Ghrelin: Much more than a hunger hormone. *Current Opinion in Clinical Nutrition & Metabolic Care, 16*(6), 619–624. https://doi.org/10.1097/MCO.0b013e328365b9be.

17. Ruhl, C. E., & Everhart, J. E. (1999). Overweight, but not high dietary fat intake, increases risk of gastroesophageal reflux disease hospitalization: The NHANES I epidemiologic follow-up study. *Annals of Epidemiology, 9*(7), 424–435. https://doi.org/10.1016/S1047-2797(99)00020-4.

18. Smolin, L. A., & Grosvenor, M. B. (2016). *Nutrition: Science and Applications* (4th ed.). Hoboken, NJ: Wiley Publishing Company. 880 pages, ISBN: 978-1-119-22469-3

19. Wallace, M. (2013). Your digestive system and how it works. *National Institute of Diabetes and Digestive and Kidney Diseases (NIDDK)*. Retrieved from: https://www.niddk.nih.gov/health-information/digestive-diseases/digestive-system-how-it-works (accessed on 23 May 2024).

20. Willet, S. G., & Mills, J. C. (2016). Stomach organ and cell lineage differentiation: From embryogenesis to adult homeostasis. *Cellular and Molecular Gastroenterology and Hepatology, 2*(5), 546–559. https://doi.org/10.1016/j.jcmgh.2016.05.006.

Chapter 3

THE PANCREAS

Contents

Introduction

An organ with glandular function, the pancreas influences how the body functions as a whole. The inability of the pancreas to biosynthesize and/or secrete digestive enzymes in sufficient amounts to aid in the digestion and absorption of food components in the intestines is known as emerging pancreatic insufficiency. The pancreas can be damaged due to a number of clinical conditions, e.g., diabetes, autoimmune disorders, chronic pancreatitis, recurrent acute pancreatitis, and pancreatectomy-related complications. It occurs that gastrointestinal or pancreatic cancer is the cause of such failure. It is most frequently linked to cystic fibrosis in children (about 90% of patients) or a rare genetic condition called Shwachman-Diamond syndrome. The typical symptoms of pancreatic insufficiency include weight loss (or failure to gain weight in children), avitaminosis, malnutrition, and malabsorption. Treating the underlying cause, stopping additional pancreatic damage, and symptom relief are the goals of treatment.

Orientation and Directional Terms

Term	Definition	Illustration
Distal pancreatectomy	The distal part of your pancreas is the body and tail ("distal" means distant, or the farthest part from the center). A distal pancreatectomy removes the tail of your pancreas, and sometimes the body if that's involved, too. The tail of your pancreas is closely connected to your spleen. A distal pancreatectomy often involves removing your spleen along with the tail of your pancreas.	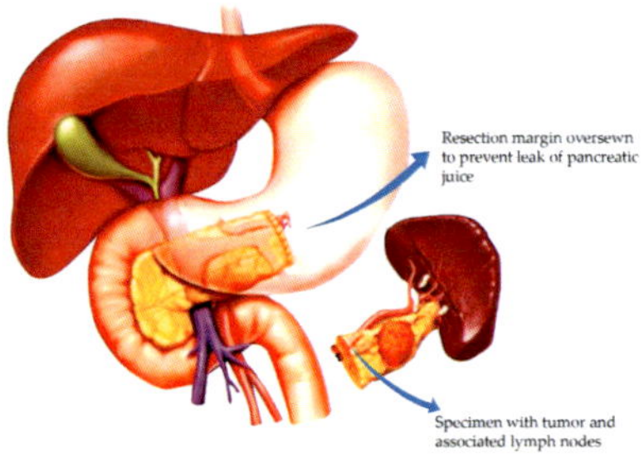
Whipple procedure	A pancreaticduodenectomy or Whipple procedure removes the head of your pancreas, along with the part of your small intestine that connects to it (your duodenum). Because the common bile duct also runs through the head of your pancreas and drains into your duodenum, your bile duct and gallbladder are also removed. The Whipple procedure concludes by reattaching your remaining pancreas, bile duct and stomach to your remaining small intestine so that digestion can continue normally.	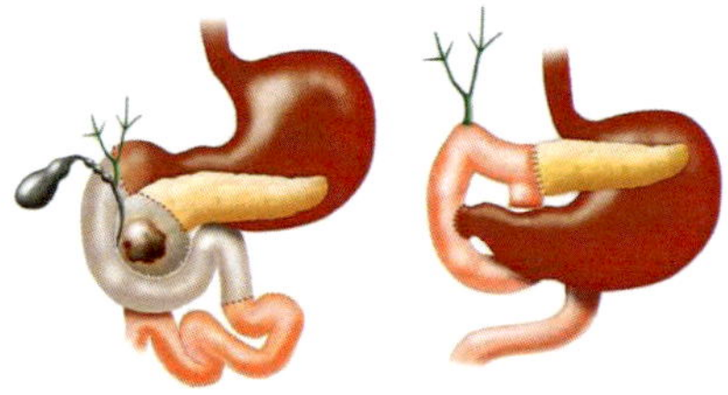
Pancreatic Cancer	Pancreatic cancer affects your pancreas, a gland in your abdomen that aids in digestion.	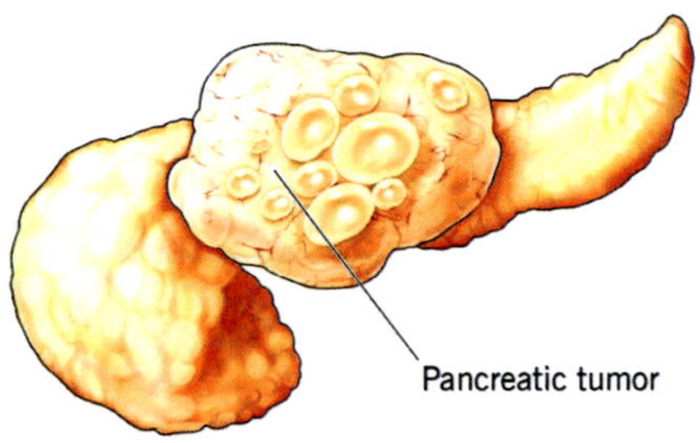
Pancreatic Cysts	A pancreatic cyst is a type of tumor that grows on or in your pancreas. It's typically liquid inside, with an outer skin.	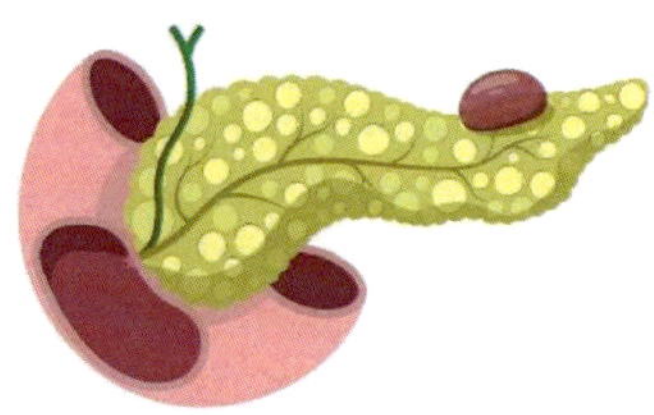

3.1. Structure and Function

The pancreas is a glandular organ located in the abdomen that performs both hormonal (endocrine) and digestive (exocrine) duties.

3.1.1. Anatomical Position

An oblong organ, the pancreas is situated at the level of the transpyloric plane (L1). It is a retroperitoneal organ, situated deep within the upper abdomen in the left hypochondrium and epigastrium regions, with the exception of the pancreatic tail. The pancreas is directly anatomically related to several structures within the abdomen.

3.1.1.1. Organs

- **Stomach:** The stomach and pylorus are located anterior to and apart from the pancreas, divided by the lesser sac.
- **Duodenum:** The duodenum, which has a "C" shape, encircles and outlines the pancreatic head. The duodenum is divided into two sections: the first portion is located anteriorly, and the second section, which includes the Vater ampulla, is located laterally and to the right of the pancreatic head.
- **Transverse Mesocolon:** Affixes to the pancreatic anterior surface.
- **Common Bile Duct:** Descends behind the pancreatic head and, via the major duodenal papilla, opens into the second section of the duodenum next to the pancreatic duct.
- **Spleen:** Situated laterally and posteriorly. The peritoneum forms the lienorenal ligament, which joins the spleen to the pancreatic tail.

3.1.1.2. Vessels

In terms of vascular anatomy, the pancreas is located close to many important vessels and landmarks.

- The pancreatic head is reached posteriorly by the aorta and inferior vena cava.
- The superior mesenteric artery is located anterior to the uncinate process and behind the pancreatic neck.
- The splenic and superior mesenteric veins combine to form the hepatic portal vein posterior to the pancreatic neck.
- The splenic artery passes through the superior border of the pancreas on its way from its source at the celiac plexus to the splenic hilum (Figure 3.1).

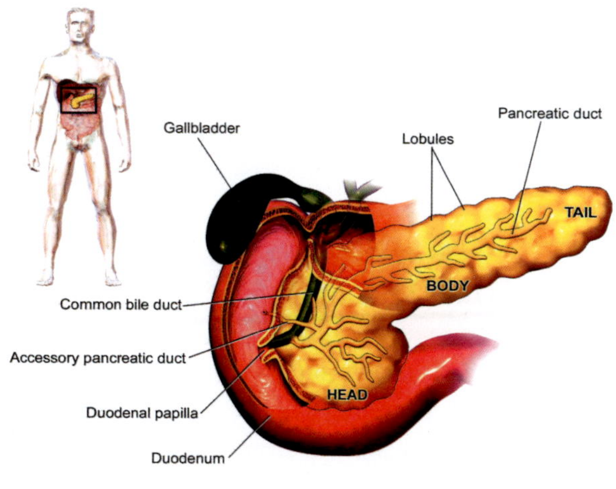

Figure 3.1. *The pancreas.*

Source: By Bruce Blaus, Own work, CC BY 3.0, https://commons.wikimedia.org/w/index.php?curid=28909219.

3.1.2. Anatomical Structure

The pancreas is typically divided into five parts:

- **Head**: the pancreatic region that is the widest. Connective tissue connects it to the duodenum, which forms a C-shaped curve around it.
- **Uncinate Process**: a protrusion that extends medially from the base of the head and rests beneath the pancreatic body. It is located behind the superior mesenteric arteries.
- **Neck**: situated halfway between the pancreatic body and head. Its posterior aspect has a groove formed by the superior mesenteric vessels, which are situated above it.
- **Body**: positioned in the center, behind the stomach and to the left of the superior mesenteric vessels, crossing the human body's midline.
- **Tail**: the portion of the pancreas on the left side that is closest to the splenic hilum. It is housed with the splenic vessels in the splenorenal ligament. There are no other intraperitoneal parts of the pancreas except this one.
- **Duct System:** The lobulated, serous exocrine pancreas is a gland that produces precursors of digestive enzymes. It is made up of roughly a million acini—clusters of cells that resemble berries—connected by brief intercalated ducts. The main pancreatic duct is reached by the intercalated ducts joining forces with those draining neighboring lobules to form a network of intralobular collecting ducts. The pancreatic duct forms the hepatopancreatic ampulla of Vater when it joins the common bile duct, which runs the entire length of the pancreas. Subsequently, this structure opens via the major duodenal papilla into the duodenum. The sphincter of Oddi is a muscular valve that regulates secretions into the duodenum. It functions as a valve by encircling Vater's ampulla.
- **Vasculature:** The pancreas receives blood supply from the pancreatic branches of the splenic artery. In addition, the head of the pancreas is supplied by the superior and inferior pancreaticoduodenal arteries, which are branches of the gastroduodenal (from the coeliac trunk) and superior mesenteric arteries, respectively. Venous drainage from the head of the pancreas goes into the superior mesenteric branches of the hepatic portal vein. The rest of the pancreas drains through the splenic vein.
- **Lymphatics:** Lymphatic vessels drain the pancreas by following the artery supply. The pyloric and pancreaticosplenal nodes, which drain into the superior mesenteric and coeliac lymph nodes, are where they empty (Table 3.1).

Table 3.1. Hormones of the Pancreas

Associated Hormones	Chemical Class	Effect
Insulin (beta cells)	Protein	Reduces blood glucose levels
Glucagon (alpha cells)	Protein	Increases blood glucose levels
Somatostatin (delta cells)	Protein	Inhibits insulin and glucagon release
Pancreatic polypeptide (PP cells)	Protein	Role in appetite

Source: https://courses.lumenlearning.com/atd-herkimer-biologyofaging/chapter/the-endocrine-pancreas/#:~:text=Although%20it%20is%20primarily%20an,and%20pancreatic%20polypeptide%20(PP).

3.1.3. Development

The pancreas is formed during development by two buds that originate from the duodenal part of the foregut, an embryonic tube that will later become the gastrointestinal tract. These buds are of endodermal origin. The development of the pancreas starts with the creation of a dorsal and ventral pancreatic bud, each connecting to the foregut through a duct. The dorsal pancreatic bud gives rise to the neck, body, and tail of the pancreas, while the ventral pancreatic bud forms the head and uncinate process (Figure 3.2).

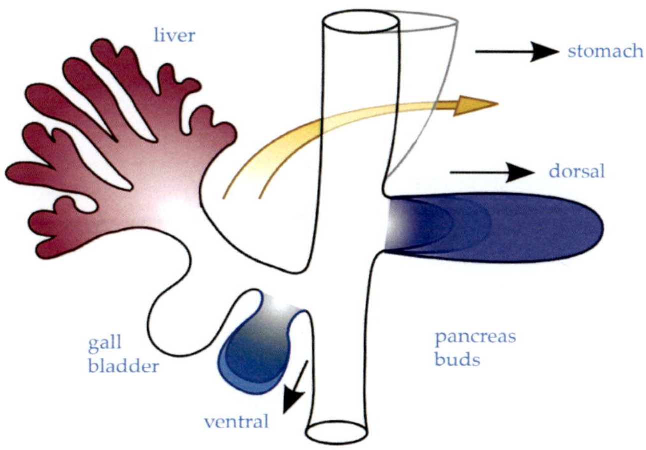

Figure 3.2. *The pancreas originates from the foregut, a precursor tube to part of the digestive tract, as a dorsal and ventral bud. As it develops, the ventral bud rotates to the other side and the two buds fuse together.*

Source: By Jakob Suckale, Michele Solimena, CC BY 3.0, https://commons.wikimedia.org/w/index.php?curid=4274618.

The rotation of the ventral bud and the union of the two buds produce the definitive pancreas. During development, the ventral bud moves to a more dorsal position as the duodenum rotates to the right along with it. The ventral pancreatic bud eventually merges with the larger dorsal bud after reaching its destination. The main pancreatic duct is formed at this point of fusion when the main ducts of the ventral and dorsal pancreatic buds unite. The dorsal bud duct typically regresses and exits the main pancreatic duct.

3.1.3.1. Cellular Development

Precursor cells known as pancreatic progenitor cells give rise to functional pancreatic cells such as ductal, endocrine islet, and exocrine acinar cells. The transcription factors PDX1 and NKX6–1 are expressed together in these progenitor cells. Molecules such as follistatin, fibroblast growth factors, and Notch receptor system activation induce differentiation in the cells of the exocrine pancreas. There are three phases that the exocrine acini go through as they develop. These represent the undetectable, low, and differentiated stages of digestive enzyme activity, respectively: proto-differentiated, differentiated, and pre-differentiated.

Pancreatic progenitor cells transform into endocrine islet cells by the actions of neurogenin-3 and ISL1, but only in the absence of notch receptor signaling. Under the guidance of a Pax gene, the endocrine precursor cells develop into alpha and gamma cells. With the help of Pax-6, the endocrine precursor cells grow into beta and delta cells. The pancreatic islets take shape as the endocrine cells move from the duct system to gather in small clusters around capillaries. This process typically occurs during the third month of development, with insulin and glucagon becoming detectable in the human fetal circulation by the fourth or fifth month of development.

3.1.4. Function

The pancreas plays a crucial role in regulating blood sugar levels and metabolism by secreting pancreatic juice for digestion. Its functions are split into two roles: endocrine, involving the release of insulin to control blood sugar, and exocrine, involving the secretion of enzymes for breaking down food in the digestive system.

3.1.4.1. Blood Glucose Regulation

Homeostasis, or the regulation of blood glucose levels, is facilitated by pancreatic cells. The pancreatic islets, which are found all over the organ, contain the cells that carry out this function. Alpha cells release glucagon when blood glucose levels are low, which raises blood glucose levels. To lower blood glucose levels, beta cells secrete insulin when blood glucose levels are high. Additionally, the islet's delta cells release somatostatin, which inhibits the release of glucagon and insulin. By encouraging the production of glucose and the conversion of glycogen to glucose in the liver, glucagon raises blood glucose levels. Moreover, it lessens the uptake of glucose by muscle and fat. Exercise and low insulin or blood glucose levels both cause the release of glucagon. Insulin lowers blood glucose levels by encouraging the uptake of glucose by cells, especially skeletal muscle, and by encouraging the breakdown of glucose into proteins, fats, and carbohydrates. Preproinsulin, the precursor form of insulin, is first produced. This is changed into proinsulin, which C-peptide then cleaves to produce insulin, which is subsequently kept in beta cell granules. Beta cells take up and break down glucose. Depolarization of the cell membrane, which results from this, ultimately triggers the release of insulin.

The concentrations of glucose in blood plasma are the primary factor influencing the secretion of glucagon and insulin. Insulin release is stimulated by high blood sugar, and glucagon release is stimulated by low blood sugar. The secretion of these hormones is also influenced by other variables. Certain amino acids, which are byproducts of breaking down protein, cause the release of glucagon and insulin. Insulin and glucagon are both inhibited by somatostatin. Additionally, the autonomic nervous system is involved. Insulin and glucagon secretion is stimulated when catecholamines released from sympathetic nerves bind to Beta-2 receptors on the sympathetic nervous system; secretion is inhibited when Alpha-1 receptors are activated. The right vagus nerve stimulates M3 receptors in the parasympathetic nervous system, which in turn causes the release of insulin from beta cells.

3.1.4.2. Digestion

In the digestive system, the pancreas is an essential organ. To accomplish this, it secretes a fluid into the duodenum, the first section of the small intestine to receive food from the stomach, which contains digestive enzymes. These enzymes aid in the digestion of proteins, lipids (fats), and carbohydrates. The pancreas plays a role known as the exocrine role. These cells are organized into groups known as acini. The main pancreatic duct empties into the duodenum directly after secretions accumulate in intralobular ducts in the middle of the acinus. In this way, between 1.5 and 3 liters of fluid are secreted daily (Figure 3.3).

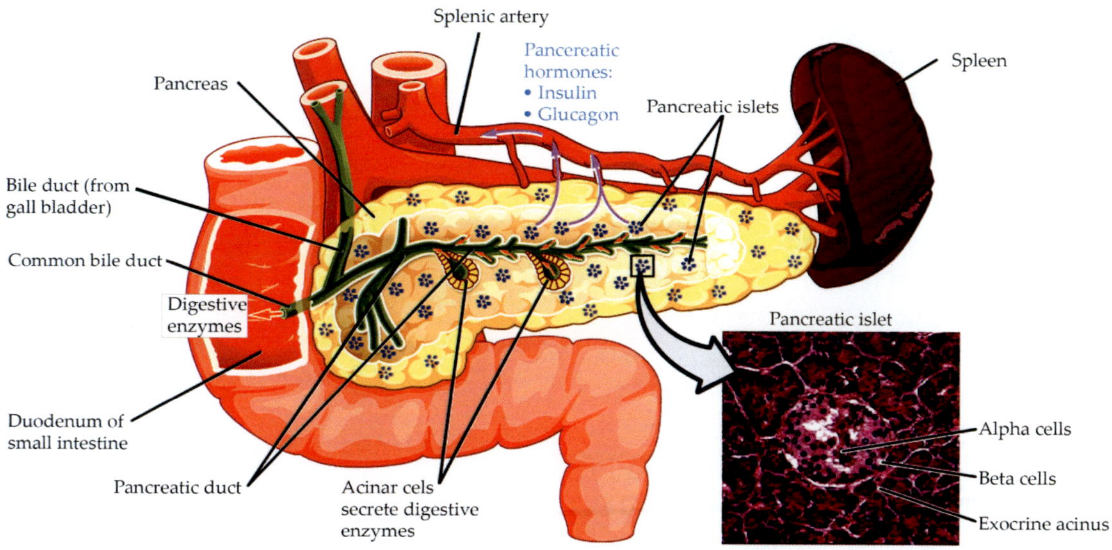

Figure 3.3. *The pancreas has a role in digestion, highlighted here. Ducts in the pancreas (green) conduct digestive enzymes into the duodenum. This image also shows a pancreatic islet, part of the endocrine pancreas, which contains cells responsible for secretion of insulin and glucagon.*

Source: By OpenStax College, CC BY 3.0, https://commons.wikimedia.org/w/index.php?curid=30148155.

The digestive enzymes are contained in granules that are inside each acinus's cells. They are called zymogens or proenzymes when they are secreted in an inactive form. The enzyme, enterokinase from the duodenum lining, activates them when they are released into the duodenum. After the proenzymes are broken down, a series of activating enzymes are produced:

- The conversion of trypsinogen to trypsin is the first step in the breakdown of proteins by enzymes. The remaining trypsinogen and chymotrypsinogen are subsequently broken down by the free trypsin to produce chymotrypsin, which is the active form.

- The secreted enzymes lipase, phospholipase A2, lysophospholipase, and cholesterol esterase are involved in the breakdown of fats.
- Amylase is one of the enzymes that breaks down starch and other carbohydrates.

These enzymes are released into a bicarbonate-rich fluid. Moreover, bicarbonate neutralizes stomach acids that enter the duodenum and helps to keep the fluid at an alkaline pH, where most enzymes function most effectively. Secretin, cholecystokinin, VIP, and acetylcholine stimulation from the vagus nerve are among the hormones that affect secretion. When gastric acid stimulates the S cells that make up the duodenum's lining, secretin is released from them. It also increases the secretion of bicarbonate and enzymes in addition to VIP. Cholecystokinin enhances the effects of secretin and is primarily released by Ito cells found in the lining of the duodenum and jejunum in response to long-chain fatty acids. Cellularly, the cystic fibrosis transmembrane conductance regulator causes membrane depolarization, which in turn causes bicarbonate to be secreted from centroacinar and ductal cells via a sodium and bicarbonate cotransporter. More membrane depolarization and bicarbonate secretion result from the action of secretin and VIP on the cystic fibrosis transmembrane conductance regulator, which widens its opening.

Numerous mechanisms work to prevent pancreatic tissue from being digested by the pancreatic digestive action. These include the release of inactive enzymes known as zymogens, the protective enzyme known as trypsin inhibitor, which secretes trypsin and inactivates it, pH changes brought on by bicarbonate secretion, which stimulates digestion only when the pancreas is stimulated, and the fact that trypsin is inactivated due to low calcium levels within cells.

3.1.4.3. Additional Functions

Pancreatic polypeptide and vasoactive intestinal peptide are other substances secreted by the pancreas. The pancreatic enterochromaffin cells secrete substance P, serotonin, and motilin.

3.2. Pancreatic Juice

The liquid that the pancreas secretes is called pancreatic juice, and it contains several digestive enzymes, such as amylase, chymotrypsinogen, elastase, carboxypeptidase, and pancreatic lipase. Situated in the visceral region, the pancreas plays a significant role in the digestive system, ensuring adequate digestion and subsequent absorption of essential macronutrients for survival. Pancreatic juice's high bicarbonate ion concentration makes it naturally alkaline. By neutralizing the acidic gastric acid, bicarbonate helps to facilitate efficient enzymatic changes. The duodenum's walls produce the hormones secretin and cholecystokinin, which in turn control pancreatic juice secretion. Autonomic innervation also plays a major role in this regulation.

The entry of the acidic chyme into the duodenum triggers the release of these hormones into the bloodstream. Their combined efforts cause the duodenum to secrete a significant amount of alkaline, high-enzyme pancreatic juice. Autonomic innervation also reaches the pancreas. Sympathetic nerve fibers control the flow of blood into the pancreas, whereas parasympathetic neurons activate the acinar and centroacinar cells (Figure 3.4).

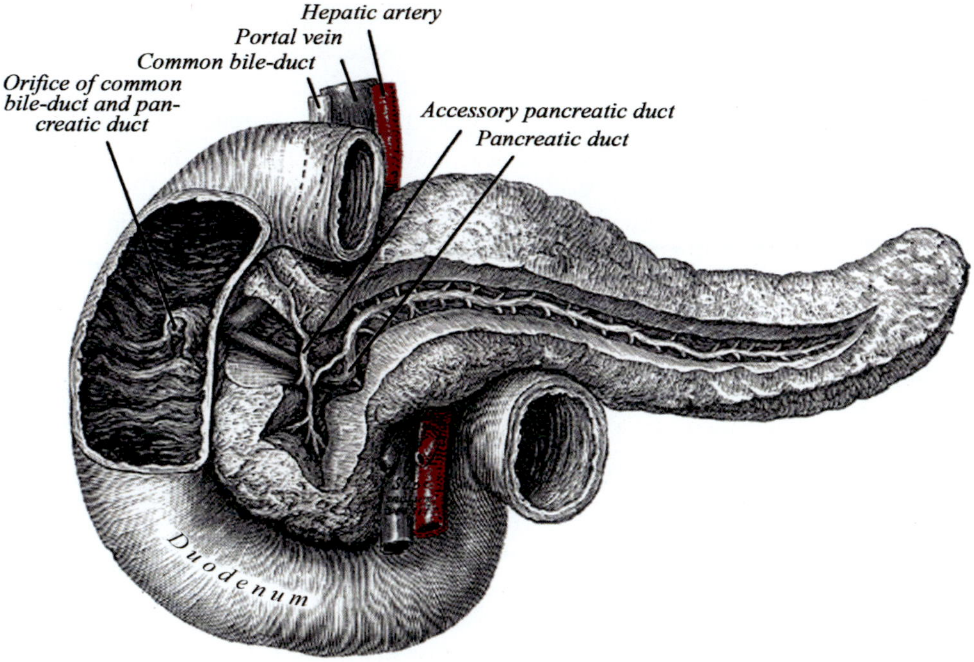

Figure 3.4. *A schematic diagram that shows pancreatic acini and the ducts where the pancreatic fluid is synthesized and released.*

Source: By Henry Vandyke Carter – Henry Gray (1918) Anatomy of the human body (See "Book" section below)Bartleby.com: Gray's Anatomy, Plate 1100, Public Domain, https://commons.wikimedia.org/w/index.php?curid=567061.

The aqueous mixture of bicarbonate from the duct cells and enzymes from the acinar cells is known as pancreatic secretion. While the enzymes help break down the proteins, fats, and carbohydrates for subsequent processing and absorption in the intestines, the bicarbonate helps balance the low pH of the stomach's chyme. During an endoscopy, secretin-stimulated pancreatic juice can be obtained. This is a valuable source of diagnostic biomarkers that enable the identification of pancreatic pathology, particularly cancer that is not yet apparent in medical imaging. Through the duodenal papillae, pancreatic juice is secreted into the duodenum. Some people also have an accessory duct called the accessory pancreatic duct. This duct can be non-functional or functional, meaning it can empty the contents of the exocrine pancreas into the duodenum.

3.3. Pancreatic Enzymes

Amylase, lipase, protease, and lactase are commercial mixtures that are known as pancreatic enzymes, or pancreases, pancrelipase, and pancreatin. They are employed to address malabsorption syndrome brought on by specific pancreatic issues. These pancreatic issues could be caused by pancreatic cancer, MODY 5, long-term pancreatitis, cystic fibrosis, or surgical pancreas removal. The preparation can be consumed orally (Figure 3.5).

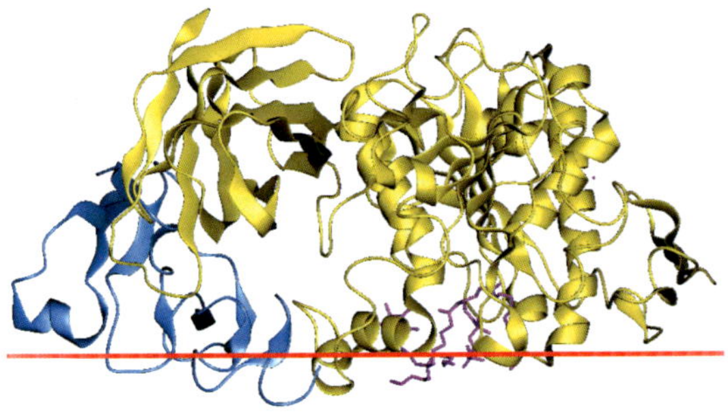

Figure 3.5. *Complex of lipase with colipase.*

Source: By Andrei Lomize – Own work, CC BY-SA 3.0, https://commons.wikimedia.org/w/index.php?curid=34115006.

Constipation, diarrhea, vomiting, and stomach pain are typical side effects. High blood uric acid and perianal irritation are additional side effects. Pigs' enzymes are used. Pregnancy is thought to be safe for use. Digestive enzymes that resemble those typically produced by the human pancreas make up the components. They aid in the body's digestion of proteins, carbohydrates, and fats. Since at least the 1800s, pancreatic enzymes have been utilized as pharmaceuticals. They are listed as essential medicines by the World Health Organization. With over a million prescriptions, it was the 243rd most frequently prescribed drug in the US in 2021.

3.3.1. Medical Uses

When treating exocrine pancreatic insufficiency and other digestive disorders that come with cystic fibrosis, complicate surgical pancreatectomy, or are the result of chronic pancreatitis, pancrelipases are typically used as a first line of treatment. The formulations are often made of granules that are resistant to stomach acid inside hard capsules. The only difference between pancreatins and pancrelipases is that the former has a higher lipase content. The exocrine cells of the pancreas produce a mixture of several digestive enzymes known as pancreatin. It is made up of lipase, protease, and amylase. This combination is used to treat diseases like cystic fibrosis, pancreatitis, and surgical pancreatectomy that are caused by insufficient pancreatic secretions. It has been touted as a treatment for autoimmune diseases, cancer, food allergies, celiac disease, and weight loss. Though it is neither an acid nor a single chemical, pancreatin is sometimes referred to as pancreatic acid.

The pancreatic enzymes lipase, amylase, and trypsin are found in pancreatin. Pancrelipase, a similar blend of enzymes, is marketed with higher active lipase enzyme content than pancreatin. Pancreatin's trypsin breaks down proteins into oligopeptides, while lipase breaks down triglycerides into fatty acids and glycerols and amylase breaks down starches into oligosaccharides and the disaccharide maltose. In cases of pancreatic insufficiency, pancreatin is a useful enzyme supplement that helps with food digestion and substitutes missing pancreatic enzymes. During digestion, pancreatin lessens the amount of iron that is absorbed from food in the duodenum. Porcine pancreatin extractives are added to some contact lens cleaning solutions to help with the targeted protein removal process.

3.3.1.1. Dosing of Pancreatic Enzymes

The package insert authorized by the FDA for a standard commercial product (e.g., Creon®) says that "clinical symptoms, the degree of steatorrhea present, and the fat content of the diet should be the basis for individualized diagnosis and adjustments in the initial starting dose [of pancreatic enzymes]." Citing the Cystic Fibrosis Foundation Consensus Conferences Guidelines, which recommend 500 lipase units/kg of body weight per meal as the lowest starting dose, they point to a clinical trial in which patients were given 72,000 lipase units per meal while consuming at least 100 g of fat daily. In addition, they state that "further research is warranted if doses exceed 2,500 lipase units/kg of body weight per meal, as there is great inter-individual variation in response to enzymes." Patients who are currently receiving higher doses than 6000 lipase units/kg of body weight per meal should be examined, and the dosage should either be immediately decreased or titrated downward to a lower range. Doses greater than 2500 lipase units/kg of body weight per meal (or greater than 10,000 lipase units/kg of body weight per day) should be used with caution.

In contrast, Forsmark in Sleisenger and Fordtran's Gastrointestinal and Liver Disease textbook suggests that 90,000 USP units of lipase are needed with each meal. Because clinicians rarely have access to patients' degrees of steatorrhea, the recommendation forces clinicians to rely on symptoms and diet fat content. Broad recommendations, such as therapy being individualized based on clinical symptoms, the degree of steatorrhea present, and the diet's fat content, do not identify which of the variables is best or whether all three are equivalent. Nevertheless, the patient receives no advice regarding what metrics to use to assess the diet's fat content or what modifications to make. Resolving malabsorption or the nutritional effects of pancreatic insufficiency is not a reliable goal that can be attained in real life by following the instructions provided in textbooks or package inserts. Here, we try to offer a useful strategy to help clinicians and patients. First, we discuss the evidence for the amount of lipase needed to treat steatorrhea. Although recommendations are made in terms of lipase concentration, this can be confusing because different countries use different units to describe lipase. USP lipase units (1IU=3USPunits) are used to describe FDA-approved products in the US. We'll discuss the findings of several studies in USP units. The range of pancreatic enzyme products that are currently approved by the FDA is 3000 USP lipase units to 36,000 USP units per pill. There are many different kinds of preparations available outside of the US (Table 3.2).

able 3.2. List of Studies Investigating the Effect of Pancreatic Enzyme Replacement Therapy (Pert) in Metastatic Pancreatic Patients

References	Study Type	Treatment	Outcome
[50]	Randomised	Panzytrat * 50,000 U.Ph.Eur/meal–25,000 U.Ph.Eur/snack	Improved nutritional status in Panzytrat-group: increase body weight (1.2% vs. body weight loss of 3.7%), increased CFA (12%). The daily total energy intake was 8.42 MJ and 6.66 MJ in pancreatic enzymes-treated group and in placebo patients, respectively ($p = 0.04$, 95% CI 0.08–3.44).
		Placebo	
[51]	Randomised	Norzyme® ** 2 capsules/meal–1 capsule/snack	No significant difference in body weight change, PG-SGA score, QoL or OS.
		Placebo	

[52]	Randomised	Creon®£	Greater weight loss in placebo-group, no statistical difference in BMI, nutrition score, QoL, mOS (mOS was 67.6 (95% CI 14.1–98.4) weeks and 17 (95% CI 8.1–48.7))
		Placebo	
[53]	Retrospective	Creon®£ 50,000 U.Ph.Eur/ meal–25,000 U.Ph. Eur/snack	Significant longer survival in Creon-group than placebo (189 days (95% CI 167.0–211.0 days) vs. 95.0 days (95% CI 75.4–114.6 days respectively (HR: 2.117, 95% CI 1.493–3.002; $p < 0.001$))
		Placebo	
[54]	Prospective	50,000 IU Creon/ meal–25,000 IU Creon/snack 1 extra 25,000 IU Creon per 16–20 g of extra fat/meal or snack	Significant reduction of pancreatic and hepatic pain compared before the treatment (47 vs. 33 and 24 vs. 11, respectively, $p < 0.05$) and diarrhea scores (26 vs. 8, $p < 0.005$). Significant improvement of QoL.
[55]	Retrospective population-based	PERT–dosage not specified	Longer survival in PERT-group respect placebo group in both patients chemotherapy treated (328 days and 226 days, respectively, $p < 0.0006$) or in best supportive care (171 days and 71 days, respectively, $p < 0.001$).

Source: Pezzilli R, Caccialanza R, Capurso G, Brunetti O, Milella M, Falconi M. Pancreatic enzyme replacement therapy in pancreatic cancer. Cancers. 2020; 12(2):275. https://doi.org/10.3390/cancers12020275.

** Panzytrat: 25,000 U.Ph.Eur lipase + 1250 U.Ph.Eur proteases + 22,500 U.Ph.Eur amylase/capsule. ** Norzyme: 25,000 U.Ph.Eur lipase + 1250 U.Ph.Eur proteases + 22,500 U.Ph.Eur amylase/capsule. £ Creon: 25,000 BP U lipase + 18,000 BP U amylase + 1000 U.Ph.Eur protease/capsule. BMI: body mass index; CFA: coefficient of fat absorption; CI: confidence interval; CT: chemotherapy; HR: hazard ratio; mOS: median overall survival; MJ: Megajoule; PERT: pancreatic enzyme replacement therapy; PG-SGA: patient-generated subjective global assessment; and QoL: quality of life.*

Postprandial lipase secretion has been estimated to occur under normal physiological conditions at a rate of 9000–18,000 USP units/min, resulting in a total of 120,000–2,196,000 USP units in the 3-hour postprandial period. It has also been proposed that normal fat absorption requires only 5–10% of normal pancreatic output, based on human intubation studies. After taking pancreatic enzymes orally, the following conditions must be met for steatorrhea to stop: (a) the enzyme must stay active; (b) it must mix and empty with food; (c) it must be coordinated with the entry of bile into the duodenum; and (d) it must have normal small intestinal motility and absorptive function. Studies have indicated that individuals with low or absent acid secretion can be cured of steatorrhea by administering approximately 30,000 USP lipase units/meal of unprotected pancreatic enzymes. It was also demonstrated that the average duodenal pH and the duration of the postprandial gastric pH ~4 correlated with the percentage reduction in steatorrhea (i.e., the average duodenal pH increased and steatorrhea reduction was greater the longer the gastric pH stayed below 4.

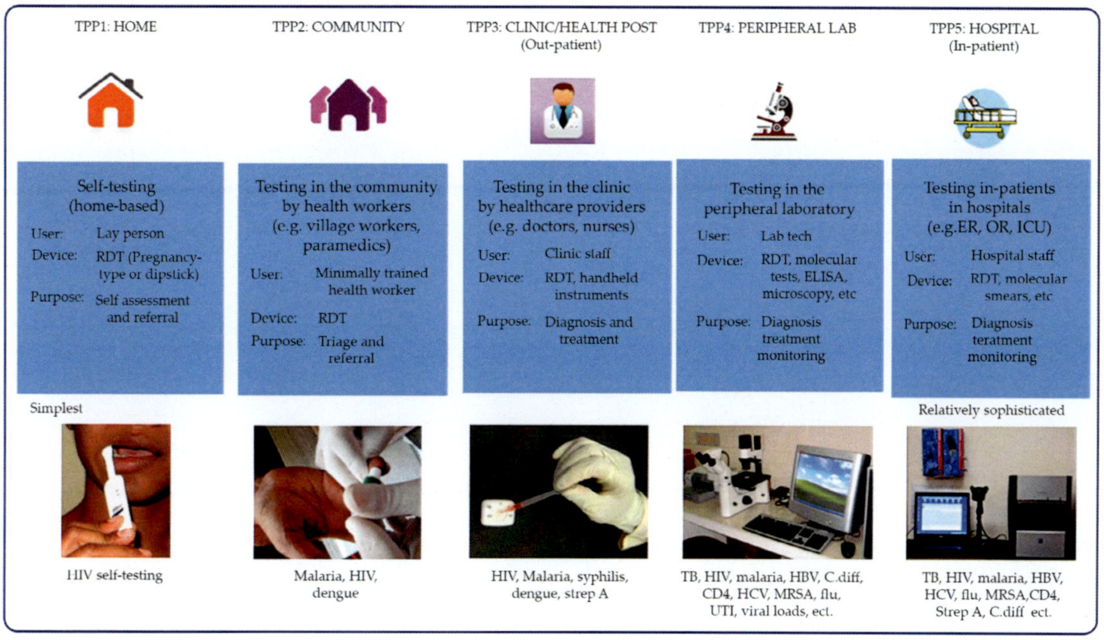

Figure 3.6. *Point-of-Care testing (POCT),*

Source: Yin J, Cui T, Yang Y, Ren T-L. Sensing of digestive enzymes—diagnosis and monitoring of pancreatitis. Chemosensors. 2023; 11(9):469. https://doi.org/10.3390/chemosensors11090469.

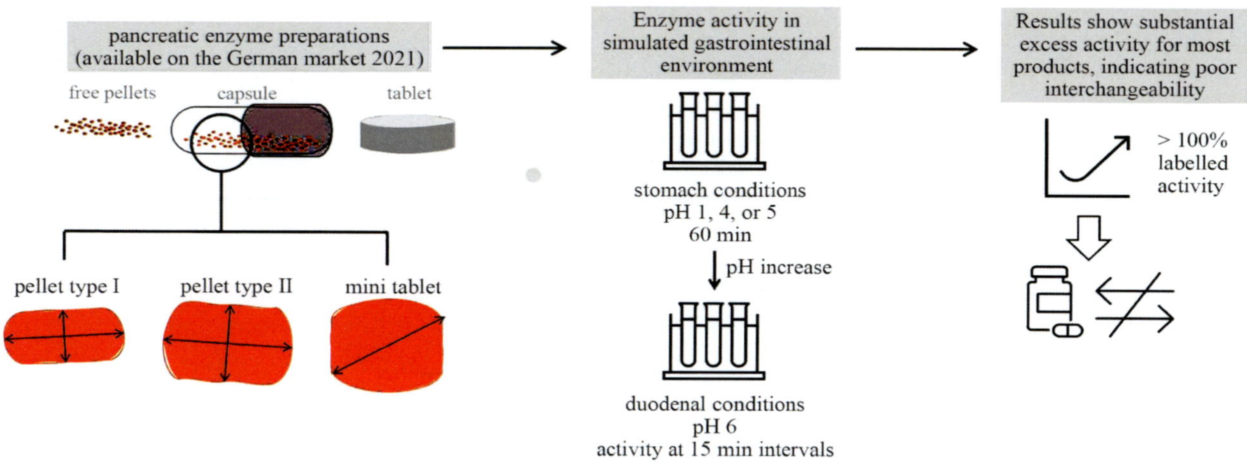

Figure 3.7. *Pancreatic enzyme preparations.*

Source: Todd A, Bennett-Huntley E, Rosendahl J, Schnekenburger J, Uhl W. Comparative investigation of pH–dependent availability of pancreatic enzyme preparations in vitro. Pharmaceuticals. 2024; 17(5):552. https://doi.org/10.3390/ph17050552.

In two of the six patients in another study, enteric-coated microspheres containing 18,000 USP lipase units per meal resulted in total resolution of steatorrhea. This leads one to the conclusion that 18,000–30,000 USP units of lipase per meal are adequate to cure pancreatic steatorrhea in adults. The challenge is knowing how to "administer an adequate quantity of active lipase at the appropriate location, i.e., proximal jejunum, duodenum, and when it's appropriate, i.e., concurrently with the emptying of nutrients from the stomach (Figures 3.6 and 3.7).

3.3.1.2. Side Effects

Fibrosing colonopathy is linked to high doses administered over an extended period of time. Owing to this correlation, a daily lipase dosage of no more than 10,000 IU per kilogram is advised. Although it has never been documented, since they come from pigs, there is a chance of a viral infection.

3.4. Regulation of Pancreatic Secretion

When food is consumed, the exocrine pancreas secretes bicarbonate, fluid, and digestive enzymes. This is an important digestive function controlled by ingested nutrients, gastrointestinal hormones, and neural reflexes. To ensure proper digestion of a meal, secretion is tightly controlled by stimulatory and inhibitory factors that synchronize the delivery of digestive enzymes with food emptying into the intestine. Maldigestion and poor nutrient absorption can result in malnutrition and related problems when there is insufficient pancreatic secretion. The physiological mechanisms that control pancreatic exocrine secretion are discussed in this review.

3.4.1. Phases of Meal Response

Four separate but overlapping phases of pancreatic secretion follow a meal, and they are called after the location of the food that is ingested. Pancreatic secretion occurs in four stages: intestinal, gastric, cephalic, and absorbed nutrition. Significant inter-phase cross-talk and regulation are linked to sufficient, but not excessive, enzyme and bicarbonate secretion. A complex network of humoral, paracrine, and neural feedback mechanisms controls each phase, assisting in the preservation of the ideal conditions for food absorption and digestion.

3.4.1.1. Cephalic Phase

Anxiety about food is a result of sensory inputs like sight, smell, taste, and mastication (before swallowing). The cephalic phase, which is the initial stage of pancreatic secretion, is started by these feelings. The receptors oral cavity for specific food molecules, like long-chain fatty acids (but not triglycerides or medium-chain fatty acids), interact with one another to cause the cephalic phase in addition to sensory input. The cephalic phase accounts for 20–25% of the total exocrine secretion in the pancreas. This estimate is based on information gathered through sham feeding, which involves anticipating food by taste, smell, and sight without actually eating it. When people sham feed, they chew but do not swallow. In humans, the pancreatic reaction to simulated feeding lasts for about sixty minutes. Sham feeding causes an increase in pancreatic secretion that is high in enzymes but low in bicarbonate, indicating that pancreatic acinar cells—rather than ductal cells—are stimulated during this stage.

The vagus nerve regulates exocrine secretion during its cephalic phase. The dorsal vagal complex, situated in the brainstem, integrates sensory inputs related to food anticipation, which are then sent to the exocrine pancreas through the vagus nerve. While vagotomy blocks the cephalic responses, cholinergic agonists produce secretory responses akin to those produced by cephalic stimulation. This suggests that the primary mechanism by which sensory inputs result in exocrine secretion is the release of acetylcholine from vagal efferents. Pancreatic polypeptide (PP), an islet hormone, is secreted more during simulated feeding and is a sign of vagal innervation of the pancreas because cholinergic blockers prevent PP from being secreted. The pancreatic secretory and PP responses are significantly higher during sham feeding when swallowing occurs, suggesting that cholinergic mechanisms are responsible for stimulating PP secretion during chewing and swallowing.

Peptidergic nerve terminals are found in the exocrine pancreas, and there is some evidence that neuropeptides like gastrin-releasing peptide (GRP) and vasoactive intestinal peptide (VIP) may have an impact on the cephalic phase. Furthermore, muscarinic and VIP receptors are involved in the process by which thyrotropin-releasing hormone triggers the pancreatic exocrine secretion of protein and bicarbonate through vagal efferents. In contrast, sympathetic noradrenergic efferents acting upon α-adrenergic receptors mediate the effects of inhibitory cerebral calcitonin gene-related peptide (CGRP). In humans, sham feeding and electrical vagus nerve stimulation might not exist. In humans, endogenous CCK has been demonstrated to increase PP release during simulated feeding. Thus, acetylcholine is thought to be the primary neurotransmitter that controls the cephalic phase, even though peptidergic neurotransmitters are released during vagal stimulation. Acinar cells contain several G protein-coupled receptors (GPCRs) that mediate the cephalic phase of enzyme secretion. It has been demonstrated that the interaction of CCK with CCK-1 receptors causes newborn calves to secrete proteins. Since cephalic stimulation does not raise blood levels of CCK, this response may be dependent on neural CCK release. Therefore, the regulation of the cephalic phase of pancreatic secretion is influenced by both neural and hormonal mechanisms.

3.4.1.2. Gastric Phase

Pancreatic secretion begins its gastric phase when food enters the stomach. Because the presence of food in the stomach triggers hormone releases and neural reflexes, studying this phase has proven challenging. As a result, physiological information about this stage has been gathered through the instillation of inert substances in the antrum or gastric distention caused by balloon dilation. The gastric phase accounted for about 10% of pancreatic secretion, according to experiments where the stomach's contents were prevented from emptying into the duodenum. This phase is mostly induced by enzyme-releasing secretions, with little bicarbonate released, indicating that acinar cells play a major role in inducing this phase.

It's still unknown what part gastrin plays in this stage of pancreatic secretion. Gradual distension of the antrum in an alkaline manner was shown to cause the release of pancreatic enzymes and gastrin. During the gastric phase of pancreatic secretion, the vagus nerve is crucial. This phase is also mediated by the antropancreatic short reflex pathway, which is inhibited by atropine and hexamethonium. Further proof that the stomach's vagovagal cholinergic reflexes, which end in the pancreas, mediate the contributions of the stomach to pancreatic secretion comes from the blocking of the gastric phase by atropine and vagotomy. Sham feeding experiments suggest that CCK release is important for human antral motility and gastrin release.

Salivary amylase aids in the ongoing breakdown of carbohydrates while pepsin and gastric lipases catabolize proteins and fats in the stomach into peptides and triglycerides plus fatty acids, respectively. Protein digests in the peptic state are useful for inducing the intestinal phase. Therefore, the intestinal phase of pancreatic secretion is stimulated when gastric chyme enters the duodenum. Pancreatic secretion is decreased in clinical settings by surgical techniques that slow the rate of stomach emptying. Thus, through neural and hormonal pathways, the rate of gastric emptying controls the release of nutrients into the intestine and, in turn, the activation of the intestinal phase.

3.4.1.3. Intestinal Phase

As previously indicated, the breakdown of food in the stomach results in the release of acidic chyme of duodenum, which starts the intestinal phase of pancreatic secretion. Cephalic and gastric factors, which improve blood flow and start exocrine secretion, have already primed the pancreas by this point. Most of the pancreatic secretory response (between 50 and 80%) happens in the intestinal phase and is controlled by neurological and hormonal systems. Since food can be injected directly into the intestinal lumen without worrying about the stomach emptying, the intestinal phase is easier to study than the gastric phase. Enzyme and bicarbonate secretion are produced in response to stimulation of both acinar and ductal cells. Food molecules like sodium oleate, monoglycerides, peptides, and amino acids (especially tryptophan and phenylalanine) stimulate the secretion of pancreatic amylase. The duodenum produces a large amount of bicarbonate, which balances the acidity of the gastric chyme. Meanwhile, pancreatic enzymes break down partially digested food into molecules that intestinal enterocytes can readily absorb.

The hormones secretin and CCK, as well as neural influences such as the enteropancreatic reflex, which is mediated by the enteric nervous system and increases the pancreatic secretory response, are the main regulators of the pancreatic response during the intestinal phase. Secretin released from S cells into the blood is stimulated upon entry of low-pH gastric chyme into the intestine. Secretin primarily stimulates the release of bicarbonate from pancreatic duct cells, but it also directly affects acinar cells and increases the secretion of enzymes. Peptides and fatty acids, which are the byproducts of partial digestion of proteins and fats, release CCK. Antagonism to the CCK receptor in humans decreased the secretion of pancreatic enzymes during the intestinal phase. During this stage of pancreatic secretion, cholinergic regulation is essential. Atropine partially inhibits pancreatic bicarbonate secretion stimulated by low pH resulting from acidic chyme in the duodenum when secretin is not present. Furthermore, the quantity of bicarbonate generated by secretin infusion is less than that produced by food entering the duodenum, indicating that additional factors play a role in meal-stimulated pancreatic bicarbonate secretion. Atropine suppressed the release of pancreatic enzymes between 30 and 120 minutes after eating, suggesting cholinergic processes. During the intestinal phase of secretion, vagovagal enteropancreatic reflexes, which are mediated by M1 and M3 muscarinic receptors and CCK receptors, are crucial. The dorsal motor nucleus of the vagus nerve, which projects into the pancreas, provides input that modulates these vagovagal enteropancreatic reflexes. Thus, both cholinergic muscarinic and noncholinergic transmission are involved in the activation of pancreatic bicarbonate secretion by vagal stimulation.

3.4.1.3.1. Role of Gastric Acid

Numerous techniques, including the implantation of acidic solutions into the duodenum and the diversion of gastric and pancreatic contents through fistulae, have been used to assess the physiological effects of acid on pancreatic secretion. The physiological effects of gastric acid are attributed to its pH, as both gastric acid and exogenous HCl are potent regulators of postprandial pancreatic bicarbonate secretion. Their effects are further amplified by intrapancreatic and vagovagal neural pathways, as well as by hormones like secretin and CCK.

The amount of bicarbonate and volume of pancreatic secretion increased in a concentration-dependent manner upon intraduodenal infusion of hydrochloric acid. The amount of secretion was comparable to what was obtained with an intravenous infusion of exogenous secretin, indicating that the entry of acidic contents into the duodenum and the subsequent pH changes play a significant role in stimulating pancreatic secretion. A maximal secretory response at pH 3.0 was produced by administering a peptone meal with varying pH levels (pH 1 to 5), and this response was similar in size to that obtained with exogenous secretin. Pancreatic secretion was induced by acid infusion in the duodenum and upper jejunum, indicating that the proximal small intestine reacts to this stimulus.

Entry of gastric contents into the duodenum creates an acidic environment with a pH of 2.0 – 3.0 in the initial segment of the duodenum, while the pH of the distal segment remains alkaline. The cause of this pH differential is pancreatic bicarbonate release, which is largely increased by gastric acid-induced intestinal mucosal secretin release. Diversion through a gastric fistula resulted in a slight increase in pancreatic secretion in conscious rats with gastric and pancreatic fistulae. On the other hand, pancreatic secretion was increased by introducing hydrochloric acid into the duodenum through an open gastric fistula. Furthermore, when pancreatic juice was removed from the intestine, there was a significant increase in pancreatic bicarbonate secretion, indicating a relationship between the amount of pancreatic bicarbonate released and intestinal pH.

Rather than the total amount of buffered acid entering the duodenum, the concentration of free, unbuffered hydrogen ions determines the pancreatic bicarbonate response. The pancreatic bicarbonate response to a meal was significantly decreased when the histamine H2 receptor blocker cimetidine or the H^+/K^+ ATPase inhibitor omeprazole inhibited the production of gastric acid. The secretion of pancreatic bicarbonate is also significantly influenced by the pH of a liquid gastric meal. According to this data, gastric acid plays a significant role in controlling the secretion of pancreatic bicarbonate, which balances acidity and produces an alkaline environment that is ideal for the activity of pancreatic enzymes and ongoing food digestion.

3.4.1.3.2. Role of Dietary Fat in Pancreatic Secretion

Pancreatic enzyme and bicarbonate secretion are stimulated by dietary fats. Human pancreatic enzyme secretion was stimulated by monoolein perfusion, and the potency of this effect was comparable to that of an intravenous CCK injection. Triglycerides, on the other hand, that were injected straight into the duodenum (without the presence of endogenous lipase) failed to cause pancreatic secretion. However, after fatty acids were broken down by lipase, pancreatic secretion was stimulated by monoglycerides but not by glycerol, suggesting that fatty acids make up the majority of ingested fats that do this.

While some studies indicate that fatty acids, both free and saponified, can stimulate pancreatic secretion, others only show that they work when in the form of micellar aggregates. It has been demonstrated that the length of the fatty acid chain affects secretion, with C4 being the least effective and C18 being the most effective. It's unclear why there is a difference in potency, but it's not thought to have anything to do with absorption efficiency. Additional research has shown that propionate (C3), when administered intraduodenally, was a more effective way to stimulate acinar cell secretion than oleate (C18).

Although it is unclear why the two studies differ, they may be related to different species because rats, humans, and rabbits were used in the experiments. While only neutral fats stimulate the secretion of pancreatic enzymes, oleate and neutral fats both promote the secretion of bicarbonate and fluid. When conscious rats were given fat emulsions, their pancreatic protein secretion increased threefold. Pancreatic secretion is also impacted by the fat administration route. While intraduodenal administration of fat resulted in increased secretion of protein, bicarbonate, and fluid, intravenous administration of fat did not cause pancreatic secretion.

When fat emulsions are administered, secretin and plasma CCK levels rise. Proglumide, a CCK receptor antagonist, inhibited fat-mediated pancreatic secretion, indicating the significance of CCK in promoting pancreatic secretion. The effects of bicarbonate secretion induced by secretin are enhanced by both C12 and C18 fatty acids.

Humans can stimulate pancreatic secretion by introducing varying concentrations of oleic acid into the duodenum; however, the threshold for CCK stimulation is significantly lower than that of secretin. Since the injection of anti-secretin antibodies significantly reduces fat-mediated protein and bicarbonate secretion in conscious rats, secretin release is physiologically significant. A neuroendocrine tumor cell line called STC-1 required a critical fatty acid chain length of C12 for CCK to be released. Less than ten carbon fatty acids did not increase secretion. This fatty acid chain length dependence is comparable to that previously noted for human in vivo CCK release. Apart from the length of the fatty acid carbon chain, another factor that matters is the presence of a free carboxyl terminus. This is because altering the methyl terminus did not affect CCK secretion, whereas esterification of the carboxylic terminus impacted it.

3.4.1.3.3. Contributions of Proteins, Peptides and Amino Acids to Pancreatic Secretion

Research has demonstrated that amino acids, proteins, and peptides increase pancreatic secretion; however, the extent of this effect may vary depending on the species under consideration. Pancreatic secretion is only stimulated by L-amino acids, which is consistent with the stereoisomers' overall physiological significance.

Tryptophan and phenylalanine are examples of aromatic amino acids, which are the most potent of all the amino acids. Peptides may be more physiologically significant than aromatic amino acids because they are more prevalent in the intestinal lumen and can stimulate pancreatic secretion more effectively. Prolonged peptides and oligopeptides that contain tryptophan and phenylalanine are potent pancreatic secretion stimulants. The bicarbonate response is enhanced when amino acid and peptide preparations are acidified with hydrochloric acid; however, pancreatic enzyme secretion remains unchanged from when acid is not present. Since potentiation of pancreatic enzyme secretion is not observed when amino acids or peptides are administered concurrently with lipid molecules like oleate or monoolein, aromatic amino acids can induce maximal secretory response.

When amino acids are administered intraduodenally, the pancreatic secretory response seems to be concentration-dependent. Most amino acids require a minimum concentration of 8 mM to stimulate secretion, but some of the more powerful aromatic amino acids, like tryptophan, can do so at as low as 3 mM. The duration of intestinal exposure to amino acids is a crucial factor in the production of pancreatic secretions. The proximal small intestine is the source of most of the stimuli that cause pancreatic stimulation. Amino acids in humans only increased pancreatic secretion when they were perfused into the duodenum; an ileum perfusion produced no noticeable effects. As a result, just like with fats, the main mechanisms triggering pancreatic secretion are restricted to the small intestine's proximal regions.

Tryptophan administered intraluminally produces bicarbonate in amounts comparable to maximal doses of exogenously infused CCK, suggesting that tryptophan-induced release of CCK causes pancreatic secretion. It is possible to considerably reduce the pancreatic stimulation brought on by intraluminal amino acids by releasing bile acids from the gallbladder. Bile acids appear to inhibit CCK release, which in turn inhibits pancreatic secretion. This feedback mechanism controls pancreatic and gallbladder function.

Through the use of a sensitive bioassay for CCK measurement, it was demonstrated that the inhibition of intraluminal trypsin activity is one of the mechanisms by which proteins stimulate CCK release. An additional way that aromatic amino acids influence CCK release is by stimulating the well-known nutrient sensor, the calcium-sensing receptor (CaSR). Aside from inducing the release of hormones like CCK and secretin, amino acids also trigger cholinergic neural mechanisms that control the secretion of pancreatic bicarbonate. Thus, pancreatic secretion is stimulated by proteins, peptides, and amino acids; however, the degree of stimulation varies depending on the species under consideration and the mode of administration.

3.4.1.3.4. Role of Bile and Bile Acids in Pancreatic Secretion

Hepatocytes create bile, which is a complex mixture of organic molecules, cholesterol, and bile acids. When chyme enters the gall bladder, it is concentrated and stored there before being released into the duodenum. Glycine or taurine amino acids are conjugated with bile acids, such as cholate, deoxycholate, and chenodeoxycholate, to increase their solubility. Bile acids aid in the emulsification and absorption of lipids, monoacylglycerols, and fatty acids in the intestine.

They also promote lipolysis by aiding in the binding of pancreatic lipase with its co-lipase. Intraduodenal injection of physiological bile concentrations or the bile salt sodium taurocholate increased plasma secretin and stimulated pancreatic fluid secretion in basal conditions. Secretin was only secreted in reaction to the duodenum's sodium taurocholate perfusion.

An ileal perfusion resulted in no response, whereas perfusion in the upper jejunum markedly reduced the pancreatic response. The free ionized form of taurocholate stimulated pancreatic fluid secretion; its detergent qualities had no effect. In humans, pancreatic exocrine secretions of fluid, bicarbonate, and enzymes were increased when bovine bile was infused.

Human bile acids and bovine bile have been shown to stimulate the release of multiple hormones and neuropeptides, including somatostatin, PP, VIP, CCK, neurotensin, and gastric inhibitory peptide (GIP), in addition to secretin. Elevated levels of VIP in the plasma increased the release of fluid and bicarbonate, indicating that bile stimulates peptidergic nerves to cause pancreatic secretion. Furthermore, atropine inhibited taurocholate- and bile-stimulated exocrine pancreatic secretion, indicating the importance of cholinergic mechanisms. Given that administration of bile differs from that of different bile acids in terms of hydrokinetic and ecbolic responses, the makeup of bile plays a significant role in the mechanisms controlling this secretory response. Bile acids did not, however, appear to stimulate pancreatic fluid secretion when the intraluminal contents of the digestive system were present.

The administration of bile acids alongside fat or amino acids has been shown in certain studies to inhibit the secretion of pancreatic enzymes. Although the exact mechanism underlying this observation is unknown, it is plausible that bile acids function as a negative feedback mechanism to help relax and refill the gallbladder by inhibiting the release of CCK.

According to other research, the bile salt chenodeoxycholate inhibited gallbladder emptying induced by bombesin and CCK in humans while also raising plasma CCK levels. Based on these findings, the authors postulated that chenodeoxycholate decreased the gall bladder's sensitivity to stimulation by bombesin and CCK through an as-yet-unidentified mechanism.

3.4.1.4. Absorbed Nutrient Phase

The absorbed nutrient phase can be initiated by directly stimulating pancreatic secretion after nutrients have been absorbed from the intestinal lumen. To further control exocrine secretion, nutrients can either directly or indirectly activate the hormonal and neural pathways that drive pancreatic acinar cells.

There isn't much solid proof that intravenous lipids and glucose can increase pancreatic secretion. On the other hand, trypsin and chymotrypsin secretion are increased upon intravenous administration of amino acids, but not lipase or amylase. Given that intraduodenal amino acid administration results in significant increases in pancreatic secretion, amino acids appear to have a significant indirect effect on pancreatic secretion. It is unclear how nutrients that are absorbed after being absorbed affect pancreatic secretion, and more research is required to properly explore these implications. One result is to increase the pancreatic supply of digestive enzymes by stimulating the synthesis of new ones.

3.4.1.5. Feedback Regulation of Pancreatic Secretion

The idea that pancreatic secretion is regulated by feedback originated with a number of studies showing that pancreatic enzyme secretion was stimulated by introducing a trypsin inhibitor into the upper small intestine or by surgically diverting the bile-pancreatic duct to remove pancreatic juice and bile from the duodenum of rats.

On the other hand, pancreatic enzyme release was suppressed when trypsin was infused into the duodenum during bile-pancreatic juice diversion. Thus, through a negative feedback system in which active proteases within the duodenum limit pancreatic secretion but reduced protease activity stimulates pancreatic secretion, the concentration of proteases in the upper small intestine appears to be closely linked to pancreatic secretion.

Upon the development of CCK assays, it was demonstrated that CCK, via protease-sensitive CCK-releasing factors, mediated the effects of proteases on pancreatic secretion. CCK releasing factor can activate CCK cells when proteases are not present, but when proteases are present, the releasing factors are inactivated and CCK secretion is reduced. Numerous species have demonstrated negative feedback regulation of pancreatic secretion; however, other proteases, like elastase, may play a more significant role in controlling pancreatic secretion in humans (Figure 3.8).

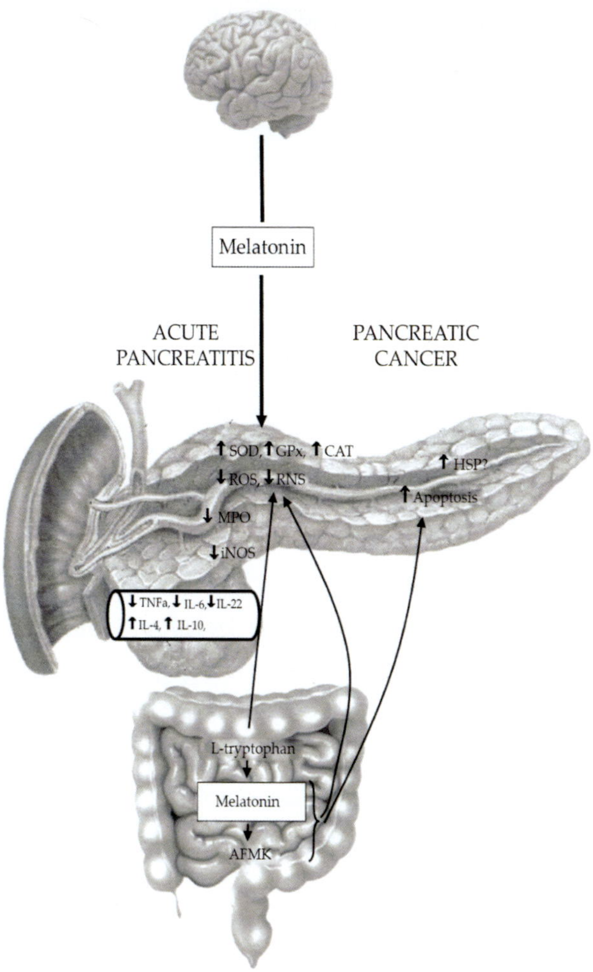

Figure 3.8. *Feedback regulation of pancreatic exocrine secretion is mediated by positive and negative mechanisms. Positive feedback: Monitor peptide is secreted by acinar cells and directly stimulates CCK cells in the small intestine and amplifies pancreatic secretion once it has been initiated. Negative feedback: Trypsin-sensitive CCK releasing factors are produced by the intestine and stimulate CCK secretion when trypsin is temporarily consumed by ingested protein or other trypsin "inhibitors."*

Source: Jaworek J, Leja-Szpak A, Nawrot-Porąbka K, Szklarczyk J, Kot M, Pierzchalski P, Góralska M, Ceranowicz P, Warzecha Z, Dembinski A, et al. Effects of melatonin and its analogs on pancreatic inflammation, enzyme secretion, and tumorigenesis. International Journal of Molecular Sciences. 2017; 18(5):1014. https://doi.org/10.3390/ijms18051014.

A positive feedback mechanism also influences the secretion of pancreatic exocrine hormones. Pancreatic acinar cells produce the 61 amino acid peptide known as "monitoring peptide," which has the ability to release CCK. Monitor peptide can directly stimulate CCK secretion from isolated CCK cells in vitro, despite having a modest trypsin inhibitory capacity. This means that monitor the ability of the peptide to stimulate CCK is independent of this action. Since monitor peptide is secreted in pancreatic juice, it cannot induce CCK secretion in the absence of pancreatic secretion. Therefore, monitoring peptides may help to support pancreatic secretion once the process has begun, but it cannot explain the rise in CCK during bile-pancreatic juice diversion.

3.4.2. Pancreatic Exocrine Secretion

After food is consumed, the exocrine pancreas secretes fluid, bicarbonate ions, and digestive enzymes into the duodenum. Endocrine and exocrine components make up the pancreas. The α, β, δ, ε, and PP (F) cells, which are found in the islets of Langerhans, make up the endocrine pancreas. The hormones insulin, glucagon, somatostatin, ghrelin, amylin, and pancreatic polypeptide are secreted into the bloodstream by these specialized cells, and they have both endocrine and paracrine effects on the pancreas. Acinar cells, which make up 90% of the pancreas, secrete digestive enzymes like trypsin, chymotrypsin, and amylase to aid in small intestine food digestion. The acinar cells are clustered and have a triangular shape. The apex of each cell opens into a terminal duct that is situated in the center. The interlobular ducts, which eventually come together to form the main pancreatic duct, are formed when the terminal or intercalated ducts combine. Exocrine secretions are delivered to the duodenum through the pancreatic duct. The fluid and bicarbonate ions secreted by the ductal cells balance out the acidic gastric contents that enter the duodenum and the secretions from the acinar cells. The pancreas has a dense network of blood vessels that control blood flow and alter pancreatic secretion. It is largely innervated by sympathetic and parasympathetic peripheral nerves (Table 3.3).

Table 3.3. Ontogeny of Common Pancreatic Enzymes in Humans

Pancreatic enzyme	Prenatal development (Gestational week)	Postnatal activities	Adult level	References
Amylase	39 weeks	<1% of adult values or absent levels until 6 weeks	6 months to 2 years	(22, 29–32)
Pancreatic triglyceride lipase	13–21 weeks	5–10% of adult values	2 years	(29, 33–35)
Trypsin *	14–16 weeks	90–100% of adult values	<1month	(22, 23, 29, 30)
Chymotrypsin*	14–16 weeks	50–60% of adult values	2 years	(22, 23, 29, 30, 36)
Elastase	14–16 weeks	25% of adult values	2 weeks	(22, 37)

Source: Mehta V, Hopson PE, Smadi Y, Patel SB, Horvath K and Mehta DI (2022) Development of the human pancreas and its exocrine function. Front. Pediatr. 10:909648. doi: 10.3389/fped.2022.909648.

The highly coordinated process of pancreatic exocrine secretion is regulated by hormones secreted from the pancreatic islets, factors secreted by other tissues, and neural and hormonal signals originating from the gut. The secretory pathways are a highly regulated system that reacts to ingestive signals. They can be stimulatory or inhibitory in nature. The following section discusses the substances that alter pancreatic exocrine secretion.

3.4.2.1. Neural Mechanisms

3.4.2.1.1. Neural Innervation

The pancreas is innervated by a network of intrapancreatic nerves, postganglionic sympathetic neurons, and parasympathetic nerve fibers. Together, these nerves release neuropeptides like VIP, GRP, serotonin, and neuropeptide Y (NPY), as well as neurotransmitters like acetylcholine, to regulate pancreatic exocrine function. Pre- and post-ganglionic nerve fibers provide information to the pancreatic ganglia, which in turn control endocrine and exocrine secretion. Intrapancreatic postganglionic neurons are stimulated during the gastric and intestinal phases of stimulation by vagovagal responses, while central input occurs during the cephalic phase. They mainly release acetylcholine, which activates muscarinic receptors on acinar and duct cells, to stimulate the secretion of bicarbonates and enzymes.

3.4.2.1.2. Vagal Innervation

The nucleus of the solitary tract and the dorsal motor nucleus of the vagus (DMV) make up the dorsal vagal complex in the brainstem, which regulates pancreatic secretion parasympathetically. The nucleus of the solitary tract processes information sent by sensory vagal afferent nerves that innervate the pancreas before projecting it onto the DMV's preganglionic motor neurons. The vagus nerve's afferent limb provides the DMV with inputs from various hormones and neuropeptides as well as from other brain regions like the hypothalamus. The DMV is the primary source of the parasympathetic preganglionic efferent vagal nerves that innervate the pancreas, which end in the pancreatic ganglion. Pancreatic secretion is triggered by electrical and chemical stimulation of the DMV and can be blocked by vagotomy or atropine blockade of muscarinic receptors. It has been proposed that when intestinal stimulants are present in low concentrations, vagal cholinergic neurons mediate pancreatic secretion, while hormones mediate the response when intestinal stimulants are present in high concentrations.

Through its direct impact on pancreatic acinar cells as well as its indirect effect on the vagus nerve, CCK influences pancreatic secretion. The effects on the vagus nerve, however, are complex, and it appears that the spatial location of the neurons in the DMV complex controls their firing response. In one study, a direct action of CCK inhibited neurons in the intermediate region while activating those in the caudal region and leaving the rostral region unaffected. It seems that the entire pancreatic secretory response is influenced by the effects of CCK on the vagus nerve, though this is not entirely understood. Group II metabotropic glutamate receptors, which couple primarily to Gi/o, are also present in the vagus nerve. These receptors are found on the excitatory and inhibitory pre-synaptic terminals of DMV neurons that project the pancreas and are triggered by pancreatic polypeptide and CCK. Thus, through different vagal neurons, glutamate also modulates pancreatic exocrine secretion in addition to γ-amino butyric acid.

3.4.2.1.3. Vasoactive Intestinal Peptide

The body contains the 28 amino acid neuropeptide known as VIP. According to immunocytochemical evidence, VIP is a vagal neurotransmitter that is localized in pancreatic nerve fibers. Acinar cells and arteriole epithelial cells are located in close proximity to VIP immunoreactive nerve endings in chicks. VIP-positive nerves contained small, transparent vesicles, suggesting that these neurons are also cholinergic in nature (Figure 3.9).

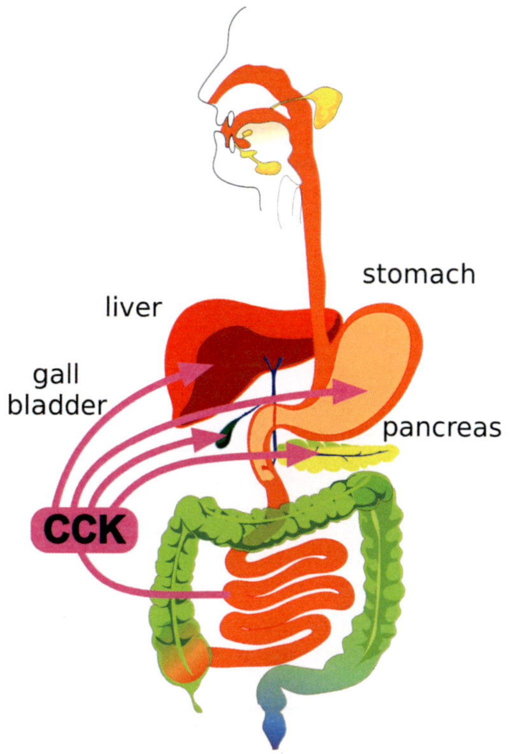

Figure 3.9. *CCK stimulates pancreatic secretion through hormonal and neuronal pathways. CCK is released from I cells of the small intestine and diffuses into the bloodstream where it is carried to the pancreas. CCK binds to receptors on acinar cells to stimulate pancreatic enzyme secretion. Secreted CCK also diffuses through the paracellular space and binds to CCK1-bearing nerves in the submucosa. Vagal afferent signals are integrated in the dorsal vagal complex which*

also receives signals from other regions of the brain (e.g., the hypothalamus). Vagal efferent fibers transmit cholinergic signals to the pancreas to stimulate pancreatic secretion.

Source: By McortNGHH – Own work, CC BY-SA 4.0, https://commons.wikimedia.org/w/index.php?curid=51666024.

In a healthy human pancreas, acinar cells, ducts, and blood vessels appear to be innervated by autonomic ganglia, which also receive a plentiful supply of VIP-positive fiber Plexi and nerves. Following atropine therapy, bicarbonate secretion was still elevated by electrical stimulation of the vagus nerve concurrent with the finding of VIP in pancreatic venous effluent, indicating a relationship between bicarbonate secretion and VIP release. Only high-affinity receptors appear to be crucial for protein secretion, as evidenced by the coupling of high-affinity receptors to cAMP-mediated amylase release and the lack of any effect on either cAMP elevation or amylase release upon activation of low-affinity receptors. Somatostatin and galanin decreased VIP-mediated fluid and protein output, which lessened the effects of VIP. Since increasing blood flow through vasodilation appears to be one of VIP's primary functions, it is challenging to assess how the substance affects pancreatic secretion in isolation from pancreatic blood flow.

3.4.2.1.4. Gastrin Releasing Peptide

The neuropeptide known as gastrin releasing peptide (GRP), which has 27 amino acids, has been found in neurons that innervate the human pancreas and is found in post-ganglionic vagal afferents. GRP-responsive receptors have been found to mediate enzyme secretion in cancer cells and the membranes of rats' pancreas. GRP can be found in the acinar and stromal areas, intrapancreatic ganglia, and on occasion the vasculature and ducts in cats. Similar to the expression pattern of VIP, GRP was localized on nerve fibers near pancreatic acini, capillaries, ductules, and arterial walls in humans. It has been shown via numerous investigations in various species that GRP regulates exocrine secretion. GRP was released upon vagal stimulation of the pig pancreas, increasing pancreatic exocrine secretion. Through a non-cholinergic pathway, electrical field-stimulated GRP release enhanced secretin-mediated fluid and amylase secretion in isolated perfused rat pancreatic preparations. γ-amino butyric acid increased the effects of GRP on rat pancreatic exocrine secretion. A GRP decapeptide called neuromedin C also increased pancreatic secretion through direct stimulation of canine acinar cells and indirect stimulation of CCK release.

3.4.2.1.5. Other Peptide Neurotransmitters

The neuropeptides listed below are present in pancreatic nerves, as indicated by immunohistochemical staining. Studies conducted in vitro and/or in vivo have demonstrated the functional significance of these neuropeptides, including their capacity to regulate pancreatic secretion. The neuropeptide known as neurotensin, which consists of 13 amino acids, is extensively expressed in the central nervous system and can also be found in the nerves that supply the pancreas. It increases the secretion of amylase and is enhanced by the cholinergic agonists carbachol, secretin, and caerulein (a CCK analog).

- **CGRP:** The 37-amino acid peptide known as CGRP is found in both peripheral and central neurons.
- **NPY:** The 36-residue peptide known as NPY is expressed in the nerve fibers that envelop exocrine pancreatic tissue as well as intrapancreatic ganglia. Its actions may be mediated by neurons

innervating the exocrine pancreas because it inhibited amylase secretion from intact pancreas and lobules that was mediated by CCK and vagally, but not from dispersed acini. Additional data points to NPY having, at most, a minor function in pancreatic exocrine secretion.

- **CCK:** It has been proposed that CCK functions as both a neurotransmitter and a hormone in pancreatic secretion due to its presence in intrapancreatic nerves. However, after vagal stimulation after a meal, CCK could not be found in the venous effluent of the isolated perfused porcine pancreas, indicating that synaptic release of CCK does not occur within the pancreas. Thus, more research is necessary to fully understand the neurotransmitter CCK functioning in pancreatic secretion.
- **Peptide Histidine Isoleucine:** Peptide histidine isoleucine (PHI) is a 27-amino acid peptide that originates from the same precursor molecule as VIP. It has an N-terminal histidine and a C-terminal isoleucine. It stimulates the secretion of fluid and bicarbonate in a cAMP-dependent manner and is found in the pancreatic nerves and ganglia.

3.4.2.1.6. Adrenergic Nerves

Adrenergic nerves have a much smaller effect on pancreatic exocrine secretion than does cholinergic stimulation. The celiac ganglion contains catecholamine-containing nerves that branch out into the intrapancreatic ganglia, blood vessels, ducts, and islets. Amylase release from superfused rat pancreatic preparations was elicited by epinephrine and norepinephrine (NE), which was comparable to the release of amylase induced by electrical stimulation in the presence of cholinergic blockade. Propranolol inhibits this process which is dependent on increased intracellular $Ca2^{+}$, indicating that β-adrenergic receptors are involved. Additionally, catecholamines suppress the secretion of amylase by interacting with α-adrenergic receptors expressed in pancreatic acini. In certain nerve fibers, NPY and NE are co-expressed, and when splanchnic nerves are stimulated, NPY and NE are released. Following electrical nerve stimulation, the pancreatoduodenal artery was infused with PACAP to increase the release of NE. It's unclear, nevertheless, how this observation relates physiologically.

Pancreatic secretion is reduced by approximately 70% upon celiac denervation, whereas blood flow is increased by 350%. The disturbance of sympathetic and stimulatory fibers that keep the pancreatic arteries' tonic constriction is most likely what causes this dissonance. It has been challenging to determine how adrenergic transmitters affect pancreatic secretion because norepinephrine has broad effects on a variety of processes, such as blood pressure, blood flow, neural reflexes, and hormone release. Although norepinephrine has been detected in rabbit pancreatic ganglia, ducts, and blood vessels at high concentrations, its effects are debatable. It has been observed that norepinephrine either stimulates, inhibits, or has no effect on pancreatic secretion. Regrettably, there has been no information provided by α- and β-adrenergic receptor agonists and antagonists to help identify key mechanisms involved in the adrenergic regulation of pancreatic secretion.

3.4.2.1.7. Dopamine

Dopamine β-hydroxylase (DBH)-positive fibers were found along the vasculature, ducts, and ganglia, indicating that dopamine may have a role in pancreatic secretion. Dopamine was also found in pancreatic ducts and ampullae. The evidence for dopamine's function in pancreatic secretion is inconclusive.

3.4.2.1.8. Serotonin

Serotonin is found in pancreatic ducts and ampullae, just like dopamine. Following tritiated serotonin uptake, autoradiography of tissue sections revealed serotonergic innervation of blood vessels in rats, but not exocrine parenchyma, indicating a restricted function in pancreatic secretion. Phenylbiguanide, a 5-HT3 receptor agonist, on the other hand, exhibited complex spatial regulation of pancreatic vagal neurons by serotonin as it activated preganglionic neurons in the caudal DMV, inhibited those in the intermediate DMV, and had no effect on rostral DMV neurons. Pancreatic amylase secretion was increased by intraduodenal infusion of melatonin, a serotonin derivative, whereas amylase release was reduced by pretreatment with ketanserin, a 5-HT2 serotonin antagonist, or MDL72222, a 5-HT3 antagonist. Bilateral vagotomy inhibited the release of amylase induced by serotonin, indicating a role for serotonergic mechanisms in exocrine secretion.

3.4.2.1.9. Nitric Oxide

When nicotinamide adenine dinucleotide hydrogen phosphate (NADPH) is present, NO synthase (NOS) converts L-arginine into nitric oxide (NO), a gaseous signaling molecule. It is a strong vasodilator that affects the pancreatic blood flow and secretory activity. The presence of NO has been determined by NOS expression or NADPH diaphorase (NADPH-d) histochemistry, as NOS and NADPH-d colocalize in neurons of the peripheral and central nervous systems since it is impractical to measure NO directly in biological tissues. The utilization of NO donors, NOS inhibitors, and inactivating agents (e.g., substances that produce superoxide) or maintain NO (e.g., oxidative dismutase). NO enters cells and activates guanylate cyclase, which produces the second messenger cGMP, in contrast to ligands that communicate through cell surface receptors.

3.4.2.2. Stimulatory Hormones

3.4.2.2.1. Cholecystokinin

Specialized enteroendocrine cells (I cells) mostly found in the upper small intestine release CCK. Dietary fats and proteins are the main boosters of CCK release. In the rat, an active feedback system allows intraluminal proteases to contribute to the release of a putative intestinal CCK releasing factor (e.g., LCRF) that ultimately results in the release of CCK. Humans have been reported to have multiple molecular forms of CCK, with sizes ranging from CCK-8 [CCK-NH2] to CCK-58. It was found that CCK-58 is the most common peptide in humans and the only form found in rats when CCK isolation methods were used to stop CCK from degrading in blood. The functional similarity between CCK-8 and CCK-58's actions suggests that CCK-8 still has the biological activity associated with this hormone. A amidated C-terminus and post-translational modification characterize CCK. One of CCK-8's key biological functions, sulfated tyrosine residues, is exocrine secretion. For CCK to bind to its receptors, C-terminal amidation is essential, and the amide group's removal reduces CCK activity. According to other research, deamidation and desulfation do not considerably reduce its capacity to induce the release of amylase; these differences might be due to species-specific variations. Longer forms of CCK, like CCK-33, are equally effective in mediating exocrine secretion as are shorter forms, like the tetrapeptide CCK-4, which is typically much less effective than CCK-8.

Through two G-coupled protein receptors, CCK-1 and CCK-2—previously known as CCK-A and CCK-B, respectively—CCK mediates its hormonal effects. To define the molecular mechanisms of CCK action, the role of these receptors in pancreatic secretion has been assessed. It has been suggested that there are two states of CCK receptors: a low affinity (nanomolar) but high capacity state and a high affinity (picomolar) but low capacity state. Autoradiography of pancreatic membranes treated with radioiodinated CCK-8 revealed that the rat pancreas has a high expression of CCK-1 receptors and a low abundance of CCK-2 receptors. Oral administration of loxiglumide, a potent CCK-1 receptor antagonist, reduces protein and fluid output in rats, suggesting that CCK-1 receptors modulate pancreatic secretion. Similar to how CCK-1 receptor antagonists prevented pancreatic amylase release induced by caerulein, the infusion of CCK, caerulein, and secretin in the presence of amino acids significantly increased fluid, bicarbonate, and enzyme output. The predominant CCK receptor subtype expressed in human pancreas is CCK-2, just like in porcine pancreas; however, it's interesting to note that CCK-1 receptor antagonists can also inhibit amylase secretion. CCK did not stimulate amylase release in dispersed human acini that responded to neuromedin C and carbamylcholine, most likely due to a lack of cellular membrane receptors. It has been suggested that CCK-1 receptors on the nerves that innervate the pancreas mediate the effects of CCK on human pancreatic secretion. Recent research, however, showed that human acinar cells treated with physiological concentrations of CCK-8 and CCK-58 elicited intracellular Ca2+ oscillations as well as normal pancreatic enzyme exocytosis, indicating the expression of functional CCK receptors on the human pancreas. Therefore, it would seem that the acinar cells of the human pancreas express CCK receptors.

Human pancreatic stellate cells have been demonstrated to express CCK receptors and release acetylcholine in response to CCK stimulation. This was more than enough acetylcholine to cause the release of amylase from acinar cells. A hitherto unidentified intrapancreatic route controlling CCK-induced pancreatic exocrine secretion may be represented by pancreatic stellate cells. CCK-mediated exocrine secretion is regulated by a number of hormones and neuropeptides. It has been demonstrated that insulin affects exocrine secretion locally. Anti-insulin antibodies were infused intraarterially into canine pancreas, inhibiting both secretin-mediated fluid and protein secretion from the pancreas and CCK stimulation.

The mechanism by which CCK induces the secretion of amylase involves a brief increase in intracellular $Ca2^{+}$. In addition, the production of diacylglycerol and inositol trisphosphate, two second messengers, and the activation of phospholipase C are needed. As evidenced by the increase in CCK-mediated amylase release in response to 8-bromo-cAMP and a phosphodiesterase inhibitor, CCK can sometimes trigger secretion by raising cAMP. Exocytosis depends on the regulation of actin cytoskeleton reorganization, which is regulated by heterotrimeric G proteins Gα13 and Gαq through their interactions with small GTP binding proteins RhoA and Rac1.

3.4.2.2.2. Secretin

The S cells of the small intestine release a hormone called secretin, which has 27 amino acids (340). During the intestinal phase, when gastric acid and ingested fatty acids enter the duodenum, secretin release is stimulated. It is one of the strongest inducers of pancreatic secretion and increases the secretion of bicarbonate and fluid. Examining the ultrastructure of the pancreas soon after secretin injection demonstrated that both duct and acinar cells secrete fluid. Even at as low as 1–2.8 pmol/kg·hr, secretin infusions have been shown to produce significant increases in pancreatic fluid and bicarbonate secretion. Secretin bolus injections as low as 0–125 pmol/kg have been shown to increase fluid and bicarbonate secretion in humans. While exogenous secretin equivalent to postprandial blood levels is thought to be the most potent stimulant of pancreatic bicarbonate secretion, it only produced 10% of the maximal pancreatic bicarbonate secretory response, indicating that other hormones and neurotransmitters are also important players in postprandial pancreatic bicarbonate secretion in humans. Through a cholinergic mechanism, secretin stimulates the release of fluid, bicarbonate, and to a lesser extent, protein from acinar cells.

Exocrine secretion mediated by secretin is facilitated by both cAMP-dependent and independent pathways. Adenylate cyclase activity increased by three to four times in response to secretin's interaction with its receptor; this increase was reversed in the presence of secretin antagonists. According to one report, secretin-mediated exocrine protein secretion was linked to phospholipase C activation. When secretin concentrations exceeded 10–8 M, acinar cells produced diacylglycerol and inositol trisphosphate. This led to the release of $Ca2^{+}$ from intracellular reserves and the activation of protein kinase C. Not every researcher has noticed this effect, though. The impact of secretin on pancreatic secretion is modulated by several hormones and peptides. By inducing acetylcholine release, CCK increased secretin-induced pancreatic fluid and protein output. Atropine or acini dispersion prevented this effect. High concentrations of islet hormones are absorbed by the exocrine pancreas through venous drainage from the pancreatic islets. A number of these hormones have strong effects on the secretion of pancreatic juice. Through an ouabain-sensitive Na^{+} K^{+}-ATPase, insulin promotes secretin-mediated fluid and protein secretion, whereas glucagon suppresses secretin-stimulated fluid and protein release.

3.4.2.2.3. Atrial Natriuretic Factor and C-Natriuretic Peptide

A peptide hormone called atrial natriuretic factor (ANF) is secreted by the atrial stretch and controls blood pressure and volume by preventing the kidneys from reabsorbing sodium. Studies using immunochemical methods revealed that acinar cells contain ANF. Early research revealed that ANF had no effect on fluid or protein secretion. G_i proteins link NPR-C, a non-guanylyl cyclase receptor, to either phospholipase C activation or adenylyl cyclase inhibition. Intracellular cAMP was elevated by secretin and VIP, but ANF attenuated this effect. Phospholipase C and protein kinase C inhibitors counteracted this effect. Secretin mediates the efflux of cAMP from intact pancreas and acinar cells in addition to increasing intracellular cAMP. ANF accelerated the removal of cAMP from cells through secretin-induced cAMP efflux. In numerous cellular systems, it has been reported that the multidrug resistance protein 4 (MRP4) is involved in the extrusion of cAMP. The pancreas also expresses MRP4, and through an NPR-C dependent mechanism and ANF, genetic knockdown of MRP4 expression decreased intracellular cAMP levels in acinar cells.

Similar in structure to ANF, C-natriuretic peptide (CNP) is expressed in both the gastrointestinal tract and central nervous system. Without changing the production of bicarbonate, CNP raises pancreatic protein, chloride, and fluid secretion, indicating that it acts on acinar rather than duct cells. Chloride secretion was reduced by truncal vagotomy, perivagal application of capsaicin, or hexamethonium, indicating that the parasympathetic nervous system regulates the effect of CNP. CNP activated NPR-C to cause protein secretion at low concentrations. PLC and PKC inhibitors inhibited CNP-induced amylase release similarly to how they did with ANF. Additionally, CNP decreased cAMP and increased intracellular cGMP concentrations, indicating that CNP may directly interact with receptors found on pancreatic acini.

3.4.2.2.4. Insulin

Insulin receptors are highly concentrated on the basolateral surfaces of acinar cells, and insulin regulates pancreatic exocrine function. CCK and secretin amplify the effects of insulin, which raises pancreatic enzyme synthesis and secretion. Given that CCK triggers the release of insulin when glucose and amino acids are present, it is plausible that these two hormones collaborate to enhance exocrine stimulation after a meal. According to the limited information available, insulin may control exocrine secretion through vagal cholinergic input and the potentiation of ouabain-sensitive Na^+ and K^+ ATPase. PP has an inhibitory effect on pancreatic secretion and modulates the action of insulin on exocrine secretion. Given their established ability to suppress insulin secretion, the peptides galanin, pancreastatin, and somatostatin may also control insulin-mediated amylase release.

3.4.2.2.5. Bombesin

Bombesin is an appetite suppressant that is a 14 amino acid peptide homolog of neuromedin B and GRP.

3.4.2.2.6. Melatonin

Melatonin is a lipophilic hormone that is produced by specific neuroendocrine cells in the gastrointestinal tract and the pineal gland. Acinar cells have melatonin receptors, and melatonin shields the pancreas from acute pancreatitis brought on by caerulein. Early research revealed that melatonin mediated the release of pancreatic amylase through the actions of CCK, vagal sensory nerves, and melatonin type 2 receptors. Melatonin did not, however, seem to directly affect pancreatic acinar cells. It is worth doing more research to determine the extent and significance of melatonin-induced pancreatic secretion.

3.4.2.2.7. Amylin

In response to nutrients, pancreatic β-cells co-secrete amylin, a 37 amino acid hormone, along with insulin. In rats, amylin increases CCK-independent pancreatic secretion. Proton pump inhibitors and atropine reverse this effect, possibly as a result of somatostatin release inhibition. By activating GPCRs and releasing Ca^{2+} from intracellular stores, amylin has also been demonstrated to increase protein secretion from pancreatic AR42J cells. Other studies have revealed that amylin does not affect the secretion of pancreatic exocrine from AR42J cells, acinar preparations, or isolated perfused pancreas. Thus, it is still unclear how amylin affects exocrine secretion.

3.4.2.2.8. Histamine

Histamine is an amino acid that may play a gender-dependent role in mediating pancreatic exocrine secretion. Increased fluid and protein secretion was observed in the rabbit pancreas upon activation of H1 receptors and inhibition of H2 receptors, indicating differential action based on regulation and coupling of the two receptors. Under normal physiological conditions, the effect of histamine on pancreatic secretion is thought to be negligible at most.

3.4.2.3. Inhibitory Hormones

3.4.2.3.1. Peptide YY and Pancreatic Peptide

The three hormones that make up the NPY family of peptides are PP, PYY, and NPY. All three peptides share the PP fold, a tertiary structural motif, and have 36 residues total, several of which are tyrosines. Peptidase activity can cleave the N-terminal amino acids of PYY and NPY to produce biologically active truncated forms, PYY_{3-36} and NPY_{3-36}. PYY and glucagon are co-expressed in α cells of the islets, while F cells of the islets of Langerhans secrete PP postprandially. The exocrine pancreas of some species contains PP immunopositive cells as well, and some of these PP cells express PYY. These three hormones work through the Y1–5 GPCR family, which is a group of five GPCRs. Similar affinities are shared by NPY and PYY for Y1, Y2, and Y5. PYY3–36 interacts preferentially with Y2, while PP is the ligand of choice for Y4.

Blood PYY levels are higher postprandially and after fatty acid infusion into the distal small intestine. PYY in the blood at physiologically relevant concentrations inhibits pancreatic secretion triggered by hormones and meals. PYY administered intravenously dramatically reduces pancreatic blood flow while simultaneously reducing secretin- and secretin plus CCK-mediated pancreatic protein and fluid secretion. PYY does not, however, suppress pancreatic secretion stimulated by 2-diacylglycerol, indicating that either protein kinase C-activated signaling or suppression of CCK-stimulated exocrine secretion occurs before 2-diacylglycerol-stimulated activation. PYY_{1-36} but not PYY_{3-36} decreased CCK-stimulated amylase release in the denervated pancreas, indicating that Y1 receptors mediate PYY's hormonal effects.

Eating a meal also increases PP secretion, which can be replicated by intraduodenal infusion of fatty acids, or aromatic amino acids. In dispersed acini, PP inhibited the release of amylase mediated by secretin and secretin plus CCK, indicating that PP may have direct effects on acinar cells. In humans, pancreatic protein output was reduced by PP infusion; however, bicarbonate secretion remained unaffected, indicating that PP action varies depending on the species. But unlike PYY, PP has an alternative mechanism to suppress exocrine secretion because it has no effect on pancreatic blood flow.

3.4.2.3.2. Somatostatin

Made up of 14 or 28 amino acids, somatostatin is generated by the δ cells found in the pancreatic islets. Additionally, the hypothalamus and some intestinal cells secrete it. After a meal, it is released into the blood, but its main mode of action is paracrine. Its wide-ranging inhibitory effects extend to the target organs and the release of multiple hormones. In a dose-dependent manner, somatostatin and its analogs suppressed secretin- and CCK-induced protein secretion. Compared to secretin-stimulated secretion, CCK-stimulated pancreatic secretion was more inhibited by low doses of somatostatin. Chloride ion secretion and the production of cAMP were the outcomes of secretin-mediated activation of slowly-activating voltage-dependent K^+ channels found on the basolateral surface of pancreatic acini. When somatostatin is added to acini, the production of intracellular cAMP is reduced, and secretin-mediated K^+ current is enhanced, indicating that somatostatin controls exocrine secretion via this pathway. Furthermore, somatostatin blocked the release of amylase that was stimulated by cAMP and Ca^{2+} by blocking exocytosis via a Gi protein-dependent mechanism.

Through a neural mechanism, somatostatin also inhibits exocrine secretion. It seems that peptidergic, but not cholinergic, and nicotinic acetylcholine receptors present on sympathetic and parasympathetic ganglia mediate somatostatin action based on atropine, hexamethonium, and tetrodotoxin sensitivities. Denervation had no effect on the somatostatin-mediated suppression of secretin-stimulated fluid and protein secretion, indicating that extrapancreatic nerves are not involved. Somatostatin's inhibitory effects were reversed by the muscarinic receptor agonist bethanechol, suggesting that intrapancreatic cholinergic neurons are primarily responsible for mediating its actions. We still don't fully understand how somatostatin prevents pancreatic secretion. Somatostatin, however, is thought to have an inhibitory effect on the hormone and neurotransmitter release that typically stimulates pancreatic secretion.

3.4.2.3.3. Galanin

The 29-amino acid peptide galanin has a variety of functions, such as preventing the pancreas from secreting PP, somatostatin, and insulin. Its presence in the secretory granules of both peripheral and central neurons points to its potential role as a neurotransmitter. Nerve fibers surrounding acini, ductules, and blood vessels exhibited galanin immunoreactivity; 73% of these fibers were dual positive for both galanin and VIP. Acinar cells contain the messenger RNA for the galanin receptor, suggesting that galanin can directly affect acini. Galanin inhibited the release of amylase from acinar cells that was stimulated by CCK and carbachol, which is consistent with this finding. Galanin suppressed the sustained phase of amylase release induced by carbachol, indicating that it may reduce cholinergic activity through a mechanism involving Gi proteins that are sensitive to pertussis toxin.

3.4.2.3.4. Pancreastatin

Numerous neuroendocrine tissues express pancreastatin, which is produced by cleaving chromogranin A. Its multiple functions include inhibiting pancreatic exocrine secretion. It has been localized to the duct cells of the exocrine pancreas.

3.4.2.3.5. Glucagon

Once a meal is consumed, the endocrine pancreas releases glucagon. Early research revealed that pancreatic protein stimulated by secretin or secretin and CCK was inhibited by glucagon, but not the secretion of bicarbonate. Glucagon, however, has been shown in other studies to inhibit the secretion of postprandial proteins and bicarbonates. Glucagon appears to have a direct and stimulatory effect rather than an inhibitory one on isolated pancreatic lobules and acini, indicating a complex action at the cellular level as opposed to the physiological level. Further research is warranted as the effects of glucagon on exocrine secretion observed in experiments are not conclusive.

3.4.2.3.6. Ghrelin

When a person fasts, their stomach endocrine cells release ghrelin, an orexigenic hormone consisting of 28 amino acids. Ghrelin increases the production of acid by the stomach's oxyntic cells, and its plasma levels rise right before a meal, indicating that it may play a part in controlling eating habits. By analyzing protein and mRNA expression, ghrelin and its receptor have been found in the pancreatic acini. Acute pancreatitis, food deprivation, and gastric acid inhibition did not change the expression of ghrelin, but they did change the expression of its receptor, which was upregulated in the former case and downregulated in the latter. In an experiment, ghrelin had no effect on the release of amylase from scattered acini when stimulated by basal or CCK.

3.4.2.3.7. Leptin

Adipocytes secrete the 16 kDa orexigenic peptide leptin, which balances energy homeostasis by decreasing food intake and increasing energy expenditure. Leptin administered intravenously or intraperitoneally decreased basal and CCK-stimulated protein output in vivo in the pancreas. Vagotomy, capsaicin pretreatment, and CCK-1 receptor blockade all lessened this effect, indicating that it suppressed pancreatic exocrine secretion via a vagal pathway that is dependent on CCK. Leptin's lack of effect on dispersed acini in vitro provides additional evidence in favor of a neural mechanism of action.

3.4.2.3.8. Adrenomedullin

In the F cells of the pancreatic islets, adrenalomedullin colocalizes with PP and inhibits insulin. It directly engages in interactions with acinar cells, potentially through modulating intracellular Ca^{2+} levels and exocytosis, to inhibit CCK-stimulated pancreatic amylase release. Adrenomedullin's mode of action is poorly understood. Food's sight and smell trigger the intricate process of pancreatic secretion, which continues until food reaches the duodenum. Food digestion is controlled at every stage by a variety of stimuli that impact hormonal and neuronal pathways. These pathways maximize the release of fluid, bicarbonate, and enzymes and are both stimulatory and inhibitory.

3.5. Pancreatectomy

The surgical removal of all or part of the pancreas is known as a pancreatectomy. For both benign and malignant pancreatic processes, there are numerous surgical techniques available, including various forms of surgical excision. Surgeons need to be well-versed in pancreatic anatomy, preoperative diagnostic modalities, and postoperative management in addition to precise surgical techniques.

Over the years, significant advancements have been made in pancreatic surgery. It is still technically difficult, though, and the surgeon must have a great deal of experience and good clinical judgment. This article will cover the anatomy, physiology, indications, contraindications, evaluation, and surgical techniques for various types of pancreatic resections. There will be a dedicated discussion about the special surgical techniques, difficulties, and management of pancreaticoduodenectomy (Whipple) elsewhere.

3.5.1. Indications

The indications for laparoscopic versus open pancreatectomy are similar, but they also largely depend on the experience and comfort level of the surgeon performing the procedure.

- Total Pancreatectomy
  - Tumors of the pancreatic head that are malignant and affect the left pancreas.
  - Unable to obtain R0 resections free of tumors at the pancreatic margin.
  - Unable to execute pancreaticoduodenectomy followed by pancreatic anastomosis.
  - In the remaining pancreas, recurrent pancreatic cancer.
  - Removal of the remaining pancreas following a leak or bleeding Whipple complication.
  - All regions of the pancreas can have multifocal intraductal papillary mucinous neoplasms (IPMN).
  - Multiple endocrine neoplasias in the past combined with multifocal neuroendocrine tumors of the pancreas.

  - Family history or hereditary pancreatic cancer (contentious).
  - Unbearable pain brought on by repeated episodes of acute pancreatitis or chronic pancreatitis.
- Distal Pancreatectomy
  - Tumors, either benign or malignant, affecting the pancreatic body or tail, which are situated on the left side of the superior mesenteric vein.
  - Body- or tail-confined chronic pancreatitis.
  - Pancreatic tail pseudocyst involved.
  - Trauma to the distal pancreas
  - Pancreatic fistula in the tail or body +/- ductal disruption or stricture.
- Central Pancreatectomy
  - Lesions in the neck or pancreatic proximal body that are benign or borderline.
  - Lesion enucleation at the neck or proximal body is not possible.
  - Injury to the neck or proximal body caused by trauma.
  - Among other things, a distal pancreatic tail longer than 5 to 6 cm is required for pancreatic conservation to be risk-worthy.

3.5.1.1. Contraindications

- Absolute Contraindications to Open and Laparoscopic
  - Medical conditions that make surgery impossible.
  - Poor functional status
  - Bleeding coagulopathy
- Laparoscopic Technique
  - Severe obesity (surgeon experience level dependent)
  - prior large abdominal surgeries due to an adhesive illness.)
  - Advanced malignancy
  - involve des structures vasculaires (surgeon experience level dependent).
  - Unable to tolerate pneumoperitoneum
- Total Pancreatectomy
  - Lesions that can be removed using a different type of resection while preserving pancreatic tissue.
- Central Pancreatectomy
  - Pancreatic cancer (involving lymph nodes and inability to eradicate cancer entirely).
- Distal Pancreatectomy

Pancreatic lesions that cannot be completely excised by a distal pancreatectomy or resected to an R0.

3.5.2. Equipment

- Sterile drapes, gowns, and gloves
- Operating room with surgical instruments, sutures, and staplers
- Cell saver machine
- Video monitors, either straight or angled camera lenses, multiple laparoscopic instruments such as scissors, graspers, and dissectors, laparoscopic staplers, energy devices, and sutures are all part of a

laparoscopic case.

- Ultrasound
- Code cart
- Anesthesia
- Arterial and Venous lines
- Foley catheter
- Closed suction drains
- Surgical loupes

3.5.3. Personnel

- Anesthesia team
- OR personnel (nurses and scrub techs)
- Surgeon
- First assistant
- competent ultrasonographer (should the surgeon not have instant access to an ultrasound in the operating room).
- Cell saver technician

3.5.4. Preparation

A stringent preoperative evaluation is required of any candidate for elective pancreatic surgery. Every patient needs to have a complete physical examination and history taken. When making surgical plans, past surgical procedures and current medical conditions must be considered. The evaluation needs to take into account the patient's past family history of cancer as well as any current symptoms or signs. Every pancreatic surgery procedure ought to be carried out on carefully chosen patients. Reviewing preoperative labs, imaging, and general status is recommended. For three reasons, patients having cancer resections should have preoperative access to your local emergency numbers.

- If elevated, indicating a malignancy.
- If extremely high, consider the possibility of a widespread illness.
- A point of departure to serve as a guide for post-operative observation.

Most patients will have preoperative endoscopic ultrasound combined with a biopsy. Following pancreatic disease diagnosis, appropriate measures need to be implemented to assess the patient's suitability for surgery. Preoperative cardiac and medical clearance should be performed by the surgical planning team. To help prevent any postoperative morbidity or mortality, the patient's cardiac and respiratory function should be medically optimized during the preoperative planning phase. Following major abdominal surgery, these two body systems have some of the highest risk factors for postoperative complications. It is important to assess the patient's nutritional status because it has been linked to positive postoperative outcomes. Patients with pancreatic cancer and chronic pancreatitis frequently exhibit varying degrees of malnourishment. Although a number of formulas and lab measurements are employed, the most crucial element should always be the clinician's clinical assessment of the patient. Any indications of malnutrition before surgery should be taken seriously and treated appropriately.

3.5.4.1. Imaging

- A very useful tool for assessing pancreatic lesions is CT imaging. The CT scan can reveal the exact location, size, and—most importantly—whether any nearby structures are affected by the lesion. Determining whether a tumor is resectable is aided greatly by CT imaging. Triphasic cross-sectional imaging with arterial, late arterial, and venous phases is part of a pancreatic CT protocol. Because many pancreatic cancers are hypovascular in nature, this type of imaging allows the identification of the majority of cases in the delayed arterial phase/venous phase. Nonetheless, numerous additional pancreatic lesions can also be detected by the arterial phase. According to reports, CT imaging can detect pancreatic cancer with a sensitivity of 76–92% and a surgical resectability of up to 90%.

- Both the preoperative and operating rooms can benefit from the use of endoscopic ultrasound. Utilizing ultrasound technology, one can check for vascular invasion and the mass's resectability. The best method for taking a tissue sample is endoscopic. When it comes to tiny pancreatic lesions like cysts, endoscopic ultrasound is quite helpful. The application of ultrasonography to assist in the diagnosis of nodal involvement and metastatic diseases, such as those involving large lymph nodes in the mediastinal or celiac positions, is another helpful benefit.
- Pancreatic lesions can also be diagnosed with MRI. When determining pancreaticobiliary anatomy and pathology, MRI is a highly effective modality. Pancreatic duct anomalies, such as strictures, can be detected by MRCP. Overall, it performs a better job of recognizing the pancreatic and biliary ductal systems. MRI is increasingly being used for both post-operative lesion tracking and diagnosis.
- There is conflicting evidence to support the routine use of PET scans for pancreatic disease diagnosis and staging. Due to the sensitivity's dependence on lesion size, small disease areas may go unnoticed. High blood glucose levels can lead to missed metastatic disease and false negative results. Combining CT and PET scans can improve overall accuracy as well as sensitivity and specificity, particularly for lesions that the CT imaging system missed. Overall, the CA 19–9 increase is more helpful in identifying and validating occult disease after resection (Figure 3.10).

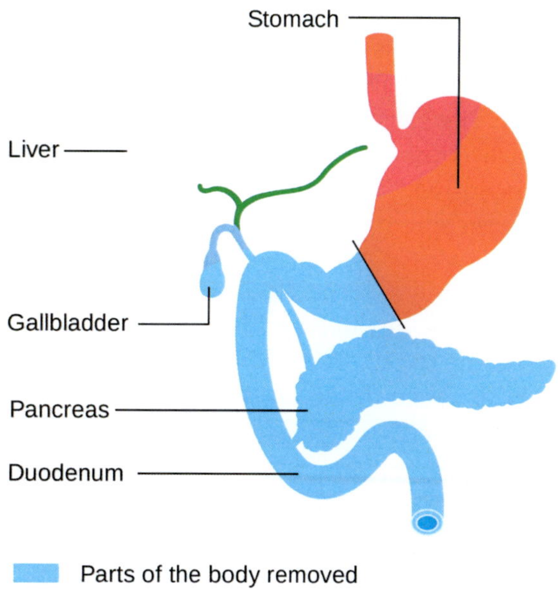

Figure 3.10. *Diagram showing the area removed for a total pancreatectomy.*

Source: By Cancer Research UK, CC BY-SA 4.0, https://commons.wikimedia.org/w/index.php?curid=34334043.

3.5.5. Technique or Treatment

3.5.5.1. Laparoscopic vs. Open Techniques

Significant progress has been made in the last ten years in the management of benign or malignant processes using minimally invasive techniques. Laparoscopic procedures were previously limited to pancreatic cancer diagnostic staging. An increasing number of surgeons are now performing distal, enucleation, or central pancreatic resections using either robotic or laparoscopic methods. Less postoperative pain, a shorter hospital stay, less intraoperative blood loss, a quicker return to normal activities, less postoperative ileus, and fewer surgical complications are all benefits of laparoscopic procedures for the patient. Because laparoscopic procedures are so complex, only highly skilled surgeons with advanced training in minimally invasive surgery should perform them. The surgeon needs to feel confident using laparoscopic staplers, laparoscopic ultrasound techniques, intracorporeal suturing, and laparoscopic bleeding control.

A diagnostic laparoscopy is typically performed on the patient prior to a pancreatic procedure if the lesion is malignant. This is accomplished by either creating a pneumoperitoneum with a Veress needle or using the Hasson technique to cut down to the fascia and place the trocar under direct visualization of the fascia. With direct visualization of the anatomy, the camera can be inserted into the abdomen following the implantation of an infraumbilical or supraumbilical trocar. After that, distinct trocars can be positioned so that the camera can see them clearly. Grabbers can be used to examine the abdomen after the other 5mm working ports are positioned to ensure that no hidden metastatic disease has affected the peritoneum, liver, or nearby structures. At this point, additional biopsies or peritoneal washings can be performed. The team may choose to proceed with minimally invasive surgery if that is their usual method, switch to an open procedure for the resection, or continue with the laparoscopic technique if no evidence of metastatic disease has been found.

3.5.5.2. Open Techniques

The standard setup for an open pancreatic surgical procedure is outlined below. The remaining methods will outline the precise actions needed to close the case. Every preoperative image was examined. Consent was obtained with knowledge. After being moved into the operating room, the patient will be put in the supine position on the operating table. Most patients receive a spinal block from the anesthesia team to manage their pain after surgery. The patient will be put under general anesthesia and have their airway ventilated. An Aline and/or central line may be inserted, depending on the patient's characteristics, the judgment of the surgeon and anesthesiologist, and the patient's degree of comfort. Verifying the appropriate patient, positioning, procedure, and preoperative antibiotics is known as a formal timeout. Pre-incision antibiotic treatment will be given to the patient.

There will be a Foley catheter inserted. After that, the patient's abdomen will be cleaned and covered from the nipples to the suprapubic area in the customary sterile manner. The first procedure is a diagnostic laparoscopy, as previously mentioned. If the results are negative, make a midline incision with a 10-bladed scalpel that runs from the subxiphoid to the supraumbilical regions. Moreover, a subcostal/chevron incision may be made. The falciform ligament should be ligated once it is inside the abdomen and removed for potential future use. Many surgical retractors, like Bookwalter, Omni-Tract, or Thompson retractor sets, can be used once they have entered the abdomen.

Examining the liver, small bowel, transverse colon, mesentery, diaphragm, and peritoneum will help to definitively rule out any findings of metastatic disease. To view the pancreas, it is necessary to open the lesser sac by puncturing the gastrocolic ligament close to the transverse colon. After that, the pancreas is made visible for the planned surgical resection. The following is a list of the precise movements and methods used in the specified pancreatic surgery.

3.5.5.3. Total Pancreatectomy

The entire pancreas must be exposed during a total pancreatectomy. To enable the duodenum to fully extend to the aorta, the hepatic flexure is mobilized as necessary. With a clear view of the retroperitoneal attachments, the entire pancreatic head can be seen with this Kocher maneuver. After that, the surgeon can palpate behind the pancreatic head for any masses involving the superior mesenteric artery (which would prevent an R0 resection). The common bile duct can then be fully circumferentially exposed during the dissection of the gastrohepatic ligament. Following its dissection from the fossa and separation from the liver bed, the gallbladder can be removed. After that, the cystic artery and cystic duct can be completely divided using clip ligation. It is possible to confirm the presence of an accessory or replaced right hepatic artery after the gallbladder has been removed from the liver bed. This lymph node station can be dissected to identify the celiac axis. After that, the gastroduodenal artery can be located and clamped. The middle colic vein can then be checked in the transverse mesocolon. This can be linked to the superior mesenteric vein's location on the inferior aspect of the pancreas. A blunt, right-angled instrument can then be used to safely dissect the confluence of the superior mesenteric vein and portal vein. A Penrose drain can be positioned between the portal vein and superior mesenteric vein dissection planes following cautious dissection. The proximal jejunum is then situated 10–15 cm distal to the Treitz ligament. A linear GIA stapler can be used to divide this area. A ligature device can then be used to remove the mesentery at the bowel's edge.

The defect of the ligament of Treitz allows the newly formed jejunal limb to be inserted into the supracolic compartment. To stop the development of an internal hernia, the defect can be sealed. The hepatic duct can then be severed, directly in front of the ligated cystic duct, to identify the porta hepatis. Posteriorly, the portal vein and hepatic artery are discernible. Take care not to damage these structures. After removing the clamp, the gastroduodenal artery can be further dissected and ligated. At this point, either the standard pancreaticoduodenectomy or a pylorus-preserving one can be carried out. The duodenum can be divided 3 cm distal to the pylorus to section the second part of the duodenum for the pylorus-preserving technique. The terminal branches of the left and right gastric arteries can be divided at the stomach's body and antrum if the standard procedure is to be followed.

The vagus nerve, which is usually found at the third crossing vein proximal to the pylorus, should be identified. The stomach antrum can then be divided just distal to the vagus nerve. Then, additional mobilization of the spleen and left colon at the splenic flexure is possible. A ligature energy device can then be used to cut the short gastric arteries. Then, the retroperitoneal attachments of the pancreas and spleen, as well as the spleen and its surrounding attachments, can all be fully mobilized. Next, the dissection is moved from the pancreatic medial aspect in the direction of the spleen. It is important to locate the splenic artery's start as well as the junction between the splenic vein and the superior mesenteric vein. Next, at the point where the artery leaves the celiac trunk, the splenic vein and artery can be tied off. Then, as they enter the portal vein and superior mesenteric vein, the small draining veins from the pancreas and duodenum can be located and ligated. The posterior attachments of the portal vein, superior mesenteric artery, and superior mesenteric vein can then be freed of the uncinate process. The pancreatic head's venous vessels are then carefully dissected and ligated to remove them. The superior mesenteric artery is examined after the head has been completely removed from the portal vein and superior mesenteric vein venous branches.

The pancreaticoduodenal arteries can then be distinguished, divided, and ligated. The superior mesenteric artery attachments allow the pancreas to be skeletonized after that. After that, the pancreas can be taken out and moved off the table so that the margins can be marked and samples from the duodenal, uncinate, and bile duct margins can be sent. Reconstruction is carried out following confirmation of the margins. The distal end of the jejunum can then be used to create the biliary enteric anastomosis. From the distal common hepatic duct to the proximal loop of the jejunum, an end-to-side anastomosis is carried out. A single layer anastomosis is executed utilizing interrupted 5–0 PDS suture. The proximal stomach anastomosis can be performed using either the standard technique or the pylorus-preserving technique, which would entail wrapping the ligated falciform ligament around the biliary anastomosis.

The duodenojejunostomy could be positioned 20 cm distal to the newly formed biliary enteric anastomosis if pylorus preservation was carried out. If the standard procedure was followed, a gastrojejunostomy could be made 20 cm away from the hepaticojejunal anastomosis by hand sewing an inner layer of 3–0 PDS and an outer layer of 3–0 silk suture, or by using a stapled anastomosis. Then, each anastomosis needs to be examined for leaks. To check for bile spillage, a ray-tech can be positioned around the posterior aspect of the biliary anastomosis. The choice to implant a gastrostomy tube or a distal feeding jejunostomy tube for feeding access can be made after it has been confirmed that all anastomoses are open and undamaged. Following the creation of the anastomosis, closed suction Jackson Pratt drains can be positioned on the anterior abdominal wall. 3–0 Nylon sutures can be used to secure them in place.

3.5.5.4. Central Pancreatectomy

If the specific lesion can be operated on using this method, the surgeon can preserve pancreatic parenchyma by performing a central pancreatectomy. Compared to distal pancreatectomy patients, who experience postoperative long-term diabetes outcomes of 20 to 50%, central pancreatectomy patients experience much more pancreatic conservation. With a central pancreatectomy, the exocrine function is also preserved at a far higher rate—just 10% of patients require supplementation, compared to 27% of patients who have a distal pancreatectomy. Additionally, a central pancreatectomy prevents a splenectomy and preserves the entire biliary anatomy. For pancreatic cancer, central pancreatectomy is not recommended because lymph node harvesting is insufficient and residual margins may still contain cancer. Central pancreatectomy is probably the least common type of pancreatic resection surgery because it is only performed on benign or possibly borderline lesions. There must be 5 to 6 cm of parenchyma left in the distal pancreas. The pancreatic neck can be mobilized once the entire pancreatic body, neck, and tail have been revealed. The vessels that supply the superior spleen can stay open and do not need to be tied. To sufficiently mobilize this area, it might be necessary to ligate a few of the tiny vessels that run along the pancreatic neck. A stapler with a reinforced staple line can be used to transect the pancreatic proximal portion. Similar to other cases of pancreatic transection, two stay sutures may be inserted in the distal portion of the pancreas to aid in hemostasis before the transection. After that, the gland can be cut open using a knife or energy tool. After that, the margins are sent right away to pathology to verify a negative margin. After that, the distal remnant of the pancreas can be drained into the small intestine or the stomach. For optimal mobilization to the stomach, the pancreatic body needs to be released from the splenic vessels if a pancreaticogastrostomy is the drainage option of choice. To be delivered into the stomach, the pancreas needs to be sufficiently mobilized.

Making an anterior and posterior gastrotomy accomplishes this. After that, the pancreatic remnant is inserted into the stomach without putting further strain on either organ. After that, the posterior stomach can be stitched using either 3–0 PDS or silk sutures in a straightforward running or interrupted pattern to the pancreatic parenchyma inside the capsule. After that, the anterior part of the stomach is sutured in two layers, the outer layer being made of silk and the underlying layer of PDS suture. Next, a drain is placed next to the recently formed anastomosis. The pancreaticojejunal anastomosis for the pancreatic remnant may be performed using a jejunal limb. It is possible to transect the jejunum 15–20 cm distal to the Treitz ligament. It is possible to pass a jejunum segment that is between 35 and 40 cm long through the mesocolon opening and lay tension-free next to the pancreatic remnant.

A jejunojejunostomy anastomosis can be used to restore the continuity of the distal jejunum. An end-to-side anastomosis can be used during the pancreatic duct to jejunum anastomosis. There are two ways to create an anastomosis. The first involves running stitches to join the pancreatic capsule and the jejunal serosal layer. A tiny enterotomy is made in the jejunum before the pancreatic duct is sewn to it. After that, the pancreatic duct is sewn straight to the mucosa using vicryl or 5–0 PDS. To act as a stent for the pancreatic duct, a tiny feeding tube can be inserted through the jejunal wall and into the duct. Utilizing a running 5–0 prolene suture, the anterior pancreatic to jejunum anastomosis is subsequently accomplished. Near the pancreatic stump and anastomosis, a drain is left in place. If it is believed that this area may have a pancreatic duct stricture or if the stapled edge is too thick for a secure staple line, the proximal pancreas can also be anastomosed to this section of the jejunum. In the unlikely event that the stump breaks, this permits the pancreatic head to drain and might prevent the patient from developing a pancreatic fistula. The procedure for this anastomosis is the same as for the pancreaticojejunostomy that was previously established.

3.5.5.5. Distal Pancreatectomy

The surgeon typically recognizes whether a distal pancreatectomy is being done for a malignant process before beginning. The spleen cannot be preserved if the distal pancreas has a malignant tumor. Let's say the benign distal pancreatic lesion is the reason for the resection. It is possible to save the spleen. Below, we'll go over both strategies.

- **Distal Pancreatectomy with Splenectomy**: The splenic flexure and colon can be further mobilized after the pancreas has been exposed through entry into the lesser sac by dividing the gastrocolic ligament, as was previously discussed. There are two possible approaches for the exposure: a medial to lateral approach where the pancreas is transectioned at the confluence of the splenic and superior mesenteric veins, and the dissection is finished laterally. In the latter case, the pancreas and spleen are mobilized from the retroperitoneum and vasculature. Distal pancreatectomy can be performed using either method.

- After that, the spleen can be further mobilized by rupturing the splenocolic ligament, which will aid in further splenic flexure mobilization. To help in mobilization, the spleen can be gently retracted medially. An energy device can be used to ligate the short gastric arteries, after which the stomach can be further retracted superiorly and medially to the right upper quadrant. Notably, if there is insufficient space between the stomach and spleen, the surgeon may divide the short gastrics close to the gastroesophageal junction using a stapler to prevent heat injury to the stomach. Pancreatic transection, encompassing the distal tail to the neck, can be carried out after the entire distal pancreas and the splenic vasculature are fully visible. The middle colic vein is a great landmark for locating the superior mesenteric vein if the pancreatic transection is to be performed on the neck. After that, the superior mesenteric vein, splenic vein, and retroperitoneal attachments can be carefully removed from the pancreatic neck. After that, the pancreas can be removed with a stapler device that has reinforcement or a scalpel. To help with hemostasis, if the scalpel technique is employed, first place superior and inferior stay sutures on the pancreas. Finding the main pancreatic duct is necessary after the pancreas has been transected. Next, employing a figure-of-eight stitch with 3–0 silk sutures, the duct's end can be oversewn. After that, multiple U stitches using pledgets are used to oversee the remaining pancreatic parenchyma. After that, the splenic artery can be tied. The common hepatic artery can be palpated to make sure it hasn't been inadvertently ligated before ligation, and the splenic artery can be momentarily clamped. The splenic artery can be divided with a vascular stapler load or double ligated using a 2–0 silk or prolene suture if the hepatic artery is pulsating. The spleen can be decompressed after the splenic inflow is removed, and the pancreatic remnants that are attached to the splenic artery and vein can then be divided. After that, the splenic vein can be crossed with a stapler load or tied off with a 2–0 silk suture. To avoid thrombosis of the splenic vein remnant, caution should be taken when ligating the splenic vein and not to leave it open for longer than necessary. The small bowel may be compromised if the thrombosis migrates into the superior mesenteric vein and causes problems with outflow. The remaining attachments are removed once the spleen is mobilized to the midline. After that, the specimens can be sent from the operative field to pathology. The distal pancreatic transection site and the ligated splenic artery stump can be covered by the previously ligated falciform ligament. Hemostasis is attainable. A surgeon must decide whether to leave a drain in place.

- Distal Pancreatectomy with Spleen Preservation – When the known distal pancreatic mass is benign, it can be carried out. To prevent asplenia and sepsis following a splenectomy, the spleen should be preserved if at all possible. There are two approaches that surgeons can take when managing spleen preservation. During the initial dissection, the Warshaw technique advises against ligating the short gastric and left gastroepiploic arteries. The splenic vein and artery may be sutured if the Warshaw technique is used.
One of the most frequent side effects of using the Warshaw technique is splenic infarction with necrosis, although late-onset left-sided portal hypertension is also occasionally observed. Careful dissection is another method of splenic preservation. Less splenic infarction and the development of gastric varices are the postoperative outcomes of ligating the small splenic arteries and veins that supply and drain the pancreas while maintaining the splenic artery and vein. The distal pancreatectomy's preliminary procedures are carried out in the same way. The pancreas is divided for preservation with intact splenic vessels, and vessel loops can then be used to encircle the splenic vessels. The splenic artery and vein can then be divided using a staple load or suture ligation, after each of the small branches has been individually ligated. After that, the transected pancreas can be removed from the operating field. The vessels are split at the distal end of the pancreas, close to the splenic hilum, and at the transected portion of the organ to execute the Warshaw technique. The pancreas and vessels are on the superior aspect of the specimen as it is subsequently passed off the field. The spleen needs to be examined right away following this procedure for any indications of ischemia. Intraoperative ultrasonography is typically used to confirm adequate perfusion as well.
- Distal Pancreatectomy with islet cell autotransplantation – This method has been used far more frequently in the past ten to fifteen years following a total pancreatectomy for persistent pancreatitis. A total pancreatectomy deprives the patient of all exocrine and endocrine functions. Even after the pancreas is removed, the patient can still function as an endocrine system thanks to autotransplantation. The choice of patients and determining who will truly benefit from autotransplantation are important issues that need to be addressed. To ensure that the number and function of islet cells are sufficient, patients must undergo testing.
A total pancreatectomy with islet autotransplantation is not recommended in several situations, including those involving active

substance abuse, pancreatic cancer, or poorly managed mental health conditions. Transplantation can take place during the same surgical procedure if the patient is found to be a good candidate for islet autotransplantation combined with a total pancreatectomy. The pancreas is prepared on the back table after it has been removed. The pancreas is submerged in ice-cold water containing the preservation and antibiotic solutions. A preservation solution is subsequently injected into the splenic and gastroduodenal arteries. Next, a preservation solution containing a variety of enzymes can be injected into the cannulated pancreatic duct on the table. Until the gland is evenly distributed throughout the parenchyma, injections are made. After that, the pancreas can be divided into tiny 5 mm pieces. After that, the sections can be put inside a Ricordi digestion chamber. After that, the chamber can be shaken. After centrifugal treatment, the chamber solution can be microscopically examined to ensure an appropriate islet cell count and to apply human albumin. Once ready, the specimen can be injected into the portal vein system. Heparin injections can be administered intravenously to the specimen to prevent any complications related to portal vein thrombosis or portal hypertension. Maintaining the patient's insulin-free status is the aim of this treatment. According to studies, up to one-third of patients continue to require insulin, and another one-third will only experience a partial benefit from their islet cell transplant. The overall objectives of a total pancreatectomy combined with islet autotransplantation are to preserve the patient's endocrine function and prevent the need for long-term insulin administration.

3.5.5.6. Trauma-Related Pancreatectomy

Blunt or penetrating trauma can result in pancreatic injury. Hemorrhage control in the operating room and ductal injury are usually the determining factors for surgical intervention. For the diagnosis of pancreatic injuries, CT imaging is crucial. In most cases, patients can be treated without surgery if a ductal injury can be ruled out using MRCP or if stent placement can be done through ERCP.

Pancreatic organ injury scale (AAST) is as follows:

- **Grade 1**: Hematomas are defined as a large contusion without duct injury, a superficial laceration without duct injury, or parenchymal loss.
- **Grade 2**: Hematoma: a large gland contusion without duct damage or tissue loss; or a large laceration without either of these conditions.
- **Grade 3**: Perforation combined with distal gland transection or parenchymal damage combined with duct damage.
- **Grade 4**: A transection or parenchymal injury resulting in a laceration to the proximal gland located to the right of the superior mesenteric vein.

- **Grade 5**: Laceration accompanied by severe pancreatic head disruption.

3.5.5.7. Management

The main objective is to stop the bleeding and prevent more gastrointestinal spillage into the abdomen, just like with any trauma-related injury to the patient. The gland must be fully exposed for the surgeon to perform their work. This is explained in the section above regarding the lesser sac. To view the pancreatic head and uncinate process in their entirety, a complete Kocher maneuver should be carried out. To facilitate dissection, a ng tube may be passed post-pyloric if a significant hematoma is observed around the C loop. Hemostases on or near the gland, minor contusions, and occasionally lacerations to the capsule comprise the majority of pancreatic injuries. All that is needed for these injuries is hemostasis and drain placement. If a capsule laceration is repaired without causing damage to the duct, pseudocyst formation may result. The patient typically tolerates pancreatic drainage better. To detect fistula formation, the drains must remain in place for a minimum of 10 days.

Some of the hardest injuries to treat are grade 4 pancreatic head and neck injuries. Wide local drainage combined with post-operative ERCP should be carried out if the duct identification cannot be done in this location. You must take into account the patient's entire medical history if it is known or if the proximal neck injury is discovered. This will establish their tolerance for a longer distal pancreatectomy that involves the removal of over 80% of the gland. To give the patient enough time to consider the best overall reconstruction options, wide local drainage and resuscitation should be carried out if a large destructive injury to the head is discovered. Consultation with a subject-matter expert is advised. Among the hardest to treat are grade 4 injuries to the pancreatic head and neck. If the duct cannot be identified in this location, post-operative ERCP and wide local drainage should be carried out. If the proximal neck injury is discovered, you need to take the patient's entire medical history into account, if it is known. This will ascertain whether they are able to withstand a lengthy distal pancreatectomy that involves the removal of more than 80% of the gland. Wide local drainage and resuscitation should be carried out if a significant destructive head injury is discovered. This will give the patient time to consider their options for the best possible overall reconstruction. It is advised to have a conversation with a subject matter expert.

If not properly managed, grade 5 head of the gland injuries can result in significant patient morbidity and mortality. In the context of trauma, pancreaticoduodenectomy (Whipple) is infrequently recommended. After undergoing damage control and hemorrhage control in the operating room, patients with pancreatic injuries who are in extremis should be transferred to the surgical intensive care unit for resuscitation. Massive pancreatic head destruction, an avulsion injury to the Vater ampulla, or an intrapancreatic or proximal pancreatic bile duct injury are indications that this should be done. Upon discovery, these injuries ought to be treated gradually. Before moving forward with a major reconstruction, the patient's physiological status should be maximized.

Determining the presence of a pancreatic duct injury is the primary objective of pancreatic injury management. The duct may be stapled or oversewn. If the patient's condition permits additional time in the operating room, feeding access should be set up at the first laparotomy.

3.5.6. Complications

The following are the potential complications:

- Among the most dreaded surgical complications are postoperative pancreatic complications. If the problems are not identified and treated right away, they could have a serious negative impact on the patient.

- After a pancreatectomy, one of the most frequent complications is postoperative fistulas. Every surgical procedure mentioned above carries a potential risk of fistula development. According to some reports, the incidence of fistulas can reach 20–60%. Since most of these fistulas heal on their own, drainage is the primary form of management for the majority of reported grade A fistulas. A patient may occasionally require the insertion of a percutaneous drain into a grade B small fluid collection. Seldom do patients with grade C complications from pancreatic leaks require intensive care unit (ICU) care due to sepsis and multisystem organ failure; however, prompt surgical intervention is necessary, potentially resulting in a complete pancreatectomy to save the patient. A pancreatic fistula can have a major effect on a patient's recovery and general health. If a significant amount of parenchyma is removed during pancreatic surgery, another dangerous consequence is the development of postoperative diabetes. It usually happens in less than 10% of cases. Pancreatogenic diabetes is the term used to describe diabetes that develops following a total pancreatectomy. Additionally, exocrine insufficiency with steatorrhea, retinopathy, increased neuropathy, and increased cardiovascular disease are possible side effects of total pancreatectomy.
- After the splenic vessels are tied during the Warshaw procedure, splenic infarction may happen. An abscess may occasionally result from this. Gastritis can also arise from ligation of the splenic vessels.
- One variable post-operative complication that affects up to 50% of patients is delayed gastric emptying. When there is a noticeable nasogastric tube output, it is diagnosed. A patient's hospital stay may be extended and their quality of life may decline until the issue is resolved if emptying is delayed. Prokinetics may help with motility problems, but the results are not entirely consistent.
- One of the main causes of complications following surgery is an anastomotic leak from the newly formed anastomotic sites. Numerous investigations have demonstrated that there is a significant chance of a leak regardless of the method used to create the anastomosis.
- After pancreatic surgery, intra-abdominal hemorrhage can result from a variety of distinct causes. It is most likely the result of hemostasis failure during surgery early in the post-operative course. During the later stages of the postoperative course, pancreatic leaks can erode a vascular structure or cause an anastomotic site to break.
- Another complication that can arise after surgery is wound complications. This is a broad topic

because many patients who require pancreatic surgery do so despite having various pathologies. Wound complications are more common in patients with diabetes and obesity, as well as in those undergoing endoscopic biliary procedures or preoperative biliary stenting.

3.5.7. Clinical Significance

Surgical resections of the pancreas refer to a group of extremely complicated surgical procedures performed for various diagnoses. After correctly diagnosing the patient and their pancreatic lesion, you must carefully consider the surgical resection that best suits your patient's needs. Both benign and malignant diseases can have excellent cure rates with the right diagnosis and surgical approach. Due to the significant impact postoperative complications have on a patient's hospital stay and quality of life, pancreatic surgery must be carried out with exceptional skill and attention to detail. The last few years have seen numerous advancements in pancreatic surgery. The use of minimally invasive procedures is growing in popularity since they reduce overall pain, shorten hospital stays, and enable patients to resume their jobs more quickly.

Pancreatectomy is most commonly indicated in the presence of benign or malignant tumors, chronic pancreatitis, and pancreatic trauma. It can be performed laparoscopically or openly. It is very difficult to remove the pancreas surgically because of its distinct anatomy and intricate vasculature. It is always advisable to have interprofessional team meetings with surgeons, anesthesiologists, nurses, and other OR staff to enhance the decision-making process. A successful pancreatic surgery requires careful preoperative planning. Throughout the procedure, all members of the team must stay in close contact with one another, follow the preoperative plan, and keep an eye on the patient's vital signs to determine whether blood, fluid, or vasopressor administration is necessary. In intensive care units, the patient's assessment is ongoing during the postoperative phase because this is the time when many surgical patients awaken from anesthesia with hemodynamic problems and increased pain. As usual, interprofessional communication lowers morbidity and mortality and improves healthcare team outcomes.

A Closer Look

Diabetes Mellitus

Diabetes mellitus is a disorder that can result from malfunctions in the synthesis and secretion of insulin as well as the target cells' ability to respond to the hormone. Over 18 million adults and over 200,000 children in the US have been diagnosed with diabetes mellitus, a condition that is becoming more and more common. Up to 7 million additional adults are thought to have the illness but are not yet diagnosed. Furthermore, pre-diabetes, a condition in which blood glucose levels are abnormally high but not yet high enough to be classified as diabetes, is thought to affect 79 million people in the US. Diabetes mellitus is classified into two primary types. An autoimmune condition called type 1 diabetes affects the pancreatic beta cells. It is known that some genes make people more susceptible. Insulin cannot be produced by beta cells in people with type 1 diabetes; therefore, injections or infusions of synthetic insulin are required. Approximately 5% of cases of diabetes are of this type.

95% of all cases of diabetes are type 2. It is acquired, and a person's risk is significantly increased by lifestyle factors like a poor diet, inactivity, and the presence of pre-diabetes. 80–90% of individuals with type 2 diabetes are obese or overweight. Cells develop resistance to the effects of insulin in type 2 diabetes. The pancreas secretes more insulin in response, but the beta cells eventually run out of energy. If blood glucose levels are not controlled, type 2 diabetes can often be reversed with moderate weight loss, regular exercise, and a nutritious diet; nevertheless, the diabetic will eventually need insulin.

Excessive thirst and urination are two of the early indicators of diabetes. They illustrate the impact of elevated blood glucose levels on renal function. The removal of glucose from the bloodstream is accomplished by the kidneys. An unusually large amount of sweet urine is expelled by the person due to water being drawn into the urine by high blood sugar. The body becomes dehydrated when body water is used to dilute urine, which results in unusually persistent thirst. Additionally, because the body's cells are unable to utilize the glucose in the bloodstream, the person might feel hungry all the time.

Chronically elevated blood glucose levels damage body tissues over time, particularly blood vessel and nerve tissues. Atherosclerosis, which raises the risk of heart attacks and strokes, is brought on by inflammation and damage to the artery lining. Kidney failure may result from injury to the kidney's tiny blood vessels, which reduces renal function. Blindness may result from damage to the blood vessels that supply the eyes. Damage to the blood vessels also results in decreased circulation to the limbs, while damage to the nerves causes neuropathy, or loss of feeling, especially in the hands and feet. All of these modifications raise the possibility of harm, infection, and necrosis, or tissue death, which is one reason why amputations of the toes, feet, and lower legs are common in diabetics. Ketoacidosis is a dangerous form of metabolic acidosis that can also result from uncontrolled diabetes. As cells run out of glucose, they depend more and more on their fat reserves. But when there is not enough glucose in the blood, the liver is compelled to use a different pathway for metabolizing fat, which leads to an increase in the production of acidic ketone bodies, also known as ketones. Ketoacidosis is brought on by an accumulation of ketones in the blood and, if untreated, can result in a potentially fatal "diabetic coma." When these issues are taken into account, diabetes ranks as the seventh most common cause of death in the US.

When blood glucose levels are higher than normal—a condition known as hyperglycemia—lab tests can identify diabetes. Diabetes treatment varies according to the kind, severity, and patient's capacity for lifestyle modifications. As previously mentioned, consuming a nutritious diet, exercising frequently, and losing moderate weight can all lower blood glucose levels. Certain individuals diagnosed with type 2 diabetes might not be able to manage their condition through lifestyle modifications and will need to take medication. Insulin was once the first-line treatment for type 2 diabetes. Alternative options, such as drugs that improve pancreatic function, have become available due to advancements in research.

Summary

- The pancreas is an abdominal glandular organ with both digestive (exocrine) and hormonal(endocrine) functions.
- The pancreas is an oblong-shaped organ positioned at the level of the transpyloric plane (L1). With the exception of the tail of the pancreas, it is a retroperitoneal organ, located deep within the upper abdomen in the epigastrium and left hypochondrium regions.
- The pancreas forms during development from two buds that arise from the duodenal part of the foregut, an embryonic tube that is a precursor to the gastrointestinal tract. It is of endodermal origin. Pancreatic development begins with the formation of a dorsal and ventral pancreatic bud. Each joins with the foregut through a duct. The dorsal pancreatic bud forms the neck, body, and tail of the developed pancreas, and the ventral pancreatic bud forms the head and uncinate process.
- The pancreas is involved in blood sugar control and metabolism within the body, and also in the secretion of substances (collectively pancreatic juice) that help digestion. These are divided into an "endocrine" role, relating to the secretion of insulin and other substances within pancreatic islets that help control blood sugar levels and metabolism within the body, and an "exocrine" role, relating to the secretion of enzymes involved in digesting substances in the digestive tract.
- Pancreatic juice is a liquid secreted by the pancreas, which contains a number of digestive enzymes, including trypsinogen, chymotrypsinogen, elastase, carboxypeptidase, pancreatic lipase, nucleases and amylase.
- Pancreatic enzymes, also known as pancreases or pancrelipase and pancreatin, are commercial mixtures of amylase, lipase, protease and lactase. They are used to treat malabsorption syndrome due to certain pancreatic problems.
- Pancrelipases are generally a first-line approach in the treatment of exocrine pancreatic insufficiency and other digestive disorders, accompanying cystic fibrosis, complicating surgical pancreatectomy, or resulting from chronic pancreatitis.
- The exocrine pancreas secretes digestive enzymes, fluid, and bicarbonate in response to food ingestion. This is a critical digestive process that is regulated by neural reflexes, gastrointestinal hormones, and absorbed nutrients. Secretion is highly regulated by both stimulatory and inhibitory influences that coordinate the delivery of digestive enzymes with food emptying into the intestine to ensure adequate digestion of a meal.
- Pancreatectomy is a term for surgical removal of all or part of the pancreas.

References

1. Achkasov, E., Pugaev, A., Zabelin, M., & Posudnevskiy, V. (2019). *Acute Pancreatitis: Clinic, Diagnosis, Treatment.* INFRA-M Academic Publishing LLC. http://dx.doi.org/10.12737/995531.
2. Beger, H. G., Warshaw, A. L., Hruban, R. H., Büchler, M. W., Lerch, M. M., Neoptolemos, J. P., Shimosegawa, T., Whitcomb, D. C., & Groß, C. (Eds.). (2018). *The Pancreas.* John Wiley & Sons, Ltd. http://dx.doi.org/10.1002/9781119188421.

3. Butler, J. R., Finnie, J. W., West, S. P., & Cosgrove, A. B. (2015). Is antisecretory therapy after pancreatoduodenectomy necessary? Meta-analysis and contemporary practices of pancreatic surgeons. *Journal of Gastrointestinal Surgery, 19*(4), 604–612.

4. Cade, J. E., & Hanison, J. (2017). The pancreas. *Anaesthesia & Intensive Care Medicine, 18*(10), 527–531.

5. Duggan SN, Ní Chonchubhair HM, Lawal O, O'Connor DB, Conlon KC. Chronic pancreatitis: A diagnostic dilemma. World J Gastroenterol. 2016 Feb 21;22(7):2304-13. doi: 10.3748/wjg.v22.i7.2304. PMID: 26900292; PMCID: PMC4735004.

6. Grammatikopoulos, T. (2018). *The Pancreas*. Oxford University Press. http://dx.doi.org/10.1093/med/9780198759928.003.0050.

7. Hruban, R. H., Pitman, M. B., & Klimstra, D. S. (2007). *AFIP Atlas of Tumor Pathology, Fourth Series, Fascicle Tumors of the Pancreas*. American Registry of Pathology in collaboration with the Armed Forces Institute of Pathology.

8. Jørgensen, M. C., Ahnfelt-Rønne, J., Hald, J., Madsen, O. D., Serup, P., & Hecksher-Sørensen, J. (2007). An illustrated review of early pancreas development in the mouse. *Endocrine Reviews, 28*(6), 685–705. https://doi.org/10.1210/er.2007-0012.

9. Lee, M. G., Ohana, E., Park, H. W., Yang, D., & Muallem, S. (2012). Molecular mechanism of pancreatic and salivary gland fluid and HCO3− secretion. *Physiological Reviews, 92*(1), 39–74.

10. Love, J. A., Yi, E., & Smith, T. G. (2007). Autonomic pathways regulating pancreatic exocrine secretion. *Autonomic Neuroscience, 133*(1), 19–34.

11. Mahadevan, V. (2019). Anatomy of the pancreas and spleen. *Surgery (Oxford), 37*(6), 297–301.

12. Malfertheiner, P., Uhl, W., & Sarr, M. G. (2004). *Diseases of the Pancreas: Acute Pancreatitis, Chronic Pancreatitis, Tumours of the Pancreas* (2nd ed.). S. Karger Publishers, DOI: https://doi.org/10.1159/isbn.978-3-318-01001-5

13. Mekapogu, A. R., Pothula, S. P., Pirola, R. C., Wilson, J. S., & Apte, M. V. (2020). Pancreatic stellate cells in health and disease. *The Pancreapedia: Exocrine Pancreas Knowledge Base*. https://doi.org/10.3998/panc.2020.08.

14. Normatov, I., & Sentongo, T. (2019). Pancreatic malnutrition in children. *Pediatric Annals, 48*(11), e441–e447.

15. Owyang, C., & Williams, J. A. (2015). Pancreatic secretion. In *Yamada's Textbook of Gastroenterology* (pp. 450–473), DOI:10.1002/9781118512074.ch25.

16. Rahier, J., Guiot, Y., Goebbels, R. M., Sempoux, C., & Henquin, J. C. (2008). Pancreatic beta-cell mass in European subjects with type 2 diabetes. *Diabetes, Obesity and Metabolism, 10*(1), 32–42. https://doi.org/10.1111/j.1463-1326.2007.00776.x.

17. Yamamoto, M., Nakamura, T., Sakurai, Y., Hirota, M., Nakatani, K., Furukawa, K., & Yoshikawa, T. (2005). Water and enzyme secretion are tightly coupled in pancreatic secretion stimulated by food or CCK-58 but not by CCK-8. *American Journal of Physiology-Gastrointestinal and Liver Physiology, 288*(5), G866–G879.

Chapter

LIVER AND BILIARY SYSTEM

4

Contents

Introduction

The liver is a biological marvel from a modern standpoint. It is the defender of homeostasis, the center of the body's metabolic potential, a massive filter that purges the portal blood and releases blood that has been cleansed for systemic circulation, and a lymphoid organ that fends off infection. In addition to processing dietary fats, carbohydrates, and vitamins, the liver is also essential for the production and breakdown of most plasma proteins, as well as for the detoxification and biliary excretion of endogenous waste products and foreign substances. As a vital component of the intricate defense mechanism against foreign macromolecules, the liver serves as an organ of the innate immune system. Because the liver's metabolic processes are vital to the health of other organs, hepatic disorders can have far-reaching effects.

Orientation and Directional Terms

Term	Definition	Illustration
Bile	A green/yellow liquid containing bile salts, bilirubin and cholesterol.	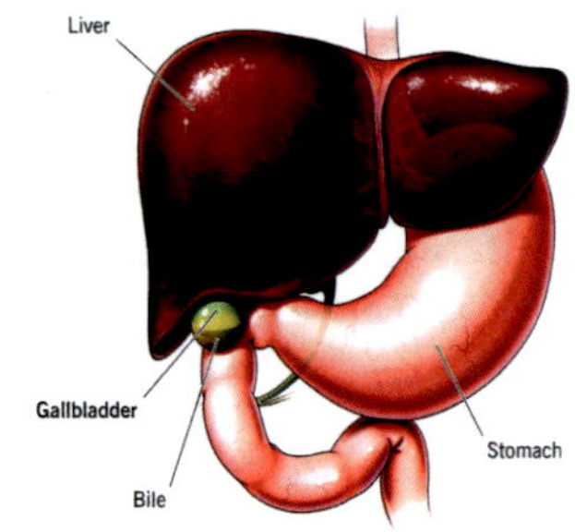
Biliary tract	The system of tubes which carry bile from the liver and gall bladder and drain into the intestine.	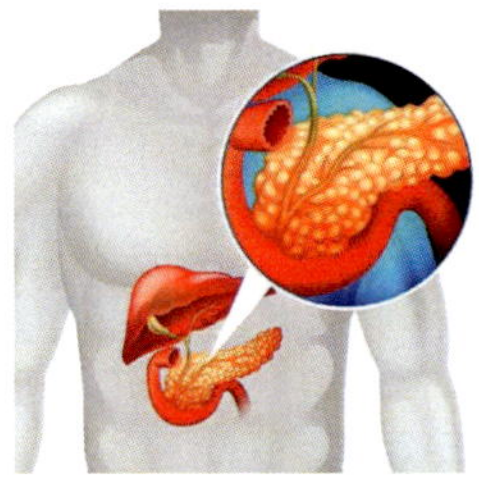
Biopsy	A procedure to take a small sample of the liver to test in the laboratory.	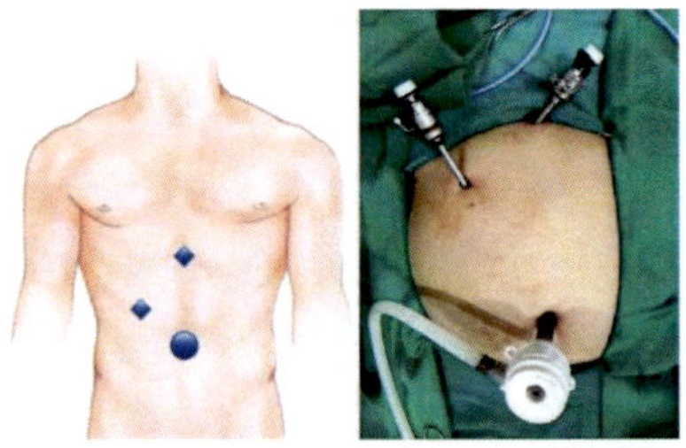
Cholangitis	Inflammation or infection of bile ducts which can cause poor bile flow from the liver and liver damage.	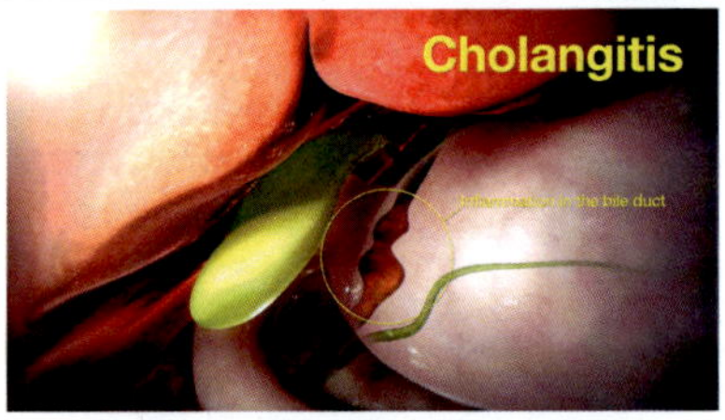
Encephalopathy	Changes in the brain which can be due to liver failure. The build-up of toxins in the blood can lead to tiredness, irritability and personality changes.	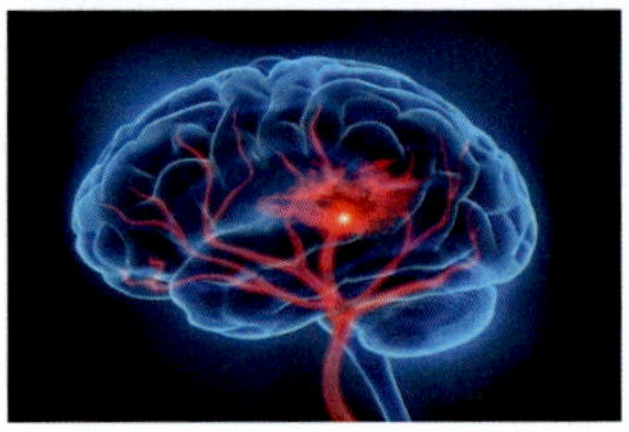

4.1. Overview of the Functioning of the Hepatobiliary System

The term "biliary tract" (also known as the "biliary tree" or "biliary system") describes the relationship between the liver, gallbladder, and bile ducts in the production, storing, and secretion of bile.

Water, electrolytes, phospholipids, cholesterol, bile acids, and conjugated bilirubin are the components of bile. Hepatocytes, or liver cells, synthesize some of the components; the liver removes the remaining substances from the blood. The liver secretes bile into tiny ducts that eventually unite to form the common hepatic duct.

The gallbladder holds secreted bile in reserve between meals. Bile is secreted into the duodenum, a portion of the small intestine, during meals to help absorb dietary fats and oils and to help the body get rid of waste that has been stored in the bile.

4.1.1. Structure

The route that the liver uses to secrete bile and then deliver it to the duodenum, the first segment of the small intestine, is known as the biliary tract.

The biliary tract, a structure shared by the majority of mammals, is frequently referred to as a tree because it starts with numerous tiny branches and ends in the common bile duct, which is also known as the biliary tree's trunk. The portal triad is composed of the duct, the hepatic artery branches, and the portal vein. The direction in which bile flows is the opposite of the blood's flow through the other two channels (Figure 4.1).

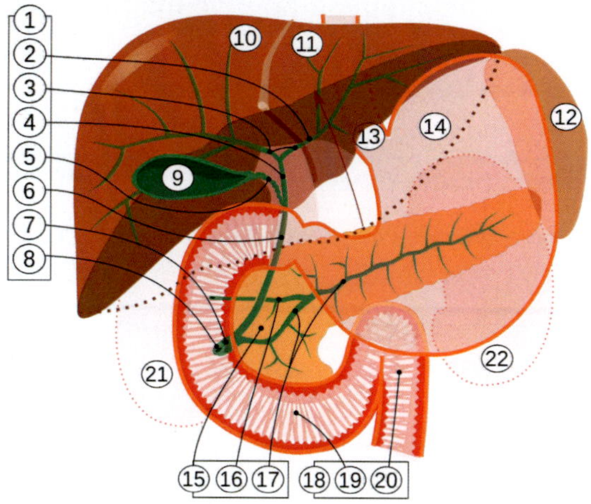

Figure 4.1. *Bile duct and pancreas, 1. Bile ducts: 2. Intrahepatic bile ducts, 3. Left and right hepatic ducts, 4. Common hepatic duct, 5. Cystic duct, 6. Common bile duct, 7. Ampulla of Vater, 8. Major duodenal papilla, 9. Gallbladder, 10–11. Right and left lobes of liver, 12. Spleen, 13. Esophagus, 14. Stomach, 15. Pancreas: 16. Accessory pancreatic duct, 17. Pancreatic duct, 18. Small intestine: 19. Duodenum, 20. Jejunum, 21–22. Right and left kidneys, the front border of the liver has been lifted up (brown arrow).*

Source: By Jmarchn – Own work, CC BY-SA 3.0, https://commons.wikimedia.org/w/index.php?curid=14612350.

When referring solely to the liver and bile ducts, the term "hepatobiliary" may be used to refer to the system, which is generally referred to as the biliary tract or system. All of the ducts, structures, and organs involved in the synthesis, storage, and secretion of bile are collectively referred to as the biliary tract.

The tract is as follows:

- Bile canaliculi >> Canals of Hering >> intrahepatic bile ductule (in portal tracts / triads) >> interlobular bile ducts >> left and right hepatic ducts

- The common hepatic duct is formed when these combine.
- The common hepatic duct leaves the liver and connects to the gall bladder's cystic duct.
- These come together to form the pancreatic and common bile ducts.
- These enter the duodenum after passing through the Vater's ampulla.

4.1.2. Function

The liver secretes bile into tiny ducts that eventually unite to form the common hepatic duct. Secreted bile is held in the gall bladder in between meals, where 80–90% of the water and electrolytes can be absorbed, leaving the cholesterol and bile acids behind. The smooth muscles in the gallbladder wall tighten during a meal, releasing bile into the duodenum to help the body eliminate waste that has been stored there and to facilitate the absorption of dietary fats and oils by solubilizing them with bile acids.

- **Nutritional Metabolic Functions:** The liver is an essential component of energy metabolism because it modifies and transports nutritional molecules. This covers the synthesis, disintegration, alteration, and storage of nutritional molecules such as proteins, fats, and glucose/glycogen.
- **Xenobiotic Metabolism:** Any substances that are "foreign" to an animal are considered xenobiotics. NSAIDs, or non-steroidal anti-inflammatory drugs, are a class of pain relievers that are an example of xenobiotics. However, non-therapeutic compounds are also included in the category of xenobiotics. Hepatocytes metabolize foreign substances through a process called biotransformation, which involves chemical modification and excretion into bile. Cytochrome P450, a metabolic enzyme involved in biotransformation, is abundant in hepatocytes. The goal of xenobiotic biotransformation is to make the foreign substance less soluble and hazardous for excretion. Although activation of the xenobiotic during biotransformation can occasionally produce an intermediate compound that is more toxic than the original form, resulting in toxicity, hepatocytes are the workhorses of xenobiotic biotransformation and, as such, play a major protective role in preventing the build-up and toxicity of xenobiotics.
- **Production of Circulating Plasma Proteins:** Many of the most prevalent circulating plasma proteins, such as albumin, lipoproteins (LDL, VLDL, and HDL), and glycoproteins, are produced by hepatocytes. These proteins made by the hepatocyte have a variety of uses, including inflammation, molecular transport, and energy. The main source of the coagulation cascade's proteins is also the liver.
- Nearly all of the clotting factors needed in the coagulation cascade—including fibrinogen, prothrombin, antithrombin III, Protein C, and Protein S—are produced by hepatocytes, except for Factor VIII, which is produced by endothelium.
- **Storage and Conversion of Vitamins and Minerals:** Iron, copper, vitamin A (retinol), vitamin D, vitamin B12, vitamin K, and other vitamins and minerals are all stored and converted in large quantities in the liver.

- **Bilirubin Metabolism:** Red blood cell fragments are transferred from the spleen to the liver, which then breaks them down for excretion or recycling. Red blood cells' hemoglobin is broken down into heme and globin. Bilirubin is produced by further processing the heme, which contains iron. Hepatocytes undergo hepatocyte-mediated bilirubin conjugation, which transforms uncojugated (insoluble) bilirubin into conjugated (soluble) bilirubin. The resulting bile is then eliminated and absorbed by the gastrointestinal tract.

4.1.3. Clinical Significance

Depending on where the stone is located in the biliary tract, gallstones can originate in the gallbladder and become lodged there, causing a variety of illnesses. Cholelithiasis, also known as gallstone disease, affects more than 20 million people in the US (Figure 4.2).

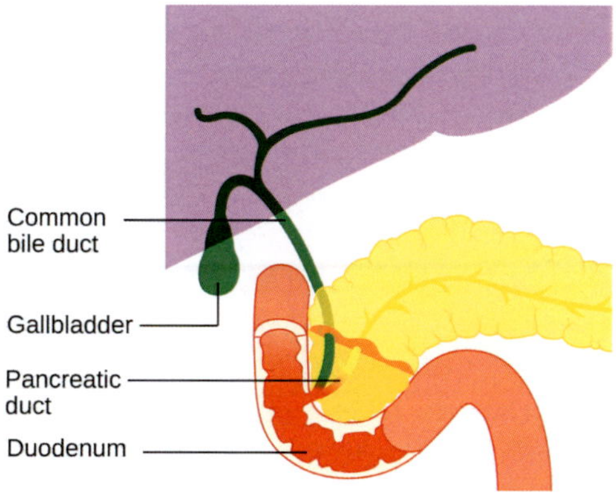

Figure 4.2. *Union of common bile duct and pancreatic duct terminating at duodenum (small intestine).*

Source: By Cancer Research UK – Original email from CRUK, CC BY-SA 4.0, https://commons.wikimedia.org/w/index.php?curid=34334066.

Gallstones often develop asymptomatic (also referred to as asymptomatic cholelithiasis). The cystic duct, which connects the gallbladder to the common bile duct, can occasionally become blocked by gallstones, which can cause inflammation in the gallbladder wall. Cholecystitis, or inflammation of the gallbladder, is a common sign that a cholecystectomy—a surgical removal of the gallbladder—is necessary. Another sign of cholecystectomy is choledocholithiasis, a condition in which gallstones lodge in the common bile duct and prevent bile from passing from the gallbladder to the small intestine. The cystic and common hepatic ducts combine to form the common bile duct, or CBD for short. It then joins the pancreatic duct and ends in the small intestine's Ampulla of Vater. The common bile duct facilitates the movement of bile from the gallbladder into the small intestine, where it combines with the digestive enzymes produced by the pancreas. An infection of the bile ducts between the liver and the gallstone lodged in the common bile duct is one potential side effect of choledocholithiasis. Acute cholangitis is the term for this illness, which is frequently accompanied by the Charcot Triad, a group of three clinical symptoms that include fever, abdominal pain in the right upper quadrant, and jaundice. Reynold's Pentad can be further defined by including hypotension and altered mental status, as this constellation of symptoms has a 96% specificity for cholangitis.

Intestinal tract infections can also be stored in the biliary tract. Biliary colic, which is caused by an infection and inflammation of the biliary tract, is not a somatic pain because the biliary tract is an internal organ and has no somatic nerve supply. Rather, luminal distension, which results in wall stretching, may be the source of pain. Bowel blockages also hurt because of the same mechanism. Hardening of the ducts in the biliary tree can result from chronic inflammatory conditions of the biliary tract, such as Primary

Sclerosing Cholangitis (PSC) and Primary Biliary Cirrhosis (PBC). Jaundice, or a yellowing of the skin and whites of the eyes, can be caused by an obstruction of the biliary tract.

4.2. Anatomy and Morphology of the Liver

Only present in vertebrate animals, the liver is a significant metabolic organ that carries out numerous vital biological processes, including the body's detoxification and the synthesis of the proteins and biochemicals required for growth and digestion. It is situated in the right upper quadrant of the abdomen in humans, mainly protected by the lower right rib cage, and beneath the diaphragm. Its other metabolic functions include the breakdown of red blood cells, the synthesis of hormones, the conversion and storage of nutrients like glucose and glycogen, and the metabolism of carbohydrates (Figure 4.3).

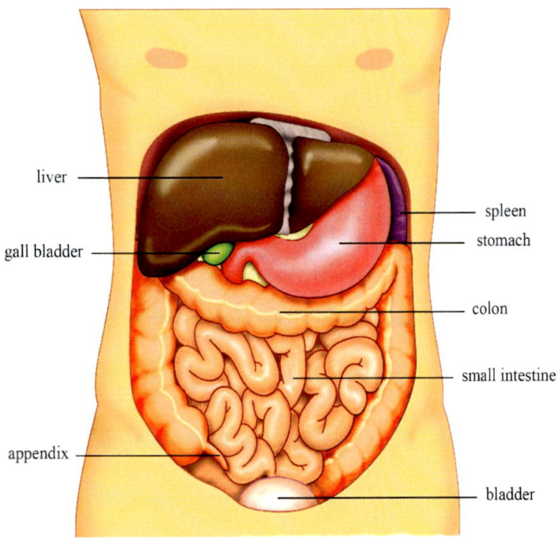

Figure 4.3. *The human liver is located in the upper right abdomen.*

Source: By Tvanbr – Own work, Public Domain, https://commons.wikimedia.org/w/index.php?curid=11625998.

Bile, an alkaline fluid with cholesterol and bile acids that the liver produces as an auxiliary digestive organ, emulsifies and facilitates the breakdown of dietary fat. The liver produces bile, which is subsequently expelled to the duodenum to aid in digestion. The bile is stored and concentrated in the gallbladder, a tiny hollow pouch located directly beneath the right lobe of the liver. The highly specialized tissue of the liver, primarily made up of hepatocytes, controls a wide range of high-volume biochemical reactions, such as the synthesis and degradation of intricate and small molecules, many of which are essential for regular bodily processes. The organ's total number of functions is estimated to be 500 or less, though figures vary widely. While liver dialysis methods can be employed in the short term, there is no known long-term solution for liver function loss. In the event that the liver is absent, artificial livers have not been synthesized to support long-term replacement. As of 2018, the only treatment available for total liver failure is liver transplantation.

4.2.1. Structure

The liver is a wedge-shaped, dark reddish brown organ with two unevenly sized and shaped lobes. A human liver typically weighs 1.5 kg (3.33 pounds) and measures approximately 15 centimeters (6 inches) in width.

The standard reference range for men is 970–1,860 grams (2.14–4.10 lb), and for women it is 600–1,770 g (1.32–3.90 lb). This indicates that there is a significant variation in size between individuals. It is the largest gland in the human body and the heaviest internal organ. It rests just below the diaphragm, to the right of the stomach, and covers the gallbladder in the right upper quadrant of the abdominal cavity (Figure 4.4).

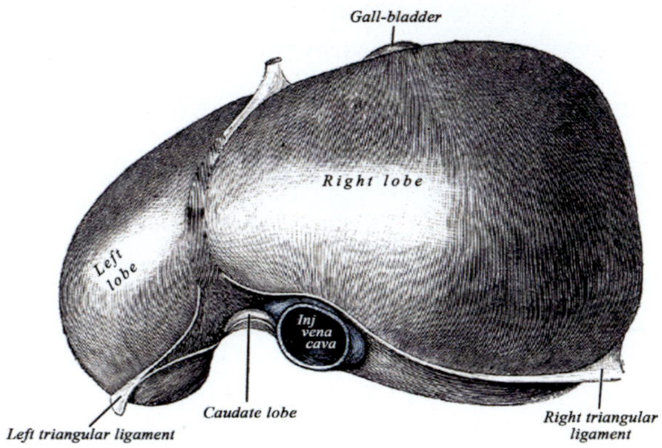

Figure 4.4. *The liver, viewed from above, showing the left and right lobes separated by the falciform ligament.*

Source: By Henry Vandyke Carter, Public Domain, https://commons.wikimedia.org/w/index.php?curid=567039.

The hepatic artery and the portal vein are two major blood vessels that supply blood to the liver. The portal vein transports blood that has been fully digested from the entire gastrointestinal tract, as well as from the pancreas and spleen, to the hepatic artery, which carries oxygen-rich blood from the aorta via the celiac trunk. These blood vessels split into liver sinusoids, which are tiny capillaries that eventually branch off to form hepatic lobules. The liver's functional units are called hepatic lobules. Millions of hepatic cells, or hepatocytes, the fundamental metabolic cells, comprise each lobule. A fine, dense, irregular, fibroelastic layer of connective tissue, called Glisson's capsule after the British physician Francis Glisson, holds the lobules together. This layer extends from the fibrous capsule that covers the entire liver. This tissue follows the ducts, nerves, and blood vessels at the hepatic hilum to extend into the structure of the liver. A serous coat derived from the peritoneum covers the entire surface of the liver, with the exception of the bare area, and it firmly adheres to the inner Glisson's capsule.

4.2.1.1. Gross Anatomy

Terminology related to the liver often starts in *hepat-*, from the Greek word for liver.

- **Lobes:** When seen from above, the liver is roughly divided into two parts: the right and left lobes; when viewed from below, the liver is roughly divided into four parts: the left, right, caudate, and quadrate lobes. The liver is superficially divided into a left and right lobe by the falciform ligament. The two extra lobes are situated between the right and left lobes, one in front of the other, as seen from below. Imagine a line dividing the liver and gallbladder into two halves, starting from the left of the vena cava and continuing forward. We refer to this as Cantlie's line.

The ligamentum venosum and the liver's round ligament, which further split the left side of the liver into two sections, are additional anatomical landmarks. This left portion is divided into four segments by the porta hepatis, an important anatomical landmark. These segments can be numbered in an anticlockwise manner, beginning at the caudate lobe, which is designated as I. Seven segments are visible from this parietal view, as the eighth segment is only visible in the visceral view.

- **Surfaces:** The peritoneum, a thin, double-layered membrane that covers the liver and helps to lessen friction against other organs, is present on the diaphragmatic surface, with the exception of a triangular bare area where it connects to the diaphragm. Where the shape of the diaphragm is accommodated, this surface covers the convex shape of the two lobes.

The right and left triangle ligaments, as well as the falciform ligament, are formed by the peritoneum folding back on itself. The right and left triangular ligaments function as surface landmarks but have no known functional significance. These peritoneal ligaments are unrelated to the anatomic ligaments in joints. The liver is attached to the posterior part of the anterior body wall by the falciform ligament. The inferior or visceral surface is concave and uneven. Aside from the points where it connects to the gallbladder and the porta hepatis, it is covered in peritoneum. The gallbladder and its cystic duct are located near the right end of the porta hepatis in the gallbladder fossa, which is located to the right of the quadrate lobe.

- **Impressions:** The liver's surface is divided into multiple impressions that house the different organs and surrounding structures. Two impressions can be found beneath the right lobe and to the right of the gallbladder fossa. They are separated by a ridge, with one impression behind the other. The hepatic flexure forms the shallow colic impression in front, while the deeper renal impression behind houses a portion of the right kidney as well as the suprarenal gland. The liver has a tiny, triangular-shaped indentation called the suprarenal impression. It is situated directly above the renal impression, between the bare region and the caudate lobe, and to the right of the fossa. The right suprarenal gland is lodged in the suprarenal impression, which is mostly free of peritoneum. A third, marginally noticeable impression is located medial to the renal impression, between it and the neck of the gall bladder. This is called the duodenal impression and is brought on by the duodenum's descending portion.

Behind and to the left of the gastric impression is the inferior surface of the liver's left lobe. This is molded over the upper front surface of the stomach. The tuber omentale, a rounded protrusion to the right of this, sits in front of the anterior layer of the lesser omentum and fits into the concavity of the stomach's lesser curvature.

4.2.1.2. Microscopic Anatomy

Hepatic lobules are visible as the constituent parts of each liver lobe under a microscope. The lobules are roughly hexagon-shaped and comprise sinusoids and hepatocyte plates that radiate from a central vein in the direction of an imaginary interlobular portal triad perimeter. To remove blood from the liver, the central vein connects to the hepatic vein. A lobule's portal triad, which runs along each of its corners, is one of its distinguishing features. The hepatic artery, portal vein, and common bile duct make up the portal triad. A liver ultrasound can reveal the triad as a Mickey Mouse sign, with the portal vein representing the head and the hepatic artery and common bile duct representing the ears (Figure 4.5).

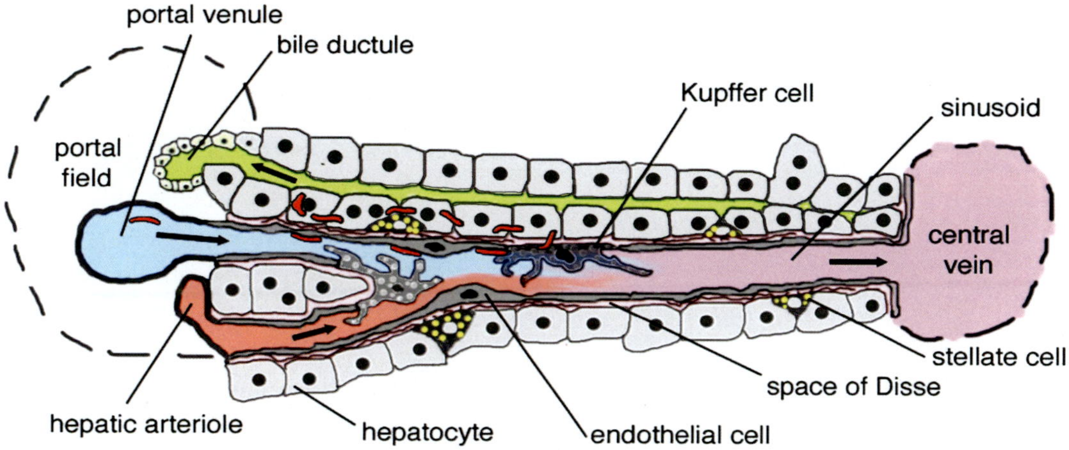

Figure 4.5. *Cells, ducts, and blood vessels.*

Source: Frevert U, Engelmann S, Zougbédé S, Stange J, Ng B, Matuschewski K, et al. (2005) Intravital Observation of Plasmodium berghei Sporozoite Infection of the Liver. PLoS Biol 3(6): e192. https://doi.org/10.1371/journal.pbio.0030192.

There are two main types of liver cells that are seen in histology, the study of microscopic anatomy: parenchymal cells and nonparenchymal cells. Parenchymal hepatocytes make up between 70 and 85% of the liver's volume. Though they make up only 6.5% of the liver's volume, nonparenchymal cells account for 40% of the total number of liver cells. Two different cell types—phagocytic Kupffer cells and sinusoidal endothelial cells—line the liver sinusoids. Nonparenchymal cells called hepatic stellate cells are situated between a sinusoid and a hepatocyte in the perisinusoidal space. In addition, the sinusoidal lumen frequently contains intrahepatic lymphocytes.

4.2.1.3. Functional Anatomy

The hepatic hilum, located in the central area of the liver, contains the porta hepatis which serves as the opening for the common bile duct, common hepatic artery, and portal vein. These structures branch out into the left and right lobes of the liver, with Cantlie's line acting as an imaginary plane dividing the liver into true right and left lobes. The middle hepatic vein and right hepatic vein further separate the right lobe into anterior and posterior segments, while the left hepatic vein divides the left lobe into medial and lateral segments (Figure 4.6).

The bile ducts and blood vessels are located on three plates that make up the liver's hilum. A sheath encloses the contents of the entire plate system. The liver's three plates—the hilar, cystic, and umbilical plates—are home to the various anatomical variations that can be observed there.

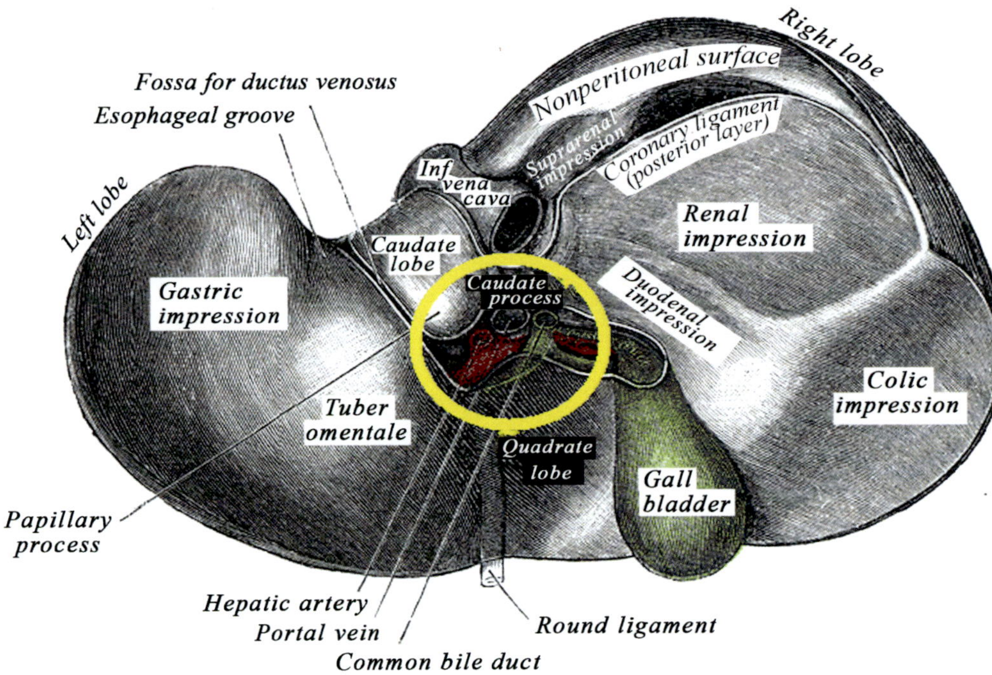

Figure 4.6. *Hilum of the liver, circled in yellow.*

Source: By Henry Vandyke Carter – en:Gray1086-liver.PNG, CC0, https://commons.wikimedia.org/w/index.php?curid=75131195.

4.2.1.4. Couinaud Classification System

The bifurcation of the main portal vein divides the functional lobes into eight subsegments based on a transverse plane in the widely used Couinaud system. Not to be confused with another structure, the caudate lobe receives blood flow from both the left and right sided vascular branches. The liver is divided into eight functionally independent liver segments according to the Couinaud classification. Every segment has a separate biliary drainage system, vascular inflow, and outflow. The hepatic artery, bile duct, and portal vein branches are located in the middle of each segment. Each segment has vascular outflow via the hepatic veins at its periphery. The caudate lobe, which receives its supply from both the left and right branches of the portal vein, is unit 1 in the classification system, which uses the vascular supply in the liver to divide the functional units (numbered I to VIII). It has one or more hepatic veins that empty into the inferior vena cava right away. The remaining units (II through VIII) have numbers that go in a clockwise direction.

4.2.1.5. Gene and Protein Expression

Human cells express about 20,000 protein-coding genes, with the liver of a healthy adult expressing 60% of these genes. The liver is the site of more specific expression for over 400 genes, of which about 150 are highly specific to liver tissue. Hepatocytes are the primary source of expression for a significant portion of the corresponding liver-specific proteins, which are then secreted into the bloodstream as hepatokines and plasma proteins. Additional proteins specific to the liver include some liver enzymes like HAO1 and RDH16, bile synthesis-related proteins like BAAT and SLC27A5, and transporter proteins that are involved in drug metabolism like ABCB11 and SLC2A2. Apolipoprotein A II, coagulation factors F2 and F9, complement factor-related proteins, and the fibrinogen beta chain protein are a few examples of highly liver-specific proteins.

4.2.2. Development

The development of the organs, or organogenesis, occurs during the third through the eighth week of embryogenesis. The components of the adjacent septum transversum mesenchyme and the ventral section of the foregut endoderm—one of the three layers of the embryonic germ layer—are where the liver originates. The endodermal tube in human embryos that projects from the foregut into the surrounding mesenchyme is known as the hepatic diverticulum. This endoderm is stimulated to multiply, branch, and form the glandular epithelium of the liver by the mesenchyme of the septum transversum. The gallbladder is produced by a branch of the hepatic diverticulum, which is the part of the liver that is closest to the digestive tube and still serves as the liver's drainage duct. Hepatic competence is also influenced by fibroblast growth factor from the developing heart and retinoic acid from the lateral plate mesoderm, in addition to signals from the septum transversum mesenchyme. The morphological change of the hepatic endodermal cells from columnar to pseudostratified leads to thickening into the early liver bud. Bipotential hepatoblasts are formed as a population by their expansion. The source of hepatic stellate cells is mesenchyme.

Hepatoblast migration into the septum transversum mesenchyme triggers the formation of the hepatic architecture, resulting in the appearance of bile canaliculi and liver sinusoids. The lobes split off from the liver bud. The right vitelline vein becomes the portal vein, and the left umbilical vein becomes the ductus venosus. Hematopoietic cells colonize the developing liver bud. The bipotential hepatoblasts start to differentiate into hepatocytes and biliary epithelial cells. Around portal veins, hepatoblasts differentiate into biliary epithelial cells, which first form a monolayer and subsequently a bilayer of cuboidal cells. Focal dilations in the ductal plate arise at bilayer points, encircled by portal mesenchyme, and tubulogenesis into intrahepatic bile ducts. Hepatoblasts that are not next to portal veins differentiate into hepatocytes and form cords that are bordered by bile canaliculi and sinusoidal epithelial cells. Hepatoblasts that are differentiated into hepatocytes and go through additional growth eventually take on the characteristics of a mature hepatocyte, which is characterized by a high degree of polarization in epithelial cells and a large accumulation of glycogen. Hepatocytes in the adult liver are not the same; the expression of metabolic genes involved in drug metabolism, carbohydrate metabolism, ammonia detoxification, and bile production and secretion is determined by the position of these cells within a liver lobule along the portocentrovenular axis. It is now known that WNT/β-catenin is essential for this phenomenon.

The liver weighs about 120 g (4 oz) on average at birth and makes up about 4% of the body weight. Over the course of further development, it increases to 1.4–1.6 kg (3.1–3.5 lb) but will only take up 2.5–3.5% of body weight. The liver weight to body weight ratio is known as the hepatosomatic index (HSI).

4.2.2.1. Fetal Blood Supply

The umbilical vein, which provides nutrients to the developing fetus, is a major source of blood to the liver in the growing fetus. The umbilical vein enters the abdomen at the umbilicus and ascends to the inferior surface of the liver along the free margin of the falciform ligament. It connects to the portal vein's left branch there.

Placental blood can avoid the liver thanks to the ductus venosus, which transports blood from the left portal vein to the left hepatic vein and finally to the inferior vena cava. Since the placenta carries nutrients directly from the mother, the fetus's liver does not carry out the typical filtration and digestion functions of an infant's liver. Some blood stem cells are released by the fetal liver and move to the fetal thymus where they develop into T cells, also known as T lymphocytes. Blood stem cell production moves to the red bone marrow after birth. The umbilical vein and ductus venosus are destroyed after two to five days; the former becomes the liver's round ligament and the latter the ligamentum venosum. The umbilical vein can reopen in cases of portal hypertension and cirrhosis.

4.2.3. Functions

Hepatocytes, or liver cells, are responsible for the liver's various functions. Up to 500 different functions are attributed to the liver, most of which it performs in concert with other organs and systems. As of right now, no artificial organ or gadget can replicate the entire range of liver functions. Liver dialysis, an experimental treatment for liver failure, can perform certain functions. Additionally, the liver is responsible for around 20% of the body's oxygen consumption at rest.

4.2.3.1. Blood Supply

The hepatic arteries and portal vein supply the liver with blood in two different ways. The hepatic portal vein transports venous blood drained from the spleen, gastrointestinal tract, and related organs, providing about 75% of the blood supply to the liver. The remaining 25% of the liver's blood flow comes from arterial blood supplied by the hepatic arteries. Both sources supply oxygen to the liver: the hepatic arteries and the hepatic portal vein supply approximately half and half of the oxygen required by the liver, respectively. Because the hepatic artery contains beta- and alpha-adrenergic receptors, the splanchnic nerves of the autonomic nervous system are partially responsible for controlling blood flow through the artery. Blood enters each lobule's central vein after passing through the liver sinusoids. Hepatic veins, which emerge from the liver and empty into the inferior vena cava, are formed when the central veins combine.

4.2.3.2. Biliary Flow

The branches of the bile ducts give rise to the biliary tract. The route by which bile is secreted by the liver and then moved to the duodenum, the first segment of the small intestine, is called the biliary tree or tract. Bile canaliculi, which are tiny grooves between the faces of nearby hepatocytes, are where the bile produced in the liver is gathered. The canaliculi branch out to form bile ducts at the edge of the liver lobule. These bile ducts are known as intrahepatic bile ducts while they are inside the liver and extrahepatic bile ducts when they are outside the liver. The intrahepatic ducts eventually empty into the left and right hepatic ducts, which combine to form the common hepatic duct after leaving the liver through the transverse fissure. The common bile duct is formed when the common hepatic duct and the cystic duct of the gallbladder combine. The hepatic artery provides the only supply to the connective tissue and biliary system. The common bile duct empties into the duodenum, while the cystic duct temporarily stores bile in the gallbladder. At the hepatopancreatic ampulla, also referred to as the ampulla of Vater, the common bile duct and the pancreatic duct combine to enter the second section of the duodenum.

4.2.3.3. Metabolism

The metabolism of lipids, proteins, amino acids, and carbohydrates is largely regulated by the liver.

- **Carbohydrate Metabolism:** The metabolism of carbohydrates involves the liver in several ways.
  - Through a process called glycogenesis, which creates glycogen from glucose, the liver produces and stores about 100g of glycogen.
  - Glycogenolysis, the process by which the liver breaks down glycogen into glucose, is how it releases glucose into the blood when needed.
  - Gluconeogenesis, the process by which glucose is made from specific amino acids, lactate, or glycerol, is also carried out by the liver. By breaking down fat, adipose and liver cells create glycerol, which the liver uses for gluconeogenesis.
  - Additionally, the liver synthesizes glycogen from lactic acid, a process known as glyconeogenesis.
- **Protein Metabolism:** The primary organ involved in protein metabolism, synthesis, and breakdown is the liver. The liver synthesizes every plasma protein except for gamma-globulins. Additionally, it plays a major role in the synthesis of amino acids. The liver contributes to both the synthesis of red blood cells and clotting factors. Coagulation factors I (fibrinogen), II (prothrombin), V, VII, VIII, IX, X, XI, XII, XIII, protein C, protein S, and antithrombin are among the proteins that the liver synthesizes. Thrombopoietin is a glycoprotein hormone that controls the bone marrow's ability to produce platelets, and it is mostly produced in the liver.
- **Lipid Metabolism:** The liver is involved in many aspects of lipid metabolism. It is where most of the body's lipoproteins are made, as well as where triglycerides, cholesterol, and lipogenesis are produced. The liver is essential to digestion because it creates and eliminates bile, (a yellowish liquid) that is needed to emulsify fats and aid in the absorption of vitamin K from food. A portion of the bile is kept in the gallbladder and some flows straight into the duodenum. Insulin-like growth factor 1 is a polypeptide protein hormone that is produced by the liver and has anabolic effects even in adulthood. It is important for childhood growth.

4.2.3.4. Breakdown

The liver breaks down insulin and other hormones, as well as bilirubin through glucuronidation for excretion in bile. It also processes and eliminates various waste products and plays a vital role in breaking down harmful substances like medications through drug metabolism. In some cases, this can lead to increased toxicity in the metabolite. Ideally, toxins are conjugated for excretion in bile or urine. The liver also converts ammonia to urea in the ornithine cycle or urea cycle, which is then excreted in urine.

4.2.3.5. Blood Reservoir

Large amounts of blood can be stored in the liver's blood vessels due to its expandable nature. Its normal blood volume is approximately 450 milliliters, or nearly 10% of the body's total blood volume, and includes blood in the hepatic sinuses as well as veins. The liver swells when the right atrium's high pressure creates backpressure in the liver, and the hepatic veins and sinuses periodically store 0.5 to 1 liter of extra blood. This is particularly common in peripherally congested heart failure. As a result, the liver functions as a sizable, expandable venous organ that can provide extra blood when needed and serve as a valuable blood reservoir when blood volume is low.

4.2.3.6. Lymph Production

Protein content in the lymph draining from the liver is typically about 6 g/dl, which is only marginally lower than the protein concentration in plasma. This is because the pores in the hepatic sinusoids are highly permeable and permit easy passage of both fluid and proteins into the perisinusoidal space. Furthermore, a lot of lymph can form because of the liver sinusoid epithelium's high permeability. As a result, the liver produces roughly half of all the lymph that the body produces while it is at rest.

4.2.3.7. Other

- The liver stores a vast array of nutrients, such as iron, copper, zinc, cobalt, molybdenum, vitamin K, vitamin E, vitamin A (one to two years' supply), vitamin D (one to four months' supply), and vitamin B_{12} (three to five years' supply).
- Haemopoiesis – The process of making blood cells is known as hemopoiesis. The liver forms WBC and RBC during the embryonic stage. The liver is the primary site of red blood cell production in the first trimester fetus. By week thirty-two of pregnancy, the bone marrow has nearly entirely assumed that function.
- The liver aids in the blood's purification. As phagocytic cells, the liver's Kupffer cells aid in the removal of bacteria and dead blood cells from the blood.
- The liver is in charge of the immune responses; the liver's mononuclear phagocyte system, which includes a large number of immunologically active cells, serves as a "sieve" for antigens that enter the liver through the portal system.
- The liver manufactures albumin, which is the most plentiful protein found in blood serum. Albumin is crucial for maintaining oncotic pressure and serves as a carrier for fatty acids and steroid hormones.
- When the kidney senses low blood pressure, the enzyme renin is released, which in turn activates the hormone angiotensinogen, which is synthesized by the liver.
- The harmful oxidizing agent hydrogen peroxide is broken down into water and oxygen by the enzyme catalase, which is produced by the liver.

4.2.3.8. With Aging

Because aging reduces the liver's ability to oxidize substances, drugs that need to be oxidized—like benzodiazepines—are more likely to build up to toxic levels. But when it comes to geriatric medicine, drugs with shorter half-lives, like oxazepam and lorazepam, are generally preferred when benzodiazepines are needed.

4.3. Bile

The liver of the majority of vertebrates produces bile, also known as gall, a yellow-green fluid that helps the small intestine break down fats. In humans, the liver continuously produces bile, which is mostly made up of water that is then stored and concentrated in the gallbladder. This bile is released into the first part of the small intestine after a person eats (Figure 4.7).

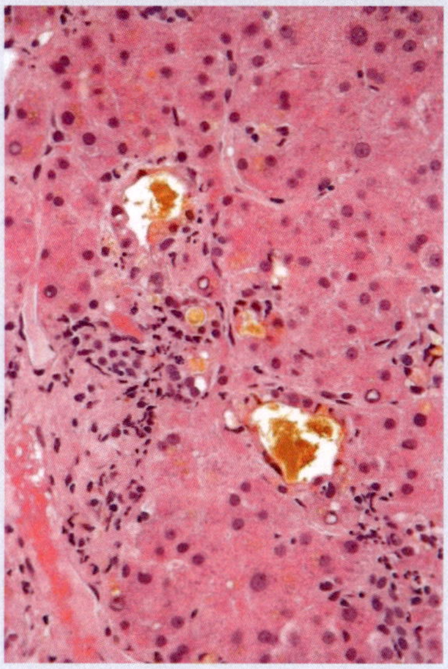

Figure 4.7. *Bile (yellow material) in a liver biopsy stained with hematoxylin-eosin in a condition called cholestasis (setting of bile stasis).*

Source: By Nephron – Own work, CC BY-SA 3.0, https://commons.wikimedia.org/w/index.php?curid=7956522.

4.3.1. Composition

The contents of bile in the human liver are as follows: 97–98% water, 0–7% bile salts, 0–2% bilirubin, 0–51% fats (fatty acids, cholesterol, and lecithin), and 200 meq/L inorganic salts. The two primary pigments of bile are the yellow bilirubin and the green biliverdin, which is the oxidized form of bilirubin. Their combination is what gives feces their brown hue. About 400 to 800 milliliters (14 to 27 U.S. fluid ounces) of bile is produced per day in adult human beings.

4.3.2. Cellular Level

Microtubules, microfilaments, and the Golgi apparatus in hepatocytes are involved in the formation of bile. The vesicles for the chemicals that will be secreted into the bile are produced by the Golgi complex. Newly synthesized ATP-binding cassettes (ABC) will be transported from the Golgi complex to the canalicular membrane, where they will serve as transporters. Microfilaments and microtubules are required for this process. The liver can be classified into three functional zones. Zone 1—also known as the periportal zone—is the zone that surrounds the portal triad (portal vein, hepatic artery, and bile duct) and is the furthest distal from the central vein. Zone 3 is the zone surrounding the central vein. Between zones 3 and 1, there is zone 2.

The average daily flow of bile in humans is estimated to be 620 mL. The osmotic force of bile acids either influences or does not affect the flow of bile. The bile-acid dependent fraction of bile (BADF) is the portion of bile flow that depends on the osmotic force of bile acids; the bile acid-independent fraction of bile (BAIF) is the portion of bile flow that is independent of the osmotic force of bile acids. Furthermore, the amount of water that osmotically follows bile acids and the bile acids themselves have a linear relationship. Some bile acids are still able to cause hypercholeresis, or an increase in bile volume. A well-known illustration is ursodeoxycholic acid. It has been suggested that ursodeoxycholic acids, which line the bile ducts, are reabsorbed into the bloodstream and subsequently into the hepatic sinusoids, which could explain the hyperocholeresis. The hepatocytes will take up these hypercholeretic bile acids from the hepatic sinusoids. The so-called hypercholeresis is caused by the hepatocytes' re-secretion of the hypercholeretic bile acids into the bile canaliculi, which raises the bile acid-dependent fraction of bile flow. The cholehepatic shunt pathway is the name given to this pathway. The bile acids found in the BADF are derived from the enterohepatic circulation or are recently synthesized in the liver. Notably, primary biliary cholangitis (previously known as cirrhosis), a disorder characterized by cholestasis and decreased bile secretion, is treated with ursodeoxycholic acid, also known as hypercholeretic bile acid.

Bile acid transporters that are both Na-dependent and Na-independent mediate the uptake of bile acids from the sinusoids. Sodium taurocholate-cotransporting polypeptide is the Na-dependent bile acid transporter (NTCP). Only the basolateral membrane is where NCTP expresses; it does not do so at the canalicular membrane. The transporter of organic anion-transporting polypeptides (OATPs) is involved in the Na-independent mechanism. Bile acids are transported into hepatocytes by the OATP transporter in return for glutathione or bicarbonate. Both cholangiocytes and hepatocytes have certain Na-independent bile acid transporters (OST/beta and OST/alpha) at their basal membrane. These transporters may be involved in the cholehepatic shunt pathway in cholangiocytes, as previously mentioned, or in the bile acid efflux into the bloodstream in hepatocytes when there is bile accumulation (cholestasis). The bile salt export pump (BSEP) is a unique energy-dependent transporter that secretes both conjugated and unconjugated bile acids into the canaliculi following their uptake from the sinusoids or endogenous synthesis from cholesterol. In addition to moving bile acids into the canaliculi, BSEP also helps with the excretion of some medications. The ATP-dependent transport of glutathione via the multidrug resistance-associated protein 2 (MRP2) primarily controls the BAIF of bile flow. The ABCG5/G8 protein secretes cholesterol and sterols, while MDR1 and multidrug resistance-P glycoprotein 3 (MDR-3) secrete phospholipids and lipophilic cationic drugs, respectively.

The secretion of bile is regulated by neural and hormone systems. Whereas acetylcholine acts through the vagus nerve in the neural mechanism, secretin, somatostatin, dopamine, and gastrin are involved in the hormonal mechanism. In part, vasoactive intestinal polypeptide (VIP) also promotes bile flow mediated by secretin. By attaching itself to receptors on the basolateral side of cholangiocytes, secretin promotes the secretion of fluid rich in sodium bicarbonate. Secretin-mediated sodium bicarbonate-rich fluid secretion is inhibited by dopamine, gastrin, and somatostatin. The role of the cholangiocytes is to secrete an alkaline fluid.

4.3.3. Development

The ventral foregut endoderm gives rise to a diverticulum, which is the liver tissue. The cranial and caudal portions comprise the two sections of the ventral foregut endoderm. The caudal region of the ventral foregut endoderm gives rise to the extrahepatic bile ducts, whereas the cranial portion gives rise to the intrahepatic duct. The intrahepatic duct's epithelium starts to form around the eighth week of pregnancy, and it moves centrifugally from the hilum to the liver borderborders. Only the first year of life marks the full maturity of the intrahepatic biliary epithelium. Prior to the intrahepatic duct, the extrahepatic biliary epithelium develops. At the level of the hepatic hilum, the two ducts will merge.

4.3.4. Organ Systems Involved

The gastrointestinal (GI), hepatobiliary, and hematologic systems are the organ systems in question. The hematologic system contributes by converting biliverdin into bilirubin. The reticuloendothelial system's oxidation of heme in aged red blood cells produces biliverdin. The GI system is in charge of controlling the alkaline bile secretions, excreting cholesterol, secreting stercobilin, which is bilirubin in the form of bilirubin, and secreting CCK, which causes the gallbladder to contract. The colonic bacterial flora transforms urobilinogen into stercobilin, which is how stercobilin is formed. Hepatobiliary system: in charge of bile production, secretion, and storage.

4.3.5. Function

In certain ways, bile or gall functions as a surfactant, aiding in the emulsification of lipids in food. Because bile salt anions have two sides, one hydrophilic and the other hydrophobic, they tend to group together around lipid droplets (phospholipids and triglycerides) to form micelles, with the hydrophilic side facing outward and the hydrophobic side facing the fat. Because the hydrophilic sides have a negative charge, bile-coated fat droplets are unable to re-aggregate into larger fat particles. In humans, the normal diameter of the micelles in the duodenum is between 1 and 50 μm. The breakdown of triglycerides by the enzyme pancreatic lipase is facilitated by the dispersion of food fat into micelles, which increases its surface area and allows it to pass through gaps in the bile salts to the fatty core. The intestinal walls' villi absorb two fatty acids and a monoglyceride that are produced when a triglyceride is broken down. The fatty acids are absorbed into the lymphatic system through lacteals after crossing the intestinal membrane and reforming into triglycerides (re-esterified). The majority of lipids in food would be eliminated undigested in feces in the absence of bile salts. Bile plays a significant role in the absorption of fat-soluble substances, including vitamins A, D, E, and K, because it enhances the absorption of fats. In addition to aiding in digestion, bile facilitates the excretion of bilirubin, a byproduct of red blood cell recycling by the liver. Hemoglobin undergoes glucuronidation to produce bilirubin.

Bile generally has an alkaline pH. The corresponding gallbladder bile (6.80 to 7.65) has a lower pH than common duct bile (7.50 to 8.05). The longer a person goes without food, the more acidic the gallbladder's bile becomes; however, this pH decline is slowed by rest. It also serves as an alkali, balancing out excess stomach acid before it reaches the duodenum, the first part of the small intestine. Additionally, bile salts have bactericidal properties that eliminate a large number of potential microorganisms from food.

4.3.6. Mechanism

Hepatocytes produce bile, which is then secreted into bile canaliculi and eventually the sphincter of Oddi. The bile is refluxed back up into the gallbladder to be concentrated and stored there if the sphincter closes. The reabsorption of bile salts and, to a lesser extent, water and electrolytes concentrates the bile. When food—especially fatty food—enters the duodenum, it stimulates the I cells to release CCK, which causes the sphincter of Oddi to relax and the gallbladder wall to contract. After that, the bile enters the duodenum's second section, where it emulsifies large fat droplets into smaller ones. The absorption of fat and fat-soluble particles is aided by the formation of micelles. This is a result of the hydrophilic outer form and hydrophobic core of a micelle. For reabsorption, the fat and fat-soluble vitamins will be incorporated into the micelle's central hydrophobic region.

4.3.7. Related Testing

Imaging and blood tests are two methods of testing for bile pathology. Ultrasonography is one imaging test for gallbladder pathology (e.g., cholecystitis and gallstones), biliary tree visualization using magnetic resonance cholangiopancreatography (MRCP) (e.g., primary sclerosing cholangitis), hepatobiliary iminodiacetic acid (HIDA) scan, abdominal magnetic resonance imaging (MRI), and abdominal computed tomography (CT). When ultrasonography cannot definitively diagnose acute cholecystitis, an HIDA scan can be especially helpful. Acute cholecystitis is suggested by the gallbladder not being visible on an HIDA scan.

Liver function tests (LFT) and CBC are among the blood tests.

CBC may reveal leukocytosis, which is common in many liver and gallbladder conditions such as cholecystitis and ascending cholangitis. Liver function tests (LFTs) include measurements of alkaline phosphatase (ALP), gamma-glutamyltransferase (GGT), aspartate aminotransferase (AST), alanine aminotransferase (ALT), prothrombin time (INR), indirect (unconjugated) bilirubin, direct (conjugated) bilirubin, total bilirubin, and serum albumin levels. A significant increase in GGT and ALP, along with direct hyperbilirubinemia and possibly only a slight elevation in AST and ALT, could suggest a cholestatic liver issue. If ALP is high but the rest of the LFT is normal, it may indicate a bone problem rather than a liver or bile duct issue. A greatly elevated GGT with only slightly abnormal LFT results may point to an infiltrative liver problem like metastasis.

4.3.8. Pathophysiology

Autoimmune disorders, obstructive and non-obstructive cholestasis, infections, and cancer are among the biliary system pathologies. Primary sclerosing cholangitis and primary biliary cholangitis (PBC) are autoimmune diseases. Impaired bile secretion and intrahepatic cholestasis are the outcomes of the autoimmune-mediated progressive destruction of intrahepatic small-medium sized bile ducts in primary biliary cholangitis. The bile ducts are destroyed both intrahepatic and extrahepatic in primary sclerosing cholangitis. PSC and ulcerative colitis have a close relationship. Both PBC and PSC have an autoimmune basis, which is evident in the histologic findings and the presence of particular antibodies in the patients. Furthermore, the autoimmune basis is further supported by the fact that both conditions are frequently linked to other autoimmune diseases.

Anytime there is a blockage to the bile flow or poor hepatocyte bile secretion, cholestasis results. The most frequent cause of the obstruction is gallstones, but it can also result from any other cause, including external compression of the biliary tree or biliary tree narrowing, as in PSC. Adenocarcinoma of the pancreatic head is a major contributor to painless jaundice, as it obstructs the bile duct due to the growing pancreatic head. When cholestasis sets in, the body begins to accumulate bilirubin, which causes the skin and sclera to turn yellow. Furthermore, the pruritus observed in these patients may be caused by the build-up of bile acids as a result of cholestasis. Bile duct infections are not unusual, and symptoms may include jaundice, fever, and pain in the right upper quadrant. Cholecystitis, or gallbladder inflammation, is also frequent and typically connected to gallstones (i.e., acute cholecystitis caused by calculi).

4.3.9. Clinical Significance

Steatorrhea is the term for the condition in which fats become indigestible and are expelled in feces due to the lack of bile. Instead of being the distinctive brown color, feces are greasy and white or gray in hue. Deficiencies in fat-soluble vitamins and essential fatty acids can result from starvation. Furthermore, the gastrointestinal tract and gut flora beyond the small intestine—which is typically in charge of absorbing fat from food—are not suited to processing fats, which causes issues in the large intestine.

Gallstones are the result of cholesterol from bile occasionally accumulating into lumps in the gallbladder. The standard course of treatment for cholesterol gallstones involves surgically removing the gallbladder. On the other hand, by raising the concentration of some naturally occurring bile acids, like chenodeoxycholic acid and ursodeoxycholic acid, they can occasionally be dissolved. When someone vomits repeatedly, for example, on an empty stomach, their vomit may be very bitter and green or dark yellow in color. The greenish-bitter substance could be bile or regular stomach-derived digestive juices. Strong muscle contractions and duodenal spasms, the presence of certain drugs, such as alcohol, or a compromised valve (pylorus) can all cause bile to be forced into the stomach. We call this biliary reflux.

4.3.9.1. Obstruction

When the bile ducts that carry bile from the liver or gallbladder to the duodenum clog, it is referred to as biliary obstruction. Jaundice may arise from an accumulation of bilirubin in the bloodstream due to bile blockage. Gallstones, cancer, trauma, choledochal cysts, and other benign causes of bile duct narrowing are a few possible causes of biliary obstruction. Gallstones that become lodged in the cystic or common bile ducts after being removed from the gallbladder are the most frequent cause of bile duct obstruction. Cholecystitis may result from a gallbladder or cystic duct obstruction. Gallstone pancreatitis may result if the blockage extends past the pancreatic duct's confluence. Ascending cholangitis can occur when bacteria infect the bile in certain cases of biliary obstruction.

4.4. Bile Acid

The steroid acids known as bile acids are primarily present in the bile of mammals and other vertebrates. The liver is where different bile acids are made. Bile salts are anions synthesized when taurine or glycine residues are conjugated with bile acids. The bile acids produced by the liver are called primary bile acids. Bacteria in the colon cause secondary bile acids to form. The main bile salts in humans are taurochenodeoxycholic acid and glycochenodeoxycholic acid (derivatives of chenodeoxycholic acid), and taurocholic acid and glycocholic acid (derivatives of cholic acid). Their levels of concentration are about equal. Over 90% of human biliary bile acids are made up of derivatives of cholic, chenodeoxycholic, and deoxycholic acids. The salts of their 7-alpha-dehydroxylated derivatives, deoxycholic acid and lithocholic acid, are also present.

About 80% of the organic compounds in bile are made up of bile acids (phospholipids and cholesterol make up the remaining 20%). Bile flow increases when bile acids are secreted more frequently. Dietary fats and oils are easier to digest when bile acids are present. They function as micelle-forming surfactants, coating nutrients to aid in absorption. Before additional processing, these micelles are suspended in the chyme. Moreover, bile acids influence hormones in various parts of the body, especially via the farnesoid X receptor and GPBAR1 (also called TGR5). It should be noted that since cholesterol is the parent compound of all bile acids, the only way that humans or other mammals can excrete excess cholesterol is through bile acid synthesis (Figure 4.8).

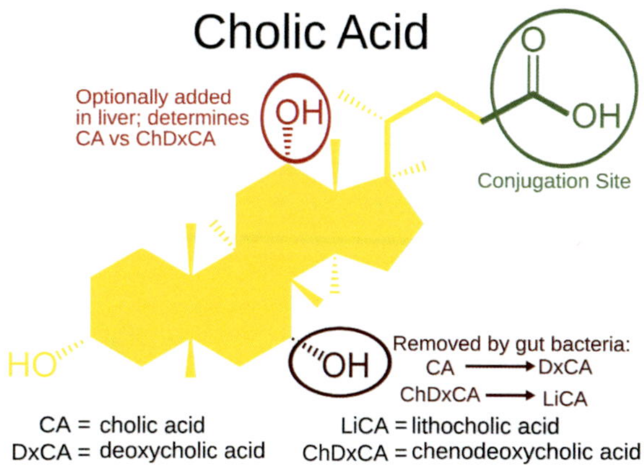

Figure 4.8. *Structure of cholic acid showing relationship to other bile acids.*

Source: By Mcstrother - Own work, CC BY 3.0, https://commons.wikimedia.org/w/index.php?curid=19888853.

4.4.1. Production

4.4.1.1. Primary Bile Acids

The production of primary bile acids, or catholic and chenodeoxycholic acids in humans, is carried out by liver cells through a multi-step process involving the oxidation of cholesterol by cytochrome P450. To replenish bile acids lost in feces, about 600 mg of bile salts are produced daily; however, much larger amounts are secreted, reabsorbed in the gut, and recycled—as will be explained below. The addition of a hydroxyl group to the seventh position of the steroid nucleus by the enzyme cholesterol 7 alpha-hydroxylase is the rate-limiting step in the synthesis process. This enzyme is inhibited by the action of the ileal hormone FGF15/19, up-regulated by cholesterol, and down-regulated by cholic acid.

Liver cells conjugate the bile acids (primary and secondary) with taurine or glycine before secreting any of them, making a total of eight possible conjugated bile acids. Bile salts are another term for these conjugated bile acids. When unconjugated bile acids are in the duodenum, they are nearly always protonated (HA form), which makes them relatively insoluble in water. The pKa of the unconjugated bile acids ranges from 5 to 6.5, and the pH of the duodenum ranges from 3 to 5. The pKa of the bile-acid/amino-acid conjugate is lowered to between 1 and 4 when bile acids are conjugated with amino acids. As a result, conjugated bile acids are nearly always found in the duodenum in their deprotonated (A-) form, which greatly increases their water solubility and improves their capacity to carry out the physiological role of emulsifying fats.

4.4.1.2. Secondary Bile Acids

Gut bacteria alter bile salts after they are secreted into the intestinal lumen. They've undergone partial dehydroxylation. Deoxycholic acid and lithocholic acid, the secondary bile acids, are obtained by removing their taurine and glycine groups. Deoxycholic acid is produced from cholic acid, and lithocholic acid is produced from chenodeoxycholic acid. The enterohepatic circulation process recycles all four of these bile acids.

4.4.2. Functions

4.4.2.1. Lipid Digestion

Conjugated bile salts are molecules that have both hydrophobic and hydrophilic regions. They are found at the lipid/water interface and, at the proper concentration, form micelles. Conjugated bile salts' increased solubility contributes to their functionality by inhibiting passive re-absorption in the small intestine. Because of this, the small intestine has a high enough concentration of bile acids and salts to form micelles and solubilize lipids. The term "*critical micellar concentration*" or CMC describes the quantity of bile acid required to participate in the spontaneous and dynamic formation of micelles as well as an intrinsic characteristic of the bile acid itself. Micelles containing bile acid help lipases break down fats and move them closer to the intestinal brush border membrane, where fat is absorbed.

In most species except humans, bile acid synthesis is a major pathway for the metabolism of cholesterol. The human body generates approximately 800 mg of cholesterol daily, of which 400–600 mg are utilized in the synthesis of bile acid. Adult humans excrete 12–18 g of bile acids into the intestine daily, primarily following meals. Because the bile acid pool is only 4–6 g in size, bile acids are recycled multiple times per day. A little over 95% of bile acids are recycled back to the liver for additional secretion into the biliary system and gallbladder through active transport in the ileum. A low rate of synthesis—roughly 0.3–0.5 grams per day—is made possible by the enterohepatic circulation of bile acids, yet a significant amount is secreted into the colon. In addition, bile acids help the body eliminate cholesterol, stimulate the flow of bile to remove some catabolites (like bilirubin), emulsify fat-soluble vitamins so that they can be absorbed, and support the motility of the bacterial flora of the small intestine and biliary tract.

4.4.2.2. Cell Signalling

Bile acids function in the body through two distinct receptors, the farnesoid X receptor and the G protein-coupled bile acid receptor/TGR5, which have metabolic effects similar to those of hormones. They have been shown to control the synthesis of various compounds, including endogenous fatty acid ethanolamides, as well as the activity of specific enzymes and ion channels. They also bind to some other receptors with less specificity.

4.4.3. Structure and Synthesis

A steroid structure with four rings, a five- or eight-carbon side chain that ends in a carboxylic acid, and numerous hydroxyl groups—the quantity and orientation of which vary depending on the particular bile salt—combine to form the broad family of molecules known as bile salts. The four rings are numbered A, B, C, and D, indicating their proximity to the side chain containing the carboxyl group from farthest to closest. Comparing the D-ring to the other three, it is one carbon smaller. Typically, the structure is depicted with D on the right and A on the left. The hydroxyl groups can be arranged in two different ways: down, called alpha (α; shown as a dashed line), or up (or out), called beta (β; frequently drawn by convention as a solid line. The 3-hydroxyl group present in all bile acids is beta in nature and is derived from the parent molecule, cholesterol (Figure 4.9).

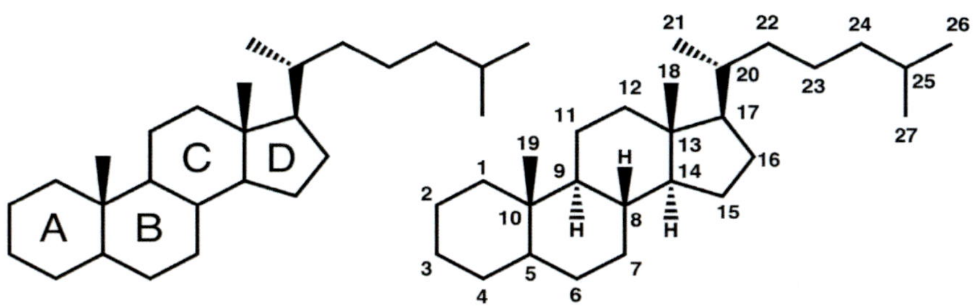

Figure 4.9. *IUPAC recommended ring lettering (left) and atom numbering (right) of the steroid skeleton. The four rings A-D form a sterane core.*

Source: By Boghog2 – Own work, Public Domain, https://commons.wikimedia.org/w/index.php?curid=5613812.

The first stage of the hepatic synthesis of bile acids follows the classical pathway, wherein cholesterol 7α-hydroxylase (CYP7A1) adds an enzymatic 7α hydroxyl group to form 7α-hydroxycholesterol. Subsequently, this is broken down into 7α-hydroxy-4-cholesten-3-one. Bile acid synthesis involves several steps and a total of 14 enzymes. These cause the molecule to become bent at the junction of the first two steroid rings (A and B), which also changes the 3-hydroxyl's orientation to the α. Positions 3α and 7α of the most basic 24-carbon bile acid contain two hydroxyl groups. This is chenodeoxycholic acid, or 3α,7α-dihydroxy-5β-cholan-24-oic acid, as it is more commonly known. The cheno part of the name was derived from the first isolation of this bile acid from domestic gooses. In the name, the 5β represents the bent orientation of the junction between rings A and B of the steroid nucleus. The term "cholan" refers to a specific 24-carbon steroid structure, and the term "24-oic acid" indicates that the carboxylic acid is located at position 24, at the end of the side-chain. Numerous species produce chenodeoxycholic acid, which is the archetypal functional bile acid.

The liver, as well as macrophages and other tissues, express mitochondrial sterol 27-hydroxylase (CYP27A1), which initiates an alternative (acidic) pathway of bile acid synthesis. By catalyzing sterol side chain oxidation, CYP27A1 plays a major role in the synthesis of total bile acid. This is followed by the cleavage of a three-carbon unit in peroxisomes, which results in the formation of a C24 bile acid. Bile acid synthesis may also be aided by minor pathways that are started by 24-hydroxylase in the brain and 25-hydroxylase in the liver. Oxysterols are produced by 7α-hydroxylase (CYP7B1) and can be further processed into CDCA in the liver. Prior to the discovery of chenodeoxycholic acid, the most abundant bile acid in humans and many other species, was identified as cholic acid, or 3α,7α,12α-trihydroxy-5β-cholan-24-oic acid. It has three hydroxyl groups (3α, 7α, and 12α) and is a tri-hydroxy bile acid. CYP8B1 performs the additional function of 12α hydroxylation during its synthesis in the liver. The discovery of chenodeoxycholic acid, which has two hydroxyl groups, as previously mentioned, turned this new bile acid into a deoxycholic acid because it contained one hydroxyl group less than cholic acid.

7-dehydroxylation converts cholic acid into deoxycholic acid, yielding two hydroxyl groups (3α and 12α). Through the use of chenodeoxycholic acid, a bile acid with just a 3α hydroxyl group is produced. This bile acid is known as lithocholic acid (litho = stone), and it was initially found in a calf gallstone. It is fairly toxic to cells and has a low solubility in water.

The majority of the positions on the steroid nucleus and side-chain of the bile acid structure have undergone modifications as different vertebrate families have evolved to use them. Most species add a third hydroxyl group to chenodeoxycholic acid to avoid the issues related to the production of lithocholic acid. A less toxic but still functional dihydroxy bile acid will be produced when intestinal bacteria remove the 7α hydroxyl group. Several sites have been selected for the third hydroxyl group's placement during the evolution of vertebrates. At first, the 16α position was preferred, especially for birds. Subsequently, many species chose the 12α position, replacing this position. Humans and other primates use 12α as their third hydroxyl group position, which results in the production of cholic acid. Muricholic acids (α or β, depending on the 7 hydroxyl position) are formed in mice and other rodents by 6β hydroxylation. Hyocholic acid (3α,6α,7α-trihydroxy-5β-cholanoic acid) has 6α hydroxylation in pigs, while other species have a hydroxyl group on position 23 of the side-chain.

Several other bile acids have been identified, often in trace amounts, as a result of bacterial enzymatic or other alterations. The iso- epimers have the 3-hydroxyl group in the β position, while the allo- epimers have the 5α configuration, leading to changes in the relative position of the A and B rings.

Ursodeoxycholic acid, originally isolated from bear bile used in traditional medicine for centuries, shares a similar structure to chenodeoxycholic acid but with the 7-hydroxyl group in the β position. Obeticholic acid, known as 6α-ethyl-chenodeoxycholic acid, is a semi-synthetic bile acid with enhanced FXR agonist activity, developed as a pharmaceutical treatment for certain liver diseases.

4.4.4. Hormonal Actions

By means of the nuclear receptor Farnesoid X receptor (FXR), also known by its gene name NR1H4, bile acids, which are also absorbed from the intestine and secreted from the liver, function as steroid hormones in the body. G protein-coupled bile acid receptor 1, or TGR5, is a cell membrane receptor that functions as an additional bile acid receptor. TGR5 may be involved in metabolic, endocrine, and neurological processes, while FXR is the primary signaling molecule in the liver and intestines, where it performs many of its functions.

- **Regulation of Synthesis:** Bile acids are surfactants or detergents, and because they may be harmful to cells, their concentrations are strictly controlled. When bile acid levels are too high, one mechanism of feedback control is the activation of FXR in the liver, which inhibits the synthesis of bile acids. Second, when bile acids activate FXR during intestinal absorption, they boost FGF19 synthesis and transcription, which in turn prevents the liver from producing bile acids.
- **Metabolic Functions:** There is growing evidence linking the activation of FXR to changes in the metabolism of glucose, triglycerides, and liver growth.
- **Other Interactions:** In addition to their transporters and hormone receptors (FXR and TGR5), bile acids also bind to a few other proteins. N-acyl phosphatidylethanolamine-specific phospholipase D (NAPE-PLD) is one of these protein targets that produces bioactive lipid amides (e.g., the endogenous cannabinoid anandamide) that are crucial for a number of physiological processes, such as appetite, longevity, and reactions to stress and pain. Lipid amide signals and bile acid physiology are directly correlated, and NAPE-PLD facilitates this communication.

4.5. Conjugation of Metabolites and Drugs

The majority of medications are xenobiotics, or chemicals that the body does not naturally produce. Xenobiotics are detoxified by the body through a variety of processes, which lessens their toxicity and makes them easily excreted. These processes, also referred to as drug metabolism or metabolic biotransformation, enable the chemical conversion of pharmaceuticals into their metabolites.

These metabolites, which come in three different forms—toxic, inactive, and active—are the end products of drug metabolism. Inactive metabolites are biochemically inert substances that have neither toxic nor therapeutic effects, whereas active metabolites are biochemically active substances that have therapeutic effects. Similar to active metabolites, toxic metabolites are biochemically active substances that can cause a variety of negative consequences. A low concentration of active metabolites is found in the systemic circulation as a result of drug metabolism, which takes place at a particular site in the body. First-pass metabolism is the term given to this phenomenon, which restricts the bioavailability of drugs. Enzymes that catalyze metabolism are present all over the body, but first-pass metabolism mostly takes place in the liver. It is essential to comprehend these changes in chemical activity to choose the best pharmacological intervention for each patient. Any healthcare professional who regularly administers medication to patients should be interested in this topic.

4.5.1. Function

Drugs are mainly eliminated from the body by the kidneys; however, lipophilic drugs easily pass through the renal tubules' cell membrane and are reabsorbed into the blood. Therefore, before the drug can be excreted, lipophilic drugs must first be metabolized in the liver. Phase I (modification), Phase II (conjugation), and occasionally Phase III (additional modification and excretion) are the different reactions that can occur during drug metabolism. Phase I modifications include oxidation, reduction, hydrolysis, cyclization/decyclization, and addition or subtraction of oxygen from more polar molecules to change the chemical structure of lipophilic drugs. This process can occasionally turn an inactive prodrug into a medication that is metabolically active. Most metabolites produced by oxidation still have some degree of pharmacological activity. Phase I modification, for instance, changes the popular anxiolytic medication diazepam into desmethyldiazepam and oxazepam. The physiological and psychological effects of diazepam and its metabolites are comparable. The majority of phase I reactions are catalyzed by the cytochrome P450 system also referred to as microsomal mixed function oxidase.

A drug molecule couples with another molecule in a conjugation reaction during phase II modifications. Conjugation typically makes the compound water soluble and pharmacologically inert, facilitating easy excretion. Methylation, acetylation, sulphation, glucuronidation, and glutathione or glycine conjugation are examples of conjugation mechanisms. These processes can take place in the kidneys, liver, lungs, intestines, and other organ systems, among other places. Oxazepam is an example of phase II metabolism; it conjugates with glucuronide, a different molecule. Without undergoing any additional chemical changes, the medication becomes physiologically inactive and is eliminated.

Phase II metabolism, during which conjugates and metabolites are eliminated from the cells, may also be followed by phase III metabolism. Phase I and II process enzymatic catalysis is a crucial component of drug metabolism. For drugs to be efficiently metabolized, liver enzyme composition and concentration are essential. The two enzymes that are most frequently utilized in medicine are cytochrome P450 and monoamine oxidase. Numerous biogenic and xenobiotic substances are broken down by these two enzymes. Monoamine oxidase, as its name implies, catalyzes the breakdown of monoamines, including dopamine and serotonin. Antidepressants called monoamine oxidase inhibitors (MAOI) raise dopamine and serotonin levels in the brain. The family of heme-containing isoenzymes known as the cytochrome P450 system is mainly found in the liver and gastrointestinal tract and is in charge of breaking down a wide range of medications and substances, including steroids and lipids. Amphetamines and opioids are among the many psychoactive substances whose metabolism is catalyzed by cytochrome P450.

4.5.2. Issues of Concern

Drug plasma concentrations can be impacted by drug metabolism, which needs to be taken into account. Drug interactions should worry prescribers because they can have a detrimental effect on the patient's health. For instance, imatinib's plasma concentrations may decrease if rifampin is taken concurrently with imatinib because rifampin can activate CYP3A4 and metabolize imatinib considerably more quickly. As a result, the anticancer effect of imatinib may be diminished. Similarly, imatinib's plasma concentrations rise when omeprazole is taken concurrently with imatinib to treat gastroesophageal reflux disease (GERD). This happens because imatinib is metabolized by CYP3A4, which is strongly inhibited by omeprazole. Imatinib builds up as a result of CYP3A4 inhibition, which can be toxic.

Another element that influences drug metabolism is aging. Age-related slowing of drug metabolism increases the risk of side effects in elderly patients. The patient's age should be taken into consideration by prescribers when writing prescriptions. Patients may respond differently to different medications due to genetic polymorphism in the enzymes that break down drugs.

4.5.3. Clinical Significance

The prescriber needs to take into account the drug's mode of elimination from the body as well as when to use it in any pharmacological intervention. The majority of the time, first-order kinetics govern drug clearance; in other words, the drug's plasma concentration determines the clearance rate. In other words, the drug's concentration is directly correlated with the elimination rate. The chemical in question determines the rate of this type of clearance, which is frequently expressed as a half-life. This is how long it takes for the body to get rid of 50% of the medication.

For instance, cocaine has a half-life of roughly one hour, meaning that after four hours, the body has only retained roughly 62.5% of the initial dose. On the other hand, some medications are eliminated at a steady pace that is unaffected by plasma concentrations. As an illustration, ethanol is excreted from the body at a steady rate of roughly 15 milliliters per hour, independent of bloodstream concentration. When low concentrations of an enzyme bind to its binding sites, a phenomenon known as zero-order kinetics takes place. Medicine is interested in kinetics because many medications require clinically significant drug concentration monitoring. Providers can modify patient-specific therapies by having a thorough understanding of pharmacokinetics, specifically drug elimination. The goal of therapy is to reach a steady-state plasma concentration where drug elimination and metabolism happen at the same time.

Numerous factors can impact the highly variable process of metabolism. Depot binding, or the coupling of drug molecules to inactive sites in the body so that the drug is no longer accessible for metabolism, is a major perturber of drug metabolism. This may have an impact on how long pharmacological agents that are prone to depot binding remain active. Tetrahydrocannabinol (THC), the primary psychoactive ingredient in marijuana, is one famous example. Because THC is so lipid-soluble, it binds to users' adipose tissue in the depot. Weeks after the patient's last usage, THC metabolites can be found in their urine due to this interaction, which significantly slows down the drug's metabolism. Enzyme induction is a further factor in drug metabolism. The same chemical is used repeatedly to induce enzymes. As a result of the drug's continuous presence, the body adjusts by producing more of the enzymes needed for the drug's metabolism. This leads to pharmacological tolerance, which is one of the reasons why patients require higher and higher dosages of some medications to achieve the same results.

One good example would be opioids. Long-term opioid analgesic prescription holders observe a gradual decrease in the efficacy of their medication. Notably, induction raises the rate at which all medications processed by the enzyme are metabolized; prolonged use of amphetamines, for instance, results in elevated CYP2D6 concentrations. Because this enzyme is also necessary for the metabolism of some opioids, including oxycodone, a doctor prescribing oxycodone to a patient who uses amphetamines would need to give a higher dose to achieve the intended result. On the other hand, some medications cause an enzyme-inhibiting effect that increases a patient's susceptibility to other medications that are metabolized by those enzymes. Monoamine oxidase inhibition caused by some antidepressants is a well-known example. These substances block the enzyme in the brain that breaks down "pleasure" chemicals, which has psychotherapeutic effects. But when people taking other medications while taking an MAOI, it can lead to abnormally high concentrations of these neurochemicals, which can cause issues. Cocaine, which increases serotonin, dopamine, and norepinephrine concentrations, will have a far more potent effect on a patient taking an MAOI. Numerous physiological issues, such as tachycardia, hypertension, and serotonin syndrome, can result from this interaction.

Drugs with similar metabolic pathways may also "compete" for the same binding sites on enzymes, reducing the efficiency of the enzymes' metabolism. For example, the same cytochrome P450 family member metabolizes alcohol and some sedatives. There are very few enzymes that can degrade these substances. One reason that alcohol and other sedative or hypnotic drugs can work well together when given together is that pentobarbital would not be fully metabolized if it were given to a patient who is also metabolizing alcohol because alcohol molecules would occupy the majority of the necessary enzymes.

4.5.4. Other Issues

Impairment in either of these systems can lead to serious problems, regardless of whether a drug is removed by the liver or the kidneys. These problems can include changed dosage, intervals between doses, and therapeutic effect; a patient's metabolism can dictate whether or not a given medication can be prescribed and used.

4.5.5. Enhancing Healthcare Team Outcomes

A critical clinical concern for the interdisciplinary healthcare team is drug metabolism. To avoid clinically significant drug interactions that could have an impact on patients' health, pharmacists and clinicians must collaborate. Nurses keep an eye out for any indications of a hazardous accumulation of metabolites or active medications in a hospital setting. This is particularly important in cases of hepatic or renal insufficiency. Pharmacists dose and oversee the administration of medications, including warfarin, aminoglycoside antibiotics, and fluoroquinolones, by keeping an eye on the serum levels of drugs and renal function. The best chance for achieving the best possible patient care is to use an interprofessional approach to drug dosing and administration in light of the effects of drug metabolism on patients, whether through impaired metabolism, drug-drug interactions, enzymatic induction, or other factors. With fewer unfavorable events, the interprofessional care approach produces better therapeutic outcomes.

4.5.6. Nursing, Allied Health, and Interprofessional Team Interventions

Monitoring and interprofessional interventions are essential for successful results. Research indicates that interprofessional interventions work best when teams are willing and able to work together, share decision-making, coordinate care, and communicate—all of which eventually lead to the integration of the team's competencies. An efficient method of managing medication through interventions and monitoring is through interprofessional team interventions. As previously stated, different people react differently to medications. Patients may therefore be more vulnerable to unfavorable outcomes if the right precautions are not done. When a patient is not taking their medication as prescribed by a physician or is taking it improperly, teams need to keep an eye on things and take appropriate action. Patient safety should always be the main priority. Adverse event reporting is essential to interprofessional team monitoring. Clinical teams should receive training to administer interventions and monitoring in an appropriate manner. Topics including standardizing medication dispensing, preventing adverse events by identifying medication errors, and improving team communication can all be covered in training. The goal of continuing medication credits ought to include both monitoring and intervention. An essential component of providing healthcare is communication. Interprofessional teams need to keep developing new strategies for guiding patients through the healthcare continuum.

Effective interprofessional education also fosters collaboration, interdisciplinary awareness, respect, and acceptance of the roles that various disciplines play in healthcare delivery. But one must also take the difficulties into account. Every discipline has a distinct methodology and culture. They differ in terms of professional language, qualifications, accountability, and routines as well as rules and regulations. This makes it challenging to standardize on any interventions or drug monitoring. But acknowledging these difficulties is the first step towards making a change. These issues can be resolved, and professionals in all fields—nurses, pharmacists, and doctors—will receive the necessary training to enable them to monitor medication for better health outcomes at any point during the course of treatment.

4.6. Determinants of Preferential Excretion into Bile

As a result of the development of combinatorial chemistry, more and more novel chemical entities with high molecular weight and lipophilicity are being synthesized and evaluated in the course of drug discovery. Medications with these physicochemical properties are frequently linked to substantial hepatic metabolism and/or biliary excretion. Drugs and metabolites that are excreted preferentially into bile have varying threshold molecular weights, ranging from approximately 235 in rats to 500–600 in humans. The pharmacological effect, toxicity, and systemic exposure of some medications can all be greatly impacted by biliary excretion of certain compounds. Medicines that are eliminated into bile frequently experience some degree of reabsorption throughout the digestive system (e.g., digoxin, warfarin, and mycophenolic acid). Another crucial physiological mechanism for maintaining the homeostasis of bile salts is enterohepatic recycling.

Humans have a highly efficient process of reabsorbing bile salts in the intestines, with over 95% of bile salts being reabsorbed in the distal ileum. However, obtaining bile samples from healthy human subjects has made it challenging to gather in vivo information on the biliary elimination of drugs and metabolites. Understanding biliary clearance and excretion of compounds is crucial for evaluating systemic clearance, potential hepatobiliary toxicity mechanisms, drug-drug interactions, and enterohepatic versus enteroenteric recirculation. Studies have shown that drug interactions can impact drug absorption by inhibiting transport proteins, leading to increased exposure to some drugs or improved therapeutic efficacy for others.

When other P-gp substrates or inhibitors are administered concurrently, significant changes in the pharmacokinetics and pharmacodynamics of digoxin, another P-gp substrate, have been seen. These changes are believed to result in interactions at the intestinal, biliary, and/or renal levels. However, due to technical challenges in conducting these experiments in humans, drug-drug interactions influencing biliary clearance of compounds have not been systematically investigated. The liver's capacity to remove bile salts from the bloodstream may be impacted by the inhibition of hepatobiliary transport processes, or perhaps more significantly, bile salt metabolism and excretion may be impacted. Drugs that inhibit bile salt biliary excretion have been shown to cause hepatotoxicity, despite the fact that the mechanisms underlying this condition are thought to be complex (e.g., as troglitazone and bosentan) can impact the viability of hepatocytes because of the build-up and direct toxicity of bile salts that resemble detergents.

Because there are currently no reliable methods for measuring the quantity of medication subjected to enterohepatic recirculation and because the processes involved in the hepatic excretion and reabsorption of drugs from the canalicular space, bile ducts, and intestine are poorly understood, the contribution of biliary excretion to the overall disposition and pharmacological effect of some drugs has been underestimated.

4.6.1. Mechanisms for Excretion of Endogenous and Exogenous Compounds into Bile

When it comes to the biotransformation and elimination of endogenous and xenobiotic substances from the blood, the liver is crucial. More polar and bulky molecules need transport systems to cross the sinusoidal membrane, but most small, lipophilic compounds enter the hepatocyte from the Space of Disse on the basolateral membrane by simple passive diffusion. Once inside the hepatocyte, substances can be eliminated into the blood by basolateral transport proteins, moved into bile either unaltered or as more hydrophilic metabolites following phase I and/or phase II biotransformations. Solutes are excreted into the dilated intercellular spaces known as bile canaliculi, which are caused by the presence of multiple transport proteins on the canalicular domain of hepatocytes. The liver performs a variety of tasks, including the synthesis of bile acids from cholesterol.

The main bile acids found in human bile are taurine and glycine conjugated with cholic and chenodeoxycholic acids. The bile salt export pump (BSEP/ABCB11) excretes bile salts into bile. Because of their surfactant properties, bile salts help the intestines absorb nutrients by emulsifying lipophilic molecules. Once this purpose is fulfilled, the apical sodium-dependent bile salt transport protein (ASBT/IBAT/SLC10A2) effectively reabsorbs bile salts into the distal ileum's cells, and the newly discovered organic solute transport proteins OST α and β excrete the salts into portal blood by crossing the basolateral membrane. Hepatic transport proteins play a crucial role in the clearance process by facilitating the excretion of metabolic byproducts like bilirubin and/or xenobiotics into bile for eventual removal via the intestine, in addition to facilitating the transport of bile salts.

4.6.2. Bile Formation and Excretion

The process of forming bile involves the absorption of bile components from sinusoidal blood and their subsequent secretion into the canalicular space. Because bile and the cytoplasm of hepatocytes have different osmotic pressures, water and other tiny ions also diffuse into bile. The bile then travels through the liver lobules and the biliary tree to the hepatic ducts. In humans, the gallbladder is where most of the approximately 800 mL of bile secreted daily is concentrated and stored, with a small portion of this hepatic bile being secreted continuously into the duodenum. The gallbladder has a substantially lower internal pressure than the intra-hepatic ducts, common bile duct, and the Sphincter of Oddi, which allows bile to flow freely into the organ. The gallbladder re-absorbs water and electrolytes from hepatic bile and fills to its maximum capacity (40–70 mL) in about 6 hours. Following a meal, endogenous neurohormones like cholecystokinin (CCK) and secretin are released by endocrine cells in the small intestine as fats, proteins, and acid pass into the duodenum. By stimulating smooth muscle fibers' CCK-A type receptors, CCK causes the gallbladder to contract and the Sphincter of Oddi to relax. A comparable result can be achieved by injecting physiological doses of CCK analogs (e.g., CCK-8).

Fasting causes CCK blood concentrations to drop to very low levels, which encourages the Sphincter of Oddi to contract and the gallbladder walls to relax, allowing the gallbladder to store bile. Moreover, CCK postpones stomach emptying to synchronize the postprandial digestive process. In the blood of humans, CCK-33, 8 and 58 are the predominant active forms of this polypeptide generated by differential post-translational modifications of the same gene; functional activity is dependent upon the last seven amino acids at the carboxyl terminus. Apart from its function in gallbladder contraction, CCK is also a neurotransmitter that regulates satiety in the cerebral cortex and bowel movement regulation on GI tract peripheral nerves.

4.6.3. Methods Used to Determine in Vivo Biliary Clearance

The degree of xenobiotic interaction with bile salt transport proteins and the biliary excretion of drugs can be assessed using a variety of preclinical methods using in vivo or ex vivo rodent models. Different techniques, which are detailed in detail below, can be used to determine the extent of biliary excretion in human subjects. Nevertheless, the evaluation of drug biliary clearance in humans has been limited to a small number of in vivo studies, and the contribution of biliary clearance to the total systemic clearance of most drugs remains poorly understood.

4.6.3.1. Patients as Study Subjects

The development of valid and trustworthy methods to measure the biliary excretion of pharmaceuticals or endogenous compounds in volunteers who are in good health has not been particularly successful in the past. Patients with gallbladder and biliary tract diseases who need medical procedures that allow measurements of drug concentrations in bile are a better source of this type of data. These individuals typically have cholestasis, biliary or cystic duct obstruction, and/or liver transplantation history.

- **Cholecystectomy:** Numerous teams have examined the concentrations of drugs in gallbladder bile and how they are disposed of by giving patients the compound of interest before they undergo cholecystectomy. Following removal, the drug concentrations in the gallbladder bile and tissue are measured and contrasted with the plasma concentrations. This method is very helpful, even though it only allows the drug content in bile and tissue to be determined at a single time point. It has been used to determine whether an antibiotic reaches the therapeutic concentrations required to treat bacterial infections of the biliary tract and gallbladder.
- **T-tube:** Drug excretion from the liver has been studied in patients requiring a temporary bile shunt (T-tube), which redirects a portion of the bile flow to a transcutaneous

port for external collection. T-tubes are frequently inserted following cholecystectomy and choledochotomy, and are primarily used in patients with cholangitis, distal bile duct obstruction, or edema. During the period that the shunt is in place, T-tubes allow for the partial collection of liver bile and provide an estimate of the biliary excretion of drugs administered. The fact that these patients' bile collections are incomplete poses a limitation to this technique. Furthermore, patients with underlying hepatobiliary diseases may have very different compositions of bile.

- **Nasobiliary Drainage:** A nasobiliary tube can be temporarily inserted to treat patients with bile duct stenosis. Perhaps because drug disposition studies are relatively new, fewer patients in this population have been recruited for them. In theory, this procedure enables full bile collection as long as the tube is inserted. By stopping the flow of bile into the duodenum, the nasobiliary drainage can be used to assess how enterohepatic recirculation affects the plasma concentration-time profile of the drug of interest. The enterohepatic recycling process has been restored in these studies by using the same patients as their own control after the stricture has resolved and the tube has been removed.

A smaller number of patients have had bile extracted from those who had percutaneous transhepatic cholangiodrainage or biliary-enteric diversions, two other forms of drainage devices. For the removal of common duct stones, less invasive techniques such as laparoscopic cholecystectomy with duct exploration and endoscopic retrograde cholangiopancreatography (ERCP) have largely taken the place in recent years. Because of this, there are far fewer T-tube users who are eligible to participate in research on the biliary excretion of medications. Seldom are the comparatively small number of patients receiving nasobiliary drainage well enough or able to keep the tube in place long enough to be good study subjects.

4.6.3.2. Healthy Volunteers as Study Subjects

The use of subjects with severe hepatobiliary disease is one of the main drawbacks of the methods mentioned above. The expression, function, localization, and/or bile flow of transport proteins can all be strongly impacted by disease status, which can change the patterns of drug excretion and reabsorption. It is well known that biliary obstruction causes hepatocytes to express more P-gp, MDR3 (ABCB4), and MRP3 (ABCC3) and less BSEP and MRP2 (ABCC2). Moreover, genetic variations in transport proteins may be linked to cholestatic syndromes. It may be possible to get more pertinent data by using healthy volunteers as research subjects. The hepatobiliary tract's physiology is sound and undamaged in this instance. The human hepatobiliary tract's anatomy and the gallbladder's difficulty of access make it more difficult to collect bile from the gallbladder or to immediately secrete it into the intestine.

- **Fecal Recovery:** Quantification of the drug of interest in feces is the method most frequently used to determine biliary excretion as a route for drug elimination. These investigations are frequently carried out using a radiolabeled compound to improve mass balance by improving selectivity and drug and unidentified metabolite recovery. Sensitive analytical methods, like high-performance liquid chromatography (HPLC) in conjunction with mass spectrometry, have been extensively utilized in biological matrix analysis to determine the excretion pathways of parent medications and their metabolites. Measuring drug levels in feces has a number of disadvantages.

Most importantly, this method is unable to differentiate between biliary excretion and intestinal secretion processes. For drugs taken orally, this method cannot differentiate between unabsorbed drug and drug secreted by the liver or gut back into the intestines. As a result, the percentage of the dose found in feces may not accurately reflect the amount excreted into bile. Additionally, unstable drugs or compounds that form unstable metabolites may not be detected in feces due to prolonged exposure to intestinal contents and colonic bacteria. Lastly, drugs that undergo entero-hepatic or entero-enteric recycling, such as glucuronide conjugates, may be reabsorbed in the colon after being degraded by microbial enzymes and therefore not found in feces.

- **Aspiration of Duodenal Fluids:** A perfect methodology would be flexible enough to enable studies looking at possible drug-drug interactions and would give information on the amount of parent drug and metabolites excreted into bile. When bile is discharged from the biliary tract into the small intestine, it can be collected by sampling the duodenal fluids. In terms of bile composition, duodenal bile is similar to gallbladder bile, despite being more diluted. In the medical field, it is standard procedure to remove pancreatico-biliary secretions from the duodenum using an oroenteric tube. This technique has been used to investigate the biliary excretion of endogenous compounds, including radiolabeled bile acids. To enable more thorough bile collection, some of these studies have made use of occlusive balloons. They have also evaluated any bile or duodenal fluid leakage distal to the balloon seal by perfusing a marker. Some groups have infused non-absorbable markers, like polyethylene glycol or sulphobromophthalein, into the duodenum to make up for any incomplete bile collection. These approaches have been successfully modified for the purpose of determining drug secretion and absorption from the intestines. This has improved our understanding of intestinal functions and added to our knowledge of drug excretion from the biliary system.

A cutting-edge technique to lessen the procedure's complexity by improving biliary secretion recovery and adjusting for the degree of gallbladder contraction. This technique uses an inflatable balloon to temporarily obstruct the intestine, ensuring the quantitative collection of bile secreted into the duodenum. In addition, the use of a hepatobiliary imaging agent (e.g., Tc-99m mebrofenin) is used to measure the extent of gallbladder contraction in response to pharmacological stimulation and to find any bile leakage resulting from partial intestine occlusion. Variations in the amount of bile and medication delivered into the duodenum during the collection interval are one of the main factors influencing the variability in the determination of biliary excretion in humans. During a fast, partial spontaneous contractions of the gallbladder are not unusual and can empty the intestine of more than 25% of the gallbladder's total bile. By pharmacologically stimulating gallbladder emptying, intravenous administration of CCK-8 can result in a more complete contraction of the gallbladder. It has been reported that the most complete gallbladder contraction can be achieved by slowly infusing CCK-8 at a low dose of 0.02-µg/kg over a 30 -60minute period. Nevertheless, individual responses vary and may be impacted by the method of collection. It is crucial to evaluate each subject's gallbladder contraction level as a result.

A gamma-emitting probe that rapidly accumulates in bile, such as Tc-99m mebrofenin, can be administered in trace amounts to help determine the overall gallbladder response and show when intestinal occlusion is incomplete. As an alternative, perfusion of the occluded tract using a non-absorbable marker to identify leaks and the degree of gallbladder contraction can be assessed via ultrasonography.

When estimating the volume of bile (containing medication) expelled into the duodenum and collected by aspiration, the gallbladder ejection fraction (EF), which can be computed from the volunteers' abdominal gamma images during gallbladder contraction, can be taken into account as a correction factor. It has been demonstrated that this technique adjusts fairly well for the significant variation in gallbladder contraction, which affects the quantity of medication secreted into the duodenum. To identify unknown metabolites that are unique to humans and are unstable and would not be detected after prolonged contact with intestinal enzymes, it can be very helpful to quantify the parent drug and its metabolites in bile that is aspirated directly from the duodenum rather than in feces (such as unstable glucuronides).

Lastly, an assessment of the significance of biliary excretion in systemic drug exposure and in researching the enterohepatic recirculation process is made possible by the possibility of conducting a second pharmacokinetic study in the same volunteers both with and without the balloon inflated. A possible explanation for multiple peaks in the plasma concentration-time profiles of certain drugs could be intestinal reabsorption and biliary excretion. These experimental findings have frequently been explained by pharmacokinetic modeling of these data using a model that takes enterohepatic recycling into account. Regretfully, this method is unable to precisely quantify the biliary clearance parameter and does not offer direct evidence for biliary excretion. Pharmacokinetic drug disposition and glucuronide conjugate disposition have been experimentally compared in patients prior to and following the restoration of enterohepatic recirculation following the removal of nasobiliary drainage. In other research, enterohepatic recirculation has been stopped using antibiotics to eradicate the colonic flora and/or cholestyramine, a resin that stops lipophilic compounds from being absorbed in the gut lumen. The investigation of hepatobiliary disposition mechanisms in greater detail than has been possible thus far should be made possible by improved techniques for examining drug disposition in healthy volunteers in the presence or absence of enterohepatic recirculation.

4.6.4. Methods Used to Determine In Vitro Biliary Excretion

The mechanisms controlling biliary excretion and possible drug interactions with the hepatic uptake and excretion of bile salts and other endogenous and exogenous substances can be studied using a variety of in vitro models.

These instruments include membrane vesicles made from cell lines transfected with particular transport proteins as well as the entire hepatocyte. These methods enable molecular characterization of transport processes and are a useful adjunct to human in vivo studies. Regretfully, it is challenging to compare in vitro model results to in vivo human data. This is mainly because values for a drug's intrinsic biliary clearance are determined using in vitro data generated. On the other hand, rather than focusing on pharmacokinetic parameters, in vivo studies frequently aim to obtain more imprecise estimates, like the percentage of the dose excreted into bile. Human in vivo biliary clearance values are typically not published. Due to the scarcity of viable whole human livers, whole liver perfusion—a popular method in rodent models to determine biliary clearance values—is rarely achievable in humans.

4.6.4.1. Sandwich-Cultured Hepatocytes

Because human primary hepatocytes express all of the proteins involved in hepatic metabolism and transport, they are valuable research instruments for studying these processes. After cell isolation in conventional culture, there is a progressive decrease in the expression of transport proteins and metabolizing enzymes. Moreover, the disruption of the canalicular membrane caused by the liver's collagenase digestion, which is necessary for hepatocyte isolation, leads to the cellular internalization of transport proteins expressed at this membrane. Compared to traditional hepatocyte culture, a novel in vitro model system that uses primary hepatocytes from different species—including rat and human—cultivated in a collagen-sandwich configuration (SC) offers a number of notable advantages. For instance, SC hepatocytes acquire and retain normal cell polarity, create large and functional bile canalicular networks, and permit direct access to the hepatocyte and surrounding biliary compartment.

Therefore, studying basolateral uptake and canalicular efflux transport processes is made possible by the unique opportunity provided by hepatocytes cultured under these conditions. The accumulation of substrates of interest in hepatocytes alone or in hepatocytes plus canalicular networks can be measured with straightforward modifications to buffer components. This makes it possible to calculate the intrinsic biliary clearance in vitro. Rat hepatocytes have been used in the majority of SC studies to date. Uptake and efflux transport proteins are expressed, correctly localized on the apical and basolateral membranes, and functional in SC human hepatocytes, which have also recently undergone characterization. Because SC human hepatocytes are still capable of metabolism, this model enables the study of the interactions between numerous in vivo processes. These cells can also be kept in culture for a few days, which makes it possible to research how drugs interact with induction mechanisms. Human hepatocytes are expensive and not always readily available. Moreover, every culture is conducted using cells from a single donor, which reflects the intrinsic differences in protein expression, function, and the development of canalicular networks among donors. Hepatobiliary transport mechanisms can be comprehensively studied using SC human hepatocytes, which are a unique tool.

4.6.4.2. Suspended Hepatocytes

The viability of primary hepatocytes can be sustained in suspension for multiple hours with the addition of suitable culture media and oxygen. The hepatic metabolic clearance of drugs has been extensively studied using either fresh or cryopreserved rat and human hepatocytes. Hepatocytes suspended in suspension are a valuable instrument for examining hepatic metabolism and uptake mechanisms. Studies of inhibition can be conducted using this system.

However, it is not possible to study induction processes because of the low viability of these cells. Furthermore, when transport into bile is crucial, the use of suspended hepatocytes to estimate an overall value for biliary clearance is restricted by the internalization of canalicular transport proteins during collagenase perfusion.

4.6.4.3. Vectorial Transport Using Polarized Cell Lines

The polarized Madin Darby Canine Kidney, strain II (MDCKII) cells have been widely employed for expressing different combinations of recombinant efflux and uptake transport proteins. At first, distinct combinations of a single canalicular efflux pump and a single basolateral uptake were transfected into MDCKII cells. In an effort to replicate vectorial transport processes in human liver, three basolateral uptake transport proteins (OATP1B1/SLCO1B1, OATP1B3/SLCO1B3, and OATP2B1/SLCO2B1) and a single efflux pump (MRP2/ABCC2) have been transfected into MDCKII cells more recently. To ascertain how each transport protein contributes to vectorial transport processes, the combination of quadruple, double, and single transfected cells is highly helpful. These cell lines can be grown on a permeable membrane, transfected with desired transport proteins, and utilized to investigate the transcellular transport of particular substrates. Using MDCK cells, a number of model substrates have been investigated and correlated with biliary clearance values measured in vivo in rats. The polarized transfected cell systems are effective tools for researching vectorial transport, but they don't have all the metabolic enzymes, cofactors, and transport proteins that hepatocytes have, and the expression levels of the proteins might not be similar to those of hepatocytes in vivo. These problems need to be taken into account when interpreting data and estimating hepatic or biliary clearance values in vivo. Nevertheless, transfected systems are helpful as a high-throughput screening tool and are easier to use and more widely available than primary human hepatocytes.

4.6.4.4. Whole Cells and Membrane Vesicles

When functional studies of the transport kinetics for individual transport proteins are required, whole cell expression systems like immortalized cell lines transfected with the target transporter or Xenopus laevis oocytes are ideal tools. These expression systems have been widely used in the literature to characterize the function of mutant proteins, including genetic polymorphisms, and to show substrate specificity. Oocytes are frequently used to study uptake processes, despite the fact that they are a transient expression system and that each one must be injected individually with cRNA of the desired protein. This model's commercial availability makes it easier to use for transportation-related research. Hepatobiliary clearance cannot be determined using these expression systems; instead, they are better suited for researching the effects of genetic diseases and the molecular mechanisms of transport. These models are better suited for studying uptake transport proteins due to the technical challenges of loading whole cells with an interest substrate before measuring efflux. Inside-out membrane vesicles have been used to study efflux transport processes, or the double transfected MDCKII cells have been used as a workaround for this problem. These vesicles can be made from primary hepatocytes or from cell lines that have been transfected with a desired transport protein. It is possible to isolate basolateral and apical membrane vesicles from polarized cells, such as primary hepatocytes, using different centrifugation techniques. Drug transport and transport inhibition can then be studied using membrane fractions that are enriched in basolateral or canalicular transporters. Because human hepatocytes are not as readily available, rat hepatocytes are more frequently used to prepare canalicular vesicles. Nonetheless, human hepatocyte-isolated canalicular membrane vesicles have been used in a number of recent investigations. When isolated from other cellular components, membrane vesicles made from primary hepatocytes have two distinct advantages over transfected systems: they contain all of the hepatic transport systems and the native membrane environment. Membrane vesicles can be made, frozen-stored, and used as needed; however, complete purity is never achieved and the isolation of the basolateral and canalicular fractions is labor-intensive.

Membrane vesicles derived from cell lines that both transiently and permanently express membrane proteins of interest have been widely employed in the analysis of efflux transport protein polymorphisms, substrate selectivity, and structure-function relationships. There are numerous expression systems in use (insect cells: e.g., Sf9 cells; mammalian cells: e.g., HEK293 cell line) and endogenous transporter expression can differ. Control studies in untransfected cells are necessary to account for the background activity of membrane vesicles. Moreover, the host cell's post-translational protein modifications may vary and impact the transport protein's affinity for the target substrate.

New and significant technologies are being developed for the assessment of biliary excretion and the associated toxicological and pharmacological problems resulting from drug interactions at the hepatobiliary transport level. Many in vitro models are currently employed as screening instruments in early drug development and discovery to weed out compounds that pose problems with this specific aspect of disposition. To support in vitro observations, it would be very helpful to compare the outcomes of in vitro systems with data generated in vivo in humans. Unfortunately, there is a lack of readily available information on the in vivo biliary excretion of drugs, and studies involving volunteers will remain difficult and subject-limited. However, the results of these studies can be very helpful in understanding the significance of biliary excretion and enterohepatic recirculation in the overall disposition of drugs, as well as in explaining results obtained using in vitro systems.

It's possible that in the future, a more thorough comparison between in vivo and in vitro hepatobiliary clearance will validate the precision of in vitro scaled predictions and enable the creation of precise models that can more confidently predict drug disposition in humans. In addition to enhancing our knowledge of drug disposition, this combination of tools will aid in the prediction of drug-drug interactions and/or the influence of genetic polymorphisms on drug exposure and toxicity. Mathematical modeling and simulations will also be heavily utilized.

4.7. The Gallbladder

The gallbladder is a tiny, hollow organ that resembles a pear in both size and form. It is a component of the biliary tract, sometimes referred to as the biliary tree or biliary system. The biliary system consists of a network of ducts that empty into the small intestine from the liver, gallbladder, and pancreas. There are components that are extrahepatic—found outside the liver—and intrahepatic—found inside the liver. The extrahepatic biliary system includes the gallbladder, which is where concentrated and stored bile is kept. The liver produces bile, a fluid that is necessary for cholesterol excretion, fat digestion, and even antimicrobial activity. The gallbladder is located in the upper right quadrant of the abdomen and is attached to the liver's underside at the gallbladder fossa. It is connected to the remainder of the extrahepatic biliary system through the cystic duct. Bile is produced by the liver and is stored in the gallbladder until it is required for digestion.

Gallstones are most frequently caused by abnormalities in the gallbladder's physiology. Insoluble stones may form due to imbalances in the components of bile and biliary sludge caused by gallbladder hypokinesis. The gallbladder and several other organs may sustain pain, inflammation, and infection as a result of these gallstones causing physical blockages in the biliary tree and other areas. The removal of the gallbladder, or cholecystectomy, is one of the most common surgical procedures carried out in the modern era because many gallbladder pathologies will eventually require surgical intervention.

4.7.1. Cellular Level

The right upper quadrant of the abdomen contains the large organ known as the liver. Hepatic lobules, the liver's functional units with a hexagonal shape, make up this structure. Hepatocytes, or liver cells, make up the majority of these lobules. Hepatocytes perform a variety of vital tasks, such as producing and secreting bile. A central vein and portal triads, which are made up of hepatic artery, portal vein, and bile duct branches, are also present in the lobules of the liver. The peripheral vasculature is connected to the central vein by epithelial-lined sinusoids that are situated in between the hepatocytes. The Canals of Hering are tiny channels that drain the bile the hepatocytes produce to the lobule's periphery in the opposite direction of blood flow. They eventually drain the bile into the bile ductule of the portal triad, which then drains into the bile duct. They are lined by simple cuboidal epithelium. There are multiple layers that make up the gallbladder wall. The columnar epithelium with microvilli makes up the innermost layer of the mucosa. Bile can be concentrated thanks to the increased surface area provided by the microvilli. Because it is located intraperitoneally, the mucosa is layered beneath smooth muscle, the lamina propria, and the outer serosal layer.

4.7.2. Development

The foregut is where the gallbladder and biliary system develop. The hepatic diverticulum emerges at the conclusion of the fourth week of development. The extrahepatic biliary system, the liver, and a portion of the pancreas develop from the hepatic diverticulum. The diverticulum's superior bud gives rise to the gallbladder. The pancreas and common bile duct begin to revolve around the duodenum at week six. The common bile duct and cystic duct connect by week seven after the bile ducts are filled with epithelial cells and their lumens are recanalized. By week twelve, the liver is secreting fluid through the patent bile ducts, which now empty into the duodenum, and the gallbladder has dissolved. The biliary system's development is incredibly intricate and can result in a wide range of structural variations.

4.7.3. Organ Systems Involved

Related organ systems that impact the physiology of the gallbladder include the pancreas, liver, and small intestine. The liver produces bile, which the gallbladder stores and concentrates. The gallbladder empties the bile into the duodenum in response to stimulation of the small intestine by fatty meals and proteins. The gallbladder's cystic duct joins the common bile duct after emptying it. At the pancreatic ampulla of Vater, the common bile duct merges with the main pancreatic duct. Pancreatitis is primarily caused by a gallstone that gets stuck in the pancreatic ducts. An uncommon type of small bowel obstruction can result from a cholecysto-enteric fistula, or an abnormal connection between the gallbladder and intestines.

4.7.4. Function

Bile is released into the duodenum during digestion and is stored and concentrated in the gallbladder. Since lipids are not soluble in water, the liver continuously produces bile, an alkaline fluid whose main purpose is to facilitate the digestion and absorption of lipids. It is made up of phospholipids, ions, water, bile salts, bilirubin, and cholesterol. The majority of the cholesterol in the body is eliminated by bile's excretion of cholesterol. I-cells are specialized enteroendocrine cells found in the jejunum and duodenum. The release of fatty and amino acids from the stomach stimulates these cells and results in the release of a peptide hormone known as cholecystokinin (CCK). There are two primary roles for CCK in relation to the gallbladder. Its primary purpose is to cause the gallbladder's smooth muscle to contract, releasing bile into the biliary tree. The second job of CCK is to concurrently induce the relaxation of the Oddi muscular sphincter. Bile travels through the common bile ducts after exiting the gallbladder and meets the ampulla of Vater, the main pancreatic duct, at this point. From there, it enters the second part of the duodenum through an aperture known as the major duodenal papilla. The sphincter of Oddi opens and closes to regulate the flow through the papilla. The gallbladder fills with bile and relaxes when it is not stimulated by CCK. Beyond the gallbladder, CCK inhibits further stomach emptying and increases pancreatic secretions that are essential for digestion. The hormone somatostatin, which stops digestion, inhibits the release of CCK.

The liver uses precursors for cholesterol to make bile acids. The enzyme known as cholesterol 7α—hydroxylase catalyzes the rate-limiting step in the production of bile acid. Glycine and taurine, two amino acids, are coupled to the bile acids to form soluble bile salts. The intestine's process of emulsifying lipids depends on these bile salts. The lipids are subsequently packed into micelles composed of bile salts that function as surfactants as they are broken down in the digestive tract into free fatty acids and monoglycerides. Bile salts' amphipathic properties allow them to accomplish this. Their hydrophobic sections keep lipids in the center while their hydrophilic portions interact with water to make them soluble. Additionally negatively charged, the hydrophilic parts repel other bile salts and maintain the lipids' small size and ease of digestion. The micelle's structure also includes phospholipids and cholesterol. Through a process known as the enterohepatic circulation, the bile salts are recycled back to the liver from the distal ileum of the small intestine.

Bilirubin is a yellow pigment that is synthesized when red blood cells break down heme. Initially, bilirubin is not soluble in water and is known as unconjugated or indirect bilirubin. The liver takes up this unconjugated bilirubin and processes it with glucuronate using the enzyme UDP-glucuronosyltransferase, turning it into conjugated or direct bilirubin. This form of bilirubin is then removed from the body through bile in a soluble form. As bile travels through the digestive system, it gives urine its yellow color and stool its brown color through the breakdown products urobilin and stercobilin. If bile is unable to enter the duodenum, a buildup of bilirubin can cause jaundice, which results in yellowing of the skin, eyes, and mucus membranes, as well as pale stools.

4.7.5. Related Testing

An abdominal ultrasound is the first test of choice for diagnosing the majority of gallbladder disorders. This test is noninvasive and can be used to assess the gallbladder for inflammation, sludge, and stones. Because calcified gallstones are only visible on plain abdominal x-rays in roughly 10% of cholelithiasis patients, X-rays are less sensitive. When a patient visits the emergency room, a CT scan is frequently performed to assess abdominal pain. Radiation exposure is incurred by the patient, but the diagnosis of gallbladder disease is extremely accurate. The hepatobiliary iminodiacetic acid

(HIDA) scan, also referred to as cholescintigraphy, is the most sensitive and specific diagnostic test to confirm cholecystitis. In this radionuclide scan, an intravenous tracer is administered, and the liver hepatocytes absorb it. If the cystic duct is open, the tracer then concentrates in the gallbladder.

It is usually carried out in conjunction with a clinical suspicion of gallbladder pathology and an equivocal abdominal ultrasound. The gallbladder's ejection fraction (EF) can be measured with the use of CCK. It is deemed abnormal and suggestive of a functional gallbladder disorder when the EF is less than 35%. When acute gallbladder disease is suspected, a complete metabolic panel (CMP) and a complete blood count (CBC) are likely to be requested. In the context of inflammation, an increased leukocytosis, or white blood cell count, would be anticipated. Different enzyme levels can be increased depending on the location of a gallstone. This includes, in the event that the pancreas is obstructed, the pancreatic enzymes lipase and amylase as well as the liver enzymes aspartate transaminase (AST), alanine transaminase (ALT), and alkaline phosphatase (ALP). Bilirubin levels may also be raised. Since gamma-glutamyltransferase (GGT) is present in both hepatocytes and the gallbladder's epithelial cells, it is likely to be elevated if it is normal.

4.7.6. Pathophysiology

4.7.6.1. Cholelithiasis and Biliary Colic

Gallstones in the gallbladder are known as cholelithiasis. Unbalances in the components of bile and biliary stasis—a condition in which bile is not flowing—can cause stones to form. Gallstones are typically categorized as pigmented or cholesterol stones. About 80% of stones are caused by cholesterol buildup. The risk factors that are most frequently linked to them are those that the four Fs stand for: female, fat, fertile, and forty. This indicates that risk factors include multiparity, aging, obesity, and estrogen. Brown and black stones are the result of the breakdown of pigmented stones. The calcium bilirubinate-containing black stones are more likely to be visible on radiography. These stones frequently result from secondary pathologies that break down red blood cells (RBCs), a process known as hemolysis. The higher bilirubin concentration in bile is due to the heme from RBCs that has been metabolized. Brown stones develop as a result of an infection. Gallstones typically don't cause any symptoms, but if a stone gets stuck in the cystic duct, a person with cholelithiasis may suffer from biliary colic. Right upper quadrant pain is a common symptom of biliary colic, which is brought on by fatty meals that trigger the secretion of CCK, which in turn causes excruciating contractions against the stone.

When a gallstone becomes stuck in the common bile duct, choledocholithiasis happens. The location of the lodged stone affects the effects and consequent changes in laboratory values. Liver enzymes including ALP, GGT, AST/ALT, and bilirubin are likely to be elevated if the stone has not traveled very far. Amylase and lipase levels will rise due to pancreatitis if the stone has made it all the way to the pancreas.

4.7.6.2. Cholecystitis

To put it simply, gallbladder inflammation is known as cholecystitis. Calculous cholecystitis, as this condition is known, is most frequently caused by gallstones in the cystic duct. Anytime a duct becomes blocked, inflammation may result from the stasis that follows. Acute cholecystitis is more likely to result in prolonged abdominal pain, fever, and leukocytosis than biliary colic. Infection is the most common side effect of untreated acute cholecystitis. In addition to infection, recurrent episodes of acute cholecystitis in the gallbladder can lead to chronic cholecystitis. The calcification and scarring that follow raise the risk of developing cancer. Acalculous cholecystitis is a different kind of cholecystitis that occurs in critically ill patients who do not have gallstones. Infection, low perfusion, or biliary stasis can all lead to this.

4.7.6.3. Cholangitis

An inflammation of the bile ducts is called cholangiosis. This most frequently refers to ascending cholangitis, an infection-related secondary condition. Bacterial overgrowth may result from bile stasis caused by obstruction of the biliary tree. This kind of cholangitis is characterized by a set of symptoms known as the Charcot triad. The triad consists of fever, right upper quadrant pain, and jaundice (caused by elevated bilirubin). A set of symptoms known as Reynolds pentad occurs when a patient exhibits shock and altered mental status.

4.7.7. Clinical Significance

The normal physiology of the gallbladder can be upset, which can have serious medical consequences. With over 20 million Americans suffering from gallbladder disease, the most common surgical procedure is a cholecystectomy. Gallbladder disease and gallstone formation are both made more likely by a number of factors, and their frequency rises with age.

Women make up roughly 14 million of the cases in the US, putting them at a higher risk. Understanding the physiology of the gallbladder can help with gallbladder disease understanding, prevention, and treatment. In clinical settings, patients may receive weight-loss counseling because obesity raises the risk of gallbladder disease. People with asymptomatic cholelithiasis can be informed about the benefits of low-fat diets to lower their risk of developing biliary colic. Many medications have the potential to raise the risk of gallstone development, so understanding the underlying mechanisms is crucial. For instance, estrogen-containing hormone replacement treatment raises cholesterol levels.

Octreotide and other somatostatin analogs prevent the release of CCK, which causes biliary sludge to accumulate. Fibrates cause a reduction in the production of bile acid and an increase in cholesterol by blocking the rate-limiting enzyme 7-alpha-hydroxylase. Understanding these processes has also aided in the development of medications that have a favorable effect on a patient's health. Bile acid sequestrants, for instance, force the body to use cholesterol as a substrate to produce new bile acids by preventing bile acids from being reabsorbed in the ileum.

This lowers cholesterol levels. Healthcare professionals who treat patients undergoing extended fasts or receiving total parenteral nutrition are aware that, in addition to medication side effects, these patients have an elevated risk of biliary stasis because of the reduced stimulation of CCK.

The majority of cholecystectomies carried out today are outpatient laparoscopic procedures. With a quick recovery, this procedure offers a very low rate of complications. Expected intraoperative risks like bleeding and perforation persist in spite of this. Post-cholecystectomy syndrome is an uncommon complication that can manifest as ongoing abdominal pain after surgery.

4.8. Liver Procedures

4.8.1. Open Liver Resection

A portion of the liver is removed during surgery, known as a liver resection. The liver can be removed up to two thirds of the way through the body. The liver can regenerate itself as well. The remaining portion of your liver will have grown back to almost normal size in three months following your operation. For many metastatic liver tumors (metastatic colorectal cancer, neuroendocrine carcinoma, sarcoma, ovarian cancer, kidney cancer, etc.), liver resection is the only treatment option left. It is also a curative treatment for primary liver tumors (hepatocellular carcinoma, cholangiocarcinoma, gallbladder cancer (+/- involving the liver), liver angiosarcoma, etc.). With advances in surgical instruments, postoperative care, and comprehension of liver anatomy over the last ten years, the safety of liver resection has improved dramatically. Less than 1% of patients die after a major liver resection today. Liver resection is now a common and safe procedure.

The conventional open technique is used in more than 70% of liver resections performed in Europe and the US. After surgery, most patients stay in the hospital for five to seven days. A minimally invasive technique for liver surgery was developed with the goal of reducing postoperative complications and shortening the recovery period. The first description of laparoscopic liver resection for a small liver tumor in the periphery appeared in 1992. Major liver resections (removal of three or more liver segments) for liver cancers are now possible thanks to the progressive advancement of laparoscopic liver resection technique. However, depending on the features of their tumors, not every patient is a candidate for the minimally invasive liver surgery. Due to the size of the tumor, its proximity to important biliary and vascular structures, and the requirement for a vascular resection with reconstruction, about 20% of patients who come to our liver surgery center need an open liver resection. For instance, the standard open technique is used during a liver tumor operation if the tumor involves a major blood vessel that supplies the liver (the main portal vein, hepatic artery, and inferior vena cava), and vascular resection is required to achieve cure.

To appropriately expose the liver and the tumor during an open liver resection, a surgical retractor is positioned away from the stomach, intestines, and colon. The blood vessels that supply the liver lobe that has to be removed are meticulously separated and tied off. Next, the liver surface's demarcation line is found. The boundary between the tumor and the healthy liver parenchyma is often marked by liver ultrasonography. A safe liver surgery requires a thorough examination of the intrahepatic anatomy to identify the major arteries. To prevent a postoperative liver failure due to insufficient liver tissue after the resection, a computerized assessment of the liver volume (to be resected and to be preserved) is equally important. In cases of marginal liver volume, an experienced liver surgeon decides whether a preoperative portal vein embolization or portal vein ligation is required to induce future liver remnant hypertrophy. Additional variables are taken into account, including previous liver resections, obesity, portal hypertension, degree of liver steatosis, history of chemotherapy, and liver cirrhosis. This assessment procedure is extremely intricate, specialized, and exclusive to liver surgery centers.

To achieve better results, intraoperative bleeding is carefully controlled and minimized. To verify that there are no tumor cells at the liver resection margins, the removed specimen is ultimately sent to the pathology laboratory for a frozen section examination. Your liver surgeon may leave a small drain after the open liver resection is finished, and it will be removed a few days later. For the liver surgeon, an open liver resection is a physically and technically demanding procedure. Therefore, especially for major liver resections, it is crucial to consult with a liver specialist or liver surgeon who has substantial experience performing liver resections.

4.8.2. Laparoscopic Liver Resection

Most advanced high volume liver centers worldwide are quickly adopting laparoscopic liver resection (LLR), which is safe and practicable. Modern, pure laparoscopic methods are used for the great majority of liver resections.

Benefits of Laparoscopic Minimally Invasive Liver Resection:

- **Faster Postoperative Recovery:** After a major robotic liver resection, most patients are discharged from the hospital in 3–4 days, and after a minor liver resection, in 2 days. Techniques for minimally invasive liver surgery significantly lower the risk of cardiac and pulmonary complications. Patients who require additional systemic chemotherapy later on can benefit from faster recovery from liver resections and an earlier start to systemic chemotherapy.
- **Reduced Blood Loss:** Less than 100 cc of blood is lost during the majority of the laparoscopic liver resection procedures we have done. Even after extensive liver resections, blood transfusions are not always necessary.
- **Less Pain:** Even following significant liver resections, the majority of patients have little pain and require little narcotic medication.
- Minimal Risk for Wound Infection Comparing an open liver resection to a surgical wound infection, the likelihood of the latter is less than 1%.
- **Minimal Risk for Hernia Formation**: Incisional hernias are much less common in small incisions that heal. Avoiding making a large incision is the best way to prevent the formation of hernias following surgery.
- **Better Cosmetic Outcome**: Tiny wounds healed leaving hardly noticeable, frequently undetectable scars.
- **Less Intra-Abdominal Adhesions**: In the event that additional liver surgery is needed, laparoscopic surgery reduces the amount of scarring (adhesions) surrounding the liver, making it easier to access and approach the organ.

4.8.2.1. Procedure of Laparoscopic Liver Operations for Benign and Malignant Liver Tumors

The procedure of laparoscopic liver resection involves four or five small (5–12 mm) incisions made in the upper abdomen. A high-definition camera visualizes and magnifies the liver. Even in the most superior and posterior regions of the liver, lesions can be fully visualized and identified with its full mobilization. The liver resection procedure adheres to the same guidelines when using the open technique. The specimen is typically removed through the pfannenstiel incision, a tiny incision in the lower abdomen.

4.8.3. Robotic Liver Resection

Like laparoscopic liver resection, robotic liver resection is a type of minimally invasive liver surgery. Similar safety and viability are shown for hepatectomies between laparoscopic and robotic liver resection. Robotic and laparoscopic liver surgery yield comparable results in skilled hands, and new research has not demonstrated any advantages of either technique over the other. Compared to laparoscopic liver surgery, robotic liver surgery has a few technical advantages, such as easier dissection and suturing. In contrast, compared to the laparoscopic method, robotic liver surgery is linked to a considerably higher cost and a longer operating duration.

4.8.4. Laparoscopic Liver Cyst Fenestration (Unroofing)

Patients frequently experience pain in the right upper quadrant, shoulder discomfort, nausea, epigastric fullness, and symptoms similar to acid reflux when a large hepatic cyst becomes symptomatic. The symptoms are brought on by either mechanical compression of the surrounding organs, including the diaphragm, stomach, intestines, and chest wall, or mechanical stretching of the Glissonean capsule that covers the liver. In this case, a large liver cyst fenestration or surgical unroofing is required. Liver dysfunction is typically not linked to the existence of a liver cyst. An MRI or CT scan can be used to quickly make a diagnosis. A premalignant cystic mass or lesion of the liver, such as a parasitic hydatid cyst or mucinous cystic neoplasm, should be excluded and should be surgically removed. An interventional radiologist's false performance and discussion of a percutaneous liver cyst aspiration are frequent, but the procedure is known to fail in over 95% of patients because of the hepatic cyst's rapid fluid re-accumulation. Thus, the pointless percutaneous liver cyst aspiration is not advised.

Laparoscopic liver cyst fenestration has emerged as the gold standard for treating symptomatic large hepatic cysts in the modern era of liver surgery. It is a very simple procedure in terms of technology, and the results last for a long time. For this disease, an open liver operation is no longer necessary. Resection or removal of a significant portion of the cyst wall is required to treat symptomatic large hepatic cysts permanently. This could involve removing a portion of the nearby attenuated liver parenchyma. A properly executed operation reduces the likelihood of a cyst recurrence. It's critical to understand the intrahepatic biliary and vascular anatomy to prevent intraoperative bleeding or bile leaks. After the cyst wall is removed, it is sent to pathology for a frozen-section analysis to check for the presence of any malignant or premalignant cells. To obtain negative margins, a formal oncologic liver resection is required when premalignant or malignant cells are found.

On the same day as the procedure, the majority of patients are able to return home. After this procedure, placing an abdominal drain is usually not necessary. A minor proportion of patients necessitate an overnight hospital stay, primarily because of health issues. Seeing a skilled liver surgeon is crucial when treating large, symptomatic hepatic cysts.

4.8.5. Repeat Liver Resection

During the surveillance phase following a liver resection, new tumors may develop using open, laparoscopic, or robotic liver surgery techniques. Usually, new liver cancers are discovered elsewhere in the liver, not where previous liver resections were performed. The recurrent potentials of each type of liver cancer varies. Many years following the initial liver surgery, metastatic colon and rectal cancers can recur in the liver. Monitoring the level of tumor markers is not as important as detecting an early tumor recurrence using imaging modalities like CT scan or MRI. To verify the recurrence of liver cancer, a liver biopsy is frequently required. To rule out other distant metastases, such as metastases to the brain, lung, bone, or retroperitoneal lymph nodes, a PET scan can be helpful. Upon diagnosis of liver cancer recurrence, prompt consultation with a liver surgeon or specialist is imperative.

Over the past ten years, there has been a significant change in the management of recurrent liver cancer. The indication for repeat liver resection is expanded by advancements in the safety profile of liver resection/liver surgery as well as the refinement of the minimally invasive liver surgery technique. Repeat liver resection combined with liver ablation and systemic chemotherapy administration is a viable treatment option for a large number of patients with recurrent liver tumors. Repeat liver resection has been safely shown to improve overall long-term survival in cases of colorectal cancer with liver metastases. After the initial liver resection and the diagnosis of index metastatic disease, some patients survive for over ten years. Preoperative assessment for a reoperation on the liver is essentially the same as for the first resection. A repeat liver resection is anticipated to present a greater technical challenge, primarily because of the volume of liver remnant and the formation of scar tissue surrounding the liver, diaphragm, and intestines. Repeat liver resections, however, can be performed safely by a skilled liver surgeon and have results that are comparable to those of the first procedure in the short- and long-term. Repeat liver resections are made simpler when minimally invasive liver surgery is used for the initial liver resection. This is partly due to the fact that less scar tissue forms following minimally invasive liver surgery. Skilled liver surgeons can also safely perform the repeat liver resections with minimally invasive surgery.

For patients with recurrent liver tumors or liver cancers, the liver surgery unit offers both robotic and laparoscopic liver resection options. With minimally invasive liver surgery, a large open incision is not necessary to perform a repeat liver resection, reducing the risk of complications after surgery and promoting a quicker recovery. Additionally, it produces a great reduction in intra-abdominal adhesions, which makes it possible to perform a minimally invasive follow-up procedure in the future if another tumor in the liver recurs. Every liver resection is performed using parenchymal sparing liver surgery to preserve as much non-cancerous liver parenchyma as possible. In this case, advanced interventional radiology techniques like preoperative portal vein embolization or portal vein ligation—which cause the future liver to swell—are also commonly used. For patients whose cancer has returned and spread to their liver, a liver transplant is not a viable option.

Depending on the location, number, and proximity of the tumor to the major biliovascular structures, liver tumor ablation (either radiofrequency ablation or microwave ablation) may also be combined with additional liver resections. The liver surgeon will decide this after examining the CT and/or MRI scan results before the procedure. When a patient with metastatic liver cancer becomes tumor-free, their overall survival benefits are noticeably longer.

4.8.6. Laparoscopic & Robotic Bile Duct Repair

A large gallstone impinging on the bile duct wall and causing a pressure necrosis phenomenon (known as Mirizzi syndrome) are among the numerous causes of bile duct leaks. Other causes include abdominal trauma from gunshot or stabbing wounds, or an unintentional injury to the bile duct during a challenging laparoscopic cholecystectomy. As for bile duct leaks, iatrogenic laparoscopic cholecystectomy is the most frequent cause. Being a highly specialized procedure, biliary surgery calls for education and experience. The majority of general surgeons lack the necessary technical proficiency for biliary surgery. Patients can have different biliary tract anatomy, and identifying this abnormality is essential before undergoing bile duct surgery. Liver surgeons gain knowledge of subsegmental biliary anatomy through the surgical resection of bile duct cancer (Klatskin tumor resection). Accessory branches from perihilar liver segments are easily found and, if not properly identified, can cause injury.

Advanced endoscopists and interventional radiologists are members of the multidisciplinary team that treats bile duct leaks. While many patients with bile duct injury are identified during the gallbladder removal procedure, a sizable portion are identified a few days later. Due to the bile duct leak, patients typically experience fever, abdominal pain, nausea, vomiting, jaundice (yellowing of the skin and eyes), or failure to thrive. Bile duct leaks and injuries are treated non-operatively whenever possible by a percutaneous transhepatic technique or by endoscopic implantation of a biliary stent. From the index diagnosis, a surgical intervention is required for specific types of bile duct leaks or injuries, such as a complete transection of the bile duct. For whatever reason, the majority of biliary surgeries are still carried out as open procedures. Because minimally invasive bile duct repair (laparoscopic or robotic) has a lower rate of postoperative complications, less pain, a shorter recovery period, and an earlier return to work, it is preferred whenever possible. Every bile duct repair usually involves the installation of a closed suction drain. This is taken out later, either in the office during the first follow-up visit or before the patient is discharged from the hospital.

4.8.7. Laparoscopic Bile Duct Exploration

When endoscopic or percutaneous methods fail, surgical exploration of the bile duct is required to remove debris or stones causing obstructive jaundice. This procedure is typically carried out using an open method. Robotic Bile Duct Exploration is a minimally invasive surgical technique that minimizes postoperative complications by avoiding a large open incision. A tiny endoscope is put into the bile duct during bile duct exploration to see the stones or debris. Using this tiny endoscope, a retrieval basket can be inserted to remove the stones or debris once they have been visualized. Many community hospitals may not have the advanced surgical and endoscopic skills needed for this procedure.

4.8.8. Two Stage Extended Liver Resection

Certain patients are referred to the practice because they have multiple large liver tumors that either completely replace or occupy the liver, necessitating the removal of more than 70% of the liver's total volume. Because of the extended resection, these patients will not have enough functioning liver parenchyma to support their metabolism, which puts them at risk of developing postoperative liver failure. After resection, at least 30% of the healthy, functioning liver parenchyma needs to be left to prevent postoperative liver failure. In the past, an interventional radiologist would embolize the ipsilateral portal vein that enters the tumor side. In roughly 6 to 8 weeks, this maneuver will cause contralateral liver hypertrophy or growth. About 70% of cases are successful with this procedure. 30% of cases have the contralateral liver failing to hypertrophy. Use a two-stage extended liver resection technique called the ALPPS procedure (Associating Liver Partition and Portal Vein Ligation for Staged Hepatectomy) to lessen this.

A laparoscopic diagnostic examination of the liver and abdominal cavity is performed in the first stage. Perform a laparoscopic liver partition (partial or full) and portal vein ligation after ruling out tumor spread within the abdomen. The contralateral liver segments hypertrophy to greater than 30% in about 2 weeks, which lowers the risk of liver failure following extended resection. To record the percentage of liver hypertrophy, a unique CT scan protocol with volumetric rendering is acquired. The second stage involves finishing the extended liver resection to cure the liver tumor or tumors.

4.8.9. Laparoscopic Liver Ablation

For patients who are not candidates for liver resection, local therapy combined with thermal ablation represents a secondary alternative treatment option for a variety of tumors. The most common reasons to recommend ablation instead of liver resection are marginal liver reserve, the need to remove excessive amounts of normal liver to clear a small tumor (<3 cm), and the patient's inability to tolerate a major operation due to medical issues. When compared to liver ablations performed percutaneously by an interventional radiologist, laparoscopically delivered ablations are linked to a decreased rate of tumor recurrence (6% vs. 14%). Additionally, a direct examination of the entire abdominal cavity and liver surface can be done using the laparoscopic or robotic approach to look for small metastatic tumors that would otherwise go undetected on high-quality CT/MRI scans (18%). After six to twelve hours of observation, many patients can be released from care. When there are additional tumors on the other liver lobe, liver ablation is also commonly performed in conjunction with tissue-preserving liver resection to achieve tumor-free status.

4.8.10. Extended Hepatectomy for Hilar Cholangiocarcinoma

In clinical practice, hilar cholangiocarcinoma detection in extrahepatic bile duct strictures remains a challenge. Most cholangiocarcinomas cause painless jaundice, or yellow discoloration of the eyes and skin when the tumor obstructs the biliary drainage system. Computed tomography is one of the first studies obtained in patients with suspected biliary tract obstruction because of its widespread availability. At the moment, the best investigative method for a suspected hilar cholangiocarcinoma is a high-quality MRI/MRCP. The majority of patients have biliary drainage done before being referred for resection. Biliary stents should ideally not be placed before resectability evaluation.

For the surgeon, heionar cholangiocarcinoma remains a challenging case. Surgery is the only effective treatment for patients with this condition, and it should only be tried in specialized facilities. More aggressive treatment has resulted from recent advancements in surgical treatment. A radical surgical approach is defined as requiring an extra hepatic resection. The Bismuth-Corlette (and/or Blumgart T-staging) classification helps determine the extent of surgery needed for hilar cholangiocarcinoma.

- **In type I and II:** the extrahepatic bile ducts and gallbladder were removed in one piece, leaving 5–10 mm bile duct margins. A Roux-en-Y hepatico-jejunostomy was performed along with a regional lymphadenectomy.
- **In type III:** trisegmentectomy or right or left hepatectomy combined with hilar resection.
- **In type IV:** right or left

In Type III and IV hilar cholangiocarcinomas, vascular recons-truction of the portal vein is frequently necessary. For these kinds of major liver surgeries, preoperative planning and volume manipulation techniques are also necessary to perform a radical resection with clear margins, prevent post-hepatetomy liver failure, and induce hypertrophy of the future liver remnant.

4.9. The Enterohepatic Circulation of Bile Acids

The movement of biliary acids, bilirubin, medications, and other substances from the liver into the bile, then into the small intestine, where they are absorbed by enterocytes and then returned to the liver, is known as enterohepatic circulation. In the field of toxicology, enterohepatic circulation is particularly crucial because many lipophilic xenobiotics cause repeated liver damage through this process.

4.9.1. Biliary Acids

- **The Circuit:** Cholesterol is broken down by hepatocytes into cholic acid and chenodeoxycholic acid. Water soluble primary conjugated bile acids, also known as bile salts, are synthesized when these lipid-soluble bile acids are conjugated (reversibly attached), primarily to taurine or glycine molecules. These bile acids pass through the major duodenal papilla of the common bile duct and into the gall bladder for storage during the interdigestive phase and digestion, respectively. The enterohepatic circulation recycles 95% of the bile acids that are transported to the duodenum.

The majority of bile acids are ionized due to the pH of the small intestine, and they primarily exist as their sodium salts, which are referred to as "primary conjugated bile salts." Bacteria dehydroxylate some of the primary bile salts in the colon and lower small intestine to create secondary conjugated bile salts, which are still soluble in water. These conjugated primary bile salts are actively reabsorbed into the hepatic portal circulation along the proximal and distal ileum. Part of the primary and secondary conjugated bile salts are deconjugated by bacteria into lipid-soluble bile acids, which enter the hepatic portal circulation passively. Ultimately, the conjugated bile acids that haven't been ionized are absorbed passively. Ileum venous blood enters the portal vein directly and subsequently the liver sinusoids. Very few bile acids leave the healthy liver and enter the bloodstream because hepatocytes there extract bile acids with extreme efficiency. Enterohepatic recirculation results in the approximate 20 times reuse of each bile salt molecule, frequently several times in a single digestive phase.

- **Function:** Biliary acids aid in the absorption of fats and other substances because they are present in the intestines.

4.9.2. Bilirubin

The liver's glucuronyltransferase enzyme conjugates bilirubin with glucuronic acid, rendering it soluble in aqueous solutions. A large portion of it enters the bile and exits through the small intestine. Conjugated bilirubin is not reabsorbed in the small intestine, despite the fact that 20% of the secreted bilirubinoid bile is. In the large intestine, colonic bacteria metabolize all conjugated bilirubin to urobilinogen, which is subsequently further oxidized to urobilin and stercobilin. Feces are brown because of uribilin, stercobilin, and the breakdown products of these substances. But some of the urobilinogen that is reabsorbed is also secreted in bile, which is a component of the enterohepatic circulation, just like bile. The residual urobilinogen is excreted in the urine, where it transforms into urobilin, the oxidized form that gives urine its distinctive yellow hue.

4.9.3. Drugs

Aspirin, paracetamol, diazepam, lorazepam, morphine, metronidazole, and chloramphenicol. This pathway is used by endogenous substrates such as thyroxine, steroidal hormones, and bilirubin in addition to medications. The process by which drugs are conjugated to glucuronic acid in the liver, eliminated into bile, metabolized back into the free drug by intestinal bacteria, and then reabsorbed into plasma is known as enterohepatic circulation of drugs. Lower dosages of medications can be therapeutically effective for many drugs that go through this process because the "recycling" of the drug reduces elimination. However, for a select few medications that are extremely harmful to the intestines (e.g., irinotecan), these molecules can undergo a process that turns them from being relatively harmless to highly toxic. As a result, blocking this step may be protective. Inhibiting this process lowers drug levels and lessens therapeutic effect for most drugs that go through enterohepatic circulation and are not toxic to the intestine. For instance, the use of antibiotics that destroy gut bacteria frequently results in a decrease in enterohepatic drug circulation, necessitating a brief increase in dosage until the antibiotic is stopped and the gut's bacterial population is restored. One kind of medication interaction is the impact of antibiotics on the enterohepatic circulation of other medications.

A Closer Look

Gallbladder: History

Images of the gallbladder and biliary tree can be seen in ancient Etruscan models from 200 BCE and Babylonian models from 2000 BCE, both of which are linked to religious devotion. Humans have been known to suffer from gallbladder diseases since ancient times; gallstones from 1500 BCE were discovered in the mummy of Princess Amenen of Thebes. According to some historians, Alexander the Great's death might have been related to a severe case of cholecystitis. Although the gallbladder has been known to exist since the fifth century, information about its diseases and function has only recently become available, especially in the last two centuries.

Perhaps as a result of a diet high in grains and vegetables and low in meat, gallstones were uncommon in earlier times, as evidenced by the Renaissance's descriptions of the condition. It was Anthonius Benevinius who first made the link between gallstones and symptoms in 1506. Gallstones are unlikely to be the cause of jaundice in an enlarged, nontender gallbladder, according to Ludwig Georg Courvoisier, who made this observation in 1890 after reviewing several cases that led to the creation of the famous Courvoisier's law.

Physician Joenisius performed the first cholecystolithotomy (surgical removal of a gallstone) in 1676, removing the stones from a biliary fistula that had developed on its own. The first known cholecystotomy was carried out by Stough Hobbs in 1867, though French surgeon Jean Louis Petit had previously written about the procedure in the middle of the eighteenth century. In 1882, German surgeon Carl Langenbuch carried out the first cholecystectomy on a cholelithiasis patient. Prior to this, the goal of surgery was to create a fistula to allow gallstones to be drained. Langenbuch reasoned that humans could live without a gallbladder because many other mammal species do not have one. In the 1920s, the question of whether surgical removal of the gallbladder or just the gallstones was preferable was resolved, with most agreeing that the former was. The gallbladder could not be seen with medical imaging methods such as contrast medium or CT scans until the middle and end of the 20th century. Erich Mühe of Germany carried out the first laparoscopic cholecystectomy in 1985, though French surgeons Phillipe Mouret and Francois Dubois are frequently given credit for their 1987 and 1988 procedures, respectively.

Summary

- The biliary tract (also biliary tree or biliary system) refers to the liver, gallbladder and bile ducts, and how they work together to make, store and secrete bile. Bile consists of water, electrolytes, bile acids, cholesterol, phospholipids and conjugated bilirubin. Some components are synthesized by hepatocytes (liver cells); the rest are extracted from the blood by the liver.
- The biliary tract refers to the path by which bile is secreted by the liver then transported to the duodenum, the first part of the small intestine.
- Bile is secreted by the liver into small ducts that join to form the common hepatic duct. Between meals, secreted bile is stored in the gall bladder, where 80–90% of the water and electrolytes can be absorbed, leaving the bile acids and cholesterol.
- The liver is a dark reddish brown, wedge-shaped organ with two lobes of unequal size and shape. A human liver normally weighs approximately 1.5 kilograms (3.3 pounds) and has a width of about 15 centimeters (6 inches).
- Organogenesis, the development of the organs, takes place from the third to the eighth week during embryogenesis. The origins of the liver lie in both the ventral portion of the foregut endoderm (endoderm being one of the three embryonic germ layers) and the constituents of the adjacent septum transversum mesenchyme.
- Bile or gall, is a yellow-green fluid produced by the liver of most vertebrates that aids the digestion of lipids in the small intestine.
- In the human liver, bile is composed of 97–98% water, 0.7% bile salts, 0.2% bilirubin, 0.51% fats (cholesterol, fatty acids, and lecithin), and 200 meq/L inorganic salts. The two main pigments of bile are bilirubin, which is yellow, and its oxidized form biliverdin, which is green.
- Bile acids are steroid acids found predominantly in the bile of mammals and other vertebrates. Diverse bile acids are synthesized in the liver. Bile acids are conjugated with taurine or glycine residues to give anions called bile salts.
- Most drugs are xenobiotics, ie, chemical substances not naturally produced by the body. Xenobiotics undergo various body processes for detoxification, thus reducing their toxicity and allowing them to be readily available for excretion. These processes allow for the chemical modification of drugs into their metabolites and are known as drug metabolism or metabolic biotransformation.
- With the advent of combinatorial chemistry, an increasing number of new chemical entities that are more lipophilic and characterized by high molecular weight are being synthesized and screened during the drug discovery process.
- The gallbladder is a small hollow organ about the size and shape of a pear. It is a part of the biliary system, also known as the biliary tree or biliary tract. The biliary system is a series of ducts within the liver, gallbladder, and pancreas that empty into the small intestine.
- Liver resection is the removal of part of the liver during an operation.

- Enterohepatic circulation is the circulation of biliary acids, bilirubin, drugs or other substances from the liver to the bile, followed by entry into the small intestine, absorption by the enterocyte and transport back to the liver. Enterohepatic circulation is an especially important concept in the field of toxicology as many lipophilic xenobiotics undergo this process causing repeated liver damage.

References

1. Ahmed, M. (2022). Functional, diagnostic and therapeutic aspects of bile. *Clinical and Experimental Gastroenterology, 15*, 105–120. https://doi.org/10.2147/CEG.S360563.
2. Alhmada, Y., Selimovic, D., Murad, F., et al. (2017). Hepatitis C virus-associated pruritus: Etiopathogenesis and therapeutic strategies. *World Journal of Gastroenterology, 23*(5), 743–750. https://doi.org/10.3748/wjg.v23.i5.743.
3. Burns, L. (Ed.). (2007). *Liver Cirrhosis Research*. New York : Nova Biomedical Books.
4. Clavien, P.-A., & Baillie, J. (Eds.). (2006). *Diseases of the Gallbladder and Bile Ducts*. Blackwell Publishing Ltd. https://doi.org/10.1002/9780470986981.
5. Di Ciaula, A., Garruti, G., Lunardi Baccetto, R., et al. (2017). Bile acid physiology. *Annals of Hepatology, 16*(Suppl 1), S4–S14. https://doi.org/10.5604/01.3001.0010.5493.
6. Dooley, J. (2011). *Sherlock's Diseases of the Liver and Biliary System*. Wiley-Blackwell, 2011 Oct; 11(5): 506, DOI:10.1002/9781444341294 .
7. Ferrell, L. D., Kakar, S. (2011). *Liver Pathology.* United States: Springer Publishing Company.
8. Gallaher, J. R., & Charles, A. (2022). Acute cholecystitis: A review. *JAMA, 327*(10), 965–975. https://doi.org/10.1001/jama.2022.2350.
9. Gu, X. X., Zhang, M. P., Zhao, Y. F., & Huang, G. M. (2020). Clinical and microbiological characteristics of patients with biliary disease. *World Journal of Gastroenterology, 26*(14), 1638–1646. https://doi.org/10.3748/wjg.v26.i14.1638.
10. Hofmann, A. F., & Hagey, L. R. (2014). Key discoveries in bile acid chemistry and biology and their clinical applications: History of the last eight decades. *Journal of Lipid Research, 55*(8), 1553–1595. https://doi.org/10.1194/jlr.R049437.
11. Karaliotas, C. C., & Papaconstantinou, T. (2006). Anatomical variations and anomalies of the biliary tree, veins and arteries. In C. C. Karaliotas, C. E. Broelsch, & N. A. Habib (Eds.), *Liver and Biliary Tract Surgery* (pp. 35–48). Springer.
12. Kostov, D. V., & Kobakov, G. L. (2011). Six rare biliary tract anatomic variations: Implications for liver surgery. *EAJM, 43*(2), 67–72. https://doi.org/10.5152/eajm.2011.16.
13. Miller MA. Book Review: Atlas of Tumor Pathology: Tumors of the Liver and Intrahepatic Bile Ducts. Veterinary Pathology. 2002;39(5):608-609. doi:10.1354/vp.39-5-608-a
14. Pan, G. (2019). Roles of hepatic drug transporters in drug disposition and liver toxicity. *Advances in Experimental Medicine and Biology, 1141*, 293–340. https://doi.org/10.1007/978-981-13-7647-4_6.
15. Maino C, Vernuccio F, Cannella R, Cortese F, Franco PN, Gaetani C, Giannini V, Inchingolo R, Ippolito D, Defeudis A, Pilato G, Tore D, Faletti R, Gatti M. Liver metastases: The role of magnetic resonance imaging. World J Gastroenterol. 2023 Sep 28;29(36):5180-5197.

16. Patel, M., Taskar, K. S., & Zamek-Gliszczynski, M. J. (2016). Importance of hepatic transporters in clinical disposition of drugs and their metabolites. *Journal of Clinical Pharmacology, 56*(Suppl 7), S23–S39. https://doi.org/10.1002/jcph.671.

17. Quinn, R. A., Melnik, A. V., Vrbanac, A., et al. (2020). Global chemical effects of the microbiome include new bile-acid conjugations. *Nature, 579*(7797), 123–129. https://doi.org/10.1038/s41586-020-2047-9.

18. Seleem, H. M., Nada, A. S., Naguib, M. A., & Abdelmaksoud, O. R. (2021). Serum immunoglobulin G4 in patients with nonmalignant common bile duct stricture. *Menoufia Medical Journal, 34*, 1275–1283.

19. Rodes J. Diseases of the Liver and Biliary System: S Sherlock, J Dooley. London: Blackwell, 2002, pp 706. ISBN 0-6320-5582- 0. Gut. 2003 Apr;52(4):615.

Chapter 5

THE SMALL INTESTINE

Contents

Introduction

The small intestine is where most food digestion and absorption occurs. It is a long, narrow, folded or coiled tube that runs from the stomach to the large intestine. It is located in the lower and central abdominal cavity and is between 22 and 25 feet (roughly 6 to 7 meters) long. It is extremely convoluted. The intestines are supported and partially suspended by a thin membrane called the mesentery. The mesentery is home to a vast network of blood vessels as well as fat regions that aid in the organs' ability to retain heat. Two divisions of the autonomic nervous system send nerves to the small intestine: sympathetic nerves suppress intestinal movements, while parasympathetic nerves cause the muscular contractions that move food along the tract (peristalsis). The duodenum, jejunum, and ileum are the three successive regions of the small intestine that are typically distinguished. These areas are one continuous tube, and while there are some distinguishable differences between each area, they are not clearly divided. The first region is the duodenum, which is next to the stomach. It is not supported by the mesentery and is only 23 to 28 cm (9 to 11 inches) long with the widest diameter. The duodenum receives juices from the pancreas, liver, and gallbladder that aid in the digestion of proteins, carbs, and fats while also neutralizing stomach acids. About two-fifths of the remaining tract is located in the second region, the jejunum, which is located in the abdomen's central section. The jejunum has a large blood supply, which gives it a deep red color. Its peristaltic movements are strong and quick, and the mesentery that supports it has little fat. The lower abdomen contains the ileum. The mesentery has more fatty regions, its walls are thinner and narrower than in the preceding section, and its blood supply is more constrained. Peristalstic movements are also slower.

The mucous membrane that lines the intestinal wall of the small intestine is folded transversely into plicae circulares, and in larger vertebrates, the cavity is punctured by tiny projections that resemble fingers and are called villi. The area of the secreting and absorbing surface is significantly increased by these structures. There are a lot of tiny glands inside the walls of the small intestine. The main purpose of the Brunner gland secretions in the duodenum's submucosa is to shield the intestinal walls from stomach acids. Within the mucous membrane, the Lieberkühn glands secrete digestive enzymes, act as Brunner gland outlet ports, and generate new cells to replace the surface-membrane cells lost from the tips of villi. Materials that are being digested are moved through the small intestine by peristaltic waves. Meanwhile, churning movements known as rhythmic segmentation mechanically break up these materials, thoroughly mix them with digestive enzymes from the intestinal wall, liver, and pancreas, and bring them into contact with the absorbing surface.

Orientation and Directional Terms

Term	Definition	Illustration
Duodenum	The duodenum is the first part of the small intestine that the stomach feeds into. It's a short, descending chute (about 10 inches long) that curves around the pancreas in a "C" shape before connecting to the rest of the coiled intestines.	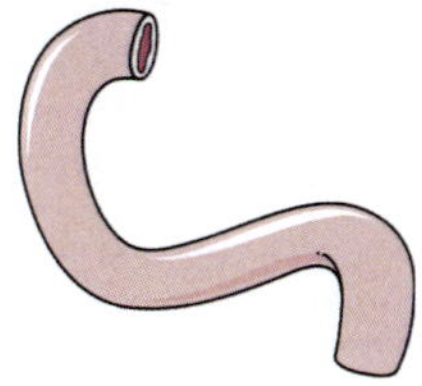
Jejunum	The remaining small intestine lays in many coils inside the lower abdominal cavity. Its middle section, called the jejunum, makes up a little less than half of this remaining length. The jejunum is characterized by many blood vessels, which give it a deep red color.	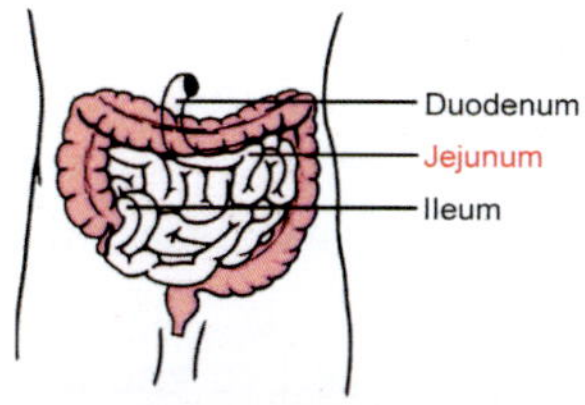
Villi	Intestinal villi are tiny, finger-like projections made up of cells that line the entire length of your small intestine.	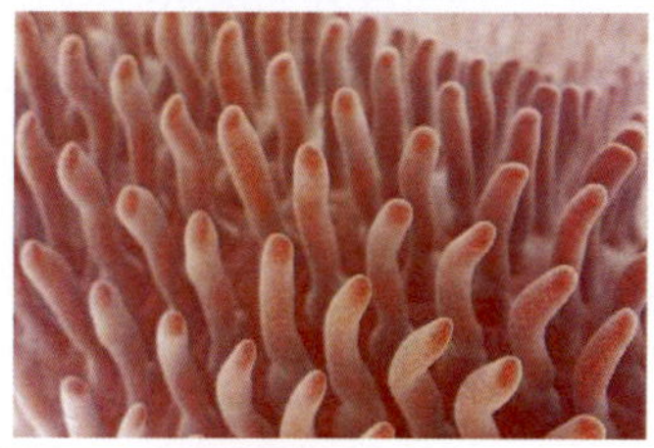
Intestinal Glands	The intestinal glands (glands of the great intestine) are minute tubular prolongations of the mucous membrane arranged perpendicularly, side by side, over its entire surface; they are longer, more numerous, and placed in much closer apposition than those of the small intestine; and they open by minute rounded orifices upon the surface, giving it a cribriform appearance. Each gland is lined by short columnar epithelium and contains numerous goblet cells.	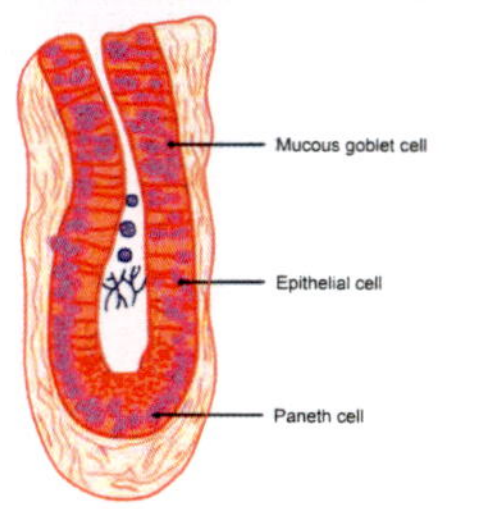

5.1. Anatomy and Structure

The small intestine, the body's main digestive organ, receives chyme that is expelled from the stomach. Not only does the majority of digestion take place here, but almost all absorption does as well. About 3:05 meters (10 feet) is the length of the small intestine in a living person, and because muscle tone is lost in cadavers, their length is approximately twice that of the alimentary canal. You may wonder why it is called "small" given that it is approximately five times longer than the large intestine. Its name actually comes from the fact that its diameter is comparatively smaller—roughly 2.54 cm (1 in) as opposed to the large intestine's 7.62 cm (3 in). As we'll see in a moment, the folds and projections of the small intestine's lining work together to give it an enormous surface area, approximately 200 m^2, which is more than 100 times the surface area of your skin, in addition to its length. The intricate processes of digestion and absorption that take place within it require this vast surface area.

5.1.1. Structure

There are three distinct regions within the coiled tube of the small intestine. The ileum, jejunum, and duodenum are arranged from proximal (at the stomach) to distal. The duodenum, which starts at the pyloric sphincter and is 25.4 cm (10 in) long, is the shortest section. It curves C-shaped around the head of the pancreas after passing the pyloric sphincter, ascends anteriorly once more to rejoin the jejunum, and bends posteriorly behind the peritoneum to become retroperitoneal. As a result, the duodenum can be separated into four segments: the ascending, descending, horizontal, and superior duodenum. The hepatopancreatic ampulla, also known as the Vater ampulla, is of special interest. The bile duct, which transports bile from the liver, and the main pancreatic duct, which transports pancreatic juice from the pancreas, converge at the ampulla, a structure in the duodenal wall that denotes the change from the anterior to the mid-region of the alimentary canal. This ampulla ends at the major duodenal papilla, a small structure resembling a volcano that connects to the duodenum. The flow of pancreatic juice and bile from the ampulla into the duodenum is controlled by the hepatopancreatic sphincter, also known as the sphincter of Oddi (Figure 5.1).

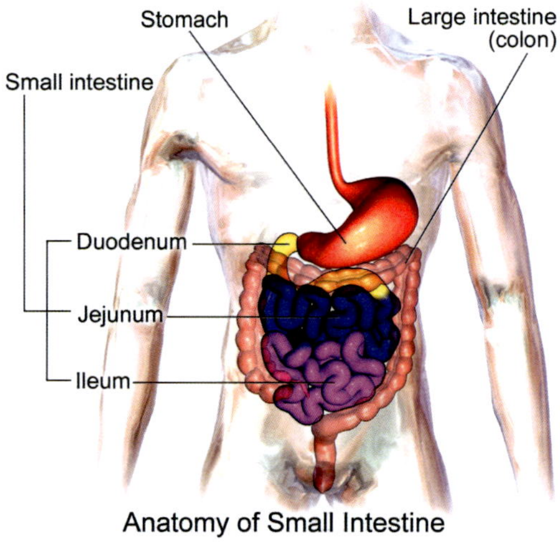

Figure 5.1. *Labeled diagram of the small intestine and its surrounding structures.*

Source: By BruceBlaus- Own work, CC BY 3.0, https://commons.wikimedia.org/w/index.php?curid=28909224.

The jejunum connects the duodenum to the ileum and is approximately 0.9 meters (3 feet) long in its entirety. The Latin word jejunum means "empty," and the ancient Greeks are said to have given it this name after observing that it was always empty after death. The ileum, the last section of the small intestine, and the jejunum do not clearly separate from one another. The longest section of the small intestine is called the ileum, and it is approximately 1.8 meters (6 feet) long. Compared to the jejunum, it is thicker, more vascular, and has more developed mucosal folds. At the ileocecal sphincter (or valve), the ileum connects to the cecum, the first segment of the large intestine. The mesentery attaches the ileum and jejunum to the posterior abdominal wall. These three sections of the small intestine are framed by the large intestine.

The small intestine is extrinsically innervated by sympathetic nerve fibers from the thoracic splanchnic nerve and parasympathetic nerve fibers from the vagus nerve. Its primary arterial supply is the superior mesenteric artery. Veins empty into the superior mesenteric vein while running parallel to the arteries. The hepatic portal vein then transports nutrient-rich blood from the small intestine to the liver.

5.1.2. Histology

The small intestine wall is made up of the four typical layers found in the digestive system, but it has three unique features in the mucosa and submucosa. These features – circular folds, villi, and microvilli – greatly increase the absorptive surface area of the small intestine by more than 600 times. These adaptations are most prominent in the upper two-thirds of the small intestine, where most absorption takes place (Figure 5.2).

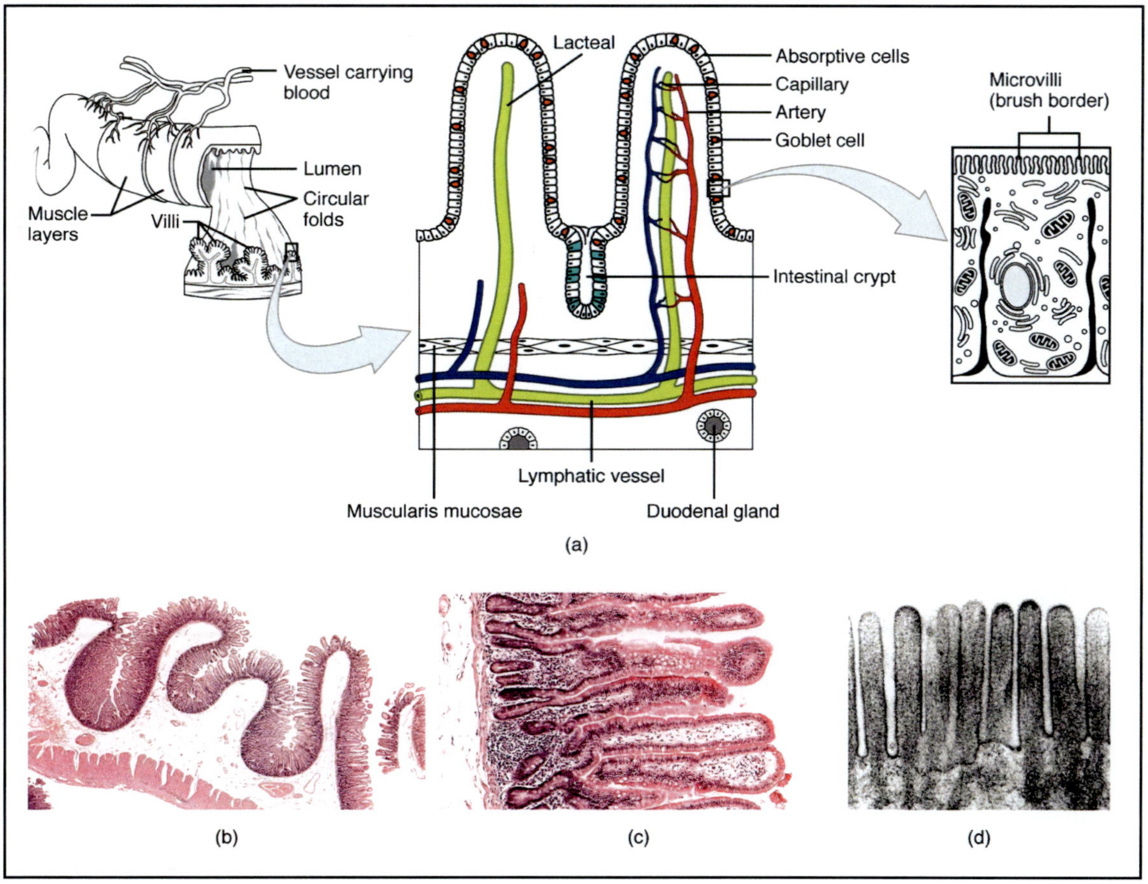

Figure 5.2. *(a) The absorptive surface of the small intestine is vastly enlarged by the presence of circular folds, villi, and microvilli. (b) Micrograph of the circular folds. (c) Micrograph of the villi. (d) Electron micrograph of the microvilli. From left to right, LM x 56, LM x 508, EM x 196,000.*

Source: https://courses.lumenlearning.com/suny-ap2/chapter/the-small-and-large-intestines/

- **Circular Folds:** A circular fold, also known as a plica circulare, is a deep ridge found in the submucosa and mucosa. These folds aid in absorption and extend from the middle of the ileum to the proximal portion of the duodenum. Because of their shape, the chyme passes through the small intestine spiraling rather than traveling straight forward. Spiraling gives nutrients time to fully absorb by slowing down their movement through the chyme.
- **Villi:** The hair-like, vascularized projections known as villi (singular: villus) that are tiny, 0.5–1 mm long, give the mucosa its furry texture within the circular folds. The surface area of the epithelium is greatly increased by the 20–40 villi that are present per square millimeter. The villi are covered in mucosal epithelium, which is mainly made up of absorptive cells. Each villus has a capillary bed made up of one venule and one arteriole, as well as a lymphatic capillary known as a lacteal, in addition to muscle and connective tissue that support its structure. While the breakdown products of fats are absorbed by the lacteals and then transferred to the bloodstream through the lymphatic system, the breakdown products of proteins and carbohydrates (sugars and amino acids) can enter the bloodstream directly.
- **Microvilli:** Microvilli, also known as microvillus, are much smaller than villi, as their name implies (1 μm). They are supported by microfilaments inside the mucosal epithelial cells, which are cylindrical extensions of the plasma membrane's apical surface. The brush border is a mass of bristles that is implied by the collective microscopic appearance of individual microvillus, despite their small size making it difficult to see them individually. Enzymes that complete the breakdown of proteins and carbohydrates are adhered to the surface of the microvilli membranes. The small intestine has an estimated 200 million microvilli per square millimeter, which significantly increases the plasma membrane's surface area and improves absorption.
- **Intestinal Glands:** The mucosa between the villi is speckled with deep fissures that each lead into a tubular intestinal gland (crypt of Lieberkühn), which is formed by cells that line the fissures, in addition to the three specialized absorptive features that were just discussed. These result in the production of intestinal juice, which is a slightly alkaline (pH 7.4–7.8) combination of mucus and water. About 0.95 to 1.9 liters (1–2 quarts) are secreted daily in response to the intestinal mucosa being irritated by chyme or the small intestine's distention. The complex mucus-secreting duodenal glands, also known as Brunner's glands, are located only in the submucosa of the duodenum. These glands produce an alkaline mucus that is rich in bicarbonate and acts as a buffer against the acidic chyme that enters from the stomach.

Table 5.1 provides a detailed overview of the functions of the cells in the small intestinal mucosa.

Table 5.1. Cells of the Small Intestinal Mucosa

Cell Type	Location in the Mucosa	Function
Absorptive	Epithelium/intestinal glands	Digestion and absorption of nutrients in chyme
Goblet	Epithelium/intestinal glands	Secretion of mucus
Paneth	Intestinal glands	Secretion of the bactericidal enzyme lysozyme; phagocytosis
G cells	Intestinal glands of duodenum	Secretion of the hormone intestinal gastrin
I cells	Intestinal glands of duodenum	Secretion of the hormone cholecystokinin, which stimulates the release of pancreatic juices and bile
K cells	Intestinal glands	Secretion of the hormone glucose-dependent insulinotropic peptide, which stimulates the release of insulin
M cells	Intestinal glands of duodenum and jejunum	Secretion of the hormone motilin, which accelerates gastric emptying, stimulates intestinal peristalsis and stimulates the production of pepsin
S cells	Intestinal glands	Secretion of the hormone secretin

Source: https://courses.lumenlearning.com/suny-ap2/chapter/the-small-and-large-intestines/.

- **Intestinal MALT:** The lamina propria of the small intestine mucosa contains a significant amount of mucosa-associated lymphoid tissue (MALT). Along with individual lymphatic nodules, clusters of intestinal MALT known as Peyer's patches are found mainly in the distal ileum. These patches work to prevent bacteria from entering the bloodstream. Peyer's patches are most noticeable in younger individuals and become less prominent with age, reflecting changes in the immune system's overall function.

5.1.3. Mechanical Digestion in the Small Intestine

Intestinal smooth muscle movement consists of segmentation as well as a type of peristalsis known as migrating motility complexes. Here, there are no peristaltic mixing waves similar to those found in the stomach (Figure 5.3).

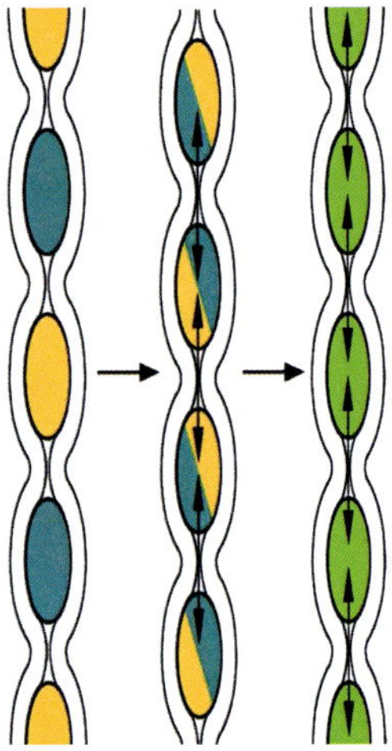

Figure 5.3. *Segmentation separates chyme and then pushes it back together, mixing it and providing time for digestion and absorption.*

Source: https://courses.lumenlearning.com/suny-ap2/chapter/the-small-and-large-intestines/.

When the small intestine is undergoing segmentation, the rings of smooth muscle contract and then relax repeatedly, giving the appearance that the contents are being moved back and forth gradually. Chyme is not forced through the digestive tract by segmentation in the small intestine. Instead, food particles are forced up against the mucosa to be absorbed by combining the chyme with digestive juices. At a rate of roughly 12 times per minute, the duodenum is the site of the fastest segmentation. There are only roughly eight segmentations in the ileum per minute. The small intestine wall shrinks when the majority of the chyme has been absorbed. At this point, transport movements take the place of the localized segmentation process. The hormone motilin, which is secreted by the duodenal mucosa, causes a migrating motility complex, which in turn triggers peristalsis. Starting in the duodenum, these complexes push chyme through a small portion of the small intestine before stopping. The second contraction starts a little bit lower than the first, pushes the chyme through the small intestine a little bit further, and then stops. It takes these complexes 90 to 120 minutes to eventually reach the end of the ileum as they travel slowly down the small intestine and force chyme along the way. The procedure is now repeated, this time beginning in the duodenum.

Food residue can pass through the ileocecal valve, a sphincter, into the cecum, the first section of the large intestine, when ileum motility increases. Normally, the sphincter is constricted. Both nerves and hormones regulate the ileocecal sphincter's ability to relax. Firstly, the force of ileal segmentation increases when the stomach's digestive activity triggers the gastroileal reflex. Second, the ileocecal sphincter relaxes as a result of the hormone gastrin being released by the stomach, which also improves ileal motility. Backward pressure aids in the closure of the sphincter after chyme passes through, preventing backflow into the ileum. By the time you eat dinner, this reflex has completely cleared your stomach and small intestine of your lunch. The entire amount of chyme needs to pass through the small intestine in 3–5 hours.

5.1.4. Chemical Digestion in the Small Intestine

Pancreatic and intestinal juices help the small intestine finish the digestion of proteins and carbohydrates, which starts in the stomach. Since lipids enter the intestine mostly undigested, a major emphasis of this discussion is on lipid digestion, which is made possible by the enzyme pancreatic lipase and bile. Additionally, pancreatic and intestinal juice mix to create a liquid medium that aids in absorption. The majority of water is also absorbed through osmosis in the intestine. Digestive enzymes are also produced by the absorptive cells of the small intestine and inserted into the plasma membranes of the microvilli. This sets the small intestine apart from the stomach because it shows that enzymatic digestion takes place on the luminal surfaces of the mucosal cell in addition to in the lumen.

For chemical digestion to work effectively, chyme needs to be released from the stomach gradually and in small portions. This is necessary because chyme is usually hypertonic when it leaves the stomach, and if large amounts were to enter the small intestine all at once, it could lead to a dangerous decrease in blood volume due to osmotic water loss. Furthermore, the process of digestion requires the stomach's acidic chyme to be neutralized and properly mixed with bile and pancreatic juices, which both take time. Therefore, the pylorus needs to regulate its pumping action carefully to avoid overwhelming the duodenum with chyme.

5.2. Blood Supply

The superior mesenteric artery and the celiac trunk supply blood to the small intestine. Both of these are aortic branches. The superior pancreaticoduodenal artery supplies blood to the duodenum from the coeliac trunk, while the inferior pancreaticoduodenal artery supplies blood from the superior mesenteric artery. The anterior and posterior branches of these two arteries meet in the midline and form an anastomose. The superior mesenteric artery provides blood to the ileum and jejunum. Arterial arcades, which can extend several layers deep in the mesentery, are formed by branches of the superior mesenteric artery. Vasa recta, or straight blood vessels, connect the arcades nearest the ileum and jejunum to the organs themselves.

5.2.1. Arterial Supply

Branches of the superior mesenteric artery and the celiac trunk supply blood to the small intestine. Since the celiac trunk normally supplies blood to the first and second segments of the duodenum, they are regarded as components of the foregut. This tissue is supplied by the superior pancreaticoduodenal and gastroduodenal arteries (posterior and posterior). The anterior and posterior branches of the inferior pancreaticoduodenal artery, which belong to the superior mesenteric artery, are usually responsible for supplying blood to the third and fourth segments of the duodenum. The fourth segment of the duodenum may also receive blood flow from branches of the first jejunal artery. The superior mesenteric artery supplies the ileum and jejunum since they are also components of the midgut. The branches that go to the ileum and the jejunum are known as the ileal and jejunal arteries, respectively. The ileocolic artery, the last branch to supply blood to the ileum, also supplies blood to the vermiform appendix and cecum.

5.2.2. Venous Drainage

The portal circulation receives the small intestine's venous drainage. Normally, the posterior superior pancreaticoduodenal vein empties blood into the portal vein after leaving the duodenum. In contrast, the superior mesenteric vein receives the drainage from the anterior superior pancreaticoduodenal vein as well as the anterior and posterior inferior pancreaticoduodenal veins. The superior mesenteric vein, which empties into the portal vein, receives the blood that exits the ileum and jejunum.

5.3. Intestinal Gland

According to histology, an intestinal gland is a gland located in the space between villi in the intestinal epithelium lining the small and large intestines (or colon). It is also referred to as an intestinal crypt or crypt of Lieberkühn. The epithelium covering the glands and intestinal villi is made up of several cell types, including cup cells, tuft cells, enterocytes (which absorb water and electrolytes), goblet cells (which secrete mucus), enteroendocrine cells (which secrete hormones), and stem cells at the base of the gland that secrete anti-microbial peptides.

5.3.1. Structure

Intestinal glands are located in the duodenum, jejunum, and ileum, which are the epithelia of the small intestine, and in the colon, the large intestine, where they are occasionally referred to as colonic crypts. The Paneth cells of the innate immune system, goblet cells, which produce mucus, and a base of replicating stem cells are found in the intestinal glands of the small intestine. Paneth cells are absent in crypts in the colon.

5.3.2. Function

Digestive enzymes are present in the enterocytes of the mucosa of the small intestine, where they break down particular foods as they pass through the epithelium. These enzymes consist of intestinal lipase, maltase, lactase, sucrase, and peptidase. On the other hand, the stomach's gastric glands secrete pepsinogen through chief cells. Additionally, new epithelium grows here, which is significant because food particles constantly wear down the nearby cells. Multipotent stem cells are found in the basal region of the crypt, which is located away from the intestinal lumen. One of the two daughter cells from each mitosis differentiates, moves up the side of the crypt, and eventually enters the villus, with the other daughter cell staying in the crypt as a stem cell. These stem cells have the ability to differentiate into secretory lineages such as Goblet cells, Paneth cells, and enteroendocrine cells, or absorptive lineages such as enterocytes. The Wnt and Notch signaling pathways are important regulators of intestinal morphogenesis and homeostasis as well as cell proliferation. It is believed that colorectal cancer is caused by a loss of proliferation control in the crypts.

5.3.2.1. Intestinal Juice

The clear to pale yellow, watery secretions from the glands lining the walls of the small intestine are referred to as intestinal juice (also known as succus entericus). Large volumes of alkaline mucus are secreted by the Brunner's glands in response to three main stimuli: (1) tactile or irritating sensations on the duodenal mucosa; (2) vagal stimulation, which causes the Brunner's glands to secrete more mucus at the same time that stomach secretion increases; and (3) gastrointestinal hormones, particularly secretin.

Its job is to finish the job that pancreatic juice started. Trypsin is found in pancreatic juice in the inactive form trypsinogen, and intestinal enterokinase in the intestinal juice activates it. Procolipase → colipase can then be catalyzed by trypsin, which can also activate additional protease enzymes. Lipase and bile salts are required for lipase activity to occur. Hormones, digestive enzymes, mucus, and chemicals to counteract the stomach's hydrochloric acid are also found in intestinal juice. Protein digestion is finished by a variety of exopeptidases, which further break down polypeptides into amino acids.

5.3.3. Colonic Crypts

Colonic crypts are the common term for the intestinal glands found in the colon. Colonic crypts, or invaginations, are spaces punctuated in the epithelial inner surface of the colon. The colon crypts have a central hole that runs the length of the tube, resembling tiny test tubes with thick walls (the crypt lumen). This image displays four tissue sections: two (A and B) that are cut parallel to the long axes of the crypts, and two (C and D) that are cut across them (Figure 5.4).

If the cells produce cytochrome c oxidase subunit I (CCOI or COX-1) a mitochondrial protein, the cells in these images have been stained to appear brown-orange.

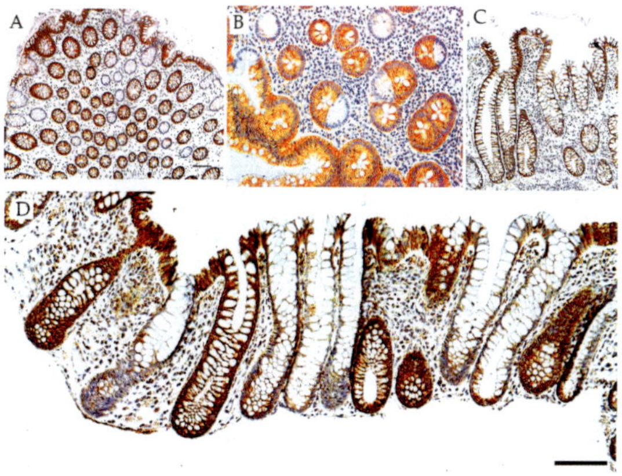

Figure 5.4. *Colonic crypts (intestinal glands) within four tissue sections. In panel A, the bar shows 100 μm and allows an estimate of the frequency of crypts in the colonic epithelium. Panel B includes three crypts in cross-section, each with one segment deficient for CCOI expression and at least one crypt, on the right side, undergoing fission into two crypts. Panel C shows, on the left side, a crypt fissioning into two crypts. Panel D shows typical small clusters of two and three CCOI deficient crypts (the bar shows 50 μm).*

Source: By Chaya5260 – Own work, CC BY-SA 4.0, https://commons.wikimedia.org/w/index.php?curid=40542376.

Haematoxylin is used to stain the cell nuclei, which are found at the outer edges of the cells lining the crypt walls. The color of the nuclei is blue-gray. As can be seen in panels C and D, crypts range in length from roughly 75 to 110 cells. A crypt's circumference is typically 23 cells. An average of 1,725 to 2530 cells per colonic crypt can be seen in the images. A further measure was obtained, resulting in a colonic crypt with between 1500 and 4900 cells. Days later, cells shed into the colonic lumen after being generated at the base of the crypt and migrating upward along the crypt axis. At the bases of the crypts are five to six stem cells.

There are roughly 100 colonic crypts per square millimeter of the colonic epithelium, based on estimates from the image in panel A. Measuring from the bottom of the cecum to the colorectal junction, the human colon's average length is 160.25 cm, with a range of 80 to 313 cm. The colon's average inner circumference is 6.2 cm. The human colon's inner surface epithelium, which comprises 9,950,000 (almost 10 million) crypts, has an average area of 995 cm^2. The blue-gray staining of the nuclei gives the intestinal glands in the four tissue sections displayed here their primary color, which is white, due to the presence of cells containing a mitochondrial DNA mutation in the CCOI gene. A section of the stem cells from three crypts, as shown in panel B, seem to have a mutation in CCOI, causing 40–50% of the cells that develop from those stem cells to form a white segment in the cross-cut area.

Generally, before the age of 40, the percentage of crypts deficient for CCOI is less than 1%, but it rises linearly with age. By the time they are 80–84 years old, the average percentage of men and women with colonic crypts deficient for CCOI is 23%. Colon crypts can proliferate through fission, as demonstrated by the crypts in panels C and B, where at least one crypt appears to be fissioning and another is splitting into two crypts. As seen in panel D, the majority of CCOI-deficient crypts are found in clusters of crypts, or clones of crypts, where two or more of these crypts are next to one another.

5.4. Physiology of Intestinal Absorption and Secretion

The highly polarized layer of epithelial cells that makes up the mucosa of the small and large intestine allows almost all nutrients from the diet to be absorbed into the blood. Through both passive and active mechanisms, the gastrointestinal tract's anatomical, histological, and functional specializations are in charge of the efficient and controlled transport of nutrients.

5.4.1. Functional Anatomy of the GI Tract

The GI tract developed to make it easier for nutrients to travel along it. The small intestine has a diameter of 2.5–3.0 cm and a length of about 6 m. The colon measures approximately 1.5 m in length with a diameter of 6–7.5 cm. The presence of villi and microvilli, which increase the intestinal surface area by 30–600 fold, respectively, greatly increases the surface area of the small intestine. The tips of villi, which range in length from 0 to 11.6 mm, are covered in columnar epithelial cells. While crypt cells are typically thought of as secretory, these are primarily absorptive cells. The colon is principally in charge of water and electrolyte transport, while the small intestine handles the majority of nutrient transport. Every day, about 8–10 L of fluid pass through the intestinal lumen and are handled by the GI tract. This fluid contains about 800 mmol of sodium (Na^+), 700 mmol of chloride (Cl^-), and 100 mmol of potassium (K^+). About 1.5 L are left for the colon to absorb and another 100 mL are lost daily through stools as the majority of these fluids and electrolytes are transported through the small intestine. Many transport proteins found at the brush border membranes of the small and large intestine are secondary to the mechanisms governing solute transport across the GI tract. The primary cause of the net fluid movement across the gastrointestinal epithelium is the active transport of various substances, including Na^+, Cl^-, and HCO_3^-

5.4.2. Intestinal Na^+ Absorption

The apical Na^+ transport in the small intestine is facilitated by three mechanisms: (a) colon-predominant electrogenic Na+ absorption by the epithelial Na+ channels (ENaC); (b) electroneutral NaCl absorption mediated primarily via the Na^+/H^+ exchange mechanism; and (c) nutrient-coupled Na+ absorption mediated by several families of Na^+-dependent nutrient transporters, such as sugar or amino acid transporters. Members of the SLC9 family of Na^+/H^+ exchangers are responsible for electroneutral NaCl absorption. NHE2, NHE3, and NHE8 are the three NHE isoforms that have been found on the enterocyte apical membrane. NHE3 is the one that affects intestinal Na^+ and water absorption the most out of the three.

Recent research has linked missense mutations in the SCL9A3 gene, which codes for NHE3, to congenital sodium diarrhea (CSD). Diarrhea in patients with microvillous inclusion disease, a rare genetic disorder linked to mutations in Myo5B or Syntaxin three, is also thought to be partially caused by reduced expression and mistargeting of NHE3 protein in enterocytes.

Inhibition of NHE3-mediated Na^+/H^+ exchange has been suggested to cause an increase in the inflammatory response, gut microbial dysbiosis, and epithelial barrier defect during intestinal inflammation. Nonetheless, there are situations in which NHE3 inhibition might have positive clinical effects. In a study, the novel oral NHE3 inhibitor tenapanor—which is poorly bioavailable—was used to treat a rat model of chronic kidney disease. The results showed that reducing NHE3-mediated intestinal Na+ absorption improved blood pressure, left ventricular hypertrophy, extracellular fluid volume, and albuminuria.

Electroneutral NaCl transport also mediates a significant portion of net Na^+ absorption in the colon, especially in the ascending segment. This process is a reflection of two parallel Na^+/H^+ – $Cl-/HCO_3-$ exchanges operating in the apical membrane, the latter mechanism mediated by PAT1 (SLC26A6) and downregulated in adenoma (DRA; SLC26A3). The apical surface of colonocytes expresses the three major Na+/H+ exchangers that are also expressed in the small intestine.

Electrogenic Na+ absorption, which is primarily found in the descending colon, sigmoid, and rectum, is primarily linked to the function of apical epithelial sodium channels (ENaC), which are regulated by mineralocorticoids. This mechanism, especially as an adaptive response following proctocolectomy, may have a limited contribution to an ileal Na^+ transport. Apical Na+ channels, consisting of three subunits (α-, β-, and γ-hENaC), mediate it. ENaC's exceptional sensitivity to the inhibitory effects of amiloride, a pyrazine diuretic, and the stimulation of aldosterone, a mineralocorticoid hormone, is one of its primary functional traits.

In the proximal colon, electrogenic but amiloride-insensitive Na+ absorption has also been reported. The physiological mechanism underlying this transport remains unclear; however, it could be associated with the role of Na^+/HCO_3 cotransporters (NBC), specifically the NBCe1B/C carrier.

5.4.3. Intestinal Anion Absorption

5.4.3.1. Chloride Absorption

A normal concentration of 10–15 mmoles/L of stool is the outcome of efficient absorption of chloride in the gut. It can surpass 90 mmoles/L in malabsorption states like congenital diarrhea. Three separate mechanisms are involved in the physiological absorption of Cl^- from the intestinal lumen: (a) the paracellular (passive) pathway; (b) the electroneutral pathways involving the coupled exchange of Cl^-/HCO_3^- and Na^+/H^+; and (c) the HCO_3–-dependent Cl^- absorption. The small intestinal epithelium primarily uses the passive pathway, which is dependent on the downhill Cl^- gradient and transmural potential difference. In the ileum and colon, the primary pathway for Cl^- absorption is the second, electroneutral exchange pathway. The coupling between Cl^-/HCO_3^- and Na^+/H^+ exchange results from H+ efflux, which is mediated by apical NHE isoforms, primarily NHE3. The Cl^-/HCO_3^- exchanger(s) are activated by NHE-driven transient alkalinization of the cytoplasm, with carbonic anhydrase serving as the primary H^+ and HCO_3^- producer. Ultimately, H^+ and HCO_3^- exit are exchanged for the absorption of Na+ and Cl^-. Anion exchangers (AEs) from the SLC26 "sulfate permease" transporter family are involved in the electroneutral exchange pathway. Congenital chloride diarrhea is caused by mutations in the DRA/CLD exchanger (SLC26A3) gene, which is expressed throughout the GI tract (predominantly in the colon). In the human small intestine and colon, PAT1 (SLC26A6), and more precisely its splice variant SLC26A6a, is expressed on the enterocyte apical membrane; however, its levels are higher in the duodenum through ileum. With the ability to exchange in multiple modes (Cl^-/oxalate, SO_4^{2-}/oxalate, SO_4^{2-}/Cl^-, Cl^-/formate, and Cl^-/OH^-), PAT1 is an especially adaptable AE.

A number of AEs from a heterogeneous SLC_4 family also aid in intestinal Cl^- absorption. Human enterocytes express AE4 (SLC4A9) on their apical membrane, whereas AE2 and AE3 (SLC4A2 and SLC4A3, respectively) are the AEs that allow HCO_3^- to enter the cell and be secreted later.

5.4.3.2. Short Chain Fatty Acid (SCFA) Absorption

The bacterial fermentation of carbohydrates and fiber results in the production of SCFAs, which are the primary regulators of colonic sodium transport (by improving Na^+/H^+ exchange), the colonic epithelium's preferred energy source, carcinogenesis-inhibiting, anti-inflammatory, oxidative stress-modulating, enhancing epithelial barrier function, and gene transcription-modifying via inhibition of histone deacetylase (HDAC) activity. About 95% of the SCFAs found in colonic fluid are composed of acetate, propionate, and butyrate; on its own, butyrate is thought to supply between 60% and 70% of the energy required by colonocytes. Monocarboxylate transporter 1 (MCT1; SLC5A8) is a specific carrier protein that is involved in this process and acts as an H^+-coupled electroneutral transporter. It has been suggested that impaired MCT1 function and intracellular butyrate oxidation play a role in the chronic nature of IBD. The primary basolateral SCFA transporter in the colon is assumed to be MCT4 isoform (SLC16A3), however research on MCT4 expression and activity in IBD is lacking.

5.4.3.3. Sulfate (SO_4^{2-}) Absorption

Inorganic anion sulfate (SO_4^{2-}) is necessary for numerous physiological functions and for the preservation of macromolecules' structure and functionality. A lack of sulfate in the diet impairs detoxification, makes the body more vulnerable to foreign substances, and changes the metabolism and functions of many internal substances, including neurotransmitters, hormones, and proteoglycans. Within the gastrointestinal tract of mammals, SO_4^{2-}– is conveyed through two distinct routes: firstly, Na^+-dependent electrogenic pH-insensitive high-affinity transport, which is facilitated by NaS1 (SLC13A1). Secondly, Na+-independent transport, which is facilitated by Sat1 (SLC26A1; electroneutral sulfate/oxalate, sulfate/bicarbonate, or oxalate/bicarbonate anion exchange) and STDST (SLC26A2). A number of other anion transporters, including DRA (SLC26A3) and PAT1 (SLC26A6), can also transfer sulfate and are probably involved in the intestinal absorption of SO_4^{2-}. NaS1 expression is limited to the kidneys in humans and is thought to have very little effect on intestinal SO_4^{2-} absorption, which is primarily controlled by mechanisms that do not require Na^+.

5.4.3.4. Oxalate Absorption and Secretion

Plants like beets, spinach, rhubarb, strawberries, nuts, chocolate, tea, wheat bran, and most dry beans—lima and green beans excluded—are the main sources of oxalate. It is also an end product of metabolism and comes from endogenous sources. In the stomach, oxalate is absorbed both passively and through carrier-mediated processes. If the luminal pH is low enough to completely protonate the anion, non-mediated non-ionic diffusion and paracellular permeability are examples of passive modes. Numerous members of the SLC26 family of anion exchangers can use oxalate as a substrate and are expressed in the gastrointestinal tract. It has been suggested that the SLC26A3 gene product known as Down Regulated in Adenoma (DRA) transports oxalate in the human duodenum, ileum, caecum, and distal colon. Oxalate can also be transported by other SLC26 transporters, including SLC26A1 (SAT1), SLC26A2 (DTDST), and SLC26A7 (SUT2). Intestinal oxalate secretion and cellular efflux are controlled by PAT1 (SLC26A6). Many factors influence the absorption of oxalate in the stomach, including angiotensin II, which raises the secretion of oxalate in the colon.

Increased influx of bile acids into the colon, stimulation of oxalate absorption, hyperoxaluria, and an increased risk of nephrolithiasis are all consequences of intestinal inflammation and/or ileum resection, which makes intestinal oxalate absorption clinically significant. Due to increased intestinal permeability to oxalate and the formation of complexes with fatty acids and calcium, fat malabsorption increases the intestinal absorption of oxalate. Hypercalcaluria following partial gastrectomy, bariatric surgery, jejunoileal bypass, and inflammatory bowel disease is most likely caused by this mechanism.

5.4.3.5. Sugar Transport Across the GI Tract

The bulk of the carbohydrates that are consumed come from sugars and starches. Among sugars are monosaccharides (e.g., glucose, fructose, and galactose) as well as disaccharides (e.g., trehalose, lactose, sucrose, and maltose). Plants store carbohydrates as starches, which are primarily made of sugars bonded together. Lactase hydrolyzes lactose while sucrase hydrolyzes sucrose to produce monosaccharides. Mucosal enzymes (such as salivary and pancreatic amylase) further break down starches after they have been initially broken down by these enzymes. isomaltase, amylase, and sucrase) are in charge of the last stage of digestion that produces glucose.

In the intestine, glucose and galactose are transported by the SGLT1 transporter. It is presently believed to be in charge of Na^+-dependent sugar transport, which propels the uphill movement of glucose and galactose from the gut lumen into the enterocyte. It is expressed on the brush border membrane of the enterocytes in the upper third of the small intestinal villi. The primary driving force is the Na^+ electrochemical gradient across the brush border membrane. The basolateral Na^+/K^+ ATPase pump sustains the Na^+ gradient. Every sugar molecule that is transported into the cells is thought to be accompanied by two Na^+ ions. To transport Na^+ and glucose at a 2:1 ratio against a glucose gradient, SGLT1 makes use of a Na^+ gradient. Every sugar molecule is co-transported across the cell with Na^+ in each cycle, along with 260 water molecules. This mechanism served as the molecular foundation for oral rehydration therapy, which aims to reduce mortality from diarrheal and cholera diseases. It was calculated to account for the human intestine's daily absorption of five liters of water. The World Health Organization's reduced osmolarity solution has a total osmolarity of 245 mOsm/L and is made up of the following components, expressed in mmol/L: Na^+ 75, Cl-65, glucose 75, K^+ 20, and citrate 10. The 20th century saw the widespread praise of oral rehydration therapy as "potentially the most important medical advance.

GLUT5, a member of the GLUT family of transporters, facilitates the diffusion process that moves fructose across the brush border membrane. GLUT2 is responsible for transporting fructose across the basolateral membrane (BLM) of the enterocyte. Seldom occurs fructose malabsorption. The clinical presentation, the existence of reducing agents in the stool, and breath hydrogen testing all play a role in the diagnosis. It is necessary to distinguish isolated fructose malabsorption from aldolase B deficiency, which results in fructose intolerance brought on by an ALDOB gene mutation.

5.4.4. Amino Acids and Peptide Absorption

In the western diet, 100 g of protein are consumed daily on average, with an additional 35 g coming from GI and salivary secretions. Pepsinogen and pepsin are activated by low pH in the stomach. Pepsin breaks down peptide bonds at aromatic amino acids, producing a mixture of amino acids, peptides, and intermediate protein moieties. These are then transported to the duodenum, where mucosal enterokinase activates pancreatic proenzymes (chymotrypsinogen, trypsinogen, proelastase, and procarboxypeptidase) to further break down these products into amino acids, dipeptides, and tripeptides. Aminations are still being released by brush border dipeptidases. However, dipeptides and tripeptides can also enter the enterocyte and pass through the BLM of the enterocytes after being hydrolyzed by cytoplasmic peptidases to release amino acids.

5.4.4.1. Apical Amino Acid Transport Systems

The intricate process of transporting amino acids involves multiple systems that work together to facilitate their uptake through the brush border membrane. Their solute specificity, dependence on Na^+, Cl^-, H^+, or K^+ ions, and potential representation of an electroneutral or electrogenic transport process vary. Table 5.2 provides an overview of the amino acid transporters expressed in the human gut as targets in cancer research.

Table 5.2. Overview of Currently Available PDB Structures of ASCT2, LAT1, and xCT, Along with their Conformation, Resolution, and Ligand, if Available. IF—Inward Facing, OF—Outward Facing

Protein	PDB	Conformation	Resolution, Å	Ligand
ASCT2	6GCT	IF (occluded)	3.85	L-Gln
	6MP6	OF (open)	3.54	
	6MPB	OF (occluded)	3.84	L-Gln
	6RVX	IF (open)	3.61	
	6RVY	IF (open)	4.13	
	7BCQ	OF (open)	3.43	Lc-BPE (position "up")
	7BCS	OF (open)	3.43	Lc-BPE (position "down")
	7BCT	OF (open)	3.37	
LAT1–4F2hc	6IRS	IF (open)	3.30	
	6IRT	IF (open)	3.50	BCH
	6JMQ	IF (open)	3.31	
	7DSK	OF (occluded)	2.90	JX-075
	7DSL	OF (occluded)	2.90	JX-078
	7DSN	OF (occluded)	3.10	JX-119
	7DSQ	OF (open/ occluded)	3.40	3,5-diiodo-L-tyrosine

xCT-4F2hc	7CCS	IF (open)	6.20	
	7EPZ	IF (open)	3.40	Erastin
	7P9U	IF (open)	3.70	L-Glu
	7P9V	IF (open)	3.40	

Source: Jakobsen S, Nielsen CU. Exploring amino acid transporters as therapeutic targets for cancer: An examination of inhibitor structures, selectivity issues, and discovery approaches. Pharmaceutics. 2024; 16(2):197. https://doi.org/10.3390/pharmaceutics16020197.

5.4.4.2. Peptide Transport

In the small intestine, dipeptides and tripeptides are absorbed very effectively. Since Na+ is required for the activity of Na+/H+ exchanger 3 (NHE3) to produce a proton gradient for H^+/peptide co-transport, the process is indirectly dependent on Na^+. The two transport processes are thus interdependent functionally. Peptides containing four or more amino acids absorb poorly through a process that is not carrier-dependent. The peptide transporter 1 (PEPT1) is the carrier in charge of peptide uptake via the intestinal wall. It is expressed in the intestinal and, to a lesser extent, renal epithelia and is encoded by the SLC15A1 gene. Due to PEPT1's great transport capacity, which is expressed throughout the small intestine, very few dietary peptides are able to bypass the terminal ileum. Though there is some debate regarding its expression in the colon, the prevailing opinion at the moment is that PEPT1 is not expressed there unless specific circumstances are met, such as inflammatory bowel disease, and in cases of short bowel syndrome (SBS), most likely as a compensatory response. This finding implies the potential application of peptide-containing nutritional formulas in clinical settings where the transport system is expressed. In conclusion, gastric pepsin and hydrochloric acid hydrolyze proteins found in food and GI secretions first, followed by pancreatic proteases and peptidases in the small intestine and the cytoplasmic domain of the enterocyte. As a result, amino acids make up 90% of the ingested proteins in the bloodstream, with the remaining 10% being tri- and dipeptides.

5.4.4.3. Basolateral Exit of Amino Acids

Through the enterocyte's BLM, amino acids are transported by a minimum of six different amino acid transporters. However, these carriers may function in either direction based on the concentration of luminal amino acids, cellular demand, and electrogenic driving forces. The six transport systems comprise of System A, which is dependent on Na^+ for the transport of all neutral amino acids and imino acids (carrier SNAT2 encoded by SLC8A2), and System GLYT1, which is dependent on Na^+ and Cl^- coupled transport of glycine (carrier SLC6A9 encoded). GLYT1 is a bidirectional transporter, but its primary function is to move glycine into the enterocyte. System L is the primary Na+-independent transport system for neutral amino acids, excluding imino acids; y^+ is the Na^+ independent transport of cationic amino acids (lysine, arginine, and ornithine; CAT1 encoded by SLC7A1).

System y^+L, though not directly Na+-dependent, forms an obligatory exchange system whereby cellular cationic amino acid is exchanged for the Na^+-coupled entry of a neutral amino acid from the blood. This transport is primarily mediated by LAT2, encoded SLC7A8, which heterodimerizes with CD98, also known as heavy chain associated with the 4F2 antigen, or 4F2hc. Two carriers, y^+LAT1 and y^+LAT2, encoded by SLC7A7 and SLC7A6, respectively, mediate the system y^+L. The y^+LAT1 and

y^+LAT2 proteins heterodimerize with 4F2hc in a manner similar to system L. Finally, system Asc: Na^+-independent transport of short chain amino acids (e.g., is principally mediated by the ASC1/4F2hc heterodimer, which also serves as a basolateral amino acid exchanger. glycine, alanine, serine, cysteine, or threonine).

5.4.5. Lipid Absorption

Gastric lipase, which is produced by chief cells, joins lingual lipase, which begins the process of breaking down fat in the mouth, to continue the process in the stomach. However, pancreatic lipase and colipase, with the help of bile acid emulsification, are primarily responsible for the digestion of fat in the duodenum. Together with phospholipids, cholesterol, and fat-soluble vitamins, the lipolysis-produced monoglycerides and long chain fatty acids form micelles with bile salts. The micelle components are then introduced into the enterocytes, where monoglycerides and long chain fatty acids undergo reesterification to become triglycerides. These triglycerides are then mixed with cholesterol, phospholipids, and protein to form chylomicrons. The chylomicrons then pass through the thoracic duct and into the intestinal lymphatics before entering the peripheral circulation. Without hydrolyzing, medium chain fatty acids can be taken up by the enterocytes. They go straight into the vein of the portal. Because of this specific characteristic, medium chain triglycerides are especially helpful in the treatment of patients suffering from disorders related to fat malabsorption, including cirrhosis, intestinal lymphangiectasia, and pancreatic insufficiency. It appears that the entry of fatty acids into the enterocyte and their intracellular movement are mediated by two transport proteins, namely CD36 and LFABP. The primary pathway for cholesterol transport is Niemann-Pick C1 like-1 (NPC1L1). Ezetimibe (also known as Zetia or Ezetrol), an authorized medication that blocks the absorption of cholesterol, targets this transporter. ABCG5 and ABCG8, two ATP-binding cassette proteins, are in charge of the cholesterol efflux from enterocytes into the lumen.

5.4.6. Water Soluble Vitamins

Since water-soluble vitamins are involved in numerous metabolic processes, they are necessary for normal growth and development. Many of these vitamins are not synthesized by humans, so they must be obtained externally.

- **Vitamin C:** Vitamin C cannot be synthesized by humans. It is transported through the intestines by a carrier-mediated, Na^+-dependent mechanism that is centered at the brush border membrane. Humans have been shown to have two distinct Na^+-dependent carriers: vitamin C transporter-1 (SVCT1) and SVCT2, which are the respective products of the SLC23A1 and SLC23A2 genes. Scurvy is caused by a vitamin C nutritional deficiency. Citrus fruits, tomatoes, cantaloupes, and strawberries are good sources of vitamin C.
- **Biotin (Vitamin H or B_7):** Two sources of biotin are available to the human gut: dietary and bacterial. Through a carrier-mediated, Na+-dependent mechanism, biotin is absorbed. Encoded by the SLC5A6 gene, the intestinal sodium-dependent multivitamin transporter (SMVT) facilitates the uptake of biotin throughout the gastrointestinal tract. A lack of biotin in the diet causes paresthesia, myalgia, alopecia, anorexia, and seborrheic dermatitis. Meat, milk, egg yolks, soybeans, liver, and soybeans are all excellent food sources.

- **Cobalamin (B_{12}):** Animal-based foods and the gut microbiota are sources of cobalamin. After being freed from the animal protein, dietary cobalamin binds to the protein haptocorrin (transcobalamin-1; TC1) in the stomach. Trypsin in the small intestine releases cobalamin from this complex, and it then attaches itself to the gastric intrinsic factor (GIF). The multi-ligand heterodimeric receptor called cubam, which is made up of cubilin (CUBL) and amnionless (AMN) and is found at the apical membrane of ileal enterocytes, binds to the B12/GIF complex. After internalization, this complex travels to the endosomes, where the IF is broken down and cubam is recycled back to the apical membrane. Meanwhile, the B_{12}/GIF complex travels to the lysosome. The multi-drug resistant associated protein-1 (MRP1) at the BLM exports and carries the released cobalamin. Transcobalamin transports cobalamin throughout the body for use and storage. Megaloblastic anemia is the main condition linked to cobalamin deficiency or malabsorption. Megaloblastic anemia is the consequence of atrophic gastritis-induced loss of GIF. Moreover, relatively uncommon hereditary abnormalities in intestinal cobalamin absorption exist (e.g., because of changes in the CUBL, AMN, or GIF genes). Meats, fish, poultry, and eggs are examples of animal foods that are dietary sources of cobalamin.
- **Folic Acid (Vitamin M or B_9):** The gut microbiota produces folate in addition to dietary sources. There are two forms of dietary folate: monoglutamate and polyglutamate. In the upper small intestine, folate is liberated from its conjugated polyglutamate form by the enzyme folate hydrolase. The reduced folate carrier (FOLT; the product of the SLC19A1 gene), the proton-coupled folate transporter (PCFT/HCP1; the product of the SLC46A1 gene), and the GPI-anchored folate receptor FOLR1 are the three carriers that are specific for folate. A multitude of conditions can lead to folate deficiency, such as long-term use of sulfasalazine, intestinal diseases like celiac disease and tropical sprue, and chronic alcohol consumption. Green veggies, liver, cantaloupes and oranges, as well as fortified breads and cereals, are dietary sources of folate.
- **Niacin (Vitamin B_3 or Nicotinic Acid):** Humans get niacin from both endogenous (found in the body) and exogenous (found in the food) sources. The latter comes from tryptophan being metabolically converted to niacin. Niacin is absorbed through the intestinal tract via a particular carrier. Its kinetic properties are similar to those of organic anion transporter 10 (OAT10, encoded by the SLC22A13 gene), despite the fact that its molecular identity is still unknown. Insufficiency of niacin is linked to dementia, dermatitis, pellagra, and diarrhea. Niacin is primarily found in whole grains, meats, fish, eggs, and dairy products.

- **Vitamin B_6 (Pyridoxine, Pyridoxal, Pyridoxamine):** Vitamin B6 is found in foods like potatoes, fish, meats, and fruits. Additionally, resident gut bacteria synthesize it. Vertebrates may have a B_6 carrier, but their identity is unknown. Alcoholism, diabetes, celiac disease, kidney disorders, and prolonged use of hydrazines or penicillamines are all linked to deficiencies in B_6. B_6 deficiency can cause microcytic anemia, peripheral neuritis, dermatitis, glossitis, cheilosis, convulsions in babies, and irritability.
- **Vitamin B_2 (Riboflavin):** Green leafy vegetables, meats, dairy products, and eggs are dietary sources of vitamin B_2. It is believed that riboflavin transporters (RFVT1 and RFVT2, encoded by SLC52A1 and SLC52A2 genes, respectively) are responsible for the intestinal transport of B_2. Mutations in the SLC52A2 gene have been connected to the Brown-Vialetto-Van Laere syndrome-2, whereas functional B2 deficiency may be linked to inflammatory bowel disorders or chronic alcoholism. Photophobia, cheilosis, glossitis, corneal vascularization, and stunted growth are linked to vitamin B_{12} deficiency.
- **Vitamin B_1 (Thiamin):** Many food sources, including whole grains, nuts, and dried legumes, are good sources of thiamin. Two human thiamin transporters, THTR1 and THTR2, which are expressed throughout the GI tract and are encoded by the SLC19A2 and SLC19A3 genes, respectively, have been linked to intestinal B_1 absorption. The main causes of dietary thiamin deficiency are inadequate dietary intake and excessive alcohol consumption, in addition to rare genetic causes (mutations in the SLC19A2 gene cause thiamin-responsive megaloblastic anemia, and in the SLC19A3 gene, thiamin-responsive Wernicke's-like encephalopathy).

5.4.7. Fat-Soluble Vitamins

5.4.7.1. Vitamin A

Pro-vitamin A carotenoids or preformed retinol or ethyl esters are the two forms of vitamin A that are found in food. Most of these forms need to be converted metabolically. There are several forms of formed vitamin A that can be found in the diet, including retinol vitamin A1, retinol vitamin A2, and retinol esters. Pro-vitamin A functions as a precursor to vitamin A and in the formation of macula pigments. Retinoids are crucial for immunological system and eye health, and they play a part in the life cycle of mammals. The intestinal absorption of Vitamin A is contingent upon its dietary form. When pro-vitamin A is consumed, retinol esters are released. Enterocytes are where carotenoids are converted to retinol. The majority of pro-vitamin A comes from animal sources, including dairy products, eggs, fish liver oil, liver, and kidneys. Because vitamin A is a fat-soluble vitamin, retinol and its esters must be re-esterified before being combined with other lipids to form chylomicrons. This process is primarily carried out by lecithin, acetyltransferase, and palmitic acid. After chylomicrons have entered the bloodstream through the lymphatics, hepatocytes internalize them in a manner dependent on apolipoprotein E. The hepatic stellate cells hydrolyze and then store retinol esters, primarily palmitate, as a byproduct. The main protein that appears to be in charge of transporting vitamin A from the liver to peripheral tissues is retinol-binding protein. Retinol-binding protein binds 95% of the retinol in plasma, with retinol esters in lipoproteins accounting for the remaining 5%. Due to inadequate diet and/or fat malabsorption, vitamin A deficiency primarily affects children. It causes xerophthalmia, keratomalacia, and irreversible corneal damage that leads to pigmentary retinopathy and night blindness. Moreover, a lack of vitamin A raises the death rate from several infections, including the measles.

5.4.7.2. Vitamin D

The terms "vitamin D" typically relate to the two main secosteroids, ergocalciferol (vitamin D_2) and cholecalciferol (vitamin D_3). The plant and fungal sources of vitamin D_2 are added to fortified cow's milk. Food naturally contains vitamin D_2, which is also found in a lot of fortified cereals. Salmon, tuna, and mackerel are among the fatty fish that are excellent providers of vitamin D. When 7-dihydrocholesterol is exposed to UVB light (270–300 nm), vitamin D_3 is produced in the skin. The resultant pre-vitamin D isomerizes spontaneously to cholecalciferol, which is then carried into the liver by the binding protein. There, CYP27A1 carries out the 25-hydroxylation of both D_2 and D_3, while CYP27B1 in the kidneys performs the 1α-hydroxylation. Among its many roles, $1,25(OH)_2D_3$ (calcitriol), the most physiologically active form of vitamin D, controls the intestinal absorption of Ca^{2+} and phosphate (Pi) as well as their reabsorption in the kidneys. In addition, $1,25(OH)_2D_3$ mobilizes Ca^{2+} and Pi from the bones when the levels of the two minerals in the blood must be maintained. Consequently, the renal-intestinal-skeletal axis, which keeps systemic mineral homeostasis and bone formation intact, depends on vitamin D.

Similar to how vitamin A is absorbed through the small intestine, vitamin D is absorbed through simple passive diffusion. The lymphatic system absorbs the majority of the absorbed vitamin D in chylomicrons. The effects of a vitamin D deficiency primarily concern Pi and Ca^{2+} homeostasis. Both adult osteomalacia and childhood rickets are associated with vitamin D deficiency. Through the vitamin D receptor (VDR), vitamin D regulates many target genes, including parathyroid hormone (PTH; downregulated), osteocalcin and RANKL (upregulated). Given its interaction with osteoblasts, VDR, which is highly expressed in intestinal and renal epithelial cells, regulates Ca^{2+} (re)absorption and the formation of bone. Immune cells and pancreatic beta cells both exhibit high expression of VDR.

5.4.7.3. Vitamin E

The two primary forms of vitamin E are tocopherol and tocotrienols (α, β, Δ, and γ). But the primary biological activity is attributed to the α-tocopherol that is found in most foods, with the exception of soy, which has a high γ-tocopherol content. As a lipid-soluble, membrane-bound, and powerful antioxidant, the primary metabolic function of vitamin E is to shield the cell from reactive oxygen species (ROS) brought on by lipid oxidation. Vegetables and grains with oil are common sources of vitamin E. Passive absorption of vitamin E occurs across the intestinal mucosa. It is then taken up by micelles, chylomicrons, and finally the lymphatics. HDL efflux provides a different pathway for vitamin E absorption by directly secreting the nutrient into the portal venous circulation from epithelial cells. In cases of pancreatic insufficiency and vitamin E absorption, pancreatic enzymes help (i.e., in cystic fibrosis) could result in a lack of vitamin E. Progressive neurological disorders such as ataxia, hyperreflexia, repressed vibratory and positional sensation, and impaired balance and coordination are caused by a vitamin E deficiency.

5.4.7.4. Vitamin K

Leafy vegetables, fruits, seeds, soybean oil, and cow's milk are good sources of vitamin K, which is primarily found as phylloquinone (also known as vitamin K1). Vitamin K1 is changed by intestinal bacteria into vitamin K2 (menaquinones), which are then synthesized from scratch. K2 is the primary form of vitamin K storage and has 60% of the activity of vitamin K1. Because of their low level of vitamin K in breast milk, limited placental permeability for vitamin K, and low colonic bacterial synthesis of menaquinones before full microbial colonization, newborns are susceptible to hemorrhagic disease and need to be supplemented via injection. Like other fat-soluble vitamins, biliary and pancreatic enzymes are required for absorption, which takes place through the lipid pathway in the terminal ileum. An indirect indicator of vitamin K status is the blood's level of gamma-carboxylated proteins. Hemorrhagic disorders and hypoprothrombinemia are caused by a vitamin K deficiency. Deficiency may result from aging, taking broad-spectrum antibiotics, small bowel damage and malabsorption, chronic kidney disease, and vitamin D deficiency.

5.4.8. Major Minerals (Calcium, Phosphate, Iron, and Magnesium)

5.4.8.1. Calcium (Ca^{2+})

One important mineral needed for many physiological and structural processes linked to health is calcium. Together, the kidney, bone, intestine, and parathyroid glands keep serum Ca^{2+} within a specific range, roughly. 2.5 mM. Most of the calcium in circulation is ionized Ca^{2+}, with the remainder bound to albumin. Dairy products are important sources of calcium; they make up about 75% of the calcium found in food. Vegetables, legumes, and cereals make up the remaining 25%. It has been demonstrated that dietary lactose improves calcium absorption even more. However, dietary fiber, phytic acid, and oxalate found in vegetables bind to calcium strongly and prevent it from being absorbed.

The consumption of calcium, the length of time it spends in each section of the small and large intestine, and the amount of soluble Ca^{2+} that is available for absorption all affect how much calcium is absorbed in the gut. The pH of each segment primarily determines the latter. Even though the colon only absorbs roughly 7% of all Ca^{2+}, in the context of short bowel syndrome, it becomes more significant. Calcium is absorbed through two complementary pathways. The paracellular diffusive pathway, which is non-saturable, is predominant at normal to high dietary calcium intake. Despite being passive, the process is regulated, primarily through the dynamics of the tight junctions in the epithelium. While Cldn-5 restricts Ca^{2+} absorption, claudins Cldn-2, Cldn-12, and Cldn-15 facilitate it. With the exception of the initial weeks following delivery, $1,25(OH)_2D_3$ increases paracellular Ca^{2+} permeability in the ileum and jejunum. It has been proposed that the downregulation of Cadherin-17 and Aquaporin-8 and the upregulation of Cldn-2 and Cldn-12 may be the underlying mechanism, though this has not been thoroughly established.

Under a concentration gradient and at lower luminal calcium levels, the saturable transcellular process takes place. It is primarily found in the duodenum and jejunum, where it is driven by TRPV6, and to a lesser extent TRPV5, non-voltage-gated Ca^{2+} channels expressed in the apical membranes of the enterocytes. It is regulated by nutritional and physiological factors, primarily vitamin D. It is believed that Cav1.3, another L-type channel in the apical membrane, offers an additional mechanism of active Ca^{2+} transport in depolarizing circumstances, such as during digestion, when luminal Ca^{2+} is abundant. After passing through the apical membrane of the enterocyte, Ca^{2+} binds to calbindin-D9k (S100G). This has two functions: it transports Ca^{2+} to the BLM and buffers it, keeping intracellular Ca^{2+} concentrations below 10–7 mol/L to stop epithelial cell apoptosis. Calcium exits the enterocyte at the BLM by two mechanisms: via Ca^{2+} ATPase PMCA1b (ca. 80% contribution), and through the Na^{+}/Ca^{2+} exchanger NCX1 (*SLC8A1*; ca. 20% contribution). Vitamin D_3 increases each of these carriers' expression.

5.4.8.2. Phosphate

Phosphate is essential for energy metabolism and bone formation in addition to Ca^{2+}. Phosphate is found in cells, where it is necessary for cellular metabolism, and in bones, where it makes up 14% of the total. Phosphate is necessary for cell physiology and metabolism because it is converted to creatinine, phosphate, and ATP, which is energy for a number of metabolic processes. Dairy products, cereals, and meats are the main dietary sources of phosphate. In nature, phosphate is widely distributed and can reach intracellular concentrations of 1–2 mmol/L.

The duodenum, jejunum, and ileum have the highest relative phosphate absorption efficiency, with small intestines being the primary sites of absorption. Because the jejunum is longer than the other, it absorbs most phosphate. Two mechanisms are involved: firstly, the apical Na+ phosphate transporter NaPi-IIb, which is part of the SLC34A2 family of solute carriers, drives Na+ and 1,25-$(OH)_2D_3$-dependent co-transport. Secondly, passive diffusion occurs through the paracellular pathway, which functions when there is a high phosphate intake. It is most likely that phosphate will leave the BLM through enhanced diffusion via unidentified phosphate transporters. The enterocyte's BLM is also home to type III Na+ phosphate transporters PIT1 and PIT2, which move phosphate from the serosal site into the cell when the diet is insufficient for the cell's phosphate metabolism. Phosphate transport is regulated by several factors, including age. To meet the demands of growth, early life involves rapid phosphate absorption. By acting on NaPi-IIb, 1,25-$(OH)_2D_3$ increases phosphate absorption. Although they don't directly affect NaPi-IIb expression and activity, estrogens have a similar effect. Systemic phosphate levels are unaffected by metabolic acidosis, which causes phosphaturia. This is probably because intestinal NaPi-IIb-mediated absorption is upregulated. EGF, glucocorticoids, and FGF23 all reduce the absorption of intestinal phosphate that is dependent on Na^{+} (the latter due to modified vitamin D_3 metabolism).

5.4.8.3. Magnesium (Mg)

The body's fourth most common cation is magnesium. About 25–28 g of Mg^{2+} are found in an adult human, with the majority of that mass being deposited in the bones. As a co-factor for a range of enzymatic reactions, including phosphate group transfer from high-energy nucleotide triphosphates, magnesium is necessary for several biological processes. Mg2+ is mainly absorbed in the jejunum and ileum of humans, where both passive and active transport pathways are involved. The "solvent drag effect" and concentration gradient both contribute to the paracellular migration of Mg^{2+}, which also happens across a much "tighter" colonic epithelium. Transient potential ion channels TRPM6 and TRPM7, which heterotetramerize and permit Mg^{2+} to be transported through the apical membrane, mediate active transport and facilitate facilitated diffusion, which are the primary mechanisms behind transcellular Mg^{2+} absorption. Human Na^{+}/Mg^{2+} exchange or Mg^{2+} ATPase have been hypothesized but not proven.

5.4.8.4. Iron (Fe)

Numerous physiological processes, such as oxygen binding and transport, cellular respiration, control over gene expression, regulation of cell growth and differentiation, and electron transfer reactions, depend on iron, an essential mineral. Humans are thought to consume 20–30 mg of iron daily, but only 1.5 mg of that is absorbed by adult males. To make up for losses from menstrual bleeding and fetal needs during pregnancy, adult females need an extra 1–2 mg per day. The human body is thought to contain 3–5 grams of iron, primarily in the form of hemoglobin or myoglobin.

Iron balance needs to be strictly regulated by means of several regulatory mechanisms. Since the body lacks a mechanism for excreting iron, the primary mechanism for regulating the amount of iron present in the body is absorption. The majority of iron in food comes in the insoluble ferric form (Fe^{3+}). In addition to dietary ascorbic acid, duodenal brush border cytochrome b reductase 1 (DCYTB; CYBRD1) reduces Fe^{3+} to its absorbable ferrous Fe^{2+} form. After it is in the ferrous state, iron is moved through the brush border membranes by the adaptable divalent metal transporter 1 (DMT1), which can also move magnesium, copper, zinc, cobalt, and cadmium alongside iron. Proton-coupled symporter DMT1 is upregulated in anemia and hypoxic environments. Through Fe-responsive elements in the 3′-untranslated regions of the DMT1 transcript, iron deficiency affects the stability of the mRNA, which in turn controls DMT1 expression and activity. Heme iron transport in the gastrointestinal tract happens through a different mechanism than DMT1, which involves the low affinity heme transporter known as HCP1 (SLC46A1). The expression of HCP1 is upregulated in response to hypoxia and is expressed at the brush border membrane, just like DMT1. In addition, HCP1 is a high-affinity transporter of folate.

Ferroportin (FPN1, SLC40A1) allows iron to leave the enterocyte by crossing its basolateral membrane. To allow oxidized iron to bind to transferrin in the interstitial fluid and plasma for body distribution, this process is linked to Fe^{2+} oxidation at the BLM. The basolateral iron oxidase hephaestin (HEPH) performs this function. The liver hepcidin antimicrobial peptide (HAMP), which acts upon FPN1 to reduce iron export from the cells, regulates (reduces) cellular iron export. Inflammation (via IL-6) and elevated Fe body stores also cause HAMP. Mutations in the HFE gene are the secondary cause of hereditary hemochromatosis. The duodenal crypt cells that are linked to transferrin receptors and β-2 microglobin are home to the HFE protein. Due to HFE mutations, there is a relative Fe deficiency in the duodenal crypt cells because Fe cannot enter the crypt cells. This ultimately causes DMT1 expression and activity to rise, which causes abnormally high iron absorption. Type 4 hemochromatosis, or ferroportin disease, is an autosomal dominant hemochromatosis caused by mutations in FPN1 (SLC40A1). Hypochromic microcytic anemia has been linked to an absorptive defect caused by rare mutations in DMT1 (SLC11A2). When intestinal disorders such as celiac disease damage the structure of the duodenum villus, it can interfere with DMT1 function secondary to the damage and prevent the patient from absorbing iron. Therefore, celiac disease needs to be looked into in patients who are Fe-deficient and do not respond to iron supplementation.

5.4.9. Trace Elements (Micronutrients)

5.4.9.1. Zinc (Zn) Absorption

Zinc is a necessary mineral for many cellular processes, such as immune system function, taste, smell, and cell growth and development. It is also found in many enzymes that are necessary for critical biological processes. The diet's source affects how much zinc is included in it. For instance, the availability of zinc in red meat is roughly 55%, while that in high-fiber cereal is only 15%. Human milk has a higher bioavailability of zinc than does cow's milk. The body contains about 2 grams of zinc, which is found in many different types of enzymes. It seems that enterohepatic circulation occurs for zinc. Because of their chelating qualities, phytate and oxalate in the diet hinder the absorption of zinc. While the majority of zinc absorption takes place in the duodenum and proximal jejunum, zinc is absorbed throughout the GI tract, including the colon. Homeostasis keeps plasma concentrations between 11 and 25 μmol/L (0.7–1.6 mg/L) and intracellular zinc concentrations steady. Transport is upregulated when there is a low dietary Zn supply, which increases absorption efficiency to nearly 100%. Numerous zinc transport proteins have been identified, one of which is Zip4 (SLC39A4), which seems to be the main zinc transporter located at the apex of the enterocyte. In fact, acrodermatitis enertopathica, a disorder that causes diarrhea, skin rashes, and failure to thrive, is caused by mutations in the Zip4 gene. It appears that the basolateral transport protein is Zip5 (SLC39A5). Zip11 (SLC39A11) might be involved in the secretion of gastric acid because it seems to be expressed in parietal cells. In different tissues, Zip10, 11, and 14 seem to be in charge of membrane transport. ZnT1 (SLC30A1), one of the other transporters, is engaged in both vesicular and basolateral transport. ZnT2, 4, 5, 6, and 7 are also involved in the trans-Golgi network membrane and vesicular Zn transport. The ZnT transport proteins appear to be in charge of vesicular transport inside the enterocyte after transit across the apical membrane via Zip4. They subsequently exit through Zip5 to the basolateral membrane. An intracellular metal-binding protein called metallothionein (MT) responds quickly to the zinc status. Elevated intake levels cause changes in binding capacity, zinc sequestration, and intestinal MT synthesis. Thus, it would seem that MT is involved in the regulation and storage of zinc.

5.4.9.2. Copper (Cu) Absorption

An important mineral called copper is needed for several metabolic processes. The brain, liver, and kidneys have the highest concentrations of Cu stored in the body when compared to other trace elements. Several food sources, such as fish and green vegetables, contain copper. 1–3 mg are included in the typical diet each day. The duodenum, which is the main organ in the small intestine, is where copper is absorbed. Because zinc prevents the absorption of copper, Zn is used in Wilson's disease patients, a condition marked by an accumulation of Cu. The process of absorbing copper is saturable. The six-transmembrane epithelial antigen of the prostate (STEAP) family proteins and cytochrome B reductase 1 (CYPBR1) first reduce the luminal copper from the cupric (Cu^{2+}) state to the cuprous (Cu^{+}) form. The apical high-affinity copper transporter 1 (CTR1; SLC31A1) then absorbs Cu+. Copper may also be transported by the DMT1 iron transporter, particularly in cases of iron deficiency. As a result of free cytosolic copper's extreme toxicity, a number of intracellular chaperones (e.g., COX17 or ATOX1), which transport it to ATP7A P-type ATPase located at the basolateral membrane (for extrusion) or in the trans-Golgi network (for cuproenzyme synthesis). Menkes disease is a terminal, progressive neurological disorder caused by Cu accumulation in the enterocytes as a result of mutations in ATP7A. ATP7A is not the same as ATP7B, a Cu transporter found in hepatocytes harboring Wilson's disease-causing mutations.

5.4.9.3. Manganese (Mn) and Cadmium (Cd) Absorption

Both passive diffusion and DMT1-mediated active transport are involved in the absorption of Mn and Cd in the colon. Alternate splice variants of the SLC39A14 gene, Zip8 (SLC39A8) and Zip14A/Zip14B, may also play a role in the transport of both metals. Iron export and binding to transferrin pathways may be involved in the export of magnesium from the enterocyte. Apotransferrin is the main protein that distributes Mn in the blood.

5.4.9.4. Selenium (Se) Absorption

The two main forms of selenium in the diet are selenocysteine from animal tissue and selenomethionine from plants. Selenium is an essential trace element. Se concentrations in the soil generally determine how much is found in food in a given area. For instance, Keshan disease, also known as congestive cardiomyopathy, was initially identified in Keshan County in the Heilongjiang province of China. It is caused by a mix of a mutated strain of Coxsackievirus and dietary deficiencies in selenium. Yeast that has been enhanced with selenium is an excellent source for fortifying food. Se appears to be transported by a saturable process in the enterocyte. It is likely that the transcellular movement of selenium is similar to amino acid transport, including the use of the basolateral amino acid transporters, as recent evidence suggests that the amino acid transporters SLC3A1 and SLC1A4 may be involved in Se transport.

5.4.9.5. Chromium (Cr) Absorption

There is a lot of chromium in food. Prior to absorption, Cr must first transform into the trivalent Cr^{3+} state. Before Cr^{3+} is absorbed throughout the small intestine, particularly in the jejunum, it is solubilized and complexed with ligands in the stomach. It is thought that part of the routes taken by the iron absorption mechanism are also used by Cr absorption. Developing glucose intolerance has been linked to chromium deficiency.

5.5. Motility in the Small Intestine

Smooth muscle contractions work together in various ways to aid in the process of digestion and absorption in the small intestine.

- Foods are combined with bile salts from the biliary system and pancreatic digestive enzymes.
- Because the molecules of nutrients in the lumen are always moving, they can come into contact with the epithelium, which is where absorption takes place after enzymatic digestion is finished.
- Chyme is eliminated along with undigestable, potentially hazardous materials as it travels down the digestive tube to make room for the next load.
- The small intestine cycles through two states in the majority of animals, and each state is linked to unique motility patterns.
- After a meal, two main forms of motility are predominant in the small intestine lumen that contains chyme: segmentation contractions, which chop, mix, and roll the chyme, and peristalsis, which moves the chyme slowly toward the large intestine.
- The lumen is mostly empty during the interdigestive phase, which occurs in between meals. At these moments, the stomach triggers what are known as "housekeeping contractions," which move through the entire small intestine and remove any debris. Growling is brought on by this intricate pattern of motility, which is also referred to as the migrating motor complex.
- Similar to other regions of the digestive tube, the small intestine's motility is primarily regulated by excitatory and inhibitory signals originating from the enteric nervous

system. However, inputs from the central nervous system modulate these local nervous signals, and a variety of gastrointestinal hormones seem to influence intestinal motility to some extent.

5.6. Function

The pyloric sphincter is a muscle that permits food from the stomach to pass through the pylorus and into the duodenum.

5.6.1. Digestion

The majority of chemical digestion happens in the small intestine. The pancreas and liver secrete a large number of digestive enzymes that act in the small intestine and enter it through the pancreatic duct. The hormone cholecystokinin, which is generated in response to the presence of nutrients, causes pancreatic enzymes and gallbladder bile to enter the small intestine. Another hormone made in the small intestine called secretin affects the pancreas further by encouraging the duodenum to release bicarbonate to counteract any potentially hazardous stomach acid.

Proteins, lipids (fats), and carbs are the three main nutritional classes that are digested.

- Prior to absorption, proteins are broken down into amino acids and tiny peptides. The stomach is where chemical breakdown starts, and it continues in the small intestine. The pancreas secretes proteolytic enzymes, such as chymotrypsin and trypsin, which break down proteins into smaller peptides. One amino acid at a time is split by the pancreatic brush border enzyme carboxypeptidase. The final amino acid products are released by aminopeptidase and dipeptidase.
- Fats, or lipids, are broken down into glycerol and fatty acids. Triglycerides are broken down by pancreatic lipase into monoglycerides and free fatty acids. The salts from the bile secreted by the liver and kept in the gall bladder assist pancreatic lipase in its function. Triglycerides are emulsified by bile salts, which facilitates pancreatic lipase's access to them. This happens as a result of the hydrophobic nature of the fatty triglycerides, which cause them to gravitate toward one another and away from the wet intestinal environment, and the water-soluble nature of lipase. Till lipase is able to disintegrate the triglycerides into smaller parts that can pass through the villi for absorption, the bile salts emulsify them in the aqueous environment.
- Certain carbohydrates are broken down into monosaccharides, or simple sugars (e.g., glucose). Certain carbohydrates, most notably starch, are broken down into oligosaccharides by pancreatic amylase. Other carbohydrates enter the large intestine undigested so that intestinal bacteria can handle them further. From there, brush border enzymes take over. Dextrinase and glucoamylase are the two most significant brush border enzymes that break down oligosaccharides even further. The brush border enzymes lactase, sucrase, and maltase are also present. Some adult humans lack the enzyme lactase, which prevents the small intestine from breaking down most polysaccharides and the disaccharide

lactose. Some carbohydrates, like cellulose, are composed of several glucose units but are not broken down at all. This is because, unlike the inter-monosaccharidal bindings found in starch, which is composed of alpha-glucose, cellulose is composed of beta-glucose. The enzyme that breaks down beta-glucose bonds is exclusive to large intestine bacteria and herbivores; it is absent from humans.

5.6.2. Absorption

Now that food has been broken down, it can enter the blood vessels in the intestinal wall by either active transport or diffusion. The majority of the nutrients from food that is consumed are absorbed in the small intestine. Simple columnar intestinal epithelium lines the mucosa, or inner wall, of the small intestine. Circular folds are wrinkles or flaps that cover the mucosa structurally and are thought to be permanent characteristics of the mucosa. They are not to be confused with rugae, which are thought to be transient or non-permanent and permit distention and contraction. Microscopic finger-like pieces of tissue called villi—the Latin word for shaggy hair—protrude from the circular folds. Microvilli, which resemble fingers, are additional projections found on individual epithelial cells. The circular folds, villi, and microvilli serve to both enhance the surface area available for nutrient absorption and restrict the amount of nutrients lost to intestinal fauna.

Near the surface of every villus is a network of lacteals, which are tiny lymphatic vessels and capillaries. Amino acids, carbohydrates, and lipids are transported into these capillaries by the villi's epithelial cells from the intestinal lumen. The absorbed materials are delivered by blood vessels to various body organs, where they are utilized to assemble complex materials like the proteins that are necessary for proper bodily function. The large intestine receives the material that is not absorbed or digested (Figure 5.5).

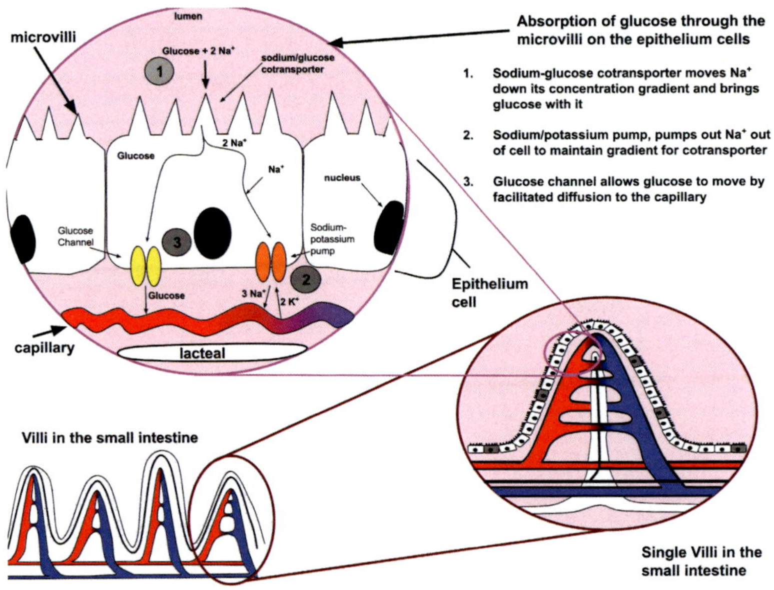

Figure 5.5. *Absorption of glucose in the small intestine.*

Source: By Allison Mason – Own work, CC BY-SA 4.0, https://commons.wikimedia.org/w/index.php?curid=118300026.

The jejunum is where most nutrients are absorbed, with the following noteworthy exceptions:

- Iron is absorbed in the duodenum.
- Vitamin B9, folate, is absorbed in the jejunum and duodenum.
- The terminal ileum is where bile salts and vitamin B12 are absorbed. The ileum won't absorb vitamin B12 until it binds to a protein called intrinsic factor.
- Lipids are absorbed throughout the small intestine by passive diffusion and water by osmosis.
- Amino acid co-transport, as well as active transport, are responsible for the absorption of sodium bicarbonate.
- Facilitated diffusion is used to absorb fructose.

5.6.3. Immunological

The immune system of the body is supported by the small intestine. The host's immune system seems to benefit from the presence of gut flora. An essential component of the local immune system in the digestive tract is Peyer's patches, which are found in the ileum of the small intestine. They are a component of the lymphatic system and offer a location for the sampling of antigens from bacteria or other microorganisms in the digestive tract that may be hazardous, which are then delivered to the immune system.

A Closer Look

Disorders of the Small Intestine: Lactose Intolerance

One of the symptoms of lactose intolerance is indigestion brought on by dairy products. It happens when the small intestine's absorptive cells don't make enough lactase, the enzyme that breaks down lactose, the sugar found in milk. Lactose intolerance rises with age in most mammals. On the other hand, some human populations—Caucasian people foremost among them—are able to continue producing lactase into adulthood.

The lactose in chime is not broken down by those who are lactose intolerant. Gas is produced when bacteria in the large intestine ferment the undigested lactose. The symptoms include diarrhea, bloating, and cramping in the abdomen in addition to gas. The intensity of the symptoms varies from moderate discomfort to excruciating pain, but they go away as soon as the lactose in the feces is removed. Lactose intolerance can be diagnosed in part by using the hydrogen breath test. People who are lactose intolerant exhale very little hydrogen. One of the gases released by the bacteria that ferments lactose in the colon is hydrogen, which is exhaled by people who are intolerant to lactose. The hydrogen enters the lungs through blood vessels after being taken up from the intestine. Grocery stores carry a variety of dairy products that are lactose free. Furthermore, dietary supplements are offered. When taken with food, they offer lactase, which aids in the digestion of lactose.

Summary

- Chyme released from the stomach enters the small intestine, which is the primary digestive organ in the body. Not only is this where most digestion occurs, it is also where practically all absorption occurs. The longest part of the alimentary canal, the small intestine is about 3.05 meters (10 feet) long in a living person (but about twice as long in a cadaver due to the loss of muscle tone).
- The coiled tube of the small intestine is subdivided into three regions. From proximal (at the stomach) to distal, these are the duodenum, jejunum, and ileum. The shortest region is the 25.4-cm (10-in) duodenum, which begins at the pyloric sphincter.
- The wall of the small intestine is composed of the same four layers typically present in the alimentary system. However, three features of the mucosa and submucosa are unique. These features, which increase the absorptive surface area of the small intestine more than 600-fold, include circular folds, villi, and microvilli. These adaptations are most abundant in the proximal two-thirds of the small intestine, where the majority of absorption occurs.
- The movement of intestinal smooth muscles includes both segmentation and a form of peristalsis called migrating motility complexes.
- The digestion of proteins and carbohydrates, which partially occurs in the stomach, is completed in the small intestine with the aid of intestinal and pancreatic juices. Lipids arrive in the intestine largely undigested, so much of the focus here is on lipid digestion, which is facilitated by bile and the enzyme pancreatic lipase.
- The small intestine receives a blood supply from the celiac trunk and the superior mesenteric artery. These are both branches of the aorta. The duodenum receives blood from the coeliac trunk via the superior pancreaticoduodenal artery and from the superior mesenteric artery via the inferior pancreaticoduodenal artery.
- The venous drainage of the small intestine is into the portal circulation. Blood draining from the duodenum via the posterior superior pancreaticoduodenal vein typically drains into the portal vein.
- Intestinal glands are found in the epithelia of the small intestine, namely the duodenum, jejunum, and ileum, and in the large intestine (colon), where they are sometimes called *colonic crypts.*
- The intestinal glands in the colon are often referred to as colonic crypts. The epithelial inner surface of the colon is punctuated by invaginations, the colonic crypts.
- Virtually all nutrients from the diet are absorbed into blood across the highly polarized epithelial cell layer forming the small and large intestinal mucosa.
- Food from the stomach is allowed into the duodenum through the pylorus by a muscle called the pyloric sphincter.

References

1. Chan, C. W., Leung, Y. K., & Chan, K. W. (2014). Microscopic anatomy of the vasculature of the human intestinal villus - A study with review. *European Journal of Anatomy, 18*(4), 291–301.

2. DeGaetani, M., Tennyson, C. A., Lebwohl, B., Lewis, S. K., Abu Daya, H., Arguelles-Grande, C., Bhagat, G., & Green, P. H. R. (2013). Villous atrophy and negative celiac serology: A diagnostic and therapeutic dilemma. *American Journal of Gastroenterology, 108*(5), 647–653. https://doi.org/10.1038/ajg.2013.45.

3. Ensari, A., & Marsh, M. N. (2018). Exploring the villus. *Gastroenterology and Hepatology from Bed to Bench, 11*(3), 181–190.

4. Gourtsoyiannis, N. C. (Ed.). (2002). *Radiological Imaging of the Small Intestine*. Springer Berlin Heidelberg. https://doi.org/10.1007/978-3-642-56231-0.

5. Gremel, G., Wanders, A., Cedernaes, J., Fagerberg, L., Hallström, B., Edlund, K., Sjöstedt, E., Uhlén, M., & Pontén, F. (2015). The human gastrointestinal tract-specific transcriptome and proteome as defined by RNA sequencing and antibody-based profiling. *Journal of Gastroenterology, 50*(1), 46–57. https://doi.org/10.1007/s00535-014-0958-7.

6. Hagen, K. D., McInally, S. G., Hilton, N. D., & Dawson, S. C. (2020). Microtubule organelles in Giardia. *Advances in Parasitology, 107*, 25–96. https://doi.org/10.1016/bs.apar.2019.11.001.

7. Hu, D., Cui, X., Ren, W., Zhang, J., Guan, X., & Jiang, X. (2021). A case of primary intestinal lymphangiectasia with non-Hodgkin lymphoma. *BMC Gastroenterology, 21*(1), 461. https://doi.org/10.1186/s12876-021-01997-x.

8. Kai, Y. (2021). Intestinal villus structure contributes to even shedding of epithelial cells. *Biophysical Journal, 120*(4), 699–710. https://doi.org/10.1016/j.bpj.2021.01.003.

9. Marcon, C. F., Ferreira, P. T. M., Franco, P. S., Ribeiro, M., Silva, R. J., Sousa, R. A. P., et al. (2020). Macrophage migration inhibitory factor (MIF) and pregnancy may impact the balance of intestinal cytokines and the development of intestinal pathology caused by *Toxoplasma gondii* infection. *Cytokine, 136*, 155283. https://doi.org/10.1016/j.cyto.2020.155283.

10. Sakai, E., Higurashi, T., Ohkubo, H., Hosono, K., Ueda, A., Matsuhashi, N., et al. (2017). Investigation of small bowel abnormalities in HIV-infected patients using capsule endoscopy. *Gastroenterology Research and Practice, 2017*, 1932647. https://doi.org/10.1155/2017/1932647.

11. Schoenwolf, G. C., Bleyl, S. B., Brauer, P. R., & Francis-West, P. H. (2009). Development of the urogenital system. In *Larsen's Human Embryology* (4th ed., p. 237). Churchill Livingstone/Elsevier. ISBN 9780443068119.

12. Sherwood, L. (2006). *Fundamentals of Physiology: A Human Perspective* (3rd ed.), International Thomson Computer Pres. ISBN 978-0-534-46697-8.

13. Solomon, E. P., Berg, L. R., & Martin, D. W. (2002). *Biology* (6th ed.). Brooks/Cole Thomson Learning. ISBN 0-03-033503-5.

14. Thomson, A., Drozdowski, L., Iordache, C., Thomson, B., Vermeire, S., Clandinin, M., & Wild, G. (2003). Small bowel review: Normal physiology, part 1. *Digestive Diseases and Sciences, 48*(8), 1546–1564. https://doi.org/10.1023/A:1024719925058.

15. Townsend, C. M., Beauchamp, R. D., Evers, B. M., & Mattox, K. L. (2004). *Sabiston Textbook of Surgery* (17th ed.). Elsevier. ISBN 0-7216-0409-9.

16. Uhlén, M., Fagerberg, L., Hallström, B. M., Lindskog, C., Oksvold, P., Mardinoglu, A., Sivertsson, Å., Kampf, C., & Sjöstedt, E. (2015). Tissue-based map of the human proteome. *Science, 347*(6220), 1260419. https://doi.org/10.1126/science.1260419.

Chapter

DIGESTION AND ABSORPTION

6

Contents

Introduction

The process of mechanically and enzymatically converting food into substances that can be absorbed into the bloodstream is called digestion. Proteins, carbs, and fats are the three macronutrients in the meal that must be digested to be absorbed. These macronutrients are converted during digestion into molecules that can pass through the intestinal epithelium and reach the circulation, where they are utilized by the body. Two distinct processes are involved in digestion, which is a type of catabolism or material breakdown: mechanical digestion and chemical digestion. Food materials are physically broken down into smaller particles during mechanical digestion to facilitate chemical digestion more effectively. Chemical digestion involves the further breakdown of the ingested compounds' molecular structure by digestive enzymes into a form that can be absorbed into the bloodstream. Both of these processes are necessary for effective digestion, and problems with chemical or mechanical digestion can result in gastrointestinal diseases and nutritional deficits. The gastrointestinal tract allows the body to absorb nutrients, vitamins, minerals, and liquids. Mostly in the small intestine, lipids, proteins, and complex carbohydrates are digested—that is, they are broken down into small, absorbable units. Digestion byproducts that pass through the mucosa and enter the lymphatic or bloodstream, such as vitamins, minerals, and water (Absorption). Numerous digestive enzymes work in an orderly manner to aid in the breakdown of the main macronutrients in food. Enzymes from the stomach break down proteins, the salivary and lingual gland enzymes break down fats and carbohydrates, and the pancreatic exocrine gland enzymes break down lipids, RNA, and DNA. The cytoplasm of the cells lining the small intestine and the luminal membranes contain additional enzymes that aid in digestion. The hydrochloric acid (HCl) secreted by the stomach and the bile from the liver enhance the enzymes' ability to work.

Enterocytes are the term for the mucosal cells found in the small intestine. They have a brush border in the small intestine, with many microvilli lining the apical surface. Enzymes abound along this border. The glycocalyx, a layer rich in neutral and amino sugars, lines its luminal side. Glycocalyx is composed partially of the carbohydrate portion of these glycoproteins that extend into the intestinal lumen. Glycoprotein enzymes hydrolyze peptides and carbohydrates and are present in the membranes of mucosal cells. A layer that is similar to the layer next to the biologic membrane but not stirred lies after the brush border and the glycocalyx. For solutes to get to the mucosal cells, they must diffuse through this layer. Significant diffusion resistance is also maintained by the mucous layer covering the cells. The majority of substances travel through the intestines' lumen, enterocytes, and finally the interstitial fluids. During food's passage through the digestive system, the digestive system breaks it down into absorbable substances through mechanical and chemical processes. An outline of the fundamental roles of the digestive organs can be found in Table 6.1.

Table 6.1. Functions of the Digestive Organs

Organ	Major Functions	Other Functions
Mouth	• Ingests food • Chews and mixes food • Begins chemical breakdown of carbohydrates • Moves food into the pharynx • Begins breakdown of lipids via lingual lipase	• Moistens and dissolves food, allowing you to taste it • Cleans and lubricates the teeth and oral cavity • Has some antimicrobial activity
Pharynx	• Propels food from the oral cavity to the esophagus	• Lubricates food and passageways
Esophagus	• Propels food to the stomach	• Lubricates food and passageways

Stomach	• Mixes and churns food with gastric juices to form chyme • Begins chemical breakdown of proteins • Releases food into the duodenum as chyme • Absorbs some fat-soluble substances (for example, alcohol, aspirin) • Possesses antimicrobial functions	• Stimulates protein-digesting enzymes • Secretes intrinsic factor required for vitamin B_{12} absorption in small intestine
Small intestine	• Mixes chyme with digestive juices • Propels food at a rate slow enough for digestion and absorption • Absorbs breakdown products of carbohydrates, proteins, lipids, and nucleic acids, along with vitamins, minerals, and water • Performs physical digestion via segmentation	• Provides optimal medium for enzymatic activity
Accessory organs	• Liver: produces bile salts, which emulsify lipids, aiding their digestion and absorption • Gallbladder: stores, concentrates, and releases bile • Pancreas: produces digestive enzymes and bicarbonate	• Bicarbonate-rich pancreatic juices help neutralize acidic chyme and provide optimal environment for enzymatic activity
Large intestine	• Further breaks down food residues • Absorbs most residual water, electrolytes, and vitamins produced by enteric bacteria • Propels feces toward rectum • Eliminates feces	• Food residue is concentrated and temporarily stored prior to defecation • Mucus eases passage of feces through colon

Source: https://courses.lumenlearning.com/suny-ap2/chapter/digestive-system-processes-and-regulation/.

Orientation and Directional Terms

Term	Definition	Illustration
Carbohydrates	Carbohydrates, or carbs, are sugar molecules. Along with proteins and fats, carbohydrates are one of three main nutrients found in foods and drinks.	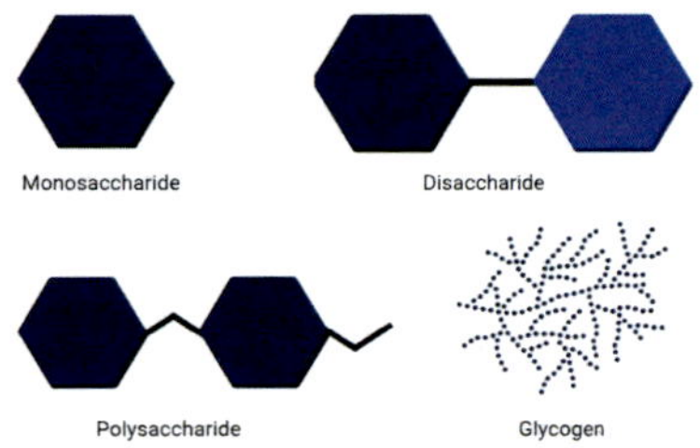
Sucrose	Sucrose, a disaccharide, is a sugar composed of glucose and fructose subunits. It is produced naturally in plants and is the main constituent of white sugar.	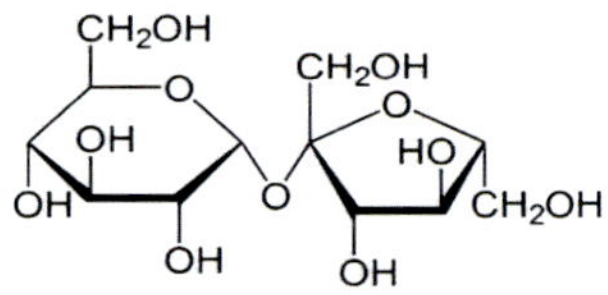
Lactose	Lactose is a sugar that is naturally found in milk and milk products, like cheese or ice cream.	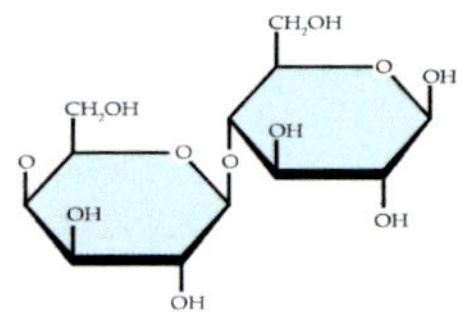
Cellulose	Cellulose is a complex carbohydrate, or polysaccharide, consisting of 3000 or more glucose units.	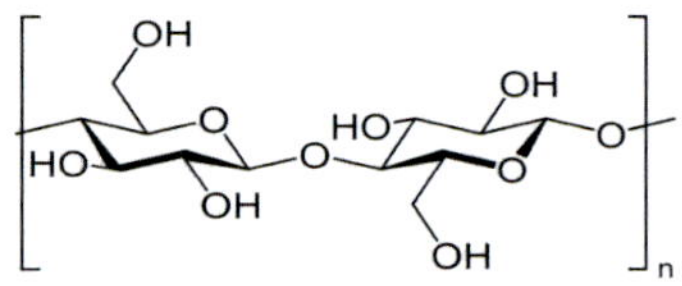
Proteolysis	Proteolysis is the breakdown of proteins into smaller polypeptides or amino acids.	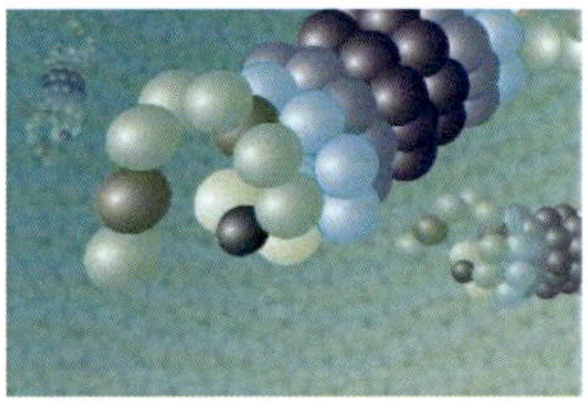
Lipids	Lipids are fatty compounds that perform a variety of functions in your body.	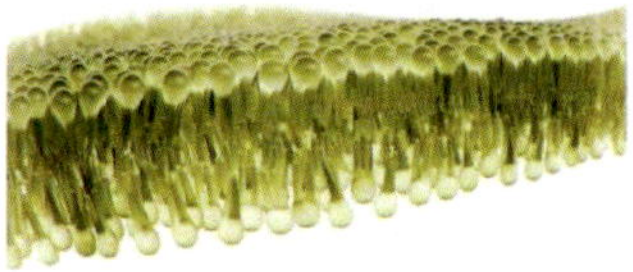

6.1. Mechanical Digestion

The process of mechanical digestion is solely physical and does not alter the chemical composition of the food. Rather, it reduces the size of the food to enhance its surface area and mobility. In addition to tongue movements that aid in breaking food into smaller pieces and combining it with saliva, it involves mastication, or chewing.

Although there may be a tendency to believe that mechanical digestion only takes place in the initial stages of the digestive process, it also happens in the stomach and intestine through segmentation and peristalsis after the food leaves the mouth. Peristalsis is the movement of food through the digestive tract to various processing stations through a series of wave-like muscular contractions. The food bolus is propelled to the stomach by peristalsis in the esophagus. Food is mashed, ground, and churned into chyme by strong peristaltic contractions that occur when food enters the stomach, an extremely muscular organ.

Chyme is a semiliquid mixture of partially broken down food and gastric secretions from stomach cells. Food is mechanically churned in the stomach to increase its surface area exposure to digestive juices and to further break it apart. Vomiting is the reverse peristaltic action of the stomach.

The brain's vomiting center, the medulla oblongata, is responsive to toxins and sudden movements of the body. Additionally receiving cortical input, the vomiting center is where certain thoughts can induce vomiting. Segmentation mostly affects the small intestine and is brought on by localized contractions of the alimentary canal's muscularis layer's circular muscle. Small sections of the intestine are isolated by these contractions, which also continuously subdivide, break up, and mix the contents as they move back and forth. Segmentation mixes food with digestive juices and promotes absorption by causing food to move back and forth in the intestinal lumen (Figure 6.1).

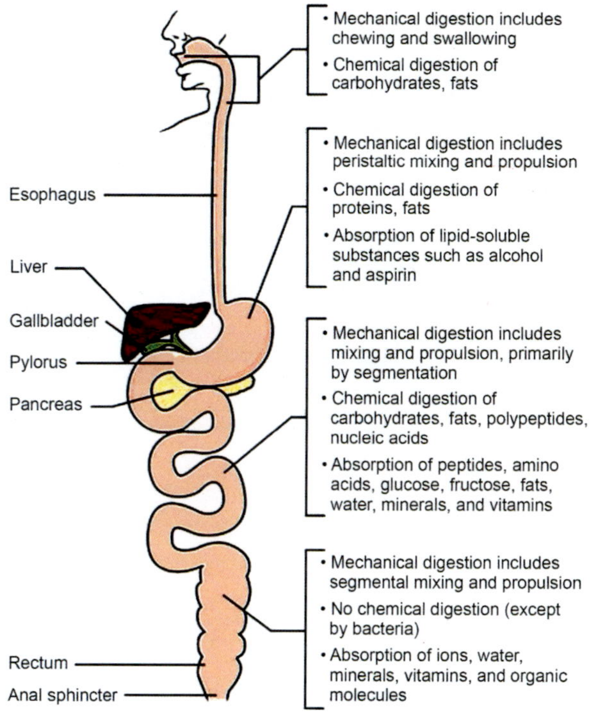

Figure 6.1. *Digestion and Absorption: Digestion begins in the mouth and continues as food travels through the small intestine. Most absorption occurs in the small intestine.*

Source: https://bio.libretexts.org/Bookshelves/Human_Biology/Human_Biology_(Wakim_and_Grewal)/18%3A_Digestive_System/18.3%3A_Digestion_and_Absorption.

6.2. Chemical Digestion

Proteins, fats, nucleic acids, and carbohydrates are examples of large food molecules that need to be broken down into smaller subunits for the lining of the alimentary canal to absorb them. Enzymes use hydrolysis to accomplish this. Table 6.2 provides an overview of the numerous enzymes used in chemical digestion.

Table 6.2. Digestive Enzymes

Enzyme Category	Enzyme Name	Source	Substrate	Product
Salivary Enzymes	Lingual lipase	Lingual glands	Triglycerides	Free fatty acids, and mono- and diglycerides
Salivary Enzymes	Salivary amylase	Salivary glands	Polysaccharides	Disaccharides and trisaccharides
Gastric enzymes	Gastric lipase	Chief cells	Triglycerides	Fatty acids and monoacylglycerides
Gastric enzymes	Pepsin*	Chief cells	Proteins	Peptides
Brush border enzymes	α-Dextrinase	Small intestine	α-Dextrins	Glucose
Brush border enzymes	Enteropeptidase	Small intestine	Trypsinogen	Trypsin
Brush border enzymes	Lactase	Small intestine	Lactose	Glucose and galactose
Brush border enzymes	Maltase	Small intestine	Maltose	Glucose
Brush border enzymes	Nucleosidases and phosphatases	Small intestine	Nucleotides	Phosphates, nitrogenous bases, and pentoses
Brush border enzymes	Peptidases	Small intestine	• Aminopeptidase: amino acids at the amino end of peptides • Dipeptidase: dipeptides	• Aminopeptidase: amino acids and peptides • Dipeptidase: amino acids
Brush border enzymes	Sucrase	Small intestine	Sucrose	Glucose and fructose
Pancreatic enzymes	Carboxy-peptidase*	Pancreatic acinar cells	Amino acids at the carboxyl end of peptides	Amino acids and peptides

Pancreatic enzymes	Chymotrypsin*	Pancreatic acinar cells	Proteins	Peptides
Pancreatic enzymes	Elastase*	Pancreatic acinar cells	Proteins	Peptides
Pancreatic enzymes	Nucleases	Pancreatic acinar cells	• Ribonuclease: ribonucleic acids • Deoxyribonuclease: deoxyribonucleic acids	Nucleotides
Pancreatic enzymes	Pancreatic amylase	Pancreatic acinar cells	Polysaccharides (starches)	α-Dextrins, disaccharides (maltose), trisaccharides (maltotriose)
Pancreatic enzymes	Pancreatic lipase	Pancreatic acinar cells	Triglycerides that have been emulsified by bile salts	Fatty acids and monoacylglycerides
Pancreatic enzymes	Trypsin*	Pancreatic acinar cells	Proteins	Peptides
*These enzymes have been activated by other substances.				

*These enzymes have been activated by other substances.

Source: https://courses.lumenlearning.com/suny-ap2/chapter/chemical-digestion-and-absorption-a-closer-look/.

6.2.1. Carbohydrate Digestion

About half of the average American diet consists of carbohydrates, which can be categorized based on how many monomers they contain of either complex (polysaccharides) or simple (monosaccharides and disaccharides) sugars. Three widely consumed and easily absorbed monosaccharides are glucose, galactose, and fructose. The polysaccharides glycogen and starch (chains of monosaccharides) as well as the disaccharides sucrose (regular table sugar: glucose + fructose), lactose (milk sugar: glucose + galactose), and maltose (grain sugar: glucose + glucose) can all be broken down by your digestive system. Enzymes needed to break down the majority of fibrous polysaccharides, including cellulose, are not produced by your bodies. Indigestible polysaccharides offer dietary fiber, which aids in moving food through the digestive tract, but they have no nutritional value (Figure 6.2).

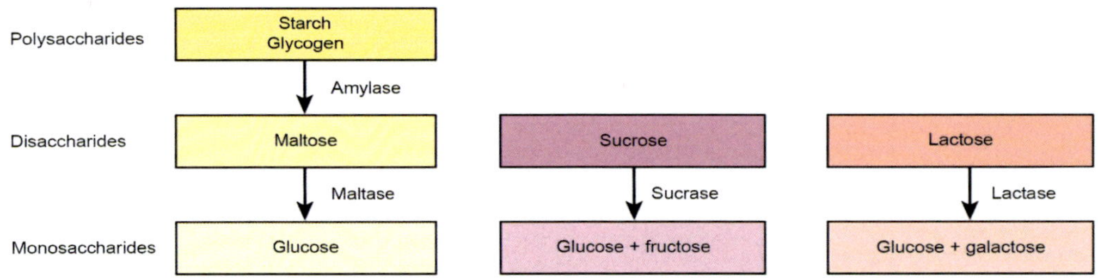

Figure 6.2. *The process of chemical digestion for some carbohydrates.*

Source: https://courses.lumenlearning.com/wm-biology2/chapter/digestive-system-processes/.

As was previously mentioned, starches are first chemically broken down in the mouth.

Pancreatic amylase performs the "heavy lifting" of starch and carbohydrate digestion in the small intestine. The brush border enzyme α-dextrinase begins working on α-dextrin, breaking off one glucose unit at a time, after amylases break down starch into smaller fragments. Lactose, maltose, and sucrose are hydrolyzed into monosaccharides by three brush border enzymes. Maltase converts maltose and maltotriose into two and three glucose molecules, respectively, while lactase breaks down lactose into one glucose molecule and one galactose molecule. Sucrase breaks down sucrose into one fructose and one glucose molecule. Lactose intolerance can result from insufficient lactase (Figure 6.3).

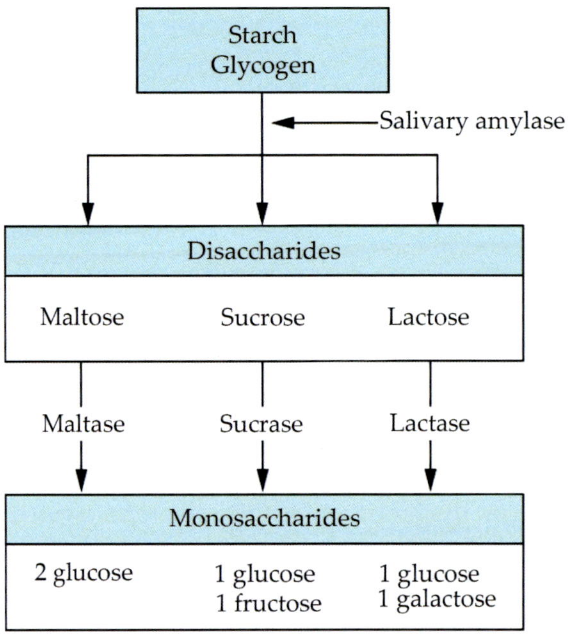

Figure 6.3. *Carbohydrate digestion flow chart: Carbohydrates are broken down into their monomers in a series of steps.*

Source: https://open.oregonstate.education/aandp/chapter/23-7-chemical-digestion-and-absorption-a-closer-look/.

6.2.2. Protein Digestion

Protein digestion begins by breaking the complex molecule into peptides, which are composed of various amino acids, before further breaking them down into individual amino acids. The stomach secretes enzymes called pepsins in the presence of acid to facilitate the breakdown of proteins (proteolysis), accounting for 10–15% of the process. Pepsins are most active in the first hour of digestion, requiring an acidic pH between 1.8 and 3.5 for optimal function. However, trypsins, powerful proteolytic enzymes secreted by the pancreas, play a more significant role in protein digestion as they are able to break down proteins more efficiently. As a result, most protein digestion occurs in the duodenum and upper jejunum rather than the stomach. Even after the stomach is removed, protein digestion is usually not impaired due to the efficiency of trypsins (Figure 6.4).

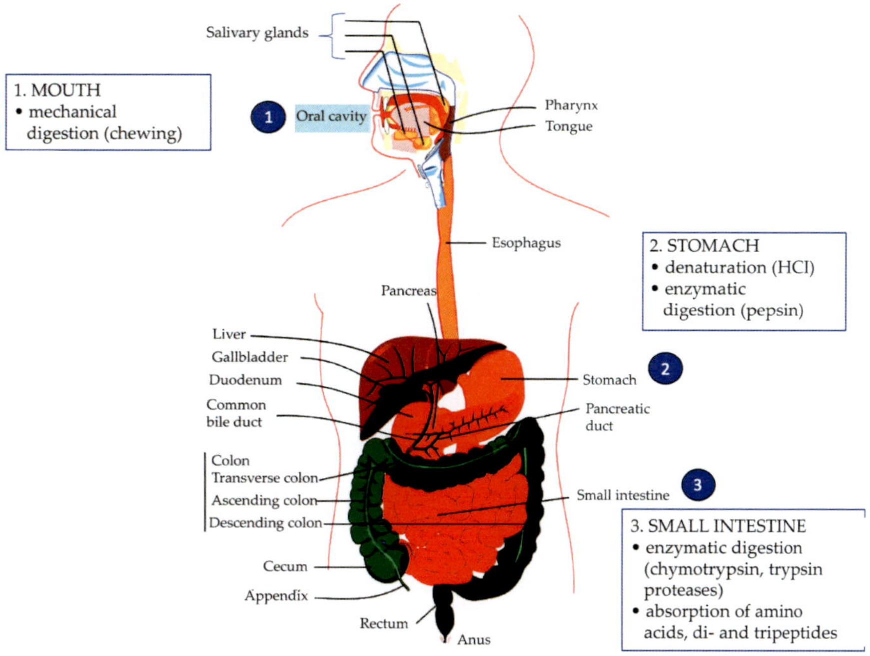

Figure 6.4. *Protein digestion in the human GI tract.*

Source: https://openoregon.pressbooks.pub/nutritionscience/chapter/6d-protein-digestion-absorption/.

Protease precursors that are inactive in pancreatic secretion can become active by interacting with another enzyme called enterokinase, which is secreted by the enterocytes' microvillous component in the mucosa of the duodenum and jejunum. Enterokinase, which is released from duodenal lining cells by the action of bile acids and CCK, activates trypsinogen in the intestine. The cleavage of six terminal amino acid residues from trypsinogen causes trypsin to activate. Free trypsin acts as an activator for the other proteases. These proteases ultimately reduce dietary proteins to single amino acids and small polypeptide chains of two to six amino acids. Chymotrypsin, elastase, and other pancreatic proteases are all activated by trypsin. Known as endopeptidases, trypsin, chymotrypsin, and elastase are in charge of hydrolyzing protein chains to peptides in the first place. The pancreas also secretes carboxypeptidases, which have the enzymatic activity responsible for breaking down these peptides into smaller molecules and eventually individual amino acids (Figure 6.5).

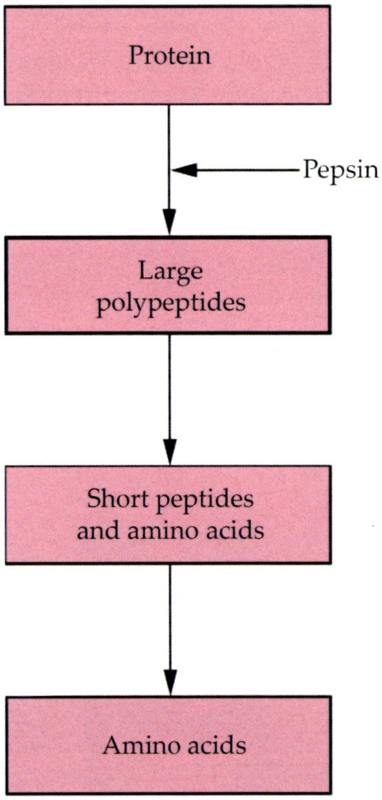

Figure 6.5. *Digestion of protein: proteins are successively broken down into their amino acid components.*

Source: https://open.oregonstate.education/aandp/chapter/23-7-chemical-digestion-and-absorption-a-closer-look/.

Peptidase activity starts in the mucus and brush border, outside the enterocytes, and continues within the cell. It appears that various peptidases are involved in the different stages of the breakdown of protein into amino acids. Similarly, distinct transport mechanisms are involved in the movement of distinct peptides. A carrier protein is involved in an energy-demanding process that transfers dipeptides—peptides that hydrolyze to release two amino acids—and tripeptides—peptides that hydrolyze to release three amino acids—from the surface brush border into the cell. As such, small peptides containing few amino acids are directly absorbed. The enterocyte is where the majority of the breakdown of peptides into amino acids occurs. It's interesting to note that small peptides absorb more quickly than amino acids. In fact, the specifics of the mechanism governing amino acid absorption remain largely unknown. It is well known that while some amino acids share a single transport system, others have unique ones (Figure 6.6).

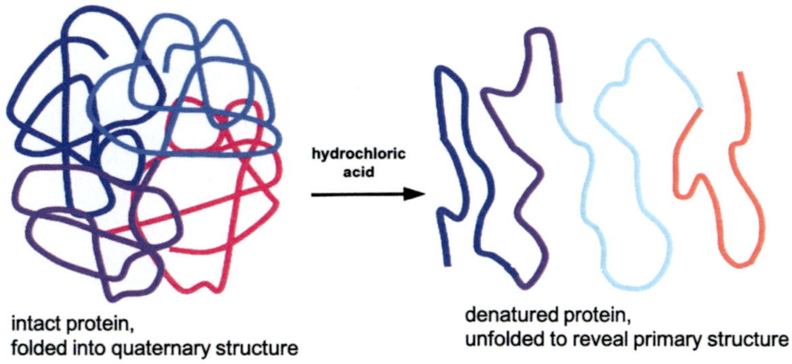

Figure 6.6. *In the stomach, proteins are denatured because of the acidity of hydrochloric acid.*

Source: https://openoregon.pressbooks.pub/nutritionscience/chapter/6d-protein-digestion-absorption/.

Groupings of amino acids can be synthesized based on the optical rotatory properties (i.e., whether they rotate polarized light in terms of reactivity, or acidity (pH), and to the left, or levo, or to the right, or dextro. Compared to dextrorotatory amino acids, levorotatory amino acids are absorbed far more quickly. Levorotatory amino acids are actually absorbed practically as fast as they are liberated from proteins or peptides. Active transport of neutral amino acids depends on specific structural arrangements; if these arrangements are broken, active transport will not take place. The rate of transportation of basic amino acids, which are acidic (pH greater than 7), is 5–10% that of neutral levorotatory amino acids.

6.2.3. Lipid Digestion

Digestion and absorption of lipids present unique difficulties. Unlike proteins and carbohydrates, triglycerides are big molecules that are not soluble in water. For this reason, in aqueous environments such as the digestive tract, they prefer to assemble in big droplets. Large fat droplets must be broken up into smaller droplets during the digestive process, and lipases are the enzymes that are used to enzymatically digest lipid molecules. The majority of the enzymatic digestion of lipids takes place in the small intestine, with minimal involvement from the mouth or stomach. Once more requiring special handling, the byproducts of lipid digestion are absorbed into circulation and moved throughout the body because lipids are not soluble in water and do not combine with the thin blood. To understand more about the movement of lipids through the digestive system, let's go back to the beginning.

6.2.3.1. Lipid Digestion in the Mouth

Lipid digestion is initiated in the mouth by a few different processes. Food is mechanically broken up into smaller pieces and combined with saliva when chewed. The tongue's cells produce an enzyme known as lingual lipase, which starts the enzymatic digestion of triglycerides by cleaving individual fatty acids from the glycerol backbone. The word "lingual" means relating to the tongue.

6.2.3.2. Lipid Digestion in the Stomach

Churning and mixing aid in the dispersal of fat molecules and food particles in the stomach. Another lipase, known as gastric lipase (the word "gastric" refers to the stomach), is produced by stomach cells and aids in the enzymatic digestion of triglycerides. In the stomach, lingual lipase that is swallowed with food and saliva is still active. However, the majority of enzymatic digestion occurs in the small intestine, so the combined action of these two lipases is negligible in the digestion of fat (apart from the case of infants, as detailed below).

6.2.3.3. Lipid Digestion in The Small Intestine

Large droplets of mostly undigested dietary lipids are passed through the stomach and into the small intestine. The duodenum, the first part of the small intestine, receives the release of bile, which is produced in the liver and kept in reserve in the gallbladder. Bile salts are drawn to both fats and water because they possess both hydrophobic and hydrophilic sides. Because of this, they function as effective emulsifiers, dissolving big fat globules into smaller droplets. Emulsification increases the surface area of lipids so that digestive enzymes have more room to act on them. Triglycerides are enzymatically broken down in the small intestine by pancreatic lipases, which are secreted by the pancreas. Fatty acids, monoglycerides (glycerol backbone with one fatty acid still attached), and some free glycerol are the byproducts of the breakdown of triglycerides. It is not necessary for fat-soluble vitamins and cholesterol to be broken down by enzymes.

6.2.3.4. Lipid Absorption from The Small Intestine

For cells all over the body to use the byproducts of fat digestion—fatty acids, monoglycerides, glycerol, cholesterol, and fat-soluble vitamins—they must next enter the circulation. Bile aids in this process once more. To help fats get close enough to the intestinal cells' microvilli for absorption, bile salts gather around the byproducts of fat digestion to form structures known as micelles. The byproducts of fat digestion permeate the intestinal cells' membranes, and bile salts are recycled back to continue the process of emulsifying fat and creating micelles (Figure 6.7).

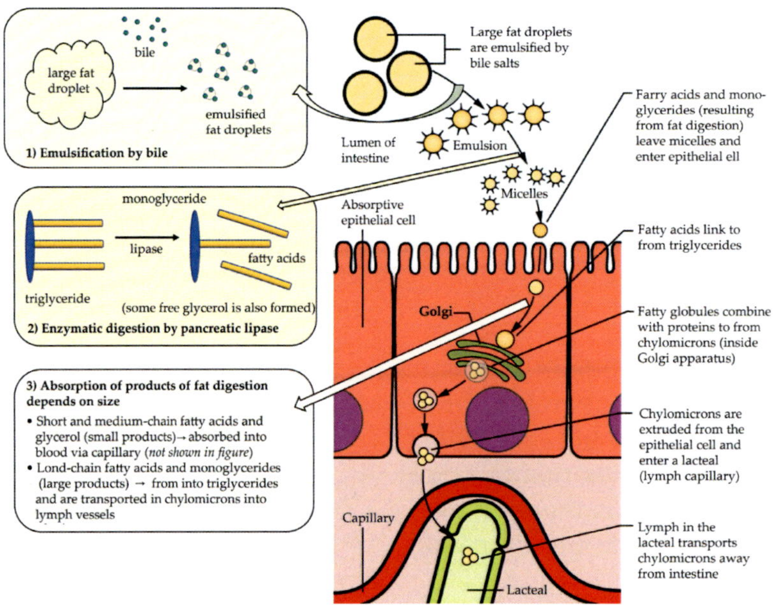

Figure 6.7. *Lipid digestion and absorption in the small intestine.*

Source: https://openoregon.pressbooks.pub/nutritionscience/chapter/5d-digestion-absorption-lipids/.

Larger lipids such as long-chain fatty acids, monoglycerides, fat-soluble vitamins, and cholesterol require assistance with absorption and transport to the bloodstream. Short- and medium-chain fatty acids, as well as glycerol, can be directly absorbed into the bloodstream once they reach the intestinal cell. Within the intestinal cell, long-chain fatty acids and monoglycerides reassemble into triglycerides. These, along with fat-soluble vitamins and cholesterol, are then integrated into transport vehicles known as chylomicrons. Chylomicrons are big structures consisting of an outer membrane composed of phospholipids and a mixture of cholesterol, triglycerides, and proteins known as apolipoproteins.

Their ability to dissolve in water thanks to their outer membrane allows them to move through the body's aqueous environment. Small intestine chylomicrons first enter lymph vessels, from where they are subsequently transported to the bloodstream. One kind of lipoprotein that carries lipids in blood and lymph is called chylomicron (Figure 6.8).

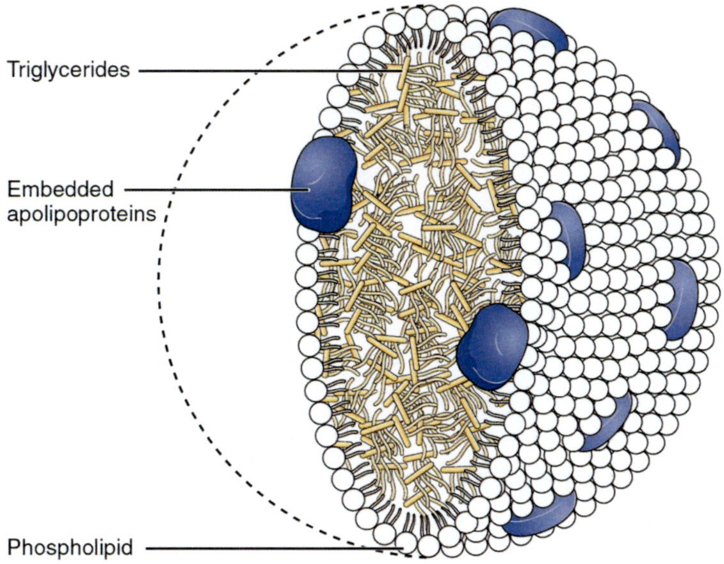

Figure 6.8. *Structure of a chylomicron. Cholesterol is not shown in this figure, but chylomicrons contain cholesterol in both the lipid core and embedded on the surface of the structure.*

Source: https://openoregon.pressbooks.pub/nutritionscience/chapter/5d-digestion-absorption-lipids/.

6.2.3.5. Special Adaptations for Lipid Digestion in Infants

An infant's diet should include a lot of lipids. Similar to whole cow's milk, breast milk has about 4% fat. Whether an infant is breastfed or fed formula, fat makes up roughly half of their calories and plays a crucial role in brain development. However, bile and pancreatic enzyme secretion are low in newborns, despite the fact that these processes are critical for the digestion of lipids in older children and adults. So how do infants process all the fat in their food?

A few unique adaptations enable infants to efficiently digest fat. First off, from birth, they have an abundance of lingual and gastric lipases. Compared to adults, babies are far more dependent on these enzymes. Second, the lipase enzymes found in breast milk are activated in the baby's small intestine. Stated differently, the mother produces lipases and secretes them into the breast milk to aid her child's digestion of the fats in it. It's amazing that young infants can effectively digest fat and benefit from its nutritional value for growth and brain development thanks to increased activity of lingual and gastric lipases and the lipases found in breast milk. Research indicates that breast milk facilitates better fat digestion in premature babies than formula does. Because heat denatures lipases, even pasteurized breast milk—which is used when breast milk is donated to feed infants in hospitals—is a little more difficult to digest. Babies are still capable of digesting pasteurized breast milk and formula; they just do so less effectively and take in less of the byproducts of the breakdown of triglycerides).

6.2.4. Nucleic Acid Digestion

The majority of the foods you eat contain the nucleic acids DNA and RNA. Their digestion is carried out by two different forms of pancreatic nuclease: ribonuclease, which breaks down RNA, and deoxyribonuclease, which breaks down DNA. Two intestinal brush border enzymes, nucleosidase and phosphatase, further break down the nucleotides produced by this digestion into pentoses, phosphates, and nitrogenous bases that can be absorbed through the alimentary canal wall. Table 6.3 summarizes the large food molecules that need to be divided into subunits.

Table 6.3. Absorbable Food Substances

Source	Substance
Carbohydrates	Monosaccharides: glucose, galactose, and fructose
Proteins	Single amino acids, dipeptides, and tripeptides
Triglycerides	Monoacylglycerides, glycerol, and free fatty acids
Nucleic acids	Pentose sugars, phosphates, and nitrogenous bases

Source: https://open.oregonstate.education/aandp/chapter/23-7-chemical-digestion-and-absorption-a-closer-look/.

6.2.5. Bacteria in the Digestive System

There is more to your large intestine than just cells. Known as the "gut flora," it is also an ecosystem that supports trillions of bacteria. Rest assured, the majority of these bacteria are beneficial. Most friendly bacteria are found in the large and partially small intestines. Bacterial growth is inhibited by the stomach's acidic environment.

The body uses gut bacteria for a variety of purposes. As an illustration, intestinal bacteria:

- Produce vitamin B12 and vitamin K.
- Control the growth of harmful bacteria.
- Poisons are broken down in the large intestine.
- Break down the fiber and certain starches and sugars in food that are indigestible. Enzymes produced by bacteria break down the carbohydrates found in plant cell walls. Without these bacteria, the majority of the nutritional value of plant material would be wasted. These aid in the digestion of plant-based foods like spinach (Figure 6.9).

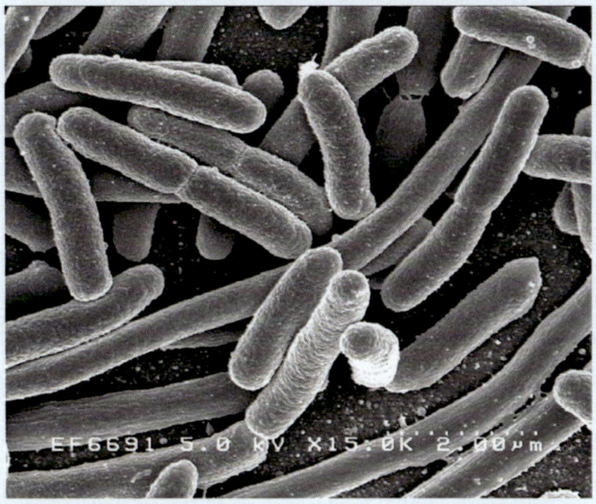

Figure 6.9. *E. coli.*

Source: By NIAID – E. coli bacteria, public domain, https://commons.wikimedia.org/w/index.php?curid=39933215.

In the gut, a diverse array of beneficial bacteria reside. The human digestive system is immediately colonized by bacteria from birth. Lactobacillus, a type of bacteria frequently found in probiotic foods like yogurt, and *E. coli* are examples of gut bacteria. Members of the Bacteroides species make up about one-third of all bacteria found in the gut. We need bacteria to aid in the digestion of plant-based diets. The gut is thought to be home to 100 trillion bacteria. You are made up of more than just human cells. Additionally, it's been calculated that the number of bacteria in your mouth surpasses the population of the planet, which stands at over 7 billion! Your digestive system contains bacteria from between 300 and 1,000 different species. Because these microorganisms are beneficial, your body does not fight them. In reality, rather than appearing as foreign invaders, they are recognized by the immune system as digestive system cells. In reality, the bacteria coat themselves in sugar molecules that have been extracted from the digestive system's actual cells. By doing this, the bacteria are hidden from the immune system and kept safe. The relationship we have with the bacteria that reside in our stomachs is known as mutualism, a type of symbiotic relationship, because the bacteria benefit us and because they have a safe place to live. Finally, remember that bacteria are tiny. The total weight of all the bacteria in your stomach could be around two pounds.

6.2.6. Control of the Digestive Process

Hormones and nerves work together to control the digestive process. Endocrine hormones secreted by stomach and small intestine lining cells are primarily responsible for controlling hormones. These hormones promote the synthesis of bile, bicarbonate, and digestive enzymes. Endocrine cells that line the duodenum in the small intestine, for instance, produce the hormone secretin. Secretin is released into the bloodstream when acidic chyme from the stomach enters the duodenum. The pancreas releases bicarbonate when secretin travels back via the bloodstream to the digestive tract. The acidic chyme is neutralized by the bicarbonate. Both the nerves inside the walls of the digestive organs and the nerves connecting the organs to the central nervous system are involved in digestion. Smooth muscles in the walls of the digestive organs contract or relax in response to changes in the presence or absence of food for digestion, thanks to nerves that connect the organs to the central nervous system. Food that enters the digestive organs and stretches their walls stimulates the nerves within. These nerves cause the secretion of digestive enzymes and the release of chemicals that alter how quickly or slowly food passes through the GI tract.

6.3. Absorption

The conversion of food into molecules small enough to be absorbed by the intestinal villi's epithelial cells is the sole objective of the mechanical and digestive processes. The alimentary canal has an almost limitless capacity for absorption. Less than one liter of the food, liquids, and GI secretions processed by the alimentary canal each day make it into the large intestine. The small intestine absorbs 90% of water, 80% of electrolytes, and nearly all food that is consumed. While the entire small intestine is involved in the absorption of fats and water, the jejunum is where most proteins and carbohydrates are absorbed. Notably, the terminal ileum is where vitamin B12 and bile salts are absorbed. Chyme is essentially indigestible food residue (mostly plant fibers like cellulose), some water, and millions of bacteria by the time it passes from the ileum into the large intestine (Figure 6.10).

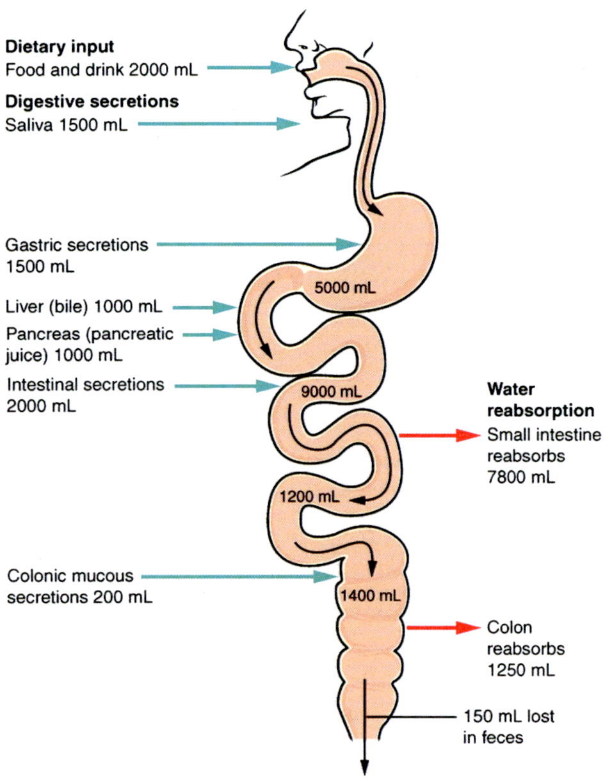

Figure 6.10. *Digestive secretions and absorption of water: Absorption is a complex process, in which nutrients from digested food are harvested.*

Source: https://open.oregonstate.education/aandp/chapter/23-7-chemical-digestion-and-absorption-a-closer-look/.

There are five different ways that absorption can happen: co-transport, also known as secondary active transport, active transport, passive diffusion, facilitated diffusion, and endocytosis. Moving a substance up the concentration gradient, or from a region of lower concentration to one of higher concentration, across a cell membrane, is referred to as active transport. This kind of transport uses cellular energy (ATP) to pump the material through proteins in the cell membrane that function as "pumps." Substances move from a higher concentration area to a lower concentration area through a process known as passive diffusion, whereas substances move from a higher concentration area to a lower concentration area with the help of a carrier protein in the cell membrane. In co-transport, one molecule moves across the membrane from a higher to a lower concentration, enabling another to move from a lower to a higher concentration. Last but not least, endocytosis is a transportation mechanism where material is absorbed by the cell membrane. It needs energy, which is usually provided by ATP.

Since the hydrophobic phospholipids that make up the cell's plasma membrane prevent water-soluble nutrients from entering the cell, they must enter through transport molecules that are embedded in the membrane. Furthermore, because the intestinal mucosa's epithelial cells are connected by tight junctions, substances cannot flow between them. Therefore, materials can only enter blood capillaries by entering the interstitial fluid and passing through the apical surfaces of epithelial cells. Water-soluble nutrients pass through the hepatic portal vein and into the capillary blood in the villi. Lipid-soluble nutrients have the ability to diffuse through the plasma membrane, in contrast to water-soluble nutrients. After entering the cell, they are packaged for transit via the cell's base and then pass through the lacteals of the villi, where they are carried by lymphatic vessels and eventually enter the thoracic duct, which connects them to the systemic circulation. The majority of nutrients must be absorbed by active transport powered by ATP to pass through the intestinal villi's mucosa. Table 6.4 summarizes the absorption pathways of each food category.

Table 6.4. Absorption in the Alimentary Canal

Food	Breakdown Products	Absorption Mechanism	Entry to Bloodstream	Destination
Carbohydrates	Glucose	Co-transport with sodium ions	Capillary blood in villi	Liver via the hepatic portal vein
Carbohydrates	Galactose	Co-transport with sodium ions	Capillary blood in villi	Liver via the hepatic portal vein
Carbohydrates	Fructose	Facilitated diffusion	Capillary blood in villi	Liver via the hepatic portal vein
Protein	Amino acids	Co-transport with sodium ions	Capillary blood in villi	Liver via the hepatic portal vein
Lipids	Long-chain fatty acids	Diffusion into intestinal cells, where they are combined with proteins to create chylomicrons	Lacteals of villi	Systemic circulation via lymph entering the thoracic duct
Lipids	Monoacylglycerides	Diffusion into intestinal cells, where they are combined with proteins to create chylomicrons	Lacteals of villi	Systemic circulation via lymph entering the thoracic duct
Lipids	Short-chain fatty acids	Simple diffusion	Capillary blood in villi	Liver via the hepatic portal vein
Lipids	Glycerol	Simple diffusion	Capillary blood in villi	Liver via the hepatic portal vein
Lipids	Nucleic acid digestion products	Active transport via membrane carriers	Capillary blood in villi	Liver via the hepatic portal vein

Source: https://open.oregonstate.education/aandp/chapter/23-7-chemical-digestion-and-absorption-a-closer-look/.

6.3.1. Carbohydrate Absorption

Monosaccharides are the only form of carbohydrates that are absorbed in the small intestine, with the estimated rate of absorption being 120 grams per hour. The small intestine efficiently absorbs all normally digested dietary carbohydrates, with indigestible fibers being excreted in the feces. Glucose and galactose are taken up by epithelial cells through secondary active transport with sodium ions, while fructose is absorbed through facilitated diffusion. After disaccharides are broken down, the monosaccharides combine with transport proteins before entering the capillaries through intercellular clefts.

6.3.2. Protein Absorption

The majority of proteins are absorbed by secondary active transport mechanisms as the amino acids produced by protein breakdown, mainly in the duodenum and jejunum. The absorptive mechanisms involved in the absorption of monosaccharides are conceptually identical to these mechanisms. The small intestine is where 95–98% of protein is broken down and absorbed. Different carriers carry different amino acids.

The majority of carriers are connected to sodium's active transport. Additionally, actively transported are short chains of two amino acids (dipeptides) or three amino acids (tripeptides). But before they exit the cell and enter the capillary blood through facilitated diffusion, they are broken down into their amino acids once they reach the absorptive epithelial cells.

6.3.3. Lipid Absorption

The small intestine absorbs about 95% of all lipids. Bile salts are necessary for the absorption of the byproducts of lipid digestion in addition to hastening the breakdown of fats. Short-chain fatty acids can directly enter enterocytes, the cells that absorb substances, due to their relative water solubility. Short-chain fatty acids are hydrophobic, but because of their small size, they can be absorbed by enterocytes through simple diffusion. From there, they enter villus blood capillaries in the same way as monosaccharides and amino acids. In the watery intestinal chyme, large, hydrophobic long-chain fatty acids and monoacylglycerides are less readily suspended. Bile salts and lecithin, on the other hand, solve this problem by encasing the long-chain fatty acids in a micelle, which is a microscopic sphere with hydrophobic tails facing inward and polar (hydrophilic) ends facing the watery environment.

Fat-soluble vitamins and cholesterol are also components of the core. Lipids wouldn't be able to interact with the absorptive surfaces of the epithelial cells; instead, they would remain on the chyme's surface in the absence of micelles. Micelles have little trouble passing through microvilli and getting very close to the luminal cell surface. Lipid materials now leave the micelle and are absorbed by straightforward diffusion.

Triglycerides are formed again from the free fatty acids and monoacylglycerides that enter the epithelial cells. Triglycerides are encased in a protein coat and combined with cholesterol and phospholipids. This new complex is a water-soluble lipoprotein known as a chylomicron. The Golgi apparatus processes chylomicrons, which are then expelled from the cell.

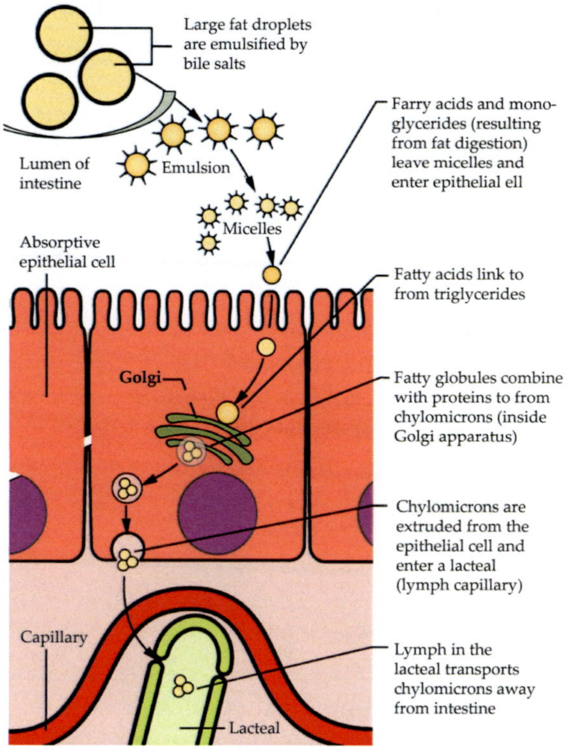

Figure 6.11. *Lipid absorption: Unlike amino acids and simple sugars, lipids are transformed as they are absorbed through epithelial cells.*

Source: https://open.oregonstate.education/aandp/chapter/23-7-chemical-digestion-and-absorption-a-closer-look/.

Chylomicrons enter the large pores of lacteals because they are too large to fit through the basement membranes of blood capillaries. The lymphatic vessels are formed by the joining of the lacteals. The lymphatic vessels carry the chylomicrons, which eventually empty into the circulatory system's subclavian vein via the thoracic duct. Once in the bloodstream, the chylomicrons' triglycerides are broken down into free fatty acids and glycerol by the enzyme lipoprotein lipase. Following breakdown, these products enter capillary walls where they are either stored as fat in adipose tissue or used by cells as an energy source. The leftover chylomicron remnants are combined with proteins by liver cells to form lipoproteins, which carry cholesterol throughout the bloodstream (Figure 6.11).

6.3.4. Nucleic Acid Absorption

Pentose sugars, nitrogenous bases, and phosphate ions—byproducts of nucleic acid digestion—are carried by carriers via active transport through the villus epithelium. The bloodstream is then exposed to these products.

6.3.5. Mineral Absorption

The small intestine absorbs electrolytes from both ingested foods and GI secretions. The majority of electrolytes are absorbed through active transport throughout the whole small intestine because they separate into ions in water. While anti-port mechanisms lower the concentration of potassium ions inside the cells during absorption, co-transport mechanisms cause an accumulation of sodium ions inside the cells.

A sodium-potassium pump that needs ATP moves potassium in and sodium out of the cell membrane to restore the sodium-potassium gradient. Whether or not you need them, minerals that enter the colon are generally absorbed. The duodenum absorbs iron and calcium in amounts that satisfy the body's present needs, but they are exceptions.

- **Iron:** Active transport is the mechanism by which mucosal cells absorb the ionic iron required for hemoglobin synthesis. Ionic iron attaches to the protein ferritin once it enters mucosal cells, forming iron-ferritin complexes that hold iron until needed. When the body stores enough iron, most of it is lost as aging epithelial cells shed their skin. The body absorbs more iron from the intestine and releases it into the bloodstream more quickly when it needs iron, such as when it is lost during acute or chronic bleeding. Women's intestinal epithelial cells contain approximately four times the amount of iron transport proteins compared to men's because they lose a significant amount of iron during menstruation.

- **Calcium:** The amount of ionic calcium in the blood controls how much dietary calcium is absorbed. The parathyroid hormone (PTH), which is secreted by the parathyroid glands, increases the kidneys' ability to reabsorb calcium and triggers the release of calcium ions from bone matrices when blood levels of ionic calcium fall. Additionally, PTH increases the kidney's activation of vitamin D, which in turn promotes intestinal calcium ion absorption.

6.3.6. Vitamin Absorption

The vitamins found in foods and supplements are absorbed in the small intestine. Dietary lipids and fat-soluble vitamins (A, D, E, and K) are absorbed in micelles through simple diffusion. For this reason, when taking fat-soluble vitamin supplements, it is recommended that you eat certain fatty foods. The majority of water-soluble vitamins, such as vitamin C and most B vitamins, are also absorbed through simple diffusion. The large molecule known as vitamin B12 is an exception. The stomach secretes an intrinsic factor that binds to vitamin B12 to stop it from being digested. This complex then binds to receptors on the mucosa of the terminal ileum, where endocytosis takes place to absorb the vitamin.

6.3.7. Water Absorption

Nine liters or so of fluid enter the small intestine every day. The remaining 2.3 liters come from GI secretions, with the remaining 2.3 liters coming from food and drink. This water is absorbed in the small intestine to the tune of about 90%. The gradient in water concentration, which is higher in chyme than in epithelial cells, is what drives water absorption. Water therefore flows from the chyme into the cells along its concentration gradient. The colon then absorbs the majority of the leftover water, as was previously mentioned.

A Closer Look

The Truth About Storing and Using Body Fat

Our ancestors struggled to find food at all before the fitness centers, weight-loss plans, and prepackaged food industry. They made plans to find food instead of trying to shed those last ten pounds to fit into a bathing suit for their vacation. That's why we can go for extended periods without eating these days, whether it's because we're ill and have lost our appetite, our level of physical activity has increased, or there's just not enough food available. Our bodies store fuel for when it rains.

The process by which the body converts carbs into glycogen, which is then stored in the muscles for energy, is one way the body stores fat. The extra glycogen is sent back to the liver to be transformed into triacylglycerols and subsequently stored as fat when the muscles have used up all of their glycogen storage capacity. Similar to this, a large portion of the triacylglycerols that the body gets from food are moved to fat storage areas if they are not needed for energy production. The body stores the triacylglycerols in adipose tissue for later use, and the chylomicrons are in charge of transporting them to different parts of the body, including the muscles, breasts, external layers beneath the skin, and internal fat layers of the abdomen, thighs, and buttocks. Remember that chylomicrons are big lipoproteins with a fatty-acid and triacylglycerol core. How is this achieved? An enzyme called lipoprotein-lipase is found in capillary walls. It breaks down the triacylglycerols in lipoproteins into glycerol and fatty acids, allowing the lipoproteins to enter adipose cells. The fatty acids and glycerol are reassembled into triacylglycerols inside the adipose cells and stored for later use. Fatty acids may also be absorbed by muscle cells, which would then use them to power their muscles and produce energy. Fat reserves are retrieved for energy utilization when an individual's energy needs surpass the quantity of fuel provided by a recent meal or prolonged physical activity that has depleted glycogen energy reserves.

Adipose tissue breaks down its triacylglycerols in response to the body's demand for more energy, releasing glycerol and fatty acids into the bloodstream. The energy-hungry cells further break these substances down into tiny fragments upon receipt. Water, carbon dioxide, and energy are produced by the chemical reactions that these fragments go through.

Summary

- Mechanical digestion is a purely physical process that does not change the chemical nature of the food. Instead, it makes the food smaller to increase both surface area and mobility. It includes mastication, or chewing, as well as tongue movements that help break food into smaller bits and mix food with saliva.
- Large food molecules (for example, proteins, lipids, nucleic acids, and starches) must be broken down into subunits that are small enough to be absorbed by the lining of the alimentary canal. This is accomplished by enzymes through hydrolysis.
- The average American diet is about 50% carbohydrates, which may be classified according to the number of monomers they contain of simple sugars (monosaccharides and disaccharides) and/or complex sugars (polysaccharides).
- The digestion of protein entails breaking the complex molecule first into peptides, each having a number of amino acids, and second into individual amino acids. The pepsins are enzymes secreted by the stomach in the presence of acid that breaks down proteins (proteolysis).
- Lipid digestion and absorption pose some special challenges. Triglycerides are large molecules, and unlike carbohydrates and proteins, they're not water-soluble. Because of this, they like to cluster together in large droplets when they're in a watery environment like the digestive tract.
- The nucleic acids DNA and RNA are found in most of the foods you eat. Two types of pancreatic nuclease are responsible for their digestion: deoxyribonuclease, which digests DNA, and ribonuclease, which digests RNA.
- Your large intestine is not just made up of cells. It is also an ecosystem, home to trillions of bacteria known as the "gut flora."
- The process of digestion is controlled by both hormones and nerves. Hormonal control is mainly by endocrine hormones secreted by cells in the lining of the stomach and small intestine. These hormones stimulate the production of digestive enzymes, bicarbonate, and bile. The hormone secretin, for example, is produced by endocrine cells lining the duodenum of the small intestine.
- The mechanical and digestive processes have one goal: to convert food into molecules small enough to be absorbed by the epithelial cells of the intestinal villi. The absorptive capacity of the alimentary canal is almost endless.

References

1. Boland, G. W. (2013). *Gastrointestinal Imaging: The Requisites* (4th ed.). Philadelphia, PA: Elsevier/Saunders. ISBN: 978-0-323-10199-8
2. Boron, W. G., & Boulpaep, E. L. (2005). *Medical Physiology*. Elsevier Saunders. ISBN: 9781455743773
3. Borowitz, D. (2015). CFTR, bicarbonate, and the pathophysiology of cystic fibrosis. *Pediatric Pulmonology, 50*(Suppl 40), S24–S30.

4. Bradbury, J. (2004). Taste perception: cracking the code. *PLOS Biology, 2*(3), E64. https://doi.org/10.1371/journal.pbio.0020064.

5. Canning, B. J., & Spina, D. (2009). *Sensory Nerves*. Handbook of Experimental Pharmacology (Vol. 194). Springer. 624 pages, ISBN-13: 978-3540790891

6. Costa, M., Brookes, S. J., & Hennig, G. W. (2000). Anatomy and physiology of the enteric nervous system. *Gut, 47*(Suppl 4), iv15–iv19. https://doi.org/10.1136/gut.47.suppl_4.iv15.

7. Cotran, R. S., Kumar, V., Fausto, N., Nelson, F., Robbins, S. L., & Abbas, A. K. (2005). *Robbins and Cotran Pathologic Basis of Disease*. Elsevier Saunders. ISBN-13 : 978-8181475282

8. Danese, S., & Fiocchi, C. (2011). Ulcerative colitis. *The New England Journal of Medicine, 365*(18), 1713–1725. https://doi.org/10.1056/NEJMra1102942.

9. Dorland, W. A. (2011). *Dorland's Illustrated Medical Dictionary* (32nd ed.). Philadelphia, PA: Saunders/Elsevier. 2176 pages, ISBN: 1455709859, 9781455709854

10. Dosch, A. R., Imagawa, D. K., & Jutric, Z. (2019). Bile Metabolism and Lithogenesis: An Update. *Surgical Clinics of North America, 99*(2), 215–229.

11. Drake, R. L., Vogl, W., Mitchell, A. W., & Richardson, P. (2004). *Gray's Anatomy for Students*. Philadelphia, PA: Elsevier/Churchill Livingstone. ISBN-13 : 978-0808923060

12. Esch, K. J., & Petersen, C. A. (2013). Transmission and epidemiology of zoonotic protozoal diseases of companion animals. *Clinical Microbiology Reviews, 26*(1), 58–85. https://doi.org/10.1128/CMR.00067-12.

13. Furness JB, Callaghan BP, Rivera LR, Cho HJ. The enteric nervous system and gastrointestinal innervation: integrated local and central control. Adv Exp Med Biol. 2014;817:39-71.

14. Făgărăşan, S., & Honjo, T. (2003). Intestinal IgA synthesis: regulation of front-line body defenses. *Nature Reviews Immunology, 3*(1), 63–72. https://doi.org/10.1038/nri982.

15. Fejerskov, O., Kidd, E., Nyvad, B., & Baelum, V. (Eds.). (2008). *Dental Caries: The Disease and Its Clinical Management* (2nd ed.). Oxford: Blackwell Munksgaard. 640 pages, ISBN: 1444309285, 9781444309287

16. Forsgård, R. A. (2019). Lactose digestion in humans: intestinal lactase appears to be constitutive whereas the colonic microbiome is adaptable. *American Journal of Clinical Nutrition, 110*(2), 273–279.

17. Frenkel, E. S., & Ribbeck, K. (2015). Salivary mucins protect surfaces from colonization by cariogenic bacteria. *Applied and Environmental Microbiology, 81*(1), 332–338. https://doi.org/10.1128/aem.02573-14.

18. Hall, J. E. (2011). General Principles of Gastrointestinal Function. In *Guyton and Hall Textbook of Medical Physiology* (12th ed., p. 755). Saunders Elsevier.

19. Kiela, P. R., & Ghishan, F. K. (2016). Physiology of Intestinal Absorption and Secretion. *Best Practice & Research Clinical Gastroenterology, 30*(2), 145–159.

20. Kong, F., & Singh, R. P. (2008). Disintegration of solid foods in human stomach. *Journal of Food Science, 73*(5), R67–R80. https://doi.org/10.1111/j.1750-3841.2008.00766.x.

21. Lai, W. Y. W., Chua, J. W. M., Gill, S., & Brownlee, I. A. (2019). Analysis of the Lipolytic Activity of Whole-Saliva and Site-Specific Secretions from the Oral Cavity of Healthy Adults. *Nutrients, 11*(1). https://doi.org/10.3390/nu11010108.

22. Mack, L. R., & Tomich, P. G. (2017). Gestational Diabetes: Diagnosis, Classification, and Clinical Care. *Obstetrics and Gynecology Clinics of North America, 44*(2), 207–217. https://doi.org/10.1016/j.ogc.2017.02.002.

23. Mattar, R., de Campos Mazo, D. F., & Carrilho, F. J. (2012). Lactose intolerance: diagnosis, genetic, and clinical factors. *Clinical and Experimental Gastroenterology, 5*, 113–121.

24. Mazzarello, P., & Harari, M. (2007). Left to digest. *Nature, 448*(7155), 753. https://doi.org/10.1038/448753a.

25. Morris, A. M., Regenbogen, S. E., Hardiman, K. M., & Hendren, S. (2014). Sigmoid diverticulitis: a systematic review. *JAMA, 311*(3), 287–297. https://doi.org/10.1001/jama.2013.282025.

26. Nanci, A. (2013). *Ten Cate's Oral Histology: Development, Structure, and Function* (8th ed.). St. Louis, MO: Elsevier. ISBN: 978-0-323-07846-7

27. Nanci, A., & Ten Cate, A. R. (2008). *Ten Cate's Oral Histology: Development, Structure, and Function* (7th ed.). St. Louis, MO: Mosby Elsevier. 432 pages, ISBN-13: 978-0323045575

28. Pandiri, A. R. (2014). Overview of exocrine pancreatic pathobiology. *Toxicologic Pathology, 42*(1), 207–216.

29. Pettit, J. D., & Moss, P. (2006). *Essential Haematology* (5th ed.). Blackwell Publishing Professional. 392 pages, ISBN: 1405136499, 9781405136495

30. Piludu, M., Lantini, M. S., Cossu, M., Piras, M., Oppenheim, F. G., Helmerhorst, E. J., et al. (2006). Salivary histatins in human deep posterior lingual glands (of von Ebner). *Archives of Oral Biology, 51*(11), 967–973. https://doi.org/10.1016/j.archoralbio.2006.05.011.

31. Sakai, D., Hirooka, Y., Kawashima, H., Ohno, E., Ishikawa, T., Suhara, H., et al. (2018). Increase in breath hydrogen concentration was correlated with the main pancreatic duct stenosis. *Journal of Breath Research, 12*(3), 036004.

32. Schoenwolf, G. C., Bleyl, S. B., Brauer, P. R., & Francis-West, P. H. (2009). *Larsen's Human Embryology* (4th Thoroughly rev. and updated ed.). Philadelphia, PA: Churchill Livingstone/Elsevier. 687 pages, ISBN: 9780443068119, 0443068119

33. Schubert, M. L. (2017). Physiologic, pathophysiologic, and pharmacologic regulation of gastric acid secretion. *Current Opinion in Gastroenterology, 33*(6), 430–438.

34. Sródka, A. (2003). The short history of gastroenterology. *Journal of Physiology and Pharmacology, 54*(Suppl 3), 9–21.

35. Stefanski, A. L., Tomiak, C., Pleyer, U., Dietrich, T., Burmester, G. R., & Dörner, T. (2017). The Diagnosis and Treatment of Sjögren's Syndrome. *Deutsches Ärzteblatt International, 114*(20), 354–361.

36. Thompson, W. G., Longstreth, G. L., Drossman, D. A., Heaton, K., Irvine, E. J., & Muller-Lissner, S. (2000). Functional Bowel Disorders. In D. A. Drossman, E. Corazziari, N. J. Talley, et al. (Eds.), *Rome II: The Functional Gastrointestinal Disorders. Diagnosis, Pathophysiology and Treatment. A Multinational Consensus.* Lawrence, KS: Allen Press.

37. Weller, P. F. (2015). Protozoal Intestinal Infections and Trichomoniasi. In D. Kasper, A. Fauci, S. Hauser, D. Longo, J. L. Jameson, & J. Loscalzo (Eds.), *Harrison's Principles of Internal Medicine* (19th ed.). McGraw-Hill.

Chapter 7

THE ABSORPTIVE AND POST-ABSORPTIVE STATES

Contents

Introduction

Whether or not food is being broken down in the digestive system affects the blood's nutritional condition. The pattern of energy metabolism known as the absorptive state occurs when nutrients like glucose and fat are being absorbed and have high concentrations in the blood. In this state, different tissues use a portion of the blood glucose to meet their short-term energy needs. The extra glucose and absorbed fat are stored as fat and glycogen, which can be used to fuel the body during fasting or in between meals. This energy metabolism pattern is referred to as the post-absorptive state. Changes in the blood concentrations of insulin and other hormones cause the absorptive state pattern to shift to the post-absorptive state pattern. The significance of preserving proper metabolic patterns can be demonstrated by examining the metabolic abnormalities found in insulin-dependent diabetes mellitus (IDDM, also known as type I diabetes), a condition marked by a significant reduction in insulin secretion.

Orientation and Directional Terms

Term	Definition	Illustration
Glycogen	Glycogen is a multibranched polysaccharide of glucose that serves as a form of energy storage in animals, fungi, and bacteria. It is the main storage form of glucose in the human body.	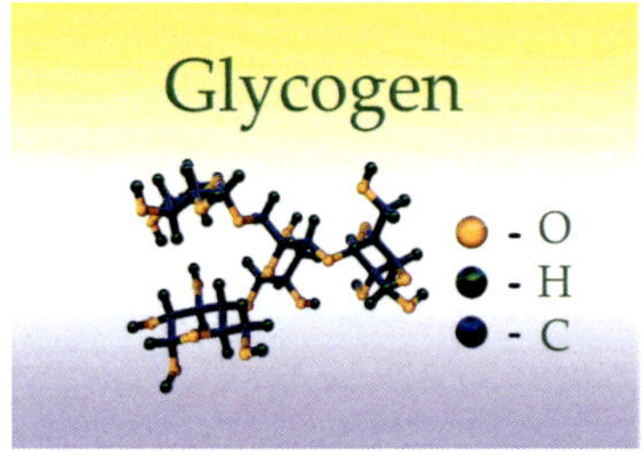
Insulin	Hormone secreted by the pancreas that stimulates the uptake of glucose into the cells.	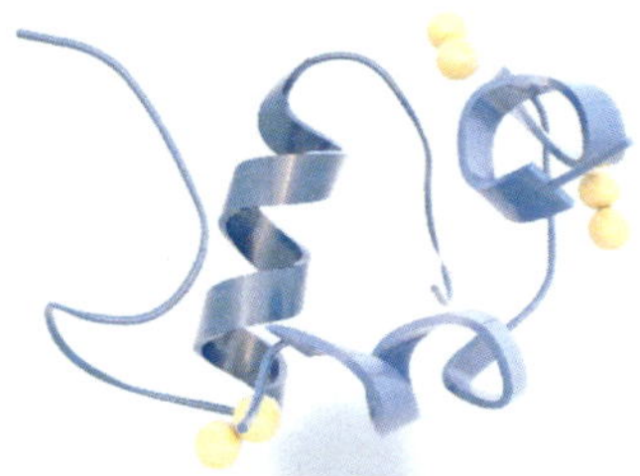
Gluconeogenesis	Gluconeogenesis is a metabolic pathway that results in the biosynthesis of glucose from certain non-carbohydrate carbon substrates.	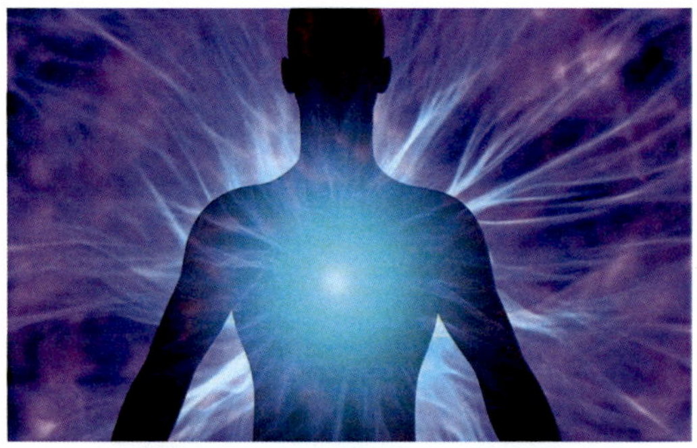
Insulin-dependent diabetes mellitus	Insulin-dependent (type I) diabetes mellitus is a chronic disease characterized by hyperglycemia, impaired metabolism and storage of important nutrients, evidence of autoimmunity, and long-term vascular and neurologic complications.	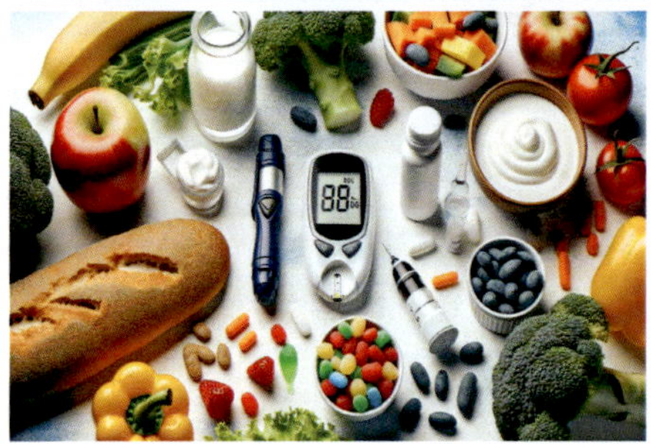

7.1. The Absorptive State

The absorptive state occurs when anabolism outpaces catabolism in the full gastrointestinal tract. When the gastrointestinal tract is full and anabolic processes outpace catabolism, this is known as the "absorptive state." Glucose serves as the process's fuel.

7.1.1. Carbohydrates

The liver receives simple sugars and transforms them into glucose. After that, the glucose is either transferred to the blood or transformed into fat (triglycerides) and glycogen for storage of energy.

As reserves for the post-absorptive state, fat and glycogen will be kept in the adipose and liver, respectively. The residual glucose is either absorbed by body cells for use as fuel or stored as glycogen in the skeletal muscle.

7.1.2. Triglycerides

Triglycerides (85–92%), phospholipids (6–12%), cholesterol (1–3%), and proteins (1–2%) make up chylomicrons, which are lipoprotein particles. Using lipoprotein lipase, this primary byproduct of fat digestion is first hydrolyzed to produce fatty acids and glycerol.

They can now freely move through capillary walls as a result. The majority of this will be stored in adipose tissue and reconstituted as triglycerides. The remainder will be utilized by skeletal muscle, hepatocytes, and adipose cells as fuel. Other body cells will start to use triglycerides as an energy source in a low-carb environment.

7.1.3. Amino Acids

To produce energy in the form of ATP, the liver deaminates amino acids to keto acids, which are then utilized in the Kreb's cycle. They could also be transformed into fat to store energy. While some go through the liver sinusoids to be used by body cells to make proteins, the majority are used to make plasma proteins (Figure 7.1).

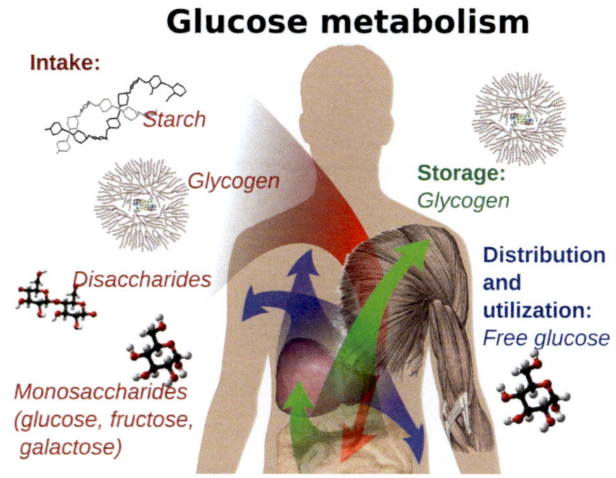

Figure 7.1. *Glucose metabolism: Glucose metabolism and various forms of it in the process.*

Source: https://university.pressbooks.pub/test456/chapter/metabolic-body-states/.

7.2. Glycogen Storage Disorders

A metabolic condition known as glycogen storage disease (GSD), also known as glycogenosis and dextrinosis, is brought on by a lack of an enzyme or transport protein that affects the synthesis, breakdown, or breakdown of glycogen, usually in the muscles and/or liver cells. There are two categories of causes of GSD: environmental and genetic. Any inborn error in the metabolism of carbohydrates (genetically defective transport proteins or enzymes) results in genetic GSD. Castanospermine intoxication is the cause of environmental GSD in livestock. Even though some inborn errors of carbohydrate metabolism are known to impact the liver or muscles, not all of them have been given a GSD number. For instance, there is a myopathic form of phosphoglycerate kinase deficiency (gene PGK1) (Figure 7.2).

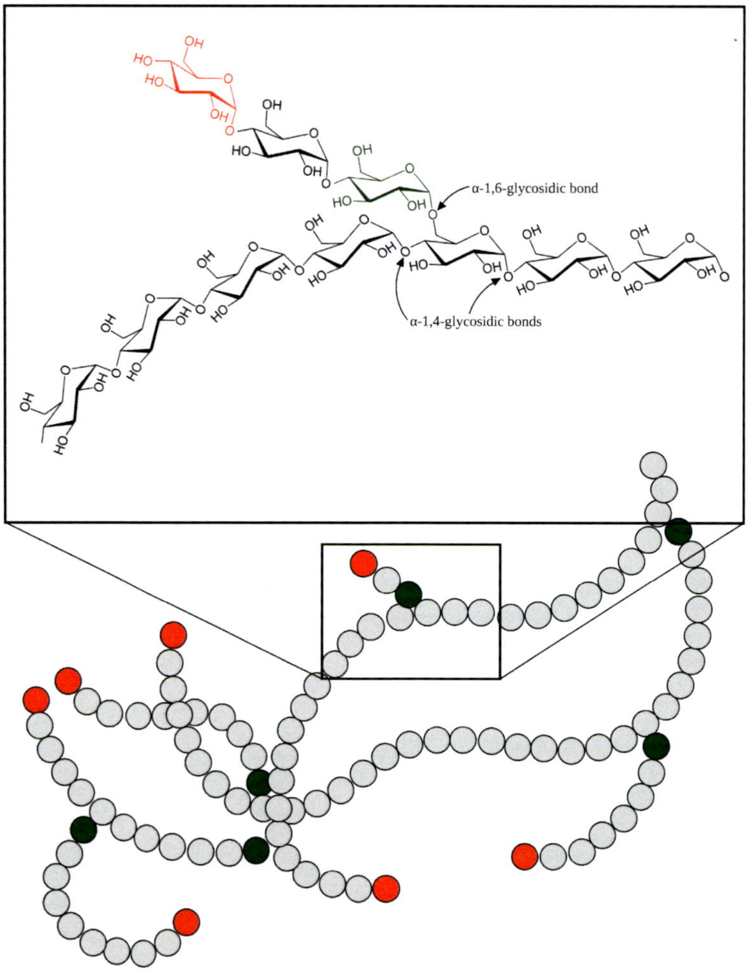

Figure 7.2. *Diagram of the structure of glycogen.*

Source: By GKFXtalk 12:08, 5 September 2017 (UTC) – vector version of file: Glycogen.png. Uses File: Alpha-D-Glucose.svg., Public Domain, https://commons.wikimedia.org/w/index.php?curid=62200406.

However, GSD-1 subtypes b, c, and d are still classified as GSDs even though they are caused by defects of transport proteins (genes SLC37A4, SLC17A3). Fanconi-Bickel syndrome (gene SLC2A2) and Danon disease (gene LAMP2) were also declassified as GSDs because they are defects of transport proteins rather than enzymes. Because it also affects the formation of N-glycans, phosphoglucomutase deficiency (gene PGM1) was reclassified as a GSD, but it should really be called GSD-XIV because it affects both glycogenolysis and glycosylation.

7.2.1. Types of GSD

The enzyme that is absent from each type of GSD is used to categorize them. Every GSD is unique and requires a different course of care. Although there are various forms of GSD, types I, III, and IV are the most prevalent. These kinds go by additional names as well:

- **Type I or Von Gierke Disease:** The most prevalent type of GSD is this one. Individuals with type I diabetes lack the enzyme necessary for the liver to convert glycogen to glucose. Liver glycogen stores accumulate. Babies who are three to four months old frequently exhibit symptoms. These could include hypoglycemia, or low blood sugar, and hepatic enlargement-related abdominal swelling.
- **Type III, Cori Disease, or Forbes Disease:** Individuals with type III diabetes have insufficient levels of the debranching enzyme, an enzyme that aids in the breakdown of glycogen. Glycogen cannot decompose completely. It gathers in the tissues of the muscles and liver. Weak muscles, delayed growth, and an enlarged abdomen are among the symptoms.
- **Type IV or Andersen Disease:** Type IV diabetics produce aberrant glycogen. Experts believe that the aberrant glycogen sets off the immune system, which fights infection in the body. This results in cirrhosis, or scarring, of the liver as well as other organs like the heart and muscles.

Table 7.1. Genetic and Epidemiologic Characteristics of the Hepatic GSDs

Type	Gene	OMIM	Location	Enzyme Deficiency	Inheritance	Incidence
0a	*GYS2*	240600	12p12.1	Liver glycogen synthase	AR	-
Ia	*G6PC*	232200	17q21	Glucose-6-phosphatase	AR	1 in 50,000–100,000
Ib	*SLC37A4*	232220	11q23.3	Glucose-6-phosphate transporter	AR	-
III	*AGL*	232400	1p21.2	Glycogen debranching enzyme	AR	1 in 83,000–100,000
IV	*GBE1*	232500	3p12.3	Glycogen branching enzyme	AR	1 to 600,000–800,000
VI	*PYGL*	232700	14q22.1	Liver glycogen phosphorylase	AR	1 in 65,000–85,000
IXa	*PHKA2*	306000	Xp22.13	Phosphorylase kinase, α subunit	XL	1 in 100,000
IXb	*PHKB*	261750	16q12.1	Phosphorylase kinase, β subunit	AR	-

IXc	*PHKG2*	613027	16p11.2	Phosphorylase kinase, γ subunit	AR	-
FBS [1]	*SLC2A2*	227810	3q26.2	Facilitated glucose transporter 2	AR	-
XII	*ALDOA*	611881	16q22-q24	Aldolase A [2]	AR	-

Key: – = unavailable data; AR = autosomal recessive; XL = X-linked; [1] Fanconi–Bickel syndrome; [2] or Fructose 1,6-biphosphate Aldolase A.

Source: de Marchi R, Nalin T, Sperb-Ludwig F, Pinheiro FC, Schwartz IVD, Steiner CE. Glycogen storage disease: Expert opinion on clinical diagnosis revisited after molecular testing. Genes. 2023; 14(12):2219. https://doi.org/10.3390/genes14122219.

7.2.2. Diagnosis

Blood tests for related metabolic disturbances, genetic testing for potential mutations, and history and physical examination for associated symptoms are methods used to diagnose glycogen storage diseases. A 12-minute walk test (12MWT), an exercise stress test, or a non-ischemic forearm test may also be included. Genetic testing is gradually reducing the need for biopsy; nevertheless, a biopsy would still be required to confirm diagnosis in the event of a VUS and inconclusive exercise tests.

7.2.3. Differential Diagnoses

7.2.3.1. Muscle

Skeletal muscle glycogen storage diseases usually present with exercise-induced (dynamic) symptoms, like fatigue, as opposed to fixed weakness (static) symptoms. The differential diagnosis of limb-girdle muscular dystrophy or inflammatory myopathy would be made in cases of glycogen storage diseases involving fixed muscle weakness, especially of the proximal muscles. Endocrinopathies should be taken into consideration for individuals who have proximal muscle weakness and/or exercise intolerance. Exercise intolerance can be distinguished from other metabolic myopathies, such as disorders of fatty acid metabolism, by timing the onset of symptoms such as muscle fatigue and cramping.

Muscle fatigue, pain, and cramping that are brought on by exercise but go away with rest can be caused by issues with the circulatory system rather than the muscles themselves. This is known as ischemia or inadequate blood flow to the muscles. Chronic venous insufficiency, popliteal artery entrapment syndrome, and intermittent claudication are examples of ischemia that frequently results in symptoms in the leg muscles. Abnormal muscle fatigue can be brought on by diseases that interfere with the neuromuscular junction, such as the autoimmune condition myasthenia gravis. The congenital myasthenic syndromes (genetic) and Lambert-Eaton myasthenic syndrome (auto-immune) are comparable.

Glycogen metabolism can be affected by diseases as a secondary effect of the main illness. Hypo- and hyperthyroidism, or abnormal thyroid function, can cause myopathy, which is characterized by proximal weakness or hypertrophy of the muscles, especially in the calves, as well as symptoms of exercise-induced muscle fatigue, cramping, and pain. In contrast, hyperthyroidism does the opposite, up-regulating glycogenolysis and glycolysis while down-regulating glycogen synthesis. Hypothyroidism increases glycogen synthesis while down-regulating glycogenolysis and glycolysis.

Long-term hypo- and hyperthyroid myopathy results in a preponderance of type I (slow-twitch/oxidative) muscle fibers and atrophy of type II (fast-twitch/glycolytic) muscle fibers. Muscle glycogen accumulation is aberrant in muscle biopsy results, with low accumulation in hyperthyroidism and high accumulation in hypothyroidism. Atrophic form, adult-onset Hoffman syndrome, childhood-onset Kocher-Debre-Semelaigne syndrome, and myasthenic syndrome are examples of hypothyroid myopathy.

Glycogen deposition in excess is one of the features of muscle biopsy in patients with increased growth hormone. Interestingly, McArdle disease (GSD-V), the most frequently diagnosed and therefore most studied of the muscle GSDs, has the second highest comorbidity of endocrine disease (primarily hypothyroidism), and some of its patients also have hypertrophy of the calf muscles. This is in contrast to hypothyroid myopathy. Comorbidities of late-onset Pompe disease (GSD-II) include hypothyroidism and calf hypertrophy.

Inadequate nutrition and disorders causing malabsorption, like celiac disease, can result in insufficient intake of vital vitamins required for the metabolism of glycogen in muscle tissue. Though malnutrition rarely results in myopathy alone, it usually manifests as systemic symptoms. Because of the interaction between vitamin D and calcium, vitamin D deficiency myopathy, also known as osteomalic myopathy, causes muscle weakness, primarily in the proximal muscles. Muscle biopsy results reveal abnormal glycogen accumulation, atrophy of type II (fast-twitch/glycolytic) muscle fibers, and decreased sarcoplasmic reticulum (which is necessary for muscle contraction) calcium uptake. While calf muscle hypertrophy has sporadically been documented, muscle atrophy is the usual symptom of Vitamin D deficiency myopathy.

Along with GSD types V, VII, IXd, X, XI, XII, and XIII, other conditions that cause exercise-induced, electrically silent muscle cramping and stiffness include Brody disease, types 1 and 2 of Rippling muscle disease, and hyper CKemia (Elevated serum creatine phosphokinase) associated with CAV3. In contrast to other myopathies, Brody's disease causes painless muscle cramps. Similar to GSD types II, III, and V, some cases of Brody disease and Rippling muscle disease also exhibit a pseudoathletic appearance of muscle hypertrophy.

Exercise-induced, electrically silent, painful muscle cramps and transient contractures, as well as exercise-induced muscle fatigue, are all associated with erythrocyte lactate transporter defect (previously known as Lactate transporter defect, myopathy due to). EMG and muscle biopsy results are normal, though, because the problem lies in the red blood cells that are supposed to remove lactate accumulation from working muscles, not the muscle itself. There are a few exceptions, but most muscular dystrophies are characterized by fixed muscle weakness as opposed to exercise-induced muscle fatigue and/or cramping.

Exercise-induced cramping and calf hypertrophy are characteristics of limb-girdle muscular dystrophy autosomal recessive 23 (LGMD R23). Myofibrillar myopathy 10 (MFM10) is characterized by hypertrophic neck and shoulder girdle muscles, exercise-induced muscle fatigue, cramping, and stiffness. Calf hypertrophy and exercise-induced muscle soreness and exhaustion are present in LGMD R28. Calf pseudohypertrophy, exercise-induced weakness (fatigue), and pain are present in LGMD R8. Muscle fatigue, proximal muscle weakness, and hypertrophy are present in an MDDGC3.

In addition to fixed muscle weakness and pseudohypertrophic calf muscles, DMD-related myopathies of Duchenne and Becker muscular dystrophy also cause low ATP production due to secondary muscular mitochondrial impairment and decreased type II (fast-twitch/glycolytic) muscle fibers, which results in a predominance of type I (slow-twitch/oxidative) muscle fibers. Milder phenotypes of DMD associated with childhood-onset exhibit fatigue, increased CK, stiffness, pain, and cramping in the muscles during exercise. Elevated CK and adult-onset exercise-induced muscle cramps and pain are characteristics of Becker muscular dystrophy. Exercise-induced muscle pain, exhaustion, stiffness, proximal muscle weakness, and calf muscle pseudohypertrophy are symptoms of tubular aggregate myopathy (TAM) types 1 and 2. TAM2 experiences cramps during exercise, whereas TAM1 experiences them at rest. The symptoms of TAM are present in Stormorken syndrome as well, but they are more severe and include short stature and other anomalies.

Short stature, painful muscle cramps brought on by exercise, and muscle hypertrophy are characteristics of Satoyoshi syndrome. The symptoms of dimethylglycine dehydrogenase deficiency include fishy body odor, elevated CK, and muscle fatigue. Exercise-induced muscle cramps, pain, and exhaustion are symptoms of myopathy with myalgia, and elevated serum creatine kinase, with or without episodic rhabdomyolysis (MMCKR); some patients also show proximal muscle weakness.

7.2.4. Treatment

The type of glycogen storage disease determines the course of treatment. Modified cornstarch therapy, or frequent small meals of carbohydrates and cornstarch, is the standard treatment for Von Gierke disease (GSD-I). Other possible treatments include human granulocyte colony-stimulating factor and allopurinol. Treatment for Cori/Forbes disease (GSD-III) may involve a high-protein diet that prioritizes complex carbohydrates, also known as modified cornstarch therapy. But unlike GSD-I, simple sugars (lactose, fructose, and sucrose) are allowed because gluconeogenesis is functional. Since ketones quickly convert to acetyl CoA for oxidative phosphorylation while free fatty acids take several minutes to do so, a ketogenic diet has shown promise in treating McArdle disease (GSD-V).

Exercise training combined with D-galactose supplements has demonstrated a favorable improvement in the signs and symptoms of phosphoglucomutase deficiency (previously known as GSD-XIV). Some patients with phosphoglucomutase deficiency also get a second wind during exercise training.

Regular aerobic exercise using second wind to help the muscles become aerobically conditioned and anaerobic exercise (strength training) that adheres to the activity adaptations to prevent muscle injury are beneficial in managing the symptoms of exercise intolerance and maintaining general health in patients with McArdle disease (GSD-V). According to studies, people with McArdle disease benefit from regular low-to-moderate aerobic exercise because it reduces heart rate, raises peak power output, increases peak oxygen uptake (VO2peak), and lowers serum CK levels.

The phenomenon of achieving a second wind can be observed by the patient in the form of a decreased heart rate while maintaining the same speed on the treadmill, even in the absence of symptoms such as cramping, muscle pain, or fatigue. During low-to-moderate aerobic exercise (walking or brisk walking), inactive patients experienced a second wind, as evidenced by the relief of typical symptoms and the signs of an increased heart rate decreasing. On the other hand, individuals who engaged in regular physical activity did not exhibit the usual symptoms associated with low-to-moderate aerobic exercise, such as walking or brisk walking, but they did exhibit second wind in the form of a decreased heart rate. It required more intense exercise (very brisk walking/ jogging or cycling) for the patients who were already regularly active to experience both the typical symptoms and their relief, as well as the indication of an elevated heart rate decreasing, which is known as second wind. Identifying the second wind phenomenon in young children (less than 10 years old) with McArdle disease (GSD-V) may present challenges. Their heart rate may be normal, and their peak cardio-respiratory capacity (VO2 max) may be normal or higher than normal. Nevertheless, exercise intolerance usually manifests in McArdle disease patients before the age of ten, with a median symptomatic age of three years.

Patients with Tarui disease (GSD-VII) are considered to be out-of-wind; they do not experience the second wind phenomenon. However, during aerobic exercise after a warm-up, they can obtain sub-maximal benefit from the lipid metabolism of free fatty acids.

7.3. Insulin

The anabolic hormone insulin affects metabolism all over the body. Beta cells are found in exocrine tissue in the pancreas called the islets of Langerhans. The synthesis of insulin is carried out by beta cells. By observing the levels of glucose, amino acids, keto acids, and fatty acids in the plasma, beta cells control the amount of insulin produced. The general function of insulin is to regulate energy expenditure and conservation during feeding and fasting.

7.3.1. Cellular Level

The insulin-dependent cascade is executed by cells found in the liver, heart, vascular endothelium, and muscle tissue. The reaction that insulin causes in these cells varies depending on the tissue. The end result is glucose metabolism through glucose uptake into cells in skeletal muscle, adipose tissue, and the heart. The heart and vascular endothelium exhibit vasodilation as a result of producing nitric oxide (NO). When insulin is present, the liver responds by increasing glycogenesis and decreasing gluconeogenesis. The effects of insulin also extend to the metabolism of proteins and fats. In contrast, it suppresses lipolysis and protein breakdown while promoting lipogenesis and protein synthesis.

7.3.2. Molecular Level

The peptide hormone insulin is made up of two peptide chains, the A and B chains, which have 21 and 30 amino acid residues, respectively, and 51 amino acids total. The two chains are joined by cysteine residue disulfide bonds.

The original precursor protein of insulin was called proproinsulin. It is a single-chain polypeptide made up of signal peptide and proinsulin sequences. Preproinsulin is broken at its signal peptide upon translocation into the endoplasmic reticulum, releasing proinsulin. Proinsulin is a single-chain that continuously combines the A and B chains of insulin, joined by a section referred to as the C domain. At either end of the C domain are dibasic residues. A trypsin-like enzyme cleaves proinsulin at each dibasic residue. Finally, a C-peptide and insulin are released by this cleavage. Insulin is stored as zinc insulin hexamers in glucose-regulated secretory vesicles until it is required metabolically.

7.3.3. Function

7.3.3.1. Role in Glucose Metabolism

Two signaling cascades, insulin-mediated glucose uptake (IMGU) and glucose-stimulated insulin secretion (GSIS) maintain the homeostasis of glucose metabolism. Insulin can enhance glucose uptake from skeletal muscle and adipose tissue while inhibiting hepatic cell production of glucose through the IMGU cascade. When insulin interacts extracellularly with the alpha subunit of the insulin receptor, the downstream signaling of the insulin cascade is initiated. This interaction causes the insulin-receptor complex to change in shape, which in turn causes the phosphorylation of insulin receptor substrates by tyrosine kinase and the consequent activation of phosphatidylinositol-3-kinase. The intended translocation of the GLUT-4 transporter from intracellular to extracellular onto the plasma membrane of skeletal muscle cells is brought about by these downstream events. GLUT4 is found intracellularly in vesicles. Exercise or the effects of insulin accelerate the exocytosis rate of these GLUT4-vesicles. Therefore, insulin facilitates the entry of glucose into skeletal muscle cells for metabolism into glycogen by increasing the presence of GLUT-4 on the plasma membrane.

7.3.3.2. Role in Glycogen Metabolism

Insulin stimulates the synthesis of glycogen in the liver, which influences the metabolism of glycogen. The essential component in controlling the metabolism of glycogen is protein phosphatase I (PPI). PPI dephosphorylates phosphorylase kinase and phosphorylase A, which slows the rate of glycogenolysis. PPI, on the other hand, speeds up glycogenesis by triggering glycogen synthase B. Insulin stimulates the liver's production of glycogen from glucose by raising PPI substrate-specific activity on glycogen particles. Insulin directly regulates several hepatic metabolic enzymes through the transcription of genes. This has an impact on metabolic pathway gene expression. Insulin suppresses the expression of the genes for fructose-1,6-bisphosphatase, glucose-6-phosphatase, and phosphoenolpyruvate carboxylase, the rate-limiting step in gluconeogenesis. Pyruvate kinase and glucokinase gene expression rises during glycolysis. Acetyl-CoA carboxylase, pyruvate dehydrogenase, and fatty acid synthase all exhibit increased expression during lipogenesis.

7.3.3.3. Role in Lipid Metabolism

As was already mentioned, some lipogenic enzymes express themselves more when insulin is present. This is because adipocytes store glucose as a lipid. As a result, as fatty acid production rises, so does the cells' absorption of glucose. Insulin further controls this mechanism by dephosphorylating hormone-sensitive lipase and blocking it, which stops lipolysis. In the end, serum-free fatty acid levels are lowered by insulin.

7.3.3.4. Role in Protein Metabolism

Insulin plays a role in controlling the rate of protein turnover. Insulin increases the intracellular uptake of short-chain amino acids, such as glutamine, arginine, and alanine, as well as the expression of the genes for albumin and muscle myosin heavy chain alpha, which in turn stimulates protein synthesis. Insulin inhibits the hepatic and muscle cell enzymes that break down proteins, which has an impact on the regulation of protein breakdown. Enzymes that are affected include hydrolases, ATP-ubiquitin-dependent proteases, and ATP-independent lysosomal proteases.

7.3.3.5. Role in Inflammation and Vasodilation

Insulin reduces inflammation in the body through its effects on macrophages and endothelial cells.

Insulin promotes the expression of endothelial nitric oxide synthase (eNOS) in endothelial cells. Nitric oxide (NO), which causes vasodilation, is released by eNOS. Nuclear factor-kappa-B (NF-kB), which is present intracellularly in endothelial cells, is suppressed by insulin. Soluble cell adhesion molecules are released into the bloodstream when endothelial NF-KB stimulates the expression of adhesion molecules, E-selectin, and ICAM-1. Research has connected the development of atherosclerotic arterial plaques to the presence of cell adhesion molecules on vascular endothelium.

Insulin inhibits the production of reactive oxygen species (ROS) and O2 radicals. Insulin suppresses p47phox, one of NADPH oxidase's essential components, in the macrophage to prevent NADPH oxidase expression. The production of oxygen radicals by NADPH oxidase triggers the activation of the inhibitor of NF-kB kinase beta (IKKB). IkB is degraded as a result of IKKB phosphorylating it. NF-kB is freed from this degradation and is able to relocate into the nucleus of the macrophage. After entering the nucleus, NF-kB activates the transcription of genes that produce pro-inflammatory proteins that are released into the bloodstream. These genes include matrix metalloproteinase (MMP), interleukin-6 (IL-6), interleukin-8 (IL-8), tumor necrosis factor-alpha (TNF-alpha), and inducible nitric oxide synthase (iNOS).

7.3.4. Clinical Significance

The body encounters chronic hyperglycemia in a set of metabolic diseases. Diabetes mellitus type 1 that is insulin-dependent occurs when the pancreas produces little or no insulin. Diabetes mellitus (DM) type 2, insulin-independent, occurs when the body makes enough insulin to meet its needs for the metabolic processing of glucose, but not enough. Insulin resistance and abnormal glucose metabolism are the results of this mismatch between supply and demand. Because proper transport of glucose into cells and metabolism are disrupted in both type 1 and type 2 diabetes, blood glucose levels remain elevated. In the US, Type 2 DM has spread to epidemic proportions. Given the numerous complications brought on by DM, this is a serious cause for concern. These consist of peripheral vascular disease, neuropathy, renal failure, retinopathy, and cardiovascular disease. Although the body experiences elevated blood glucose levels in the early stages of type 2 DM development, the pancreatic beta cells generate adequate insulin to sustain euglycemia. When a portion of the insulin-mediated glucose uptake cascade is not functioning properly, insulin production is no longer sufficient for sufficient glucose metabolism. Insulin resistance specifically results in impaired glucose transport across the plasma membrane via GLUT-4 transporters, which impairs glycogenesis in muscle cells. Impaired GLUT-4 transporters can arise from either a preexisting condition or from ongoing hyperglycemia.

7.4. Post-absorptive State

After the meal has been broken down, absorbed, and stored, the body enters the postabsorptive state, also known as the fasting state. Although it's customary to fast overnight, your body also enters the postabsorptive state when you miss meals during the day. The body's primary source of energy during this state is stored glycogen. As glucose is absorbed and utilized by the cells, blood glucose levels start to decline. Insulin levels also decrease in response to a drop in glucose. Triglyceride and glycogen storage is lowered. However, blood glucose levels need to be kept within the normal range of 80–120 mg/dL due to the demands placed on the tissues and organs. The pancreatic alpha cells release the hormone glucagon in reaction to a decrease in blood glucose levels. When glucagon interacts with liver cells, it prevents glycogen from being synthesized and promotes the conversion of glycogen that has been stored back into glucose. The liver releases this glucose so that the brain and other peripheral tissues can use it. Blood glucose levels start to rise as a result. To replenish the glucose that has been utilized by the peripheral tissues, the liver will also start the process of gluconeogenesis. Proteins and fats are digested after food is consumed in the same way as previously mentioned; however, glucose processing is slightly altered. Glucose is absorbed preferentially by the peripheral tissues. After an extended fast, the liver, which normally absorbs and processes glucose, will not function.

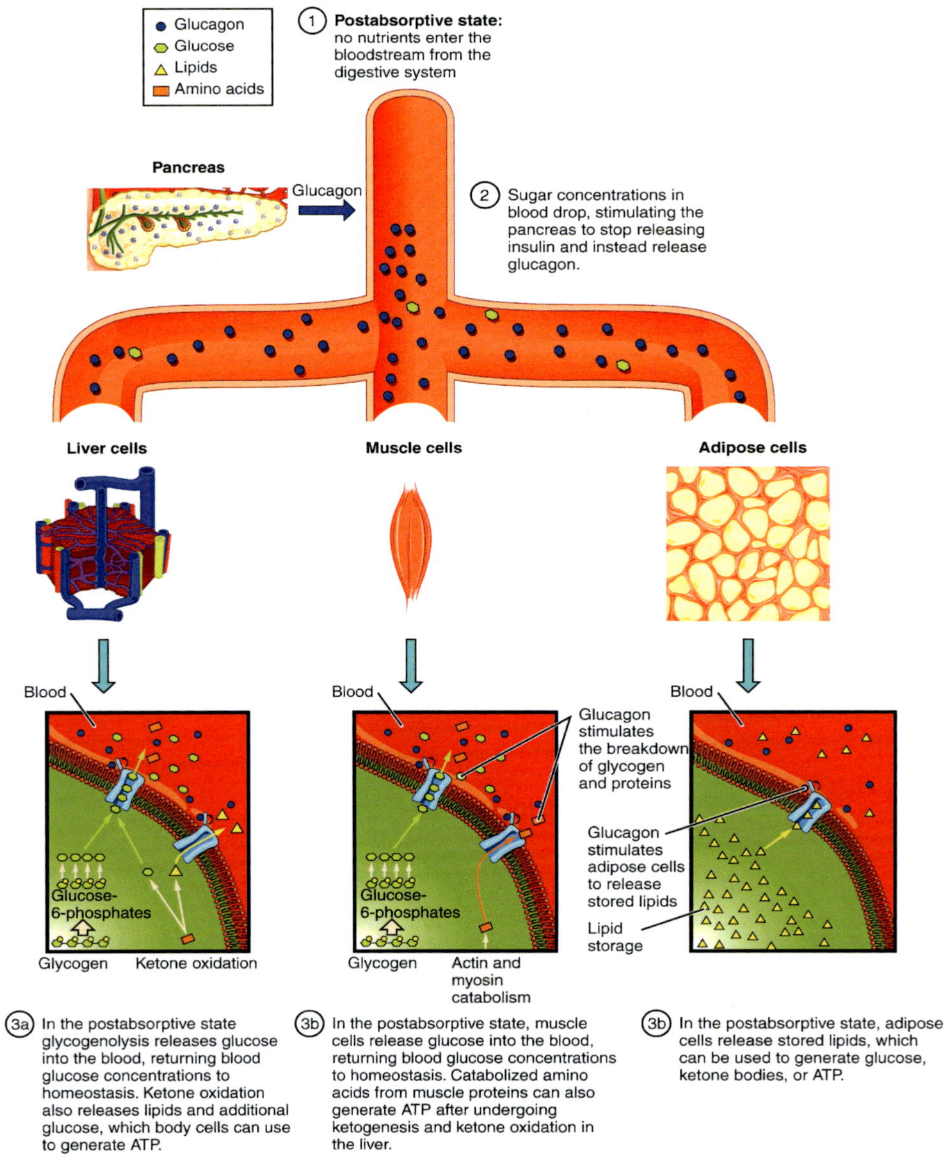

Figure 7.3. *During the postabsorptive state, the body must rely on stored glycogen for energy.*

Source: https://courses.lumenlearning.com/suny-ap2/chapter/metabolic-states-of-the-body/#:~:text=There%20are%20three%20main%20metabolic,in%20generally%20well%2Dnourished%20individuals.

After the fast, the ongoing gluconeogenesis in the liver resumes replenishing the exhausted glycogen stores. The excess glucose that is absorbed by the liver is transformed into triglycerides and fatty acids for long-term storage after these stores have been restored. The metabolic activities that take place in the body while it is in the postabsorptive state are outlined in Figure 7.3.

A Closer Look

Catabolic-Anabolic Steady State

The energy required for anabolic reactions to produce complex molecules is supplied by catabolic reactions that break complex molecules.

Energy is required for anabolic reactions. The chemical process that converts ATP to ADP provides the energy needed for this metabolic activity. Cells can create an effective energy cycle by combining anabolic and catabolic processes that release energy. Chemical fuels are converted into cellular energy by the catabolic reactions, which is then utilized to start the anabolic reactions, which need energy. The high-energy molecule ATP couples anabolism through free energy release. This energy is obtained from the hydration of the phosphate group rather than the dissolution of phosphate bonds.

The antithesis of catabolism is anabolism. For instance, the synthesis of glucose is an anabolic process, but its breakdown is a catabolic one. Energy intake, sometimes known as the "uphill" process of anabolism, is necessary for the process. As an organism uses up energy, it releases energy during the "downhill" process of catabolism. It is necessary to control anabolism and catabolism to prevent the two processes from happening at the same time. The hormones that activate and deactivate each process are unique to it. Growth hormone, testosterone, and estrogen are examples of anabolic hormones. Adrenaline, cortisol, and glucagon are examples of catabolic hormones. Circadian rhythms also control the ratio of anabolism to catabolism, causing metabolic processes like glucose metabolism to change in response to an animal's regular activity cycles. Anabolism can be understood as a collection of metabolic processes where the energy released from catabolism is used to start the synthesis of complex molecules. Small and basic precursors are converted into these complex molecules via a methodical process. One example of an anabolic reaction is the synthesis of relatively complex products like sugar, some lipids, or even DNA, which has an incredibly complex physical structure, from relatively simple precursor molecules that were first produced by catabolic reactions. The byproducts of anabolic reactions are also more energetically dense than their simpler precursors due to their increased complexity. Anabolic responses are differentiable processes. In other words, an increase in cellular size, complexity, or both results from the synthesis of a large variety of end products from a relatively small number of raw material types. Body size increases and cell differentiation are the results of anabolic processes. These processes are linked to muscle mass and bone mineralization. Peptides, proteins, polysaccharides, lipids, and nucleic acids are all produced during anabolic processes. These molecules include all the components of living cells, including chromosomes and membranes, as well as the specialized byproducts of particular cell types, including hormones, neurotransmitters, enzymes, and antibodies.

Summary

- When the gastrointestinal tract is full, anabolism exceeds catabolism; this is the absorptive state. The absorptive state is the period in which the gastrointestinal tract is full and the anabolic processes exceed catabolism. The fuel used for this process is glucose.
- Simple sugars are sent to the liver where they are converted to glucose. The glucose then travels to the blood or is converted to glycogen and fat (triglyceride) for energy storage. The glycogen and fat will be stored in the liver and adipose tissue, respectively, as reserves for the post-absorptive state. The remaining glucose is taken in for use by body cells or stored in skeletal muscle as glycogen.
- Chylomicrons are lipoprotein particles that consist of triglycerides (85–92%), phospholipids (6–12%), cholesterol (1–3%) and proteins (1–2%). This main product of fat digestion is first broken down into fatty acids and glycerol through hydrolysis using lipoprotein lipase. This allows them to pass freely through capillary walls. Most of this will be reconstituted as triglycerides and stored in adipose tissue.
- The liver deaminates amino acids to keto acids to be used in the Kreb's cycle to generate energy in the form of ATP.
- A glycogen storage disease (GSD, also glycogenosis and dextrinosis) is a metabolic disorder caused by a deficiency of an enzyme or transport protein affecting glycogen synthesis, glycogen breakdown, or glucose breakdown, typically in muscles and/or liver cells.
- Methods to diagnose glycogen storage diseases include history and physical examination for associated symptoms, blood tests for associated metabolic disturbances, and genetic testing for suspected mutations.
- Insulin is an anabolic hormone that elicits metabolic effects throughout the body. In the pancreas, exocrine tissue known as the islets of Langerhans contain beta cells. Beta cells are responsible for insulin synthesis.
- The postabsorptive state, or the fasting state, occurs when the food has been digested, absorbed, and stored. You commonly fast overnight, but skipping meals during the day puts your body in the postabsorptive state as well. During this state, the body must rely initially on stored glycogen.

References

1. Berg, J., Tymoczko, J., & Stryer, L. (2002). *Biochemistry*. W. H. Freeman Publishing, New York. ISBN 0-7167-4955-6.
2. Brock, T. D., Madigan, M. R., Martinko, J., & Parker, J. (2002). *Brock's Biology of Microorganisms*. Benjamin Cummings. ISBN 0-13-066271-2.
3. Chan, J., Desai, A. K., Kazi, Z. B., Corey, K., Austin, S., Hobson-Webb, L. D., Case, L. E., Jones, H. N., & Kishnani, P. S. (2017). The emerging phenotype of late-onset Pompe disease: A systematic literature review. *Molecular Genetics and Metabolism, 120*(3), 163–172.
4. Cox, M., & Nelson, D. L. (2004). *Lehninger Principles of Biochemistry*. Palgrave Macmillan. ISBN 0-7167-4339-6.

5. Da Silva, J. J., & Williams, R. J. (1991). *The Biological Chemistry of the Elements: The Inorganic Chemistry of Life*. Clarendon Press. ISBN 0-19-855598-9.

6. Ferreira, C. R., & Gahl, W. A. (2017). Lysosomal storage diseases. *Translational Science of Rare Diseases, 2*(1–2), 1–71.

7. Hicks, J., Wartchow, E., & Mierau, G. (2011). Glycogen storage diseases: A brief review and update on clinical features, genetic abnormalities, pathologic features, and treatment. *Ultrastructural Pathology, 35*(5), 183–196.

8. Kannourakis, G. (2002). Glycogen storage disease. *Seminars in Hematology, 39*(2), 103–106.

9. Kanungo, S., Wells, K., Tribett, T., & El-Gharbawy, A. (2018). Glycogen metabolism and glycogen storage disorders. *Annals of Translational Medicine, 6*(24), 474.

10. Koeberl, D. D., Kishnani, P. S., & Chen, Y. T. (2007). Glycogen storage disease types I and II: treatment updates. *Journal of Inherited Metabolic Disease, 30*(2), 159–164.

11. Kohler, L., Puertollano, R., & Raben, N. (2018). Pompe Disease: From Basic Science to Therapy. *Neurotherapeutics, 15*(4), 928–942.

12. Lane, N. (2004). *Oxygen: The Molecule that Made the World*. Oxford University Press. ISBN 0-19-860783-0.

13. Lefeuvre, C., Schaeffer, S., Carlier, R. Y., Fournier, M., Chapon, F., Biancalana, V., Nicolas, G., Malfatti, E., & Laforêt, P. (2020). Glycogenin-1 deficiency mimicking limb-girdle muscular dystrophy. *Molecular Genetics and Metabolism Reports, 24*, 100597.

14. Martin, A. P., Bartels, M., Schreiber, S., Buehrdel, P., Hauss, J., & Fangmann, J. (2006). Successful staged kidney and liver transplantation for glycogen storage disease type Ib: A case report. *Transplantation Proceedings, 38*(10), 3615–3619.

15. Molares-Vila, A., Corbalán-Rivas, A., Carnero-Gregorio, M., González-Cespón, J. L., & Rodríguez-Cerdeira, C. (2021). Biomarkers in Glycogen Storage Diseases: An Update. *International Journal of Molecular Sciences, 22*(9), 474.

16. Nicholls, D. G., & Ferguson, S. J. (2002). *Bioenergetics*. Biochemistry (Moscow) 69, 818–819 (2004). https://doi.org/10.1023/B:BIRY.0000040210.06512.a7

17. Oldfors, A., & DiMauro, S. (2013). New insights in the field of muscle glycogenoses. *Current Opinion in Neurology, 26*(5), 544–553.

18. Ozen, H. (2007). Glycogen storage diseases: new perspectives. *World Journal of Gastroenterology, 13*(18), 2541–2553.

19. Parikh, N. S., & Ahlawat, R. (2023). Glycogen Storage Disease Type I. In *StatPearls* [Internet]. StatPearls Publishing. Retrieved from: https://www.ncbi.nlm.nih.gov/books/NBK459277/ (accessed on 23 May 2024).

20. Saltik-Temizel, I. N., Coşkun, T., Yüce, A., & Koçak, N. (2005). Fanconi-Bickel syndrome in three Turkish patients with different homozygous mutations. *Turkish Journal of Pediatrics, 47*(2), 167–169.

21. Schreuder, A. B., Rossi, A., Grünert, S. C., & Derks, T. G. J. (2010). Glycogen Storage Disease Type III. In Adam, M. P., Feldman, J., Mirzaa, G. M., Pagon, R. A., Wallace, S. E., Bean, L. J. H., Gripp, K. W., & Amemiya, A. (Eds.), *GeneReviews®* [Internet]. University of Washington, Seattle.

22. Stone, W. L., Basit, H., & Adil, A. (2023). Glycogen Storage Disease. In *StatPearls* [Internet]. StatPearls Publishing. Retrieved from: https://www.ncbi.nlm.nih.gov/books/NBK459277/ (accessed on 23 May 2024).

23. Tarnopolsky, M. A. (2016). Metabolic Myopathies. *Continuum (Minneap Minn), 22*(6), Muscle and Neuromuscular Junction Disorders, 1829–1851.

24. Thornton, P. S., Stanley, C. A., De Leon, D. D., Harris, D., Haymond, M. W., Hussain, K., Levitsky, L. L., Murad, M. H., Rozance, P. J., Simmons, R. A., Sperling, M. A., Weinstein, D. A., White, N. H., & Wolfsdorf, J. I. (2015). Recommendations from the Pediatric Endocrine Society for Evaluation and Management of Persistent Hypoglycemia in Neonates, Infants, and Children. *Journal of Pediatrics, 167*(2), 238 Metabolic Myopathies 245.

25. Weinstein, D. A., Steuerwald, U., De Souza, C. F. M., & Derks, T. G. J. (2018). Inborn Errors of Metabolism with Hypoglycemia: Glycogen Storage Diseases and Inherited Disorders of Gluconeogenesis. *Pediatric Clinics of North America, 65*(2), 247 Metabolic Myopathies 265.

Chapter 8

THE COLON

Contents

Introduction

In tetrapods, the large intestine—also referred to as the colon—is the final segment of the digestive system and gastrointestinal tract. Here, water is absorbed, and the leftover waste is held as feces in the rectum until it is expelled through defecation. Although the terms are frequently used interchangeably, the majority of sources define the large intestine as the combination of the cecum, colon, rectum, and anal canal. The colon is the longest portion of the large intestine. The anal canal is not mentioned in some other sources. The ileocecal valve connects the human large intestine to the end of the small intestine at the cecum, located in the right iliac region of the pelvis, just below or at the waist. After that, it continues as the colon ascends the abdomen, moves as the transverse colon across the width of the abdominal cavity, descends to the rectum, and ends at the anal canal. The large intestine in humans is approximately 10.5 meters (5 feet) long overall, or roughly one-fifth of the entire length of the gastrointestinal tract.

Orientation and Directional Terms

Term	Definition	Illustration
Cecum	The cecum is the beginning of the colon. The small intestine feeds into the cecum through a small channel in the side of it (the ileocecal valve), so the end of the cecum is actually closed like a pouch. This pouch, the first 6 inches of the colon, is also the widest portion of the large intestine. This is the reservoir where food from the small intestine arrives in the large intestine. When the cecum is full, it triggers the muscle movements of the colon to begin.	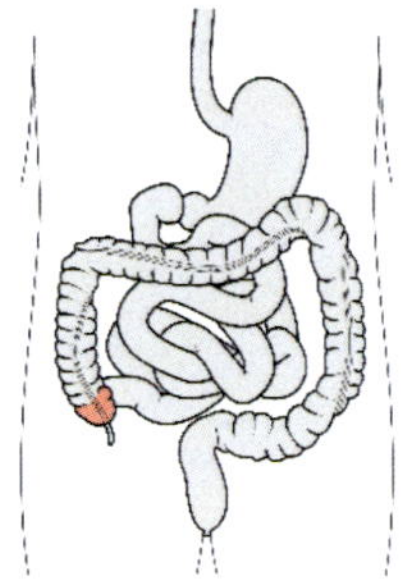
Rectum	By the time the sigmoid colon delivers the food waste to the rectum, it resembles the poop you know. The poop now consists of indigestible matter and dead cells shed from your intestinal mucosa, along with small amounts of mucus and water. If about 16 ounces of liquid food entered the large intestine, about 5 ounces of it remain as poop. When poop enters the rectum, it triggers the urge to defecate. This is the natural continuation of the mass muscle movements of the colon.	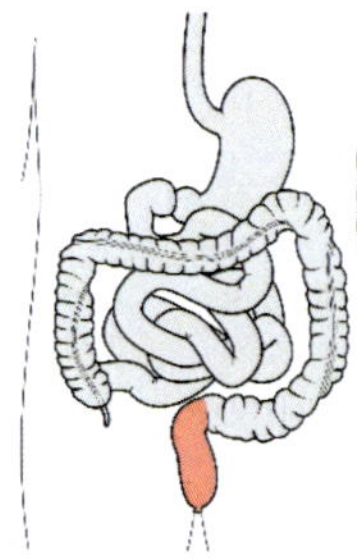
Anus	The anus is the canal your poop will travel through to leave your body. It's closed on each side by a muscle sphincter. On the inside, the internal sphincter opens automatically to let feces through. The outer sphincter is the one you control to let feces out when you're ready. When feces in the rectum triggers the urge to defecate, nerve signals cause the internal sphincter to relax. This is your cue to find a toilet where you can let the feces out through your external sphincter.	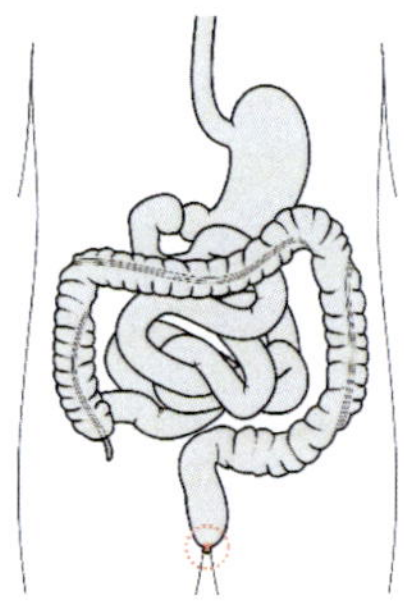
Appendix	The appendix is a vestigial organ attached to the large intestine. The inflammation of the appendix known as appendicitis requires the removal of the organ.	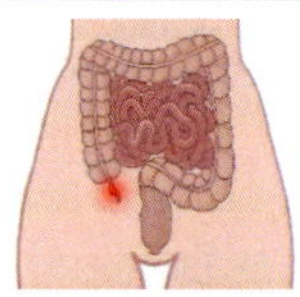
Constipation	Constipation generally means passing fewer than three stools a week or having a difficult time passing stool.	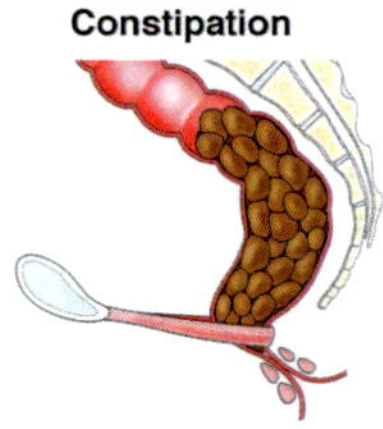

8.1. Structure

The final segment of the digestive system is the colon of the large intestine. It appears segmented because of haustra, a group of saccules. It is the site where the fermentation of unabsorbed material by the gut microbiota takes place and where it extracts water and salt from solid wastes before they are expelled from the body. The colon does not contribute significantly to food and nutrient absorption, in contrast to the small intestine. Every day, approximately 10.5 liters, or 45 ounces, of water enter the colon. The colon, which is the longest segment of the large intestine, measures 65 inches, or 166 cm, on average in adult humans (ranging from 80 to 313 cm in males), and 61 inches, or 155 cm, in females (ranging from 80 to 214 cm).

8.1.1. Sections

The colon, which is the longest portion of the large intestine in mammals, includes the appendix, the rectum, the anal canal, and the cecum (Figure 8.1).

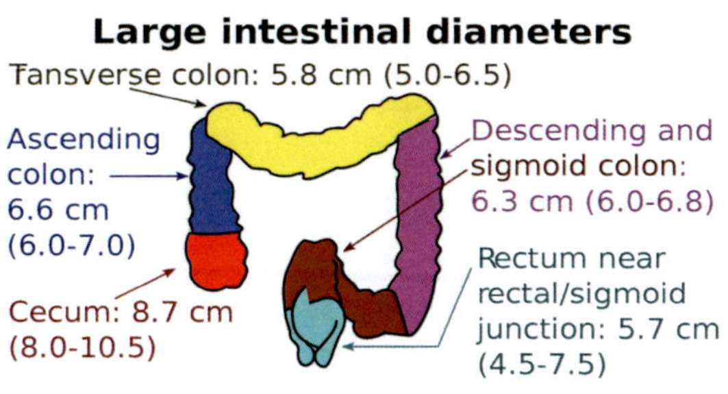

Figure 8.1. *Inner diameters of colon sections.*

Source: By Mikael Häggström, M.D., CC0, https://commons.wikimedia.org/w/index.php?curid=66530254.

The colon is divided into four sections: the sigmoid colon, descending colon, transverse colon, and ascending colon. At the colic flexures, these sections turn. Either the colon's components are located intraperitoneally or in the retroperitoneum, which is behind it. Retroperitoneal organs are fixed in place because, generally speaking, the peritoneum does not completely cover them. Because the peritoneum completely encloses intraperitoneal organs, they are mobile. The cecum of the colon, appendix, transverse colon, and sigmoid colon are intraperitoneal, but the ascending, descending, and rectum are retroperitoneal.

This matters because it influences which organs are easily accessible during procedures like laparotomies. The transverse colon has an average diameter of less than 6 cm, while the cecum has the largest diameter, averaging slightly less than 9 cm in healthy individuals. Both the sigmoid and descending colons are marginally smaller, with the sigmoid colon's average diameter measuring 4–5 cm (1.6–2.0 in). Megacolon can be diagnosed based on diameters greater than a certain threshold for each colonic section.

8.1.1.1. Cecum and Appendix

The appendix, which develops embryologically from the cecum and is thought to be a part of the gut-associated lymphoid tissue, is not involved in digestion. The cecum is the first section of the large intestine and is involved in digestion. The purpose of the appendix is unknown, but according to some sources, it serves as a repository for a sample of the gut microbiota and can replenish the microbiota in the colon if it is lost during an immunological response. It has also been demonstrated that the appendix contains a high concentration of lymphatic cells.

8.1.1.2. Ascending Colon

The portion of the colon that is situated between the transverse colon and the cecum is known as the ascending colon in human anatomy.

- **Characteristics and Structure:** The diameter of the ascending colon is lower than that of the cecum, where it originates. It travels upward, past the colic valve, and into the right lobe of the liver's underside, just to the right of the gallbladder. There, it lodges in the colic impression, a shallow depression. From there, it bends sharply left and forward to form the right colic flexure (hepatic), which is where it meets the transverse colon. Its posterior surface is connected by loose areolar tissue to the iliacus, quadratus lumborum, aponeurotic origin of the transversus abdominis, and the front of the lower and lateral part of the right kidney. The peritoneum, which covers its anterior surface and sides, keeps it in contact with the abdomen's posterior wall.

Occasionally it is fully invested by the peritoneum, forming a distinct but narrow mesocolon. It is situated in front of the abdominal walls and the ileum's convolutions. The vagus nerve provides parasympathetic innervation to the ascending colon. The thoracic splanchnic nerves supply sympathetic innervation.

- **Location:** If there are no abnormalities, the ascending colon is located on the right side of the body. In precise usage, the term "right colon" is synonymous with "ascending colon," and many remarks about the right colon informally refer primarily to the ascending colon.

8.1.1.3. Transverse Colon

The longest and most flexible portion of the colon in the human anatomy is the transverse colon.

- **Anatomical Position:** It traverses the abdomen with a downward convexity from the ascending colon at the right colic flexure (hepatic flexure) to the descending colon at the left colic flexure (splenic flexure), where it curves sharply on itself beneath the lower end of the spleen. It describes an arch along its path, with a concavity that faces both backward and slightly upward. There is frequently an abrupt U-shaped curve toward the splenic end, which may descend lower than the main curve. It is almost entirely covered in the peritoneum, and the transverse mesocolon, a broad duplication of that membrane, connects it to the pancreatic inferior border.

Its upper surface corresponds to the liver and gallbladder, the greater curvature of the stomach, and the lower end of the spleen; its lower surface corresponds to the small intestine; its anterior surface corresponds to the abdominal wall and the posterior layer of the greater omentum; its posterior surface corresponds, from right to left to the head of the pancreas, the descending portion of the duodenum, and some of the convolutions of the jejunum and ileum.

- **Function:** Salts and water are absorbed by the transverse colon.

8.1.1.4. Descending Colon

The portion of the colon that extends from the left colic flexure to the level of the iliac crest in humans and homologous primates is known as the descending colon (whereupon it transitions into the sigmoid colon). The function of descending colon in the digestive system is to hold the leftovers of food that have been broken down and emptied into the rectum. If there are no deformities, the descending colon is located on the left side of the body. In precise usage, the term "left colon" is synonymous with "descending colon," and many trite references to the left colon primarily refer to the descending colon.

- **Structure:** The left colic flexure in the upper left abdomen is the beginning of the descending colon. It continues inferiorly through the left hypochondrium and lumbar regions, along the outer border of the left kidney, and ends at the level of the iliac crest in the lower left abdomen. From that point on, it is known as the sigmoid colon. It is often retroperitoneal, with the peritoneum lining its anterior and lateral aspects. However, a small percentage of people may have suspended mesentery, which is typically short.

The left colic artery is the conduit for the arterial supply.

- **Function:** The initial section of the large intestine absorbs water and other substances from chyme, while the descending colon's main role is to retain waste until it exits the body during a bowel movement. Stools solidify as they progress through the descending colon.

8.1.1.5. Sigmoid Colon

The portion of the large intestine nearest to the rectum and anus is called the sigmoid colon, sometimes known as the pelvic colon. It creates a loop that is typically between 14 and 16 inches (35 to 40 centimeters) long. Usually, the loop has the form of the Latin letter S or the Greek letter sigma (ς), which is sigma + -oid. This portion of the colon usually rests inside the pelvis, but because of its flexibility, it could end up in the abdominal cavity.

- **Structure:** The sigmoid colon extends transversely across the front of the sacrum to the right side of the pelvis, starting at the superior aperture of the lesser pelvis, where it is continuous with the iliac colon. After that, it turns left and curves back on itself to meet the middle line at the level of the sacrum's third segment, where it bends downward and ends in the rectum. Its job is to remove gaseous and solid waste from the digestive system. It stores gas in the superior arched portion of its path toward the anus, which allows the colon to expel gas without simultaneously releasing feces.
  - **Coverings:** The peritoneum forms a mesentery (sigmoid mesocolon), which decreases in length from the loop's center toward its ends, where it disappears. As a result, the loop is fixed at its junctions with the iliac colon and rectum, but it has a significant range of motion in its central portion. The peritoneum completely encircles the sigmoid colon, making it non-retroperitoneal.
  - **Nerve Supply:** The main source of parasympathetic innervation is the pelvic splanchnic nerves. Via the inferior mesenteric ganglion, the lumbar splanchnic nerves supply sympathetic innervation.
  - **Relations:** The external iliac

vessels, ovary, obturator nerve, left piriformis, and left sacral plexus of nerves are located behind the sigmoid colon. It is divided in front by a few small intestine coils from the uterus in females and the bladder in males.

- **Clinical Significance:** Diverticulosis frequently coexists with focal weakness in the colonic wall and elevated intraluminal pressure in the sigmoid colon. It is frequently the cause of hemoptysis. A section of the colon twists around its mesentery to cause volvulus, which can cause blockage and infarction. Volvulus is more likely to occur in the midgut in infants and children, but it typically occurs in the sigmoid colon in elderly people. This could self-correct, or the rotation could keep going until the gut's blood supply is totally severed.

8.1.1.6. Rectum

In humans and certain other mammals, the rectum is the last straight segment of the large intestine; in other animals, it is the gut. The length of the adult human rectum is approximately 12 centimeters (4.7 in). Depending on the definition, it starts at the sacral promontory or the rectosigmoid junction, which is the terminus of the sigmoid colon, at the level of the third sacral vertebra. At the beginning, its diameter is comparable to that of the sigmoid colon; however, it becomes dilated near the end, where it forms the rectal ampulla. Depending on which definition is applied, it ends at either the dentate line or the level of the anorectal ring, which is the level of the puborectalis sling. The anal canal, which is roughly 4 centimeters (1.6 in) long in humans, comes after the rectum before the gastrointestinal tract ends at the anal verge. The Latin rectum intestinum, which means straight intestine, is where the word "rectum" originates.

- **Structure:** The sacrum is behind the rectum. It is located behind the uterus and vagina in females (right), and the bladder in males (left). The lower gastrointestinal tract includes the rectum. The rectum joins the anus and is the sigmoid colon's continuation. The rectum takes on the shape of the sacrum and terminates in an elongated segment known as the ampulla, which is used to hold feces until they are released through the anal canal. A Roman ampulla-shaped cavity or the dilated end of a duct is called an ampulla (from the Latin bottle). At the level of S3, the rectum joins the sigmoid colon, and as it passes through the pelvic floor muscles, it joins the anal canal.

The rectum does not have distinct taeniae coli, in contrast to other parts of the colon. Five centimeters above the rectum, in the sigmoid colon, the taeniae merge to form a single longitudinal muscle that encircles the rectum along its whole length.

- **Blood Supply and Drainage:** The top and bottom parts of the rectum receive different blood supplies. The superior rectal artery supplies the upper two-thirds. The inferior and middle rectal arteries supply the lower third. The inferior mesenteric artery continues as it crosses the pelvic brim and becomes the superior rectal artery, which is a single artery. It enters the mesorectum at the level of S3, after which it divides into two branches that run along the sides of the rectum first and the lateral back portion of the rectum second. These finally terminate as branches in the submucosa, where they anastamosely join the inferior and middle rectal artery branches.

- **Function:** Stools are temporarily stored in the rectum. Fecal material is transferred from the descending colon to the rectum employing regular contractions of the muscles, a process known as peristalsis. Defecation occurs when the urge to pass feces is stimulated by stretch receptors from the nervous system located in the rectal walls, which expand as a result of the materials filling it from the inside.

Fecal incontinence is prevented by the puborectalis muscle contraction during rest and the presence of both internal and external anal sphincters. The sphincters relax as the rectum expands, causing the contents to reflexively exit the rectum. The rectal muscles contract to facilitate expulsion. When the rectal pressure rises to more than 18 mmHg, the urge to voluntarily defecate appears, and reflex expulsion happens at 55 mmHg. During voluntary defecation, abdominal muscle contraction and puborectalis muscle relaxation take place in addition to the contraction of the rectal muscles and the relaxation of the external anal sphincter. This helps to facilitate defecation by straightening the angle formed by the rectum and anus.

- Clinical Significance
  - **Examination:** Rectal exams are utilized for diagnosing various conditions such as fecal impaction, prostatic cancer, benign prostatic hypertrophy in men, fecal incontinence, and internal hemorrhoids. Medical imaging options for examining the rectum include CT scans, MRI scans, and ultrasound probes that can be inserted for a closer look at nearby structures like the prostate. Colonoscopy and sigmoidoscopy are types of endoscopy procedures that use a camera for direct visualization of the rectal area, with the ability to perform biopsies if necessary. Additionally, a proctoscope can be used as a tool for viewing the rectum.

One can also take their body temperature in the rectum. Rectal temperature can be obtained by passing a medical thermometer through the anus and into the rectum, no more than 25 mm (1 inch). A digital thermometer should be inserted until it beeps, and a mercury thermometer should be inserted for three to five minutes. The normal range for rectal temperature is 36 to 38 °C (96.8 to 100.4 °F), which is approximately 0.5°C (1°F) higher than oral (mouth) temperature and 1.2 °C (2 °F) higher than axilla (armpit) temperature. The fact that there are less invasive ways to take a temperature, such as forehead and tympanic thermometers, has made it easier to use this method less frequently.

- **Route of Administration:** Additionally, some drugs are given via the rectum (per rectum in Latin). Enemas are injected into the rectum, and suppositories are inserted according to their definitions. Medication can be injected via the rectum to treat conditions like hemorrhoids or fissures around the rectum, relieve constipation, or administer systemically active medications when oral administration is not feasible. People generally dislike taking medications this way due to discomfort, cultural differences, and potential problems that could interfere with the medication's effectiveness, like leakage.

- **Constipation:** A dry, hard stool called faecal impaction in the rectum can be one of the causes of constipation. Though there are many possible causes, the most common ones include dietary and lifestyle choices like dehydration, immobility, and a low intake of dietary fiber. Such causes may include narrowing-related obstruction, local diseases (e.g., Crohn's disease, fissures, or hemorrhoids); diseases affecting the nervous system that control the bowel; spinal cord injury and multiple sclerosis; use of opioid medications; conditions (e.g., diabetes mellitus); and severe illness. Constipation can also result from low thyroid activity and high calcium levels.

Testing could be done to look into the reason. Blood tests for biochemistry, calcium levels, and thyroid function may be part of this. To determine whether stool is present in the rectum and whether there is an obstruction, a digital rectal examination may be carried out. If there are symptoms like pain, bleeding through the rectum, or weight loss, further tests like a CT scan might be prescribed. Testing may also involve magnetic resonance proctography, electrophysiological studies, and anal manometry to measure pressures in the anus and rectum if constipation does not improve with basic treatments.

Typically, constipation is managed by improving factors such as hydration, exercise, and dietary fiber. Laxatives can be used as well. If constipation continues, enemas or suppositories may be necessary. In some cases, manual evacuation using the fingers or hand may be needed. While laxatives like bisacodyl or senna can stimulate peristalsis in the large intestine, they do not seem to promote peristalsis in the rectum. Instead, they create a feeling of rectal fullness and contractions that often result in a bowel movement.

- Inflammation:
  - Anus and rectum inflammation is known as proctitis.
  - One type of inflammatory bowel disease that can lead to rectum ulcers is ulcerative colitis. A person's lifetime may be filled with episodes like this. These could result in blood stains in the stool. The cause is under study.
- Cancer:
  - Rectal cancer is a type of colorectal cancer that only affects the rectum.

Other diseases of the rectum include:

- Rectal prolapse is the term used to describe the prolapse of the rectum into the external area, or anus. This is frequently brought on by a postpartum weak pelvic floor.
- The upper rectum, also known as Sudeck's point in the context of mesenteric ischemia, is clinically significant as a watershed region between the inferior mesenteric artery

circulation and the internal iliac artery circulation via the middle rectal artery and is therefore susceptible to ischemia. Sudeck's point and Griffith's point at the splenic flexure are frequently mentioned as a watershed area.

8.1.2. Appearance

The cecum – the first part of the large intestine

- Taeniae coli – three bands of smooth muscle
- Haustra – swellings brought on by Taeniae coli contractions.
- Epiploic appendages – tiny fat deposits on the internal organs.

The large intestine is lined with taeniae coli. The colon becomes sacculated, forming the haustra of the colon—the shelf-like intraluminal projections—because the taenia coli are shorter than the large bowel itself.

8.1.3. Blood Supply

The colon receives its vascular supply from the branches of the inferior and superior mesenteric arteries (IMA and SMA, respectively). The colon's marginal artery, which runs the entire length of the colon parallel to it, serves as a conduit for communication between the two systems. Historically, it was believed that a structure that connected the proximal SMA to the proximal IMA was the Riolan arc or the Moskowitz meandering mesenteric artery.

This varying structure would become significant if either vessel became obstructed. Venous drainage typically follows the pattern of colonic artery supply, with the superior mesenteric vein joining the splenic vein to form the hepatic portal vein, which subsequently enters the liver, and the inferior mesenteric vein draining into the splenic vein. The exception is the middle rectal vein, which sends blood directly to the inferior vena cava instead of the liver.

8.1.4. Lymphatic Drainage

The ileocolic and superior mesenteric lymph nodes, which empty into the cisterna chyli, receive lymphatic drainage from the ascending colon and the proximal two-thirds of the transverse colon. The inferior mesenteric and colic lymph nodes receive the lymph from the distal third of the transverse colon, the descending colon, the sigmoid colon, and the upper rectum. The internal ileocolic nodes receive drainage from the lower rectum to the anal canal above the pectinate line. The superficial inguinal nodes receive the anal canal's drainage below the pectinate line. This transition is only partially indicated by the pectinate line.

8.1.5. Nerve Supply

Parasympathetic supply: vagus and pelvic nerves; sympathetic supply: superior and inferior mesenteric ganglia.

8.1.6. Development

The germ layers known as the endoderm, mesoderm, and ectoderm develop through a process known as gastrulation. Early in a person's development, gastritis happens. These layers give rise to the digestive system.

8.1.7. Variation

One deviation from the colon's typical structure is the formation of additional loops, which can cause the colon to grow up to five meters longer than it should. Known as redundant colon, this condition usually has no major health effects; however, on rare occasions, volvulus may occur, causing obstruction and necessitating immediate medical attention. When a redundant colon is present, using a standard adult colonoscope can be challenging or even impossible. However, there are specialized versions of the instrument, such as the pediatric variant, that can help with this issue. This is a significant indirect health consequence.

8.2. Histology

In vertebrate animals, the large intestine, also known as the large bowel, is the final segment of the digestive system. Its job is to remove the body's needless waste products after absorbing water from the food that is still indigestible. The colon, rectum, anal canal, and cecum make up the large intestine. It connects to the lower end of the small intestine at the right iliac region of the pelvis, which is located just below the right waist. From this point on, it travels up the abdomen, across the width of the abdominal cavity, and then descends to reach the anus, where it ends (Figure 8.2).

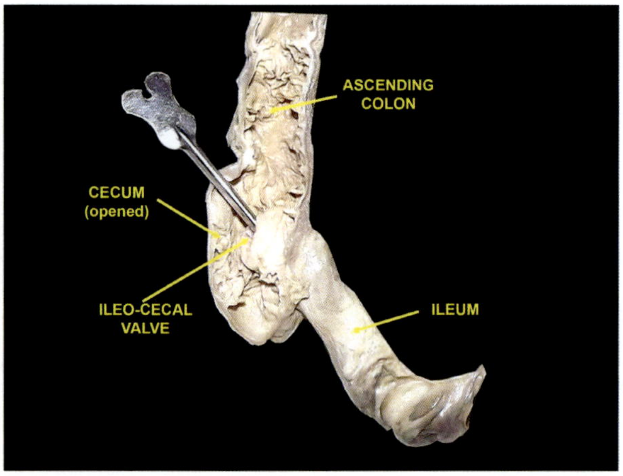

Figure 8.2. *The colon.*

Source: By Anatomist90 – Own work, CC BY-SA 3.0, https://commons.wikimedia.org/w/index.php?curid=30356294.

The large intestine is substantially wider than the small intestine, which is how they differ physically. The three strap-like structures known as the taeniae coli, or bands of longitudinal muscle fibers, each measuring roughly 1/5 of an inch in width, comprise the longitudinal layer of the muscularis. These three bands run from the cecum to the rectum, beginning at the base of the appendix. Appendices epiploicae, or epiploic appendages, are fat-filled peritoneal tags that run along the sides of the taeniae. Simple columnar epithelium lines the wall of the large intestine. The large intestine has invaginations (the intestinal glands) as opposed to the evaginations of the small intestine (villi). Goblet cells, which secrete mucin to form mucus in water, are found in both the small and large intestines; however, they are more numerous in the latter (Figure 8.3).

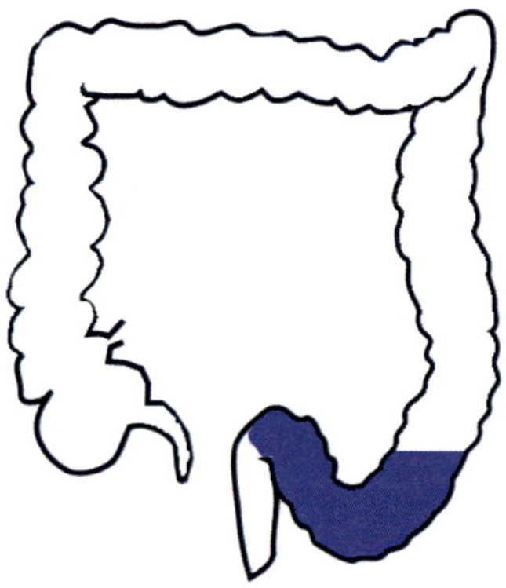

Figure 8.3. *Sigmoid colon.*

Source: By Adert – Own work, CC BY-SA 3.0, https://commons.wikimedia.org/w/index.php?curid=17963657.

An intestinal crypt, also known as the crypt of Lieberkühn, is a gland located in the colon's and small intestine's epithelial lining. The epithelium covering the crypts and intestinal villi is made up of two different cell types: enterocytes, which secrete water and electrolytes, and goblet cells, which secrete mucus. Digestive enzymes found in the mucosa's enterocytes break down particular foods as they pass through the epithelium. Peptidase, sucrase, maltase, lactase, and intestinal lipase are some of these enzymes. On the other hand, the primary cells in the stomach secrete pepsinogen. The intestinal cells do not secrete digestive enzymes within the intestine. Additionally, new epithelium grows here, which is significant because food constantly wears away at this site's cells. Multipotent stem cells are found in the basal part of the crypt, which is located farther away from the intestinal lumen.

One of the two daughter cells from each mitosis differentiates, moves up the side of the crypt, and eventually enters the villus, with the other daughter cell staying in the crypt as a stem cell. Among the cells synthesized in this way are goblet cells. Numerous genes have been demonstrated to be crucial for intestinal stem cell differentiation. The crypts' loss of ability to control proliferation is thought to be the cause of colorectal cancer.

8.3. The Appendix

The appendix develops in the embryo from the cecum, a tube with a blind end that resembles a finger. The large intestine's cecum, which resembles a pouch, is situated where the small and large intestines converge. The Latin word "vermiform" means "worm-shaped." Before the early 2000s, the appendix was thought to be a vestigial organ, but this opinion has since evolved. According to research, the appendix may have a crucial role in the body as a storehouse for good gut bacteria.

8.3.1. Structure

The length of the human appendix ranges from 5 to 35 cm (2.0 to 13.8 in), with an average of 9 cm (3.5 in). The appendix has a diameter of 6 mm (0.24 in), and anything larger is regarded as an inflammatory or thickened appendix. 26 cm (10 in) was the longest appendix ever removed. Usually found in the lower right quadrant of the abdomen, close to the right hip bone, is the appendix. The ileocecal valve, which divides the large and small intestines, is 2 cm (0.79 in) below the base of the appendix. Its location within the abdomen corresponds to McBurney's point, which is a point on the surface. The mesoappendix, a brief section of the mesocolon, connects the appendix to the mesentery in the lower part of the ileum.

8.3.1.1. Variation

The term "mirror image twins" refers to a type of identical twin where the appendix is congenitally located in the lower left quadrant of the abdomen rather than the lower right. The appendix may also be displaced to the left side due to intestinal malrotation. The appendix's tip can be found in the pelvis, outside the peritoneum, or behind the cecum, but its base is normally found 2 cm (0.79 in) below the ileocecal valve. Populations vary in the frequency of the various positions; retrocecal positions are most common in Ghana and Sudan, with 67.3% and 58.3% occurrences, respectively, while pelvic positions are more common in Iran and Bosnia, with 55.8% and 55.7% occurrences, respectively.

Rarely, there may be no appendix at all (the frequency of laparotomies performed for suspected appendicitis has been reported to be 1 in 100,000). Occasionally, the opening has a semi-circular mucous membrane fold. Gerlach's valve is another name for this vermiform appendix valve.

8.3.2. Functions

8.3.2.1. Maintaining Gut Flora

Although it has long been known that the immune tissue known as "gut-associated lymphoid tissue," which surrounds the appendix and other areas of the gut, performs a variety of vital tasks, there have never been adequate explanations for the unique shape of the appendix or its apparent lack of significance or function, as indicated by the absence of side effects after removal. As a result, it became commonly believed that the appendix is merely vestigial (Figure 8.4).

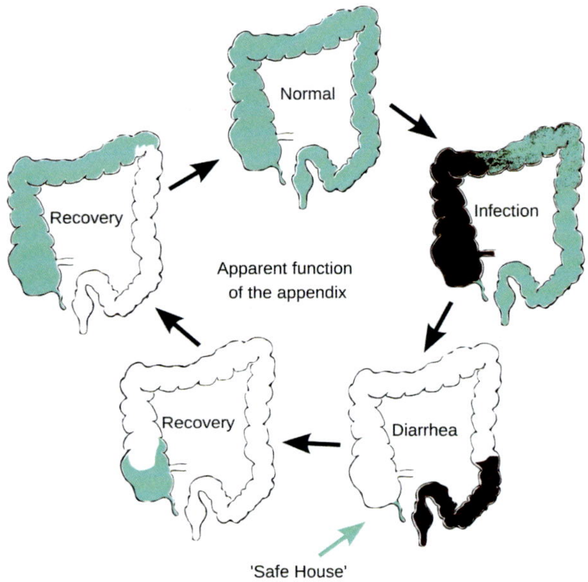

Figure 8.4. *A possible function of the human appendix is a "safe house" for beneficial bacteria in the recovery from diarrhea.*

Source: By WebHamster at English Wikipedia, CC BY-SA 3.0, https://commons.wikimedia.org/w/index.php?curid=36572266.

In 2007, William Parker, Randy Bollinger, and associates from Duke University put forth the theory that when disease clears the bacteria from the remainder of the intestines, the appendix acts as a refuge for beneficial bacteria. This idea is supported by knowledge that became available in the early 2000s about how the immune system aids in the growth of advantageous intestinal bacteria. It also takes into account many well-known characteristics of the appendix, such as its structure, location directly below the normal one-way flow of food and microbes in the large intestine, and association with a large amount of immune tissue. According to research, people without an appendix had a four times higher chance of developing *Clostridium difficile* colitis again. As a result, the appendix might serve as a haven for helpful bacteria. The gut flora in the digestive system could then be replenished or enhanced by this reservoir of bacteria after a milder gastrointestinal ailment or after a bout of dysentery or cholera.

8.3.2.2. Immune and Lymphatic Systems

It has been determined that the appendix plays a significant role in mammalian mucosal immune function, specifically in B cell-mediated immunity and T cells derived extrathymically. This structure has lymphatic vessels that control pathogens, aids in the proper movement and elimination of waste products from the digestive system, and may even develop early defenses against fatal illnesses. Furthermore, it's believed that this could boost immune defenses against invasive pathogens and train B and T cells in the lymphatic system to combat the bacteria and viruses that infect that area of the colon. This will help to target immune responses and make them more effective at warding off infections safely and reliably. Furthermore, distinct immune cells known as innate lymphoid cells work in the gut to support the appendix in maintaining digestive health. Studies also reveal a positive relationship between the concentration of cecal lymphoid tissue and the presence of the appendix, bolstering the theory that the appendix not only develops as a complex with the cecum but also provides significant immune benefits.

8.3.3. Clinical Significance

Appendicitis and carcinoid tumors (appendiceal carcinoid) are common diseases of the appendix in humans. Approximately 1 in 200 gastrointestinal cancers are appendix cancers. Adenomas can also be seen in rare instances.

8.3.3.1. Appendicitis

An inflammation of the appendix is the hallmark of appendicitis. As the appendix develops as a component of the embryonic midgut, pain frequently starts in the center of the abdomen. Usually, this pain is dull, visceral, and poorly localized.

As the inflammation worsens and the peritoneum becomes inflamed, the pain starts to more clearly localize to the right lower quadrant. Rebound tenderness, or pain experienced when pressure is removed rather than applied, is caused by this peritoneal inflammation, also known as peritonitis. It manifests specifically at McBurney's point, which is located 1/3 of the way from the anterior superior iliac spine to the umbilicus. Point (skin) pain usually does not manifest until the parietal peritoneum is also inflamed. An immune system reaction and a fever are additional features of appendicitis. Additional indications and symptoms could be vomiting and nausea, a low-grade fever that could worsen, diarrhea or constipation, bloating in the abdomen, or flatulence. The standard treatment for appendicitis is an appendectomy, which can be performed by laparotomy or laparoscopy, to remove the inflamed appendix. If left untreated, the rupture of the appendix may result in peritonitis, shock, and, in the worst case scenario, death.

8.3.3.2. Surgery

An appendectomy is the surgical removal of the appendix. In cases of acute appendicitis, this removal is typically done as an emergency procedure for the patient. Intravenous antibiotics are used to prevent or delay the onset of sepsis in situations where surgical facilities are not available. Sometimes the appendicitis goes away entirely, but more frequently a mass of inflammation develops around the appendix. Surgery is somewhat contraindicated in this case.

The appendix can be utilized for the creation of an efferent urinary conduit in a procedure called the Mitrofanoff procedure for individuals with a neurogenic bladder. Additionally, the appendix can be used as a way to reach the colon in children with paralyzed bowels or significant rectal sphincter issues. By bringing the appendix to the skin surface, a catheter can be attached by the child or parent to easily cleanse the colon with a suitable solution.

8.4. The Anal Canal

The portion of the digestive system that transports food from the rectum to the anus is called the anal canal. It is longer than it appears, usually ranging from 2.5 to 4 cm, but its complexity is surprising. The anal canal is essential for maintaining fecal continence, differentiating between solid, liquid, and gas, and protecting the body from potentially harmful organisms. Anal canal pathologies are frequently overlooked when there are no symptoms, but they can be treated in a variety of ways, from conservative measures like sitz baths to more involved procedures like radiation or surgical resection.

8.4.1. Structure and Function

The rectum and the anus, the extremity of the digestive tract, are connected by the anal canal. It is situated between the fat-filled, wedge-shaped ischioanal, or ischiorectal, fossae that allow it to expand to allow the passage of fecal material, and the anal triangle of the perineum. The anorectal junction, also known as the anorectal ring, is a bend in the gastrointestinal tract that marks the transition from the rectum to the anus. It is sustained by the puborectalis muscular sling. The superior blending of the two sphincters' muscular fibers with the puborectalis muscle occurs at the anorectal junction.

The internal and external anal sphincters are the two anatomically and functionally unique sphincters that encircle the anal canal. Involuntary is the internal anal sphincter (IAS). Its operation is reliant on the integrity of the internal anal sphincter's reflexive relaxation in the presence of rectal distension, or the rectoanal inhibitory reflex (RAIR). When there is no rectal distension, it keeps the body at resting pressure. As a result, the resting pressure of the internal anal sphincter is frequently measured when assessing a range of pathologies and is frequently used as a direct indicator of the function of the muscle. Control over the external anal sphincter (EAS) is voluntary. When a person defecates, the external anal sphincter relaxes from its maintained tone, which keeps the anal canal orifice closed. The external anal sphincter keeps stool in the anal canal until the person is ready to void, while the internal anal sphincter relaxes in response to rectal distension due to the rectoanal inhibitory reflex.

The pectinate, or dentate, line usually separates the anal canal into superior and inferior segments. The inferior aspect of longitudinal folds called the anal columns or anal valves forms the pectinate line, a noticeable zigzag pattern. The superior and inferior halves of the anal canal are separated by the pectinate line. Additionally, it functions as an embryologic landmark that clarifies the variations in the anal canal's segments' venous, lymphatic, and arterial supplies.

8.4.2. Embryology

The embryology of the anal canal differs superiorly and inferiorly from the pectinate line, just like its structure and function. The anal canal is the endodermally derived terminal portion of the hindgut, located above the pectinate line. Columnar epithelium lines the superior anal canal, just like it does the rest of the hindgut. The anal canal is ectodermally derived and lined with stratified squamous epithelium below the pectinate line. The external anal sphincter is not fully developed or completely under voluntary control at birth. Around the ages of 18 to 24 months, a person typically reaches voluntary control over the external anal sphincter.

8.4.3. Blood Supply and Lymphatics

A great way to comprehend the venous drainage, lymphatics, and arterial supply of the anal canal is to think about the supply that lies above and below the pectinate line, as well as the overlapped area.

- **Arterial Supply and Lymphatic Drainage:** The superior rectal artery, a branch of the inferior mesenteric artery, supplies the anal canal above the pectinate line. This area sends lymphatic fluid to the lymph nodes in the inferior mesentery. The inferior and middle rectal arteries supply blood to the anal canal below the pectinate line. The internal iliac artery gives rise to the inferior rectal artery, which is a branch of the internal pudendal artery. The internal iliac artery gives rise to the middle rectal artery. The superficial inguinal lymph nodes receive the majority of the lymphatic drainage that occurs below the pectinate line.
- **Venous Drainage:** The superior rectal veins, which empty into the inferior mesenteric vein, receive the venous drainage of the anal canal above the pectinate line. These veins transport nutrient-rich, oxygen-poor blood to the liver for processing. They are a component of the hepatic portal venous system. The internal pudendal veins receive the venous drainage of the anal canal below the

pectinate line, and the internal iliac vein receives the contents of these veins. The systemic venous system, which carries blood deficient in nutrients and oxygen to the heart, includes these veins. Potential collateral circulatory pathways are made possible by the portal and systemic venous anastomoses of the anorectal canal. Patients with portal hypertension may exhibit noticeable anorectal varices. These portosystemic anastomoses are not exclusive to the anal canal; they can be found throughout the body.

8.4.4. Nerves

As with lymphatics and blood supply, it is helpful to talk about the anal canal's nervous system from both the superior and inferior perspectives to the pectinate line. These two areas react differently to stimuli and have distinct innervations. The inferior hypogastric plexus provides autonomic innervation to the anal canal above the pectinate line. Defecation is made possible by the parasympathetic innervation, which suppresses the tone of the internal anal sphincter and causes a peristaltic contraction. To maintain continence and the tone of the internal anal sphincter, sympathetic innervation acts antagonistically. The superior aspect of the anal canal is the most sensitive to distention or stretch because viscerosensory signals originate from this area and return. The anal canal receives somatic innervation from branches of the pudendal nerve below the pectinate line. Because of this, the anal canal's inferior aspect is extremely sensitive to touch, temperature, and pain.

8.4.5. Physiologic Variants

The literature contains a few anatomical variations of the anal canal. Anal canal duplication, in which a newborn has an additional anal canal either superior or posterior to the main canal, has been the subject of several case reports. The accessory anal canal in people with duplicated anal canals is usually quite normal, but it terminates in a blind pouch that is disconnected from the rectum. To prevent the accessory anal canal from acting as a potential source of inflammation, fistulization, or cancer, this condition is currently treated with surgical excision.

The anal canal varies in certain ways as people age. The thickness of the internal anal sphincter rises with age in humans. Typically, the effect is more noticeable in females over 50. According to current guidelines, patients under 50 years of age should have a maximal internal anal sphincter thickness of no more than 4 mm, and those over 50 years of age should have a thickness of 5 mm. This becomes crucial in identifying patients who have internal anal sphincter hypertrophy.

8.4.6. Surgical Considerations

The surgeon can distinguish between the upper and lower portions of the anal canal using a number of different techniques when performing anal canal surgery. Understanding the vascular supply, drainage, and innervation of the various anal canal segments is essential for surgical considerations. This can be achieved by locating the pectinate line. The anal canal's narrow opening and compact anatomy make it a challenging area to operate in. For example, sphincter-saving surgery in cases of lower rectal cancer is extremely difficult due to the anatomy of the anal canal. Negative consequences from these surgeries include permanent colostomy or compromise of the anal sphincter leading to incontinence. Other methods, including transvaginal, transperineal, transsacral, and abdominal, have been investigated because surgeons have a limited window of opportunity inside the anal canal.

8.4.7. Clinical Significance

- **Incontinence:** Fecal incontinence can arise from any malfunction of the anal canal musculature, as the anal canal and its muscles are responsible for preserving fecal continence. Currently, anal manometry is recommended to evaluate sphincter tone in patients with fecal incontinence. When positive manometry indicates a sphincter tone dysfunction, anorectal imaging is typically performed to assess structural integrity.
- **Hemorrhoids:** Vein engorgement and possible prolapse in the lower anus and rectum are symptoms of a common anal disorder called hemorrhoids. Hemorrhoids can occur as a result of a number of factors, including heavy lifting, anal intercourse, age, diarrhea, chronic constipation, obesity, genetics, and prolonged sitting, especially on the toilet. Hemorrhoids can be classified into two main categories: internal and external. Because of the visceral sensations in that area, internal hemorrhoids are typically painless and located deep within the anal canal, superior to the pectinate line. When these hemorrhoids strain, they may prolapse out of the anus and frequently present with painless bleeding. External hemorrhoids are located near the anal opening and beneath the pectinate line. External hemorrhoids are often painful and itchy because they occur in the inferior anal canal and are served by somatosensory signals. Hemorrhoids usually go away on their own, but patients can ease the pain with dietary fiber, stool softeners, and regular sitz baths. It's crucial to counsel these patients to consume enough fiber, to strain less in the restroom, and to spend less time sitting on the toilet. Hemorrhoids that are large or bothersome can be surgically removed from the body in the office or banded.
- **Anal Cancer:** Anal cancer is a condition where the anus's healthy cells develop into cancerous ones. The majority of cases are associated with the human papillomavirus (HPV). Anal cancer is more likely to occur in people who smoke and have weakened immune systems. The size of the tumor and whether the cancer has spread to the lymph nodes are the main factors affecting the prognosis of anal cancer. Anal cancer is graded from 0 to 5 according to its size and spread after it has been identified, with stage 5 having the worst prognosis. Chemotherapy, radiation therapy, surgery, or a combination of these treatments are frequently used to treat anal cancer.

8.5. Functions of the Colon

Before sending the indigestible material to the rectum, the large intestine absorbs water and any nutrients that are still absorbable from the meal. Thiamine, riboflavin, and vitamin K—particularly crucial since daily consumption of this vitamin is typically insufficient to sustain appropriate blood coagulation—are among the vitamins produced by the colonic bacteria and are absorbed by the colon. Additionally, it compacts excrement and holds it in the rectum until it is ready to be expelled through the anus during defecation.

K+ and Cl- are also secreted by the large intestine. In patients with cystic fibrosis, chloride secretion rises. In the colon, different nutrients are recycled. The urea cycle, short-chain fatty acid metabolism, and carbohydrate fermentation are a few examples. The appendix has an unknown function in immunity because it contains a tiny amount of mucosa-associated lymphoid tissue. However, because it contains endocrine cells that release peptide hormones and biogenic amines necessary for homeostasis during early growth and development, the appendix is known to be significant in fetal life.

By the time the chyme reaches this tube, the body has absorbed 90% of the water and most of the nutrients. As evidenced by the widespread use of ileostomy procedures, many individuals can actually survive without having a large portion of their large intestine or even without having it at all. At this point, only some electrolytes like sodium, magnesium, and chloride are left as well as indigestible parts of ingested food (e.g., a large part of ingested amylose, starch which has been shielded from digestion heretofore, and dietary fiber, which is largely indigestible carbohydrate in either soluble or insoluble form). The chyme is combined with mucus and bacteria (known as gut flora) as it passes through the large intestine, losing most of its water content and turning into feces. Fecal material is delivered as a liquid to the ascending colon. The stools then gradually solidify as they pass into the descending colon because the colon's muscles push the watery waste material forward and gradually absorb all the extra water.

Acetate, propionate, and butyrate are waste products produced by the bacteria as they break down some of the fiber for their own nutrition. The colon's cell lining uses these substances as food. There is no protein made accessible. Perhaps 10% of the undigested carbohydrates are thus made available in humans, though this depends on diet; other animals, such as primates and other apes with proportionally larger colons, have more made available, allowing a higher percentage of plant material in the diet. Digestion is finished chemically in the small intestine before the chyme reaching the large intestine, hence the large intestine does not produce any digestive enzymes. The colon's pH ranges from 5.5 to 7. (slightly acidic to neutral).

8.5.1. Standing Gradient Osmosis

Water absorption in the colon occurs by moving against an osmotic pressure gradient. The process involves the reabsorption of water against the osmotic gradient within the intestines. Cells in the intestinal lining push sodium ions into the intercellular space, increasing the osmolarity of the fluid between cells. This hypertonic fluid creates pressure that drives water through tight junctions and neighboring cells into the spaces between cells, then across the basement membrane and into the blood vessels. Meanwhile, more sodium ions are pumped back into the intercellular fluid. Despite water moving down an osmotic gradient in each step, overall, water flows against the osmotic gradient due to the sodium ion pumping. This mechanism allows the large intestine to absorb water even when the blood in the vessels is less concentrated than the fluid in the intestines.

8.5.2. Gut Flora

The large intestine is home to fungi, protozoa, archaea, and more than 700 different species of bacteria that serve a multitude of purposes. Geographical location and diet influence species diversity. The distal gut microbes in humans can weigh up to 200 grams (0.44 pounds) and are frequently in the range of 100 trillion. It has been suggested that this collection of primarily symbiotic microbes is the forgotten organ—the most recent human organ to be found. A portion of the products produced by the bacteria residing in this area are absorbed by the large intestine. In the large intestine, bacteria convert undigested polysaccharides (fiber) into short-chain fatty acids, which are then absorbed by passive diffusion. The large intestine secretes bicarbonate, which aids in balancing the elevated acidity brought on by the fatty acid formation.

In addition, these bacteria generate a lot of vitamins, particularly the B vitamin biotin and vitamin K, which the blood can absorb. Even though this vitamin source generally only supplies a small portion of the daily requirement, it plays a major role in cases where the intake of vitamins from food is inadequate. If antibiotics are used to treat a patient who depends on the absorption of vitamins produced by bacteria in the large intestine, they may cause vitamin deficiency by inhibiting both the bacteria that cause the disease and the species that produce vitamins.

Other byproducts of bacteria include gas (flatus), a mixture of carbon dioxide and nitrogen with trace amounts of hydrogen, methane, and hydrogen sulfide. These are made by bacteria fermenting undigested polysaccharides. Tryptophan is broken down into indoles, which contribute to some of the odor associated with feces. The development of specific tissues, such as the lymphatics and cecum, depends on the normal flora.

Additionally, they contribute to the synthesis of cross-reactive antibodies. These are immune system-produced antibodies that work against related pathogens as well as the normal flora, preventing infection or invasion. Bacteroidota and Bacillota are the two phyla of the colon that are most common. According to the Human Microbiome Project, there appears to be a wide range in the ratio between the two. Both colitis and colon cancer are thought to have their origins in Bacteroides. Bifidobacteria are also widely distributed and frequently referred to as "friendly bacteria." The large intestine is shielded from colonic commensal bacteria attacks by a mucus layer.

8.6. Surgical Resection

The removal of all or a portion of the colon is known as colon resection. Arteries, veins, and lymphatic drainage are located in the mesocolon, which during the oncological surgical resections of total mesorectal excision and complete mesocolic excision gets removed in its entirety corresponding to the part of the colon to be removed.

8.6.1. Indications

Colorectal cancer is the most common reason for surgical colon resection, and oncological guidelines should be followed when performing the resection.

- For colonic cancers, the resection margin is 5 cm both proximal and distal to the tumor.
- The margin of circumferential resection for the rectum; a 2 cm distal margin is sufficient.
- At the point where the primary feeding vessel originates, remove the lymphatic drainage and vasculature.
- To cure and stage, this permits the resection of locoregional lymph node-bearing mesentery.
- The creation of a tension-free, well-vascularized anastomosis.

8.6.2. Contraindications

Since colonic resection is considered major surgery, it should not be performed on a patient who is not physically capable of enduring such a procedure. Before surgery, reversible and modifiable risk factors should be addressed. A patient may also need to stay in an intensive care unit or a high dependency facility after surgery.

8.6.3. Equipment

Colonic resection can be performed with minimal access techniques (laparotomy) or open techniques (laparotomy).

- An operating table that permits the removal of the end segment, sidebars for mounting the attachments that position the patient's legs in the Lloyd Davies position, and a sterile operating theater are necessary for the open approach. Bowel clamps are among the instruments included in a major laparotomy set.
- In addition to the setup mentioned above, the laparoscopic approach calls for instruments, a gas insufflator, display screens, and a laparoscopic camera.
- The robot is necessary for the robotic approach.
- Suture material for a hand-sewn anastomosis (absorbable braided or monofilament, strength 3/0) would be necessary equipment for bowel anastomosis.
- For a stapled anastomosis, one would need either circular or linear staplers, with the diameter ranging from 28 to 33 mm, depending on the patient's size. Linear staplers are used for side-to-side anastomoses, measuring 75 or 100 mm in length.
- To facilitate rectal washout and anastomosis during rectal surgery, a small additional table containing a proctoscope, bladder syringe, and lubricant must be set up.

8.6.4. Personnel

An anesthetist, a team of surgeons (at least one operating surgeon and one assistant), and the entire operating room staff (scrub side, anesthesia side, and patient positioning assistant) are needed for a colonic resection.

8.6.5. Preparation

The patient needs to be thoroughly assessed before surgery.

- The evaluation of the colon includes a colonoscopy to determine whether the disease requires resection and to confirm that the remaining portion of the colon is normal (e.g., no concurrent tumors) and imaging techniques like CT scans to determine the disease's proper staging and check for distant metastases.
- For small tumors undergoing laparoscopic resection, the lesion must be endoscopically tattooed prior to surgery to facilitate intraoperative identification.
- In addition to the above, rectal cancers necessitate an endorectal ultrasound or a rectum MRI scan.
- Preoperatively, get the patient ready following local protocol. The majority of facilities will administer intravenous peri-operative antibiotic prophylaxis in addition to bowel preparation.

8.6.6. Technique or Treatment

Bowel resection can be performed either through open surgery or laparoscopy while adhering to the same surgical principles. The key factor in a successful resection is ensuring proper blood supply to the colon. For benign conditions, the resection may not need to be as extensive, but when treating malignancies, the goal is to resect the colonic vessels supplying the cancerous area as closely to their origin as possible to obtain an adequate number of lymph nodes in the colonic mesentery (more than 12). The bowel segments on either side of the resected area must be mobilized to allow for tension-free anastomosis, which should also have a good blood supply. Depending on the surgeon's skill level and available equipment, the bowel anastomosis can be done by hand-sewing or using staples.

For instance, ligation of the ileocolic, right branch of the middle colic artery, and right colic (if present) is required for a formal right hemicolectomy. The transverse colon is where distal bowel division occurs, and the terminal ileum is where proximal bowel division occurs. Traditionally, the transverse colon and terminal ileum form the anastomosis side by side. Ligating the inferior mesenteric artery and inferior mesenteric vein is necessary for the excision of a sigmoid colon tumor. Distal bowel division occurs at the upper rectum, above the peritoneal reflection, while proximal bowel division occurs at the distal descending colon. An end-to-end anastomosis is typically facilitated between the upper rectum and the descending colon using a circular stapling tool that is inserted through the anal canal.

8.6.7. Complications

Complications that arise during the procedure can be separated into two categories: those that arise after the surgery and those that arise during the procedure. Bleeding is a common procedural complication that occurs from handling the mesocolon or dissecting the greater omentum; it is rarely caused by any of the vessels mentioned. An arterial bleed from the colon's named vessels, however, can be torrential and needs to be treated quickly, particularly during laparoscopic procedures when the bleeding may cover the camera and obstruct the view.

When feasible, apply direct pressure to temporarily stop the bleeding. This will give you time to plan, reposition, ask for more instruments, locate additional ports, and, if needed, stop the bleeding completely. Damage to surrounding structures is another intraoperative complication. The left ureter is the most vulnerable structure. It should always be noted in cases of left-sided surgery. If an intraoperative injury (transsection, diathermy burn) happens and is identified right away, it can be fixed, and to lower the risk of stricture, a ureteric stent should be inserted.

The management of an injury that is discovered only after surgery is contingent upon the type and location of the injury, the patient's overall health, and the level of expertise that is available. If one is available, a urological specialist should be consulted. Among the complications following surgery are infections of the wound, chest, and urinary tract. Infections can be avoided by early mobilization, physical therapy, incentive spirometry, and urinary catheter removal. Prophylactic antibiotics given within one hour of skin incision greatly reduce the risk of wound infection in clean-contaminated surgery.

All surgeons performing primary anastomosis and colonic resection dread the possibility of an astomotic leak. As signs and symptoms can be subtle at first, particularly if the leak is in the pelvis and the patient has a defuncting stoma, a high index of suspicion is recommended if a patient does not recover as planned after surgery. In addition to complaining of bloating and abdominal pain, patients may also exhibit tachycardia, cardiac arrhythmias (new-onset atrial fibrillation), pyrexia, and a distended, tender, possibly peritonitic abdomen. During the postoperative phase, there will be a greater than anticipated increase in inflammatory markers. An erect chest X-ray may not reveal free air under the diaphragm, but a

CT scan will reveal pneumoperitoneum and fluid surrounding the anastomosis. Rectal contrast should be used during the scan in patients who have had anterior resection.

The management may consist of all or some of the following, depending on the extent of the leak and the patient's overall condition.

- antimicrobial therapy;
- drainage of pus collections (percutaneously if patient stable and expertise available); and
- the possibility of performing a reexamination surgery to clean and empty the abdominal cavity, check the anastomosis, and either defunction the patient or remove the anastomosis and expose the proximal bowel as an end stoma (much like a Hartmann's procedure).

8.6.8. Clinical Significance

Prerequisites For Good Anastomosis:

- Adequate blood supply: Patient factors such as blood pressure, inotropes, peripheral vascular disease, calcified vessels, thrombosis, and plaques should be taken into account during surgery.
- Additional pathologies of the colon (diverticulosis, proximal dilatation in cases of obstruction).
- tension-free (mesentery and colon are both of sufficient length).
- The colonic conduit is long enough for anterior resection.
- Divide the peritoneum with caution so as not to damage the marginal artery, divide the IMV as high as possible (the DJ flexure serves as a landmark), and divide the cephalad to the last visible tributary.
- full splenic flexure mobilization. Make sure the conduit passes through the pubic symphysis so that it can go to the pelvis for the colorectal anastomosis.
- Make sure the conduit passes through the pubic symphysis and into the pelvis, where a colorectal anastomosis will take place.

8.6.9. Enhancing Healthcare Team Outcomes

The anesthesiologist typically oversees the patient's preoperative workup and monitoring while the surgeon performs colon resection. The nurse is essential to postoperative monitoring and bowel preparation both before and after surgery. Deep vein thrombosis prophylaxis is required, and the patient needs to learn how to use the incentive spirometer. During the post-operative phase, patients who are ambulating are typically consulted by physical therapy.

8.6.9.1. Evidence-based Outcomes

Elective colon resections now have excellent results, with patients typically staying in the hospital for around four days. Careful attention to detail helps minimize the risk of wound infections. Recent data suggests that laparoscopic colectomy is just as effective as open colectomy in preventing cancer recurrence. Additionally, clinical trials have shown that there is no increased risk of seeding at the port sites.

A Closer Look

Colonoscopy

Colonoscopy is an endoscopic procedure that involves passing a flexible tube through the anus and using a CCD or fiber optic camera to examine the large intestine and the distal portion of the small bowel. A visual diagnosis (e.g., ulceration, polyps) provides the chance to remove or biopsy lesions that may be indicative of colorectal cancer. Polyps as small as one millimeter or less can be removed with a colonoscopy. After polyps are removed, a microscope can be used to examine them and identify whether or not they are precancerous. It takes a polyp 15 years or less to become malignant.

The only distinction between sigmoidoscopy and colonoscopy is the parts of the colon that each can examine. An examination of the entire colon (length: 1200–1500 mm) is possible with a colonoscopy. Since the benefits of colonoscopy to cancer survival have been restricted to the detection of lesions in the distal portion of the colon, a sigmoidoscopy may be sufficient to examine the distal portion of the colon (roughly 600 mm).

A stool-based test, such as a fecal occult blood test (FOBT), fecal immunochemical test (FIT), multi-target stool DNA test (Cologuard), or blood-based test, SEPT9 DNA methylation test (Epi proColon), is frequently used in conjunction with a sigmoidoscopy as a screening procedure for a full colonoscopy. Of these screened patients, about 5% are recommended for a colonoscopy.

Virtual colonoscopy is another completely non-invasive medical test that is possible. It uses 2D and 3D imagery reconstructed from nuclear magnetic resonance (MR) or computed tomography (CT) scans. However, its diagnostic efficacy is still being investigated and is not yet standard. Additionally, therapeutic procedures like polyp/tumor removal, biopsy, and the visualization of lesions smaller than 5 millimeters are not possible with virtual colonoscopy. Even in cases where CT colonography identifies a growth or polyp, a conventional colonoscopy would still be necessary. Furthermore, a colonoscopy of the ileo-anal pouch is now referred to by surgeons as a "pouchoscopy."

Summary

- The colon of the large intestine is the last part of the digestive system. It has a segmented appearance due to a series of saccules called haustra. It extracts water and salt from solid wastes before they are eliminated from the body and is the site in which the fermentation of unabsorbed material by the gut microbiota occurs.
- In mammals, the large intestine consists of the cecum (including the appendix), colon (the longest part), rectum, and anal canal.
- Arterial supply to the colon comes from branches of the superior mesenteric artery (SMA) and inferior mesenteric artery (IMA). The flow between these two systems communicates via the marginal artery of the colon that runs parallel to the colon for its entire length.
- Lymphatic drainage from the ascending colon and proximal two-thirds of the transverse colon is to the ileocolic lymph nodes and the superior mesenteric lymph nodes, which drain into the cisterna chyli.
- One variation on the normal anatomy of the colon occurs when extra loops form, resulting in a colon that is up to five meters longer than normal. This condition, referred to as redundant colon, typically has no direct major health consequences, though rarely volvulus occurs, resulting in obstruction and requiring immediate medical attention.
- The large intestine, or large bowel, is the last part of the digestive system in vertebrate animals. Its function is to absorb water from the remaining indigestible food matter, and then to pass the useless waste material from the body. The large intestine consists of the cecum, colon, rectum, and anal canal.
- The appendix is a finger-like, blind-ended tube connected to the cecum, from which it develops in the embryo. The cecum is a pouch-like structure of the large intestine, located at the junction of the small and the large intestines.
- Common diseases of the appendix (in humans) are appendicitis and carcinoid tumors (appendiceal carcinoid). Appendix cancer accounts for about 1 in 200 of all gastrointestinal malignancies. In rare cases, adenomas are also present.
- The anal canal is the terminal part of the gastrointestinal tract that conveys material from the rectum to the anus. While it is typically around 2.5 to 4 cm in length, it is more complex than it seems.
- The large intestine absorbs water and any remaining absorbable nutrients from the food before sending the indigestible matter to the rectum. The colon absorbs vitamins that are synthesized by the colonic bacteria, such as thiamine, riboflavin, and vitamin K (especially important as the daily ingestion of vitamin K is not normally enough to maintain adequate blood coagulation). It also compacts feces and stores fecal matter in the rectum until it can be discharged via the anus in defecation.
- Colon resection is the removal of either a portion of or the entire colon. Arteries, veins, and lymphatic drainage are located in the mesocolon, which during the oncological surgical resections of total mesorectal excision and complete mesocolic excision gets removed in its entirety corresponding to the part of the colon to be removed.

References

1. Arakawa, T., Hwang, S. E., Kim, J. H., Wilting, J., Rodríguez-Vázquez, J. F., Murakami, G., Hwang, H. P., & Cho, B. H. (2016). Fetal growth of the anal sinus and sphincters, especially in relation to anal anomalies. *International Journal of Colorectal Disease, 31*(3), 493–502.
2. Atkins, P. (2011). Food for Thought: Enzyme Action. In *Reactions*. Oxford University Press. http://dx.doi.org/10.1093/oso/9780199695126.003.0034.
3. Aykan, N. F. (2015). Red meat and colorectal cancer. *Oncology Reviews, 9*(1), 288. doi:10.4081/oncol.2015.288.
4. Barrett, K. E., Barman, S. M., Yuan, J. X., & Brooks, H. (2019). *Ganong's Review of Medical Physiology* (26th ed.). New York, McGraw Hill / Medical. ISBN 9781260122404.
5. Carethers, J. M. (2018). Risk factors for colon location of cancer. *Translational Gastroenterology and Hepatology, 3*, 76. doi:10.21037/tgh.2018.09.15.
6. Collier, J. (2020). Investigation and management of jaundice. In J. Satsangi (Ed.), *Oxford Textbook of Medicine* (pp. 3049–3057). Oxford University Press. http://dx.doi.org/10.1093/med/9780198746690.003.0317.
7. Di Saverio, S., Birindelli, A., Kelly, M. D., Catena, F., Weber, D. G., Sartelli, M., & Andersson, R. (2016). WSES Jerusalem guidelines for diagnosis and treatment of acute appendicitis. *World Journal of Emergency Surgery, 11*, 34. https://www.ncbi.nlm.nih.gov/pmc/articles/PMC4949879/pdf/13017_2016_Article_90.pdf (accessed on 23 May 2024).
8. Durot, C., Dohan, A., Boudiaf, M., Servois, V., Soyer, P., & Hoeffel, C. (2017). Cancer of the Anal Canal: Diagnosis, Staging and Follow-Up with MRI. *Korean Journal of Radiology, 18*(6), 946–956.
9. Farne, H., Norris-Cervetto, E., & Warbrick-Smith, J. (2015). Nausea and vomiting. In *Oxford Cases in Medicine and Surgery*. Oxford University Press. http://dx.doi.org/10.1093/oso/9780198716228.003.0019.
10. Faucheron, J. L. (2008). [Anal incontinence]. *Presse Médicale, 37*(10), 1447–1462.
11. Guttenplan, M. (2017). The Evaluation and Office Management of Hemorrhoids for the Gastroenterologist. *Current Gastroenterology Reports, 19*(7), 30.
12. Kumar, L., & Emmanuel, A. (2017). Internal anal sphincter: Clinical perspective. *The Surgeon, 15*(4), 211–226.
13. Kumar, V., Abbas, A. K., Fausto, N., & Mitchell, R. N. (2007). Chapter 15. In *Robbins' Basic Pathology* (8th ed., pp. 579–586). Philadelphia, PA: Elsevier Saunders.
14. Kunzmann, A. T., Coleman, H. G., Huang, W. Y., Kitahara, C. M., Cantwell, M. M., & Berndt, S. I. (2015). Dietary fiber intake and risk of colorectal cancer and incident and recurrent adenoma in the Prostate, Lung, Colorectal, and Ovarian Cancer Screening Trial. *American Journal of Clinical Nutrition, 102*(4), 881–890. doi:10.3945/ajcn.115.113282.
15. Li, X., Zhang, J., Sang, L., Zhang, W., Chu, Z., Li, X., & Liu, Y. (2010). Laparoscopic versus conventional appendectomy: A meta-analysis of randomized controlled trials. *BMC Gastroenterology, 10*(129), 1–8. http://bmcgastroenterol.biomedcentral.com/articles/10.1186/1471-230X-10-129 (accessed on 23 May 2024).

16. Liao, Y. H., Hsia, W. T., Yung-Fang, C., & Tsai, P. P. (2016). Severe Portal Hypertension-Induced Anorectal Varices Bleeding Treated via a Transjugular Intrahepatic Portosystemic Shunt. *American Journal of Gastroenterology, 111*(1), 27.

17. Lohsiriwat, V. (2015). Treatment of hemorrhoids: A coloproctologist's view. *World Journal of Gastroenterology, 21*(31), 9245–9252.

18. Nakashima, J., & Zulfiqar, H. (2023). Embryology, Rectum and Anal Canal. In *StatPearls* [Internet]. StatPearls Publishing. Retrieved from: https://www.ncbi.nlm.nih.gov/books/NBK459277/ (accessed on 23 May 2024).

19. Palazon, P., Julia, V., Saura, L., de Haro, I., Bejarano, M., Rovira, C., & Tarrado, X. (2017). Anal canal duplication and triplication: a rare entity with different presentations. *Pediatric Surgery International, 33*(5), 609–617.

20. Ralston, S. H., Penman, I. D., Strachan, M. W., & Hobson, R. P. (2018). *Davidson's Principles and Practice of Medicine* (23rd ed.). Elsevier. ISBN 978-0-7020-7028-0.

21. Rossi, M., Jahanzaib Anwar, M., Usman, A., Keshavarzian, A., & Bishehsari, F. (2018). Colorectal cancer and alcohol consumption-populations to molecules. *Cancers (Basel), 10*(2). doi:10.3390/cancers10020038.

22. Salminen, P., Paajanen, H., Rautio, T., Nordström, P., Aarnio, M., Rantanen, T., & Grönroos, J. M. (2015). Antibiotic therapy vs. appendectomy for treatment of uncomplicated acute appendicitis: The APPAC randomized clinical trial. *JAMA, 313*(23), 2340–2348. Retrieved from: https://www.ncbi.nlm.nih.gov/pubmed/26080338 (accessed on 23 May 2024).

23. Sanders, N. L., Bollinger, R. R., Lee, R., Thomas, S., & Parker, W. (2013). Appendectomy and Clostridium difficile colitis: Relationships revealed by clinical observations and immunology. *World Journal of Gastroenterology, 19*(34), 5607–5614. https://www.ncbi.nlm.nih.gov/pmc/articles/PMC3769896/pdf/WJG-19-5607.pdf (accessed on 23 May 2024).

24. Skibber, J., Rodriguez-Bigas, M. A., & Gordon, P. H. (2004). Surgical considerations in anal cancer. *Surgical Oncology Clinics of North America, 13*(2), 321–338.

25. Standring, S. (Ed.). (2016). *Gray's Anatomy: The Anatomical Basis of Clinical Practice* (41st ed.). Philadelphia. ISBN 9780702052309.

26. Stewart, A. M., Cook, M. S., Dyer, K. Y., & Alperin, M. (2018). Structure-function relationship of the human external anal sphincter. *International Urogynecology Journal, 29*(5), 673–678.

27. Takeda, M., Miyahara, K., Akazawa, C., Lane, G. J., & Yamataka, A. (2017). Sensory innervation of the anal canal and anorectal line in Hirschsprung's disease: Histological evidence from mouse models. *Pediatric Surgery International, 33*(8), 883–886.

28. Varadhan, K. K., Neal, K. R., & Lobo, D. N. (2012). Safety and efficacy of antibiotics compared with appendectomy for treatment of uncomplicated acute appendicitis: Meta-analysis of randomised controlled trials. *BMJ, 344*, e2156. http://www.bmj.com/content/344/bmj.e2156 (accessed on 23 May 2024).

29. Wu, S. C., Chen, W. T. L., Muo, C. H., Ke, T. W., Fang, C. W., & Sung, F. C. (2015). Association between appendectomy and subsequent colorectal cancer development: An Asian population study. *PloS One, 10*(2), e0118411. https://www.ncbi.nlm.nih.gov/pmc/articles/PMC4339380/ (accessed on 23 May 2024).

30. Wu, W., Yang, J., Li, D., Huang, Q., Zhao, F., Feng, X., & others. (2021). Competitive Risk Analysis of Prognosis in Patients with Cecum Cancer: A Population-Based Study. *Cancer Control, 28*, 1073274821989316. doi:10.1177/1073274821989316.

31. Young, B., O'Dowd, G., & Woodford, P. (2013). *Wheater's Functional Histology: A Text and Color Atlas* (6th ed.). Philadelphia: Elsevier. ISBN 9780702047473.

Chapter

THE INTESTINAL MICROBIOME

9

Contents

Introduction

Microorganisms, also known as microbes, are small living organisms such as bacteria, viruses, fungi, and others. These bacteria, which number in the trillions, are mostly found on your skin and in your intestines. The majority of the microorganisms in your digestive system are known as the gut microbiome, and they are located in a "pocket" of your large intestine called the cecum. Although your body contains a wide variety of microbes, bacteria have received the most research. Your body actually contains more bacterial than human cells. Your body contains only 30 trillion human cells, compared to about 40 trillion bacterial cells. It implies that you are not so much human as bacteria. Furthermore, the human gut microbiome contains up to 1,000 different species of bacteria, each of which has a unique function in your body. Some of them may lead to illness, but the majority are vital to your well-being. These microorganisms could weigh up to 2.5 pounds (1–2 kg) in total, which is about the same as your brain. When combined, they act as an additional organ in your body and are vital to your overall well-being.

Orientation and Directional Terms

Term	Definition	Illustration
Bacteria	Bacteria are microscopic living organisms that have only one cell. Most bacteria aren't harmful, but certain types can make you sick.	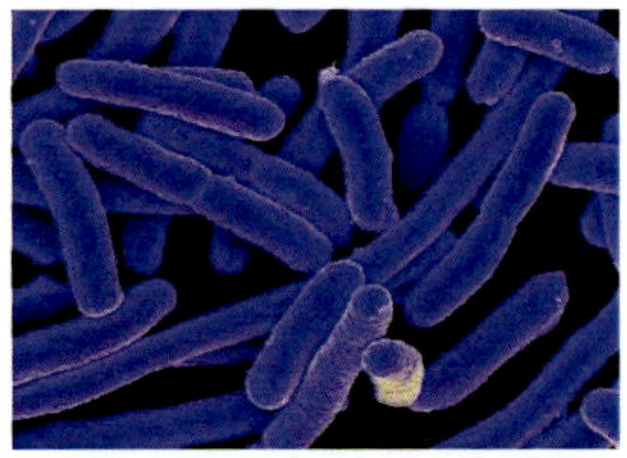
Viruses	A virus is a submicroscopic infectious agent that replicates only inside the living cells of an organism.	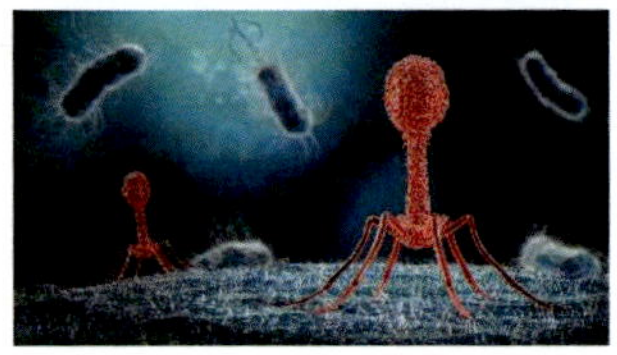
Fungi	Fungi include symbionts of plants, animals, or other fungi and also parasites. They may become noticeable when fruiting, either as mushrooms or as molds.	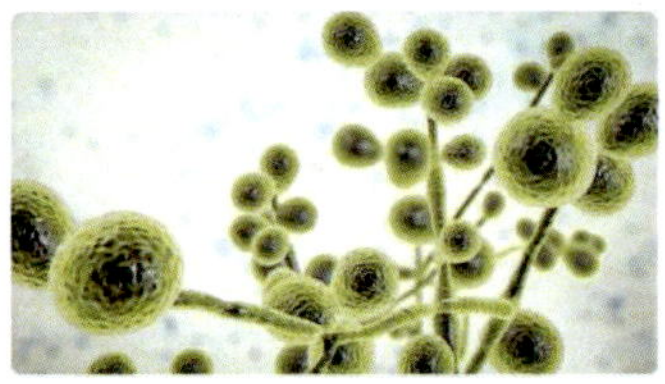
Bacteroidetes	Bacteroidetes are prevalent in soil ecosystems and are associated with various eukaryotic hosts, including plants, animals, and humans.	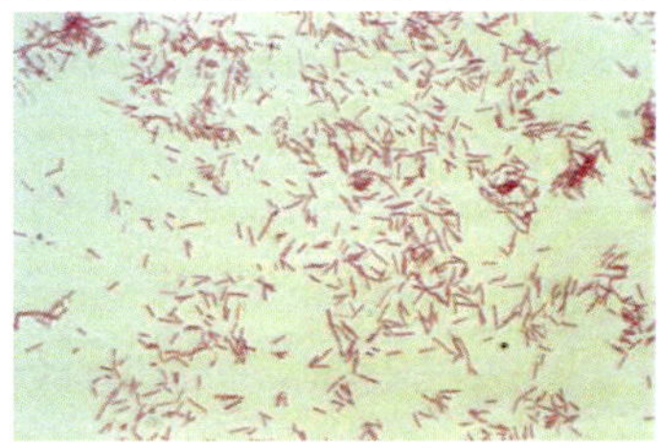
Firmicutes	The Firmicutes are a phylum of bacteria, most of which have Gram-positive cell wall structures and some of which can form endospores.	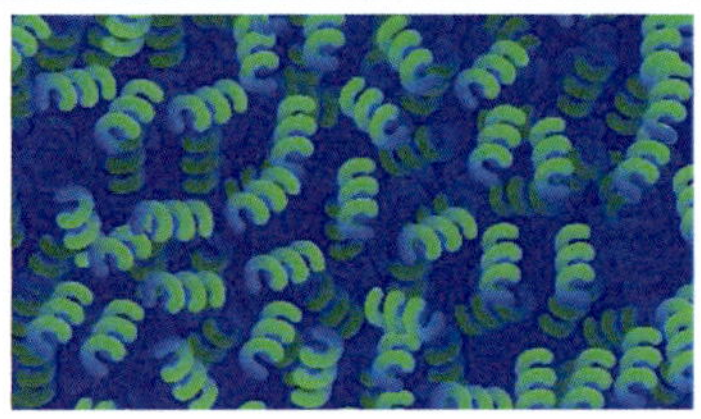

9.1. Classification and Composition of the Microbiome

Strict anaerobes make up the majority of the gut microbiota; they can outnumber facultative anaerobes—organisms with the capacity to grow both aerobically and anaerobically—by a factor of up to 100. Even though over 50 different bacterial phyla have been found in the human gut to date, only two phyla—the Firmicutes and the Bacteroidetes—dominate the microbiota. Although estimates of the number of bacterial species found in the human gut vary greatly amongst research, it is generally agreed upon that over a thousand species-level phylotypes of microbes are present in each individual.

9.1.1. Classifications

Throughout the digestive tract, the gut microbiota's microbial makeup varies. There are usually only a few types of bacteria found in the stomach and small intestine. In contrast, with between 10^{10} and 10^{11} cells per gram of intestinal content, the colon has the highest microbial density of any human-associated microbial community that has been studied to date. There are between 300 and 1000 distinct species of bacteria among them. Nonetheless, roughly 30 to 40 species account for 99% of the total bacteria. Owing to their profusion in the intestine, bacteria can account for as much as 60% of the dry mass of excrement. The gut flora also includes viruses, protists, fungi, and archaea, although little is known about their functions. While aerobic bacteria can reach high densities in the cecum, anaerobes make up over 99% of the bacteria in the gut. The total number of genes in these gut flora is thought to be approximately 100 times greater than that of the human genome. Since many species in the gut cannot be cultured, research on them outside of their hosts has not been conducted. Although most people share a limited number of core microbial species, microbe populations can differ greatly from one another. The microbial populations of an individual remain relatively constant over time, with some alterations brought about by dietary, lifestyle, and age changes. The goal of the Human Microbiome Project is to provide a more thorough description of the microbiota found in the human gut and other body parts.

In the human gut, Bacillota (*Firmicutes*), Bacteroidota, *Actinomycetota*, and Pseudomonadota are the four predominant bacterial phyla. The genera *Bacteroides*, *Clostridium*, *Faecalibacterium*, *Eubacterium*, *Ruminococcus*, *Peptococcus*, *Peptostreptococcus*, and *Bifidobacterium* are home to the majority of bacteria. To a lesser degree, other genera like Escherichia and Lactobacillus are present. About 30% of all bacteria in the gut are species from the genus Bacteroides alone, indicating that this genus is particularly significant for the host's proper functioning.

Numerous fungal genera, including *Candida*, *Saccharomyces*, *Aspergillus*, *Penicillium*, *Rhodotorula*, *Trametes*, *Pleospora*, *Sclerotinia*, *Bullera*, and *Galactomyces*, have been found in the gastrointestinal tract. People with inflammatory bowel disease are more likely to have *Rhodotorula*, whereas people with cirrhosis and chronic hepatitis B are more likely to have *Candida*. Another sizable class of gut flora that plays a significant role in the metabolism of fermentation-related bacterial products is called Archaea. Research from 2018 suggested the creation of a human microbiota biobank repository. Industrialization is linked to changes in the microbiota, and the loss of diversity may result in the extinction of some species.

Enterotype: An enterotype is a category of living things that is determined by the bacteriological ecosystem within the gut microbiome of humans, rather than by factors such as body weight, age, gender, or nationality. Evidence suggests that enterotype is influenced by long-term diet. Though their usefulness has been questioned, three human enterotypes have been proposed.

9.1.2. Composition and Development

The human gut is colonized by microbes from birth. A baby's intestines are thought to be sterile or to have very few bacteria when it is born, but the GIT rapidly becomes colonized during and after delivery. A newborn is exposed to the microbiota of the mother's vagina as they go through the birth canal. An infant's intestinal microbiota develops as a result of this process, and it resembles the mother's vaginal microbiota in certain ways. When compared to infants delivered vaginally, infants delivered via cesarean section had fewer microorganisms in their stomachs at one month of age; however, these differences were no longer apparent at six months of age. The gut microbiota's composition is comparatively simple and exhibits significant interindividual variation during the first year of life. It is thought that the adult gut microbiota's composition is largely shaped by the initial gut colonization. When a baby transitions from being breastfed or formula-fed to being weaned and starting solid food, their gut microbiota experiences a series of changes. Even though gut microbiomes of mothers and their children are comparatively similar, microbial succession in the GIT is also impacted by a variety of host-related internal and external factors. In addition to the makeup of the mother microbiota, external factors include the food type consumed, feeding habits, and the microbial load of the immediate environment. Additionally, stresses related to diet and temperature can affect how bacteria proliferate. Intestinal pH, microbial interactions, environmental temperature, physiological factors like peristalsis, bile acids, host secretions and immune responses, drug therapy, and bacterial mucosal receptors are just a few examples of internal factors.

Despite the many factors that can impact the makeup of the intestinal microbiota, it is interesting to note that the microbial community in the human gut remains stable at the phylum level. The Bacteroidetes and Firmicutes are consistently found in all individuals, though their proportions may differ. However, when looking at specific bacterial species, there is much more variability between individuals than at the phylum level. This variation is likely due to the functional redundancy within the gut microbiota. The host's selective pressure helps maintain important functions within the gastrointestinal tract, which can be carried out by a variety of bacterial species within the major phyla. Functional redundancy allows for different compositions of the microbiota without compromising overall function within an individual.

The GIT's length has an uneven distribution of bacterial cells. A gram of stomach and duodenal contents can contain anywhere from 10 to 10^3 bacteria, while a gram of small intestine contents can contain between 10^4 and 10^7 bacteria, and a gram of large intestine contents can contain between 10^{11} and 10^{12} bacteria. Furthermore, the microbial community's composition differs in each of these locations, with the colon and small intestine having higher concentrations of particular bacterial phyla. Upon analyzing biopsy samples from both gut regions in healthy individuals, it was discovered that specific members of the Firmicutes phyla were more abundant in the small intestine, while members of the Bacteroidetes phylum were more prevalent in the colon.

When intestines were examined in transverse sections, there were numerous differences in the microbiota's composition in addition to microbial heterogeneity throughout the length of the GIT. There were multiple microenvironments located throughout the intestine, and the microbiota in the lumen of the intestine had a very different makeup from the microbiota that was attached to the epithelium and in close proximity. For instance, the composition of the feces was representative of the luminal community because it contained the genera *Bacteroides*, *Bifidobacterium*, *Streptococcus*, *Enterococcus*, *Clostridium*, *Lactobacillus*, and *Ruminococcus*; in contrast, the mucus layer and epithelial crypts of the small intestine only contained the genera *Clostridium*, *Lactobacillus*, and *Enterococcus*.

9.2. Functions of the Intestinal Microbiome

Three main functions of gut flora were initially identified when research on the subject started in 1995: direct defense against pathogens, strengthening host defense by promoting the development and maintenance of the intestinal epithelium and producing antibodies there, and breaking down otherwise indigestible food components. Later research revealed its function in immune system development and more research concentrated on its function in the gut-brain axis.

9.2.1. Direct Inhibition of Pathogens

By completely colonizing the area, utilizing all available nutrients, and secreting substances known as cytokines that either kill or inhibit undesirable organisms that would compete with it for nutrients, the gut flora community directly contributes to the defense against pathogens. Different cytokines are produced by different strains of gut bacteria. Our immune system produces chemicals called cytokines to start the inflammatory response in response to infections. When the gut flora is disturbed, competing organisms that would otherwise be kept in check, such as *Clostridium difficile*, can establish themselves.

9.2.2. Development of Enteric Protection and Immune System

Within one to two years of birth, humans develop a gut flora that is comparable to that of an adult. The intestinal lining, including the intestinal epithelium and the intestinal mucosal barrier it secretes, develops in tandem with the establishment of the gut flora. This results in the intestinal lining being somewhat tolerant of commensalistic microorganisms and even supportive of them, while also acting as a barrier against pathogenic ones. In particular, the mucosa-producing goblet cells multiply and the mucosa layer thickens, creating an outer mucosal layer that is accessible to and hospitable for microorganisms, as well as an inner layer that is impenetrable even by these organisms. Furthermore, during the period that the gut flora is developing and establishing, the development of gut-associated lymphoid tissue (GALT), which is a component of the intestinal epithelium and which recognizes and responds to pathogens, appears and develops. The GALT that forms is resistant to other microbes but tolerant to species of the gut flora. Additionally, GALT typically develops tolerance to food that the baby is exposed to, food-derived digestive products, and metabolites—molecules formed by metabolism—produced by the gut flora (Figure 9.1).

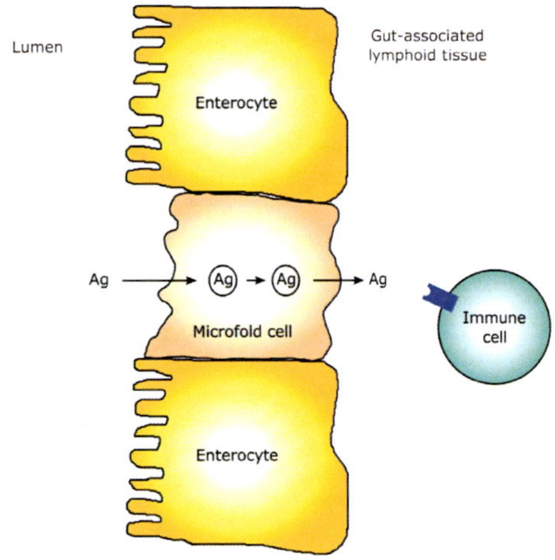

Figure 9.1. *Microfold cells transfer antigens (Ag) from the lumen of the gut to gut-associated lymphoid tissue (GALT) via transcytosis and present them to different innate and adaptive immune cells.*

Source: By 2n00b – Own work, CC BY-SA 4.0, https://commons.wikimedia.org/w/index.php?curid=45697731.

Human immune system cytokines can both stimulate the immune system to produce inflammation in self-defense and suppress the immune response to preserve homeostasis and promote healing following insult or injury. It has been demonstrated that certain bacterial species found in the gut flora can selectively stimulate the immune system to produce cytokines. For instance, certain *Clostridium* species and *Bacteroides fragilis* appear to stimulate an anti-inflammatory response, while certain segmented filamentous bacteria stimulate the production of inflammatory cytokines. Additionally, the immune system's ability to produce antibodies can be regulated by gut flora. This regulation has the effect of making B cells convert to IgA. Generally, B cells require T helper cell activation to trigger class switching; on the other hand, gut flora triggers intestinal epithelial cells to initiate NF-kB signaling, which in turn triggers the release of additional signaling molecules. By interacting with B cells, these signaling molecules cause IgA class switching. In mucosal environments such as the gut, IgA is a crucial class of antibody. IgA has been demonstrated to aid in gut community diversification and to aid in the removal of bacteria that trigger inflammatory reactions. In the end, IgA keeps the environment between the host and gut bacteria healthy. These antibodies and cytokines can affect tissues other than the stomach, such as the lungs.

The gut bacteria's capacity to generate metabolites that can impact immune system cells can also change the immune system. For instance, certain gut bacteria can ferment food to produce short-chain fatty acids (SCFA). SCFAs cause the production of innate immune cells such as neutrophils, basophils, and eosinophils to increase quickly. These cells work to stop the spread of infection as a component of the innate immune system.

9.2.3. Metabolism

Some types of gut flora contain enzymes that human cells lack for breaking down certain polysaccharides, which means that without gut flora, the human body would not be able to utilize some of the undigested carbohydrates it consumes. Certain starches, fiber, oligosaccharides, and sugars that the body was unable to break down and absorb—such as lactose in the case of lactose intolerance and sugar alcohols—as well as mucus secreted by the gut and proteins are examples of carbohydrates that humans cannot digest without the assistance of bacteria. Saccharolytic fermentation is a type of fermentation that bacteria use to convert carbohydrates into short-chain fatty acids. Among the products are butyric acid, propionic acid, and acetic acid. Host cells can utilize these substances as a major source of nutrition and energy. Fermentation also yields organic acids like lactic acid and gases that are involved in signaling and can cause flatulence. Muscle uses acetic acid, liver produces more ATP with the help of propionic acid, and gut cells get their energy from butyric acid.

Additionally, gut flora produces vitamins like biotin and folate and aid in the absorption of dietary minerals like calcium, iron, and magnesium. *Methanobrevibacter smithii* is the most prevalent methane-producing archaeal species in the human gastrointestinal microbiota. It is distinct from other bacteria species because it belongs to the domain *Archaea*. Additionally, the gut microbiota provides a source of vitamins K and B_{12}, which the body either cannot produce or only produces in small amounts.

9.2.3.1. Cellulose Degradation

Ruminococcus and other cellulose-degrading bacteria are found in great apes, prehistoric human societies, hunter-gatherer communities, and even contemporary rural populations. They are uncommon in industrialized societies, though. Genes that can break down particular plant fibers, like those found in maize, rice, and wheat, have been acquired by strains linked to humans. Numerous nonhuman primates consume insects, which contain chitin, a polymer that can be broken down by bacterial strains discovered in primates. The change to more Western lifestyles is probably what caused these bacteria in the human gut to decline.

9.2.3.2. Pharmacomicrobiomics

Metagenomes of humans (i.e., the genetic makeup of each person and every microbe that lives on or inside their body) differs greatly from person to person. Since there are many times more microbial cells in the human body than there are *Homo sapiens* cells (tens of trillions), there is a great deal of potential for interactions between drugs and a person's microbiome. These interactions could include the following: drugs changing the microbiome's composition; microbial drug metabolism changing the pharmacokinetic profile of a drug; and microbial drug metabolism influencing the toxicity and clinical efficacy of a drug. In addition to carbohydrates, medications, phytochemicals, and food poisons are among the other xenobiotics that the gut microbiota can metabolize. It has been demonstrated that the gut microbiota metabolizes over thirty medications. Sometimes a drug's microbial metabolism renders it inactive.

9.2.3.3. Contribution to Drug Metabolism

The gut microbiota is a diverse community with a wide range of genes capable of modifying drugs, particularly those taken orally. It can impact drug metabolism through both direct and indirect mechanisms. Directly, microbial enzymes can alter the chemical structure of drugs. Indirectly, microbial metabolites can affect the expression of host enzymes like cytochrome P450. The effects of the gut microbiota on drug pharmacokinetics and bioavailability have been studied for several decades. These effects can vary, from activating inactive drugs like lovastatin to inactivating active drugs like digoxin, or even causing drug toxicity as seen with irinotecan. The influence of the gut microbiota on the pharmacokinetics of many drugs has been extensively researched since then.

The human gut microbiota is essential for regulating how medications are absorbed by the body. Direct drug metabolism is possible through the synthesis and release of several enzymes by the gut microbiota, including the microbial biotransformation of L-dopa by the enzymes decarboxylase and dehydroxylase. Conversely, by modifying the host's drug metabolism, gut microbiota may also change how the medications are metabolized. Microbial metabolites or altered host metabolites, which alter host metabolizing enzyme expression, can mediate this mechanism.

Numerous studies have shown that the gut microbiota is involved in the metabolism of more than 50 medications. For instance, the human gut microbiota partially activates the lactone prodrug lovastatin, a cholesterol-lowering medication, by producing active acid hydroxylated metabolites. Conversely, digoxin (a drug used to treat congestive heart failure) is inactivated by a member of the gut microbiota (i.e., *Eggerthella lanta*). Digoxin induces upregulation of a cytochrome-encoding operon in *Eggerthella lanta*, which is linked to digoxin-inactivation. Additionally, the toxicity and effectiveness of chemotherapeutic drugs like irinotecan can be affected by gut microbiota. The β-glucuronidase enzymes, which are encoded by the microbiome, are responsible for this effect as they enable the recovery of the irinotecan's active form that causes gastrointestinal toxicity.

9.2.3.4. Secondary Metabolites

The gut's microbial community possesses a vast biochemical capacity to generate unique secondary metabolites, which are occasionally generated through the metabolic conversion of dietary items like fibers and endogenous biological substances like bile acids or indole. Microbial metabolites, particularly secondary bile acids (BAs) and SCFAs are significant for human health and disease states. Secondary bile acids (BAs) are among the most significant bacterial metabolites generated by the gut microbiota. Lithocholic acid (LCA) and deoxycholic acid (DCA), two secondary BAs, are synthesized when bacteria biotransform primary bile acids like cholic acid (CA) and chenodeoxycholic acid (CDCA) into these metabolites. Hepatocytes produce primary bile acids, which are hydrophobic substances kept in the gall bladder. The gut microbiota then transforms these metabolites into secondary metabolites that are more hydrophobic. Bile salt hydrolases (BSH) are responsible for the initial stage of the metabolism of secondary bile acids and are conserved across phyla of gut microbiota, including *Bacteroides*, *Firmicutes*, and *Actinobacteria*. It has been shown that secondary BAs like DCA and LCA prevent *Clostridium difficile* from germination and growth.

9.2.3.5. Dysbiosis

The preservation of intestinal homeostasis depends on the gut microbiota. Dysbiosis, or an unbalanced natural microbiota, is linked to the development of intestinal cancer. Increased intestinal carcinogenesis is linked to changes in the microbial community caused by the secondary bile acid deoxycholic acid. Due to dysbiosis, the colon is exposed to more secondary bile acids, which can damage DNA and result in mutations that can cause cancer in colon cells. The colon's high bacterial density (roughly 10^{12} per milliliter) that are susceptible to dysbiosis in contrast to the small intestine's comparatively low density (roughly 10^{2} per milliliter) could explain why the colon has a cancer incidence that is more than ten times higher than that of the small intestine.

9.2.4. Gut–brain Axis

The biochemical communication between the central nervous system and the gastrointestinal tract is known as the "gut-brain axis." The term "microbiome-brain axis" is occasionally used to describe paradigms that explicitly include the gut flora. However, that term has been expanded to include the role of the gut flora in the interplay. The central nervous system, neuroendocrine and neuroimmune systems, including the hypothalamic-pituitary-adrenal (HPA) axis, the sympathetic and parasympathetic arms of the autonomic nervous system, which include the enteric nervous system, the vagus nerve, and the gut microbiota, are all included in the broad definition of the gut-brain axis.

9.3. Dysbiosis of the Intestinal Microbiome

A disruption to the microbiome leading to an imbalance in the microbiota, modifications to their functional makeup and metabolic activities, or a change in their local distribution are the hallmarks of dysbiosis, also known as dysbacteriosis. For instance, a portion of the human microbiota, such as the flora on the skin, in the gut, or in the vagina, can go awry, with typically dominant species being underrepresented and typically outcompeted or contained species proliferating to fill the space. The plant rhizosphere is colonized by a variety of microbes, much like the human gut microbiome, and dysbiosis in the rhizosphere can have a detrimental effect on plant health. Most frequently, dysbiosis is described as a disease of the gastrointestinal system or the rhizosphere of plants.

The majority of microbial colonies that are found on or in the body are helpful or benign. These suitably sized microbial colonies perform many beneficial and essential tasks, including assisting with digestion. They also aid in preventing harmful bacteria from entering the body. These advantageous microbial communities fight for resources and available space. But when this equilibrium is upset, these colonies show a diminished capacity to restrain one another's expansion. This can then result in the overgrowth of one or more of the upset colonies, which can further harm some of the other smaller but helpful ones in a vicious cycle. More overgrowth problems arise as a result of the imbalance becoming more apparent as more beneficial colonies sustain damage that reduces their ability to control the growth of the overgrowing colonies. If this is allowed to continue unchecked for an extended period of time, a persistent and widespread imbalance between colonies will develop, which will ultimately reduce the overall beneficial nature of these colonies.

9.3.1. Function, Composition, and the Dysbiosis of the Gut Microbiota

Numerous microbial communities, including viruses, fungi, bacteria, and archaea, can be found in the GI tract. With about 10^3 bacteria per milliliter of aspirate in the upper gut (stomach, duodenum, and jejunum), the microbe population is more sparse there than in the lower gut (ileum and proximal colon), where there are roughly 10^7–10^{12} bacteria per milliliter of aspirate.

In addition to helping with food digestion, the gut microbiota also produce vital vitamins, synthesize metabolites, inhibit the growth of pathogenic bacteria, regulate the gut-immune system, metabolize drugs, aid in detoxification, and maintain gastrointestinal physiological homeostasis (Fig. 9.2). Therefore, it is crucial for human health to maintain a healthy proportion of beneficial microbes, also known as eubiosis (Figure 9.2).

The term dysbiosis refers to an imbalance of gut microbes that can include colonic bacteria translocation, an increase in the fraction of small intestine bacteria, and a change in the ratio of beneficial to pathogenic microbes. Fundamentally, a variety of factors, such as diet, the host environment, host immunological response, microbial metabolites, host physiology, and interactions between microbes, contribute to the development of diseased states.

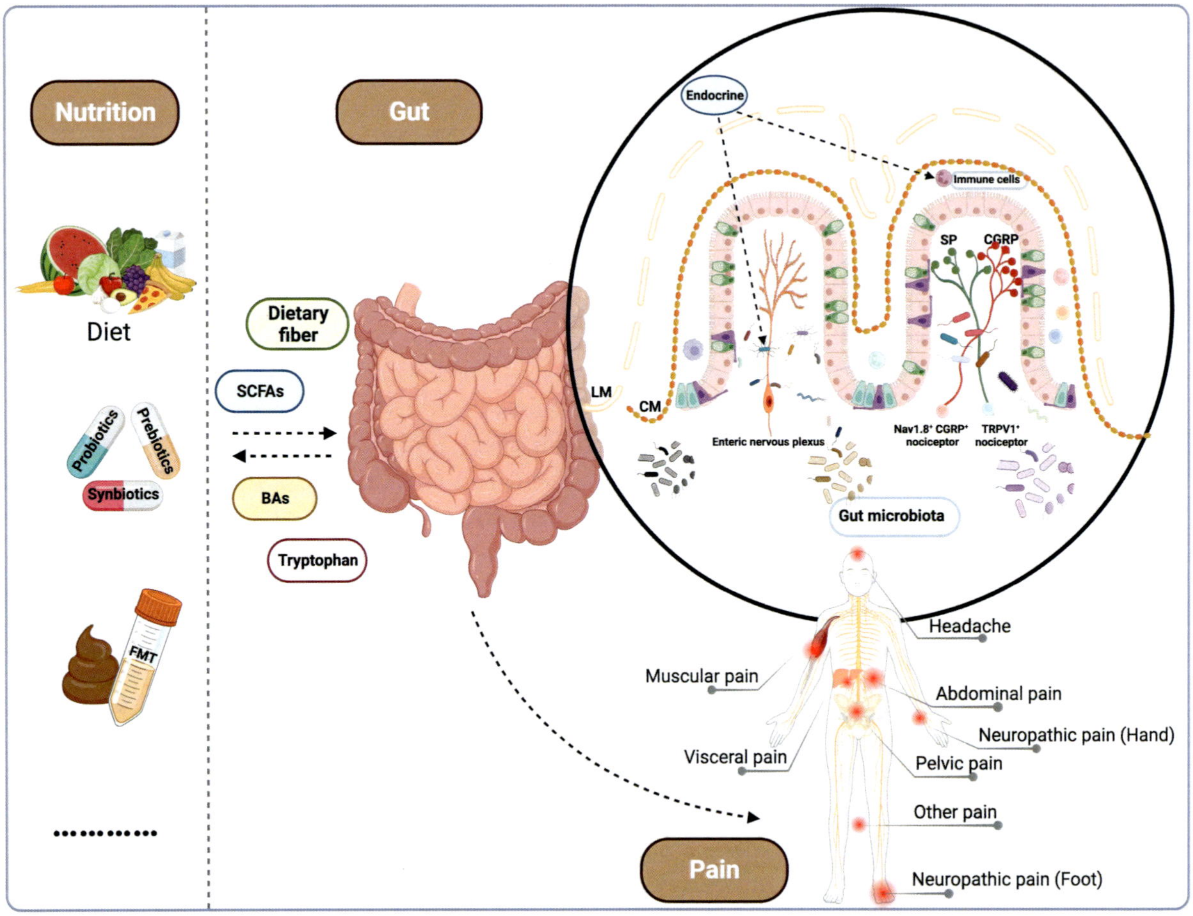

Figure 9.2. *Functions of gut microbiota.*

Source: Lu G, Zhang S, Wang R, Zhang Z, Wang W, Wen Q, Zhang F, Li P. Global trends in research of pain–gut-microbiota relationship and how nutrition can modulate this link. Nutrients. 2023; 15(17):3704. https://doi.org/10.3390/nu15173704.

Throughout the various GI tract microenvironments, the composition and relative abundance of the gut microbiota vary, and more than 50 bacterial phyla have been found in the human GI tract to date. Bacteroidetes and Firmicutes are the two phyla that are most commonly found in the gut of a healthy host, with much smaller amounts of *Proteobacteria*, *Verrucomicrobia*, Actinobacteria, Fusobacteria, and *Cyanobacteria*. Different microbial communities typically colonize the different sections of the GI tract; in the small intestine, Gram-positive bacteria are more common than Gram-negative bacteria. Depending on the nutrients available, about 95% of the bacteria living in the colon are strict anaerobes. Both internal and external factors play a major role in determining small intestinal bacterial overgrowth (SIBO). The production of mucin, gut antibacterial peptides, peristaltic movement, normal gut defense mechanisms, gastric acid and bile acid (BA) secretion, and prevention of bacterial retrograde translocation from the lower gut to the upper gut via the ileocecal valve are the most prominent intrinsic factors preventing this overgrowth of bacteria. Extrinsic factors encompass dietary habits and nutrient intake, infections caused by bacteria and viruses, drugs that modify motility (prokinetics), and medications that modify the gut microbiota, such as antibiotics, proton pump inhibitors, H2 blockers, and prebiotics and probiotics. Dysbiosis may result from commensal and pathogenic gut microbiota colonizing disproportionately if any one of the extrinsic factors causes imbalance to offset the numerous protective mechanisms put in place. The onset of SIBO, which is defined as total bacterial overgrowth equal to or greater than 10^5 CFU per mL of upper gut (e.g., jejunal) aspirate culture, is one example of dysbiosis. However, the diagnosis of SIBO now includes the overgrowth of bacteria equal to or greater than 10^3 CFU/mL of upper gut aspirate. One study found that *Streptococcus species* (spp.), *Escherichia coli*, and jejunal aspirate cultures. *Staphylococcus* species, *Pseudomonas aeruginosa*, etc. *Enterococcus faecium*, *Klebsiella pneumoniae*, *Acinetobacter baumannii*, *Acinetobacter lwoffii*, and *Enterococcus faecalis* were primarily detected in SIBO patients with impaired GI motility.

9.3.2. Gut Microbiota Affect Host Physiology

Mainly through preserving gut homeostasis, the gut microbiota offers vital health benefits to its host. Researchers are currently examining the components of a healthy gut microbiome as well as the molecular processes and signaling pathways that permit communication between the host and gut microorganisms. Numerous investigations have demonstrated the capacity of pathogens to compromise the function of the epithelial barrier. On the other hand, it has been discovered that commensal gut microbiota function as gatekeepers to safeguard the integrity of epithelial cells against pathogen-induced disease and penetration.

Micronutrient synthesis, including the production of vitamin K and folate, is another advantageous consequence of commensal gut microbiota. Short-chain fatty acids (SCFAs), which are produced when unabsorbed carbohydrates are fermented by colonic bacteria, can then be absorbed through the colonic mucosa and utilized as an extra energy source. Above all, commensal gut microbiota are necessary to stop pathogenic bacteria from colonizing and migrating across the intestinal epithelial barrier.

In afflicted hosts, SIBO has been linked to a number of problems, such as the death of microvilli and an increased epithelial inflammatory response, which frequently impairs absorption. Aerobes are frequently the bacteria that cause SIBO to have negative effects; however, facultative anaerobes predominate in the small intestine of a healthy gut. Patients with SIBO experience malabsorption of fat and a deficiency in fat-soluble vitamins D, E, A, and K as a result of this microbial shift. Frequent signs of SIBO include bloating, gas, distension, and discomfort in the abdomen. These symptoms are most likely brought on by bacteria colonizing the small intestine and fermenting carbohydrates in an uncontrolled manner, producing hydrogen, carbon dioxide, and methane.

9.3.3. Potential Causes of Dysbiosis

Dysbiosis can result from any disturbance of the microbiota within the body. An imbalance of bacteria in the gastrointestinal tract results in dysbiosis in the gut. The gut's dysbiosis has numerous causes. Among the causes are a few, though not all of them are:

- dietary changes
- antibiotics have an impact on gut flora
- physical and psychological stress (depresses immunity)
- application of hormone therapy, radiation, chemotherapy, antiviral

medications, and radioactive isotopes
- intestinal helminths (human parasites) are present
- uncontrolled use of enemas for rectal cleaning
- intestinal inflammatory process
- chronic and acute infections (HIV, Hepatitis C & B, herpes, etc.)

9.3.3.1. Gut/intestinal Dysbiosis

The most varied bacteria in the human body are found in the intestines of the human gut, and they are essential to human health. SIBO, which is frequently brought on by a decrease in the flow of food and waste through the gastrointestinal tract after surgery or other pre-existing conditions, is one condition in which dysbiosis in the gastrointestinal tract is most noticeable. The symptoms of SIBO include diarrhea, discomfort after eating, malnourishment, and abdominal pain. Similar to this, dysbiosis appears when there is small intestinal fungal overgrowth (SIFO), which is brought on by an overabundance of fungi in the bowel. GI symptoms (diarrhea, vomiting) in individuals who have previously had immunocompromised status are indicative of SIFO. One of the biggest influences on the gut microbiota of a consumer may be their eating habits. Diets heavy in refined sugars and carbohydrates are frequently associated with dysbiosis in the gut, while diets high in fruits, vegetables, and fish oils are thought to be better for the gut because of their anti-inflammatory qualities. Numerous illnesses, including Crohn's disease, Type 2 Diabetes, IBD, and even allergies, are thought to be partially caused by changes in the gut microbiome. When taking probiotics for the first time, especially in large doses, people may experience mild gas and bloating while their bodies adjust to the new gut bacteria.

9.3.3.2. Oral Dysbiosis

Microbial disruptions in the mouth, stomach, and intestines can result from the mouth's frequent exposure to new microbes from the environment. Because altered microbial communities in the oral cavity are linked to oral diseases like cavities, gingivitis, and tooth decay, prevention through good hygiene and dietary modification is essential. Oral pathogens have the ability to impact various microbiota compartments within the body and modify systemic functions, including immune system modifications and digestive problems. Oral intercourse, drinking, smoking, and getting older are all linked to oral dysbiosis.

9.3.3.3. Skin Dysbiosis

The term "skin flora" refers to the various kinds of microorganisms that live in and on human skin. Regular, healthy microbial communities might provide some advantages. Atopic dermatitis, psoriasis, rosacea, and acne are examples of non-infectious skin conditions that may be influenced by altered microbial diversity and composition, or dysbiosis. Pathogenic bacteria, most commonly Streptococci species and Staphylococcus aureus, can infect the skin in more severe cases, like cellulitis.

9.3.3.4. Vaginal Dysbiosis

Bacterial vaginosis is one condition that can arise from disruptions in the microbiome (vaginal flora) of the vagina. Changes in the vaginal flora can also impact the health of the vagina during reproduction, as well as an individual's risk of contracting an STD and the severity of the infection that follows.

9.3.3.5. Role of Antibiotics in Promoting Dysbiosis

Dysbiosis can develop at various phases of life and be brought on by a variety of factors. For instance, antibiotics frequently play a major role in the disruption of microbiomes. This happens because different types of microbes will respond differently to antibiotics, which means that the antibiotic may alter both the overall population of microbes and their balance. The use of antibiotics during early childhood development can cause dysbiosis, or adverse gut problems, in later life. Antibiotics change the gut microbiome and are associated with the development of future gut diseases, i.e., IBD, obesity, ulcerative colitis, and so forth. The gut microbiota has a direct impact on the intestinal immune system, which is why antibiotic damage can make it difficult to heal. Dermatological and intestinal dysbiosis have been linked to minocycline treatment for acne vulgaris.

9.3.4. Effects

Disorders affecting the intestines and extraintestinal tract have been related to the pathogenesis of gut dysbiosis. Dysbiosis can impact extra-intestinal conditions like allergies, asthma, metabolic syndrome, cardiovascular disease, and obesity in addition to intestinal disorders like IBD, IBS, and celiac disease. Because age-related dysbiosis and inflammation are linked, gut dysbiosis may also play a role in neurodegenerative and cerebrovascular diseases. Many age-related pathologies share an inflammatory component, including neurological disorders. It could be possible to stop the onset of neurodegenerative diseases in elderly patients by treating their dysbiosis. Dysbiosis has been implicated in the etiology or progression of neurological disorders, such as autism, pain, anxiety, depression, and stroke. Because of interactions with the gut-brain axis, which allows the gut microbiome to affect neural development, cognition, and behavior, dysbiosis is linked to neurological conditions. Additionally, there is evidence that behavioral changes can also affect the composition of the gut microbiota and that depressive-like behaviors can also result from modifications to the microbiome.

Additionally, microbial colonies release a wide variety of waste byproducts. Under normal circumstances, the body efficiently removes these byproducts with little to no difficulty using various waste removal mechanisms. Regrettably, because of their increased population, oversized and inappropriately large colonies excrete more of these byproducts. Higher levels of waste byproducts can overwhelm the body's waste elimination systems as microbial byproduct production rises. Inflammatory processes, including host- and cell-mediated inflammation, as well as "driver" bacteria that induce or exacerbate inflammation, can alter a person's microbiome. This alteration makes the microbial community more vulnerable to infections. Once successfully established, the pathogens produce genotoxins and other potentially cancer-causing microbial metabolites in addition to contributing to dysbiosis. Another potential consequence of dysbiosis is the evolution of pathogens, which may raise the risk of cancer.

The colon has a high bacterial density—(roughly 10^{12} per milliliter), and dysbiosis affects these bacteria. The small intestine, on the other hand, has a comparatively low density of bacteria (about 10^2 per ml). So dysbiosis probably poses less of an issue. The greater than 10-fold higher incidence of cancer in the colon compared to the small intestine may be explained by this difference. Western diets high in fat are linked to an increased risk of secondary bile acid-induced dysbiosis and therefore, intestinal cancer. Dysbiosis-induced elevation of secondary bile acids in the colon can damage DNA, and this damage can lead to cancer-causing mutations in colon cells. The cardiovascular system may be impacted by gut dysbiosis "through signaling molecules and bioactive metabolites." Neuro-entero-endocrine hormones from this may result in diseases like heart failure and other ailments like diabetes, obesity, hypertension, and chronic kidney disease.

9.3.5. Associated Illnesses

In healthy individuals, there is a homeostatic equilibrium of bacteria that maintains the gastrointestinal tract free of potentially pathogenic bacteria due to cross-regulation between the host and the gut microbiota. Loss of advantageous organisms, excessive growth of potentially hazardous microorganisms, and loss of total microbial diversity are the three main types of dysbiosis. Microbiome disruptions can give pathogenic microbiota members or external factors access to the gut environment. Numerous diseases, including multiple chemical sensitivity, colitis, inflammatory bowel disease, periodontal disease, obesity, cancer, and bacterial vaginosis, have been linked to dysbiosis.

9.3.5.1. Inflammatory Bowel Disease

Although the exact microbial cause of Crohn's disease is unknown, three major pathogens have been linked to the condition: adherent-invasive *Escherichia coli* (AIEC), *Clostridium difficile*, and *Mycobacteriumavium paratuberculosis* (MAP). It is unknown what, if any, causative role these bacteria play. Some believe that Crohn's disease is caused by an imbalance of commensal microflora linked to more intricate interactions between the host and the entire intestinal microbiota, as opposed to the one microbe, one disease theory.

9.3.5.2. Obesity

A metabolic disorder called obesity occurs when the body holds onto an excessive amount of fat. Just like in inflammatory bowel disease, obesity seems to be associated with a particular microbiota. In obese people, the diversity of microbes is significantly reduced. Obesity has been linked in studies on both humans and animals to changes in the ratios of Bacteroidetes to Firmicutes, with Firmicutes increasing as Bacteriodetes decrease. This ratio has been connected to fat accumulation and body weight, suggesting that obese individuals have a higher-than-normal ratio of these bacteria.

9.3.5.3. Diabetes Mellitus

Diabetes mellitus (DM) is a disorder of the metabolism of carbohydrates that is characterized by inadequate production or utilization of insulin, which is necessary for the body to convert carbohydrates and sugars into energy. In the US, there are approximately 29.1 million cases of DM, and 11.7 million new cases are diagnosed with the disease each year. Type 1 and Type 2 diabetes are the two types that exist. Insulin-Dependent Diabetes Mellitus is another name for type 1 diabetes (IDDM). An autoimmune disease called type 1 diabetes damages the pancreatic beta cells, which reduces the ability to produce insulin. The majority of cases are diagnosed in young adults and children. Insulin resistance, or decreased tissue sensitivity to insulin, is a feature of type 2 diabetes mellitus, also referred to as non-insulin-dependent diabetes mellitus (NIDDM), which affects adults. This reduces the body's sensitivity to the insulin that is released. Studies have indicated that dysbiosis of the intestinal microbiota could be a factor in diabetes mellitus. A decrease in mucin-degrading bacteria like Bifidobacteria, Lactobacillus, and Prevotella and an increase in Bacteroidetes and Clostridium are the hallmarks of the dysbiosis associated with type 1 diabetes mellitus.

9.3.5.4. Cancer

Prolonged periods of dysbiosis cause the gut microbiota to experience high levels of stress and inflammation, which can encourage the synthesis of metabolites that cause cancer. Colorectal cancer (CRC) has been linked to intestinal dysbiosis. The American Cancer Society reports that colorectal cancer ranks second in the country for cancer-related deaths and is the third most common type of cancer. A general dysbiosis pattern has been identified in CRC patients, characterized by an increase in the proportion of several potentially pathogenic bacteria and a decrease in butyrate-producing bacteria.

- **Clostridium Difficile:** *C. difficile* is an opportunistic bacterium that typically infects patients after the microbiome is disturbed, as happens when receiving antibiotic treatment. A number of symptoms, such as watery diarrhea, fever, appetite loss, nausea, and abdominal pain, can be brought on by an infection. Severe or persistent *C. difficile* infections may result in colitis, an inflammatory disease of the colon.

9.3.5.5. Periodontitis

An oral infection called periodontitis can harm the bones that support teeth and cause tooth loss. Disruption of the oral microbiome leading to an accumulation of pathogenic bacteria is one of the main risk factors for periodontitis. Research indicates that when periodontitis worsens, the oral microbiota shifts from gram-positive aerobes to gram-negative anaerobes. It is likely that oral dysbiosis will develop, changing the beneficial host-microbe relationship to a harmful one. The host experiences a decline in oral health during this period, which ultimately results in clinical illness.

9.3.5.6. Acne Vulgaris

Dermatological and intestinal dysbiosis have been linked to minocycline use for acne vulgaris.

9.3.5.7. Cardiovascular Disease

Intestinal microbiota dysbiosis may hasten the development of cardiovascular disease. An imbalance in the species and quantity of microorganisms in the adult intestine can be brought on by dietary practices, high levels of stress, intestinal infections, and the use of antibiotics. Dysbiosis in the gut can cause inflammation and metabolic problems that accelerate the onset of cardiovascular disease.

9.3.6. Treatments

9.3.6.1. Antibiotics

There is little information on the effectiveness of using antibiotics to treat dysbiosis due to the intricate interactions in the microbiome. Rifaximin, a broad-spectrum antibiotic, has been demonstrated to respond well to treatment in several dysbiosis-related illnesses, including irritable bowel syndrome. Some antibiotics cause long-lasting changes in the gut microbiota, while most only affect it temporarily during treatment. The gut microbiome can become unstable as a result of repeated antibiotic exposure, which can have the opposite effect of what is intended and encourage the "outgrowth of antibiotic-resistant pathogenic bacteria" and worsen gut dysbiosis.

9.3.6.2. Fecal Microbiota Transplant (FMT)

An experimental therapy called fecal microbiota transplantation (FMT) has successfully treated 80–90% of infections linked to dysbiosis that are brought on by recurrent *C. difficile* infections in randomized, controlled clinical trials that are resistant to antibiotics. When a patient undergoes FMT, their colon is transplanted using feces prepared from a carefully chosen, healthy stool donor. Repopulating the patient's microbiome with different microorganisms that are competitive with *C. difficile* is theorized to be how FMT functions.

Similar to probiotics, FMTs work by introducing beneficial microbes into the environment to restore the microbiome's natural balance of microbiota. FMT does this by using a healthy person's donated feces, diluting, straining, and giving them to a patient who is ill. A patient's colon is transplanted during FMT with a fecal preparation from a carefully screened, healthy stool donor. FMT is thought to work by repopulating the patient's microbiome with various microorganisms that compete with *C. difficile* for space. FMT is being researched for use in treating mental health issues as well. There is a push to isolate important microbiota and culture them separately because the procedure is not sterile and contaminations can transfer from donor to patient.

9.3.6.3. Probiotics

Probiotics are defined by the World Health Organization as live microorganisms that, when given in sufficient quantities, benefit the host's health. Probiotics are beneficial for treating dysbiosis-related illnesses because they can address the underlying cause of these conditions. Among their advantages are their capacity to inhibit pathogen colonization and reduce inflammation in the microbiome. Dysbiosis, or disruptions in the microbiome, is linked to many illnesses, including obesity, diabetes, cardiovascular disease, IBD, and excessive antibiotic use. This is especially true in the human gut. By introducing or reintroducing beneficial bacteria to strengthen the weaknesses found in a dysbiotic microbiome, probiotics can support healthier microbial function. It is critical to understand that under these conditions, beneficial bacteria predominate over harmful ones. Probiotics have anti-inflammatory qualities and enhance immune cell function, which can be used to treat current ailments and prevent diseases of this kind.

The bacteria in the human gut are highly diverse and are easily disturbed by a variety of factors, including food, medications, illnesses, and other conditions. Probiotics have been shown to be effective in restoring the homeostatic balance of the gut microbiota and enhancing intestinal health. Because of their anti-inflammatory qualities, probiotics can help prevent and treat intestinal diseases brought on by microbial dysbiosis. To fully comprehend the numerous advantages probiotics can provide for various types of dysbiosis, more research is required. The probiotic bacterium strain that has been studied the most is Lactobacillus. Customers can purchase it as part of a multi-strain formulation or as a single strain for gut health.

9.4. Factors Shaping the GI Microbiota

Selection pressures from both the host and the environment can shape the composition of the microbiota. The GI tract recruits a multifactorial and dynamic intestinal barrier to limit exposure of the host immune system to the microbiota, protecting against injury and preserving homeostasis. The barrier is made up of a number of interconnected parts, including immunological (IgA and epithelia-associated immune cells), biochemical (enzymes and antimicrobial proteins), and physical (mucus and epithelial layers). The lifespan of a single microbe is defined by how much it contributes to the variety of vital processes that host fitness depends on. It is suggested that organisms that do not perform advantageous tasks are subject to control and may occasionally be eliminated, for instance, when the microbiota is transferred to a new host.

Compared to other microbially rich environments, the gut has comparatively fewer biochemical niches, so gut microbes have to adapt to a specific lifestyle. Energy can typically be obtained in the gut by procedures like fermentation and the sulfate reduction of host and dietary carbohydrates. Therefore, the phenotypic traits of the organisms are what determine their ability to survive in the gut. According to recent studies, diet has a significant impact on gut microbiota. The ability of the microbial members to metabolize simple sugars is what drives the ileal microbiota, according to meta-transcriptomic studies. This indicates that the microbiota has adapted to the small intestine's nutrient availability. The availability of dietary fiber's microbiota-accessible carbohydrates (MACs) affects how the colonic microbiota is shaped. Severe "plant-based" or "animal-based" diets cause profound changes in human gut microbiota. A crossover study that showed the impact of fiber produced a significant and consistent enrichment of various bacterial species in the human gut when otherwise matched diets high in resistant starch or non-starch polysaccharide fiber (wheat bran) were consumed. The quantity of particular bacterial groups in an infant's gut microbiota can also be influenced by their feeding techniques. For example, fucosylated oligosaccharides present in human milk can be utilized by *Bifidobacterium longum* and several species of *Bacteroides* allowing them to outcompete other bacteria such as *E. coli* and *Clostridium perfringens*. Although the quantity of Bifidobacterium spp. The microbiota of breastfed infants is usually higher than that of formula-fed infants.

Furthermore, formula-fed infant microbiota has increased diversity and altered levels of other groups such as *E. coli*, *Clostridium difficile*, *Bacteroides fragilis* and lactobacilli. Babies who are malnourished have dysbiotic, immature microbiota that is higher in enteropathogens like Enterobacteriaceae. With a diet high in starch, fiber, and plant polysaccharides, infants from rural Africa have a microbiota rich in Actinobacteria (10%) and Bacteroidetes (57%) phyla. In comparison, the abundance of these groups is only 6.7 and 22.4% in children from Europe, whose diet is high in sugar, starch, and animal protein. Certain SCFA producers, like *Prevotella*, were unique to the microbiota in African children. This pattern was also seen in healthy people who consumed large quantities of simple sugars and carbohydrates. People who follow a low-MAC diet also exhibit a decreased SCFA output, which is noteworthy because SCFAs are crucial for host health through functions like anti-inflammatory pathways. The Western diet significantly lowers the abundance of MACs.

The gut microbiota obtains carbohydrates from intestinal mucus as well. The massive, highly glycosylated mucin MUC2, which forms a gel and is secreted by goblet cells, serves as the foundation for the intestinal mucus layers. Mucins are composed of four core mucin-type O-glycans that contain N-acetylgalactosamine, galactose, and N-acetylglucosamine. These glycan structures are diverse and complex. Fucose and sialic acid sugar residues further extend and often terminate these core structures. O-glycans together make up as much as 80% of Muc2/MUC2's total molecular mass. The GI tract is filled with mucus, which is thickest in the colon and plays a critical role in mediating the host-microbiota relationship there. Long-term microbial colonization is necessary for the host's intestinal mucus layers to return to normal. Colonic mucus is made up of two layers: a loose outer layer that bacteria can penetrate and an inner layer that is dense and impermeable. The outer layer's mucin proteins, which are adorned with a wide variety of O-glycans, give commensal bacteria a source of energy and preferred binding sites, while the inner layer is essentially sterile. When compared to their counterparts in the lumen, bacterial species exhibit distinct patterns of resource utilization and proliferation within the specific niche created by the arrangement of the outer mucus layer. The expression of glycosyltransferases and their location within the Golgi apparatus determine the type of mucin O-glycosylation, which in turn influences the composition of the microbiota. For instance, the abundance of numerous bacterial groups is influenced by the presence (secretor) or lack (non-secretor) of H and ABO antigens in GI mucosa, which is determined by the FUT2 genotype (a gene expressing an α1,2-fucosyltransferase). Therefore, the glycosylation of mucus and mucin is essential for forming the microbiota and enabling the selection of the best microbial species to mediate host health.

The repertoire of glycoside hydrolases (GHs) and polysaccharide lyases (PLs) encoded by the genomes of gut bacteria determines their ability to utilize dietary or mucin glycans. While some species are specialists that only target particular glycans, others function as generalists that can break down a broad variety of polysaccharides. Compared to members of Firmicutes, which encode 39.6 GH and PL genes per genome, Bacteroidetes encode significantly more glycan-cleaving enzymes (137.1 GH and PL genes per genome). The 260 GHs found in the *Bacteroides thetaiotaomicron* genome contrast with the 97 hydrolases encoded in the human genome. The most abundant family in the gut microbiota is the GH13 family, which includes enzymes involved in the digestion of starch. Recently, the detailed biochemical and structural characterization of the extensive degrading apparatus of prominent gut species such as *B. thetaiotaomicron* or *Bacteroides ovatus* revealed that the recognition and breakdown of complex carbohydrates, such as Xylan, mannan, xyloglucan or starch, by the human gut microbiota is significantly more complex than previously suggested. Although less studied, members of Firmicutes also show some unique and complex features such as the recent discovery of amylosomes in the resistant starch-utilizing bacterium *Ruminococcus bromii*.

A microbial population can become more diverse through lateral gene transfer or mutation, for example. More diversity can arise as a result of the introduction of novel bacterial functions, which encourage niche variation and establish a positive feedback loop. Collaboration among gut microbes facilitates the colonization of a wider range of organisms, thereby influencing the composition of the gut microbiota community. It has been suggested that microbial cross-feeding mediates this effect. Certain byproducts of the fermentation of carbohydrates, such as lactate, succinate, and 1,2-propanediol, can act as substrates for other bacteria that produce butyrate and propionate, so they typically do not build up to high concentrations in the colons of healthy adults. For example, acetate produced by fermentation of resistant starch by *R. bromii* or lactate produced by lactic acid bacteria such as lactobacilli and bifidobacteria provides substrate for other microbiota members such as *Eubacterium hallii* and *Anaerostipes caccae* which convert it into butyrate. Further, *B. ovatus* has been demonstrated to perform extracellular digestion of inulin at its own cost, but at an advantage to other species which provides reciprocal benefits. This kind of cooperation is especially noticeable in the outer mucus layer, where bacteria that break down mucin supply mono- or oligosaccharides to bacteria that lack specialized mucolytic activity. For instance, only bacterial species expressing GH33 sialidases can cleave sialic acid off mucins. Many bacteria, including pathogens such as *Salmonella typhimurium* or *C. difficile*, which are deficient in sialidase but have a "nan cluster" devoted to sialic acid metabolism, are dependent on other gut microbiota members for this carbon source. A novel class of sialidase called intramolecular trans-sialidase was recently discovered in strains of *Ruminococcus gnavus*, and it may be involved in the gut commensal bacteria's adaptation to the mucosal niche. Given that the gut mucosal environment is rich in short, sialylated mucin glycans, this activity may give these bacteria a competitive nutritional advantage over other species in inflammatory bowel diseases in particular.

The availability of sulfated compounds in the colon, either of inorganic (e.g., sulfates and sulfites) or organic (e.g., dietary amino acids and host mucins) origin, can influence specific groups of bacteria such as sulfate-reducing bacteria, which are residents of the gut microbiota that have been implicated in the etiology of intestinal disorders such as IBD, IBS or colorectal cancer.

As has been extensively reviewed, the dynamics of the bacterial community in the gut can also be impacted by the distribution of bile acids in the small and large intestines. Primary bile acids, like taurocholate, can help spores germinate and give homing signals to gut bacteria. They can also help the microbiota recover from dysbiosis brought on by antibiotics or toxins. Furthermore, the expansion of pro-inflammatory microbial taxa may be significantly facilitated by decreased bile acid concentration in the gut. The GI microbiota is shaped by bile acids, as these studies demonstrate.

The host immune system can also influence the microbiota. Because of the high degree of functional redundancy within the microbiota, species-specific effects are less likely. This effect is primarily restricted to the stratification and compartmentalization of bacteria to prevent opportunistic invasion of host tissue. The gut microbiota is significantly shaped by antimicrobials that are administered and derived from the host. Paneth cells in the GI tract generate antimicrobials like lectins like REGIIIα/γ, α-defensins, cathelicidins, collectins, histatins, lysozymes, lipopolysaccharide (LPS)-binding protein, and angiogenin 4. These proteins are primarily found in the mucus layer and are essentially nonexistent in the lumen, most likely as a result of luminal degradation or inadequate mucus diffusion. Numerous secreted antimicrobial proteins (AMPs) destroy bacteria by interacting directly with them and by enzymatically attacking their inner membrane or cell wall. The significance of these proteins is highlighted by the observation that patients with ileal Crohn's disease (CD) have reduced mucosal α-defensin expression. Another immune system component, secretory IgA (SIgA), co-localizes in the outer mucus layer with gut bacteria and helps to prevent bacteria from penetrating the surface of epithelial cells. It has been suggested that SIgA binds to SIgA receptors on bacteria to mediate the formation of bacterial biofilms. In people with low IgA levels, bacteria express fewer SIgA receptors.

Numerous environmental factors, such as geographic location, surgery, smoking, depression, and living arrangements (rural vs. urban), have been linked to the shaping of the microbiota. Antibiotics and other xenobiotics, which do not target the host, influence the physiology and gene expression of the human gut microbiome in action. Both the short- and long-term microbial balance are severely upset by antibiotic treatment, with the community's richness and diversity declining along with it. It has been shown that the microbiota structure is impacted by ciproflaxin, clarithromycin, and metronidazole for differing periods of time. Due to inter-individual variation in the microbiota before treatment, the precise effects and recovery time of the microbiota after antibiotic administration seem to be individual-dependent. An exploratory study conducted on humans revealed that the microbial ecology and the production of important metabolites, like acetyl phosphate and acetyl-CoA, which are involved in important cellular functions, are both impacted by the administration of β-lactam intravenous therapy consisting of ampicillin, sulbactam, and cefazolin. A deeper comprehension of the processes causing the bacterial blooms brought on by antibiotics, as well as the impacted biochemical processes and metabolites, will aid in the development of supplementary and/or alternative approaches needed to preserve human health.

9.5. Role of the GI Microbiota in Health and Nutrition

Due to its extensive genomic makeup and metabolic diversity, the gut microbiota offers several advantageous characteristics to the host. Among these microbes' most significant functions are their assistance in preserving the mucosal barrier's integrity, their provision of nutrients like vitamins, and their defense against infections. Furthermore, for optimal immune function, commensal microbiota and the mucosal immune system must interact.

The ability to ferment complex carbohydrates and produce metabolites like SCFAs is attributed to the expression of carbohydrate-active enzymes by colonic bacteria. In the GI tract, the three main SCFAs—propionate, butyrate, and acetate—are normally present in a 1:1:3 ratio. The GI tract's epithelial cells quickly absorb these SCFAs, and they play a role in the control of several biological processes, including gene expression, chemotaxis, differentiation, proliferation, and apoptosis. Most gut anaerobes produce acetate, but different subsets of gut bacteria use different molecular pathways to produce propionate and butyrate. Glycolysis and acetoacetyl-CoA are the processes that convert carbohydrates into butyrate, while the formation of propionate can occur through either the succinate or propanediol pathway, depending on the type of sugar. In the human gut, Firmicutes are primarily responsible for producing butyrate, while Bacteroidetes are primarily responsible for producing propionate. For instance, starch fermentation by specialized Firmicutes and Actinobacteria, e.g., *Eubacterium*, also known as *E. hallii* is believed to have a major direct and indirect role in the colon's production of butyrate through metabolic cross-feeding. *A. muciniphila* is a key propionate producer specialized in mucin degradation. Acetate is released into peripheral tissues, whereas propionate is mainly absorbed by the liver.

A review of the impact of SCFAs on human metabolism was published. Butyrate has a reputation for being anti-inflammatory and anti-tumorous. For colonocytes, butyrate is a crucial source of energy. It is proposed that intestinal epithelial turnover and homeostasis are regulated by a decreasing gradient of butyrate from the lumen to the crypt, which increases apoptosis and exfoliation of cells closer to the lumen and promotes colonocyte proliferation at the bottom of crypts. Through its effects on tight-junction assembly and mucin synthesis, butyrate can reduce bacterial translocation and improve the function of the gut barrier. Additionally, hepatic lipid and glucose homeostasis appear to be regulated by SCFAs through complementary mechanisms. Acetate and butyrate are lipogenic substances in the liver, whereas propionate can stimulate gluconeogenesis. Additionally, SCFAs are involved in immune system and inflammatory response regulation. They have an impact on cytokine production; for instance, they can promote the synthesis of IL-18, an interleukin that helps to preserve and repair epithelial integrity. Histone deacetylase inhibitors that epigenetically control gene expression include butyrate and propionate. Through receptor-mediated mechanisms, SCFAs have also been demonstrated to modify the regulation of appetite and energy intake. Propionate has been shown to have positive effects on human health by modulating β-cell activity and decreasing reward-driven eating through striatal pathways. It has been documented that microbial metabolites other than SCFAs affect the immune system, epithelium proliferation, and intestinal barrier functions.

Additionally, the de novo synthesis of vital vitamins—which the host is unable to produce—depends on the GI microbiota. Animals, plants, or fungi are unable to synthesize vitamin B12, which is primarily produced by lactic acid bacteria. The primary source of folate, a vitamin essential to host metabolic processes like DNA synthesis and repair, is bifidobacteria. Additional vitamins, such as vitamin K, riboflavin, biotin, nicotinic acid, pantothenic acid, pyridoxine, and thiamine, have been demonstrated to be synthesized by gut microbiota in humans. Bile acids that are not reabsorbed can also be biotransformed into secondary bile acids by colonic bacteria. Each of these elements has an impact on the host's health. A change in the co-metabolism of branched fatty acids, choline, vitamins is known. Metabolic disorders like type 2 diabetes and obesity have been linked to niacin, purines, and phenolic compounds.

In addition to producing antimicrobial compounds and competing for attachment sites or nutrient sources, the physical presence of the microbiota in the GI tract affects pathogen colonization. Antibiotics have a significant effect on the microbiota, which changes the gut's nutritional environment and promotes the growth of pathogenic populations. As an illustration, *S. typhimurium* and *C. difficile* make use of the fucose and sialic acid that the gut microbiota releases, and sialic acid levels that are higher after antibiotic treatment encourage the growth of *C. difficile* in the gut. It has also been demonstrated that *E.coli* can access sialic acid or fucose that the gut microbiota has released from mucins. Through its structural elements and metabolites, the GI microbiota also encourages the host to produce a range of antimicrobial substances. These include AMPs produced by the host Paneth cells through a PRR-mediated mechanism, such as cathelicidins, C-type lectins, and (pro)defensins.

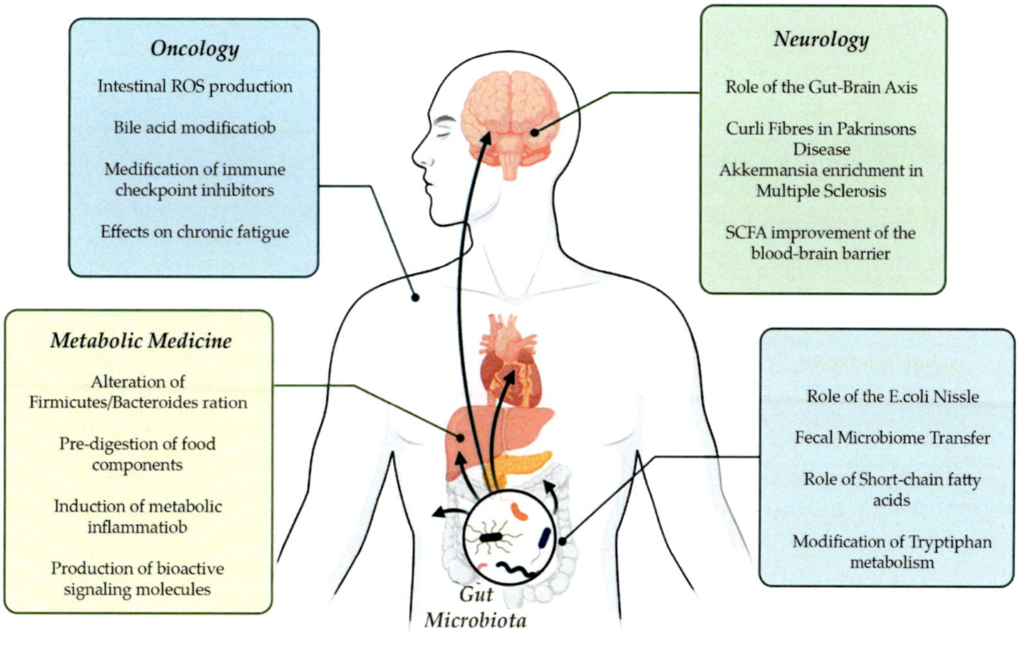

Figure 9.3. *Schematic representation of the role of the gut microbiota in health and disease giving some examples of inputs and outputs. SCFA=short chain fatty acids.*

Source: Laudes M, Geisler C, Rohmann N, Bouwman J, Pischon T, Schlicht K. Microbiota in health and disease—potential clinical applications. Nutrients. 2021; 13(11):3866. https://doi.org/10.3390/nu13113866.

Inducing mucosal SIgA is another way that the gut microbiota can prevent pathogen overgrowth. Via an M-cell-mediated sampling mechanism, SIgAs directed against gut commensal bacteria are induced. Through their combined interactions with mucins and gut bacteria, SIgAs are then anchored in the outer layer of colonic mucus, where they provide immune protection against pathogens while preserving a mutually beneficial relationship with commensals. Pattern recognition receptor–microbe-associated molecular patterns, or PRR–MAMP—cross-talk activates a number of signaling pathways that are critical for enhancing the function of the mucosal barrier and AMP, mucin, and IgA production. These pathways also help the host defend against invasive pathogens and stop the overgrowth of commensals (Figure 9.3).

9.5.1. Metabolic Functions of the Gut Microbiota Relevant to Human Nutrition

There are multiple sources of nutrition for the gut microbiota (Table 9.1). These include substances that are obtained from the host, such as mucus and shed epithelial cells, as well as ingested food components like proteins, carbohydrates, and fat. These substrates are used by the gut microbiota to produce energy for growth and cellular functions. The utilization of these substrates by the microbiota results in the production of various metabolites that have an impact on human metabolism and health. Short-chain fatty acids (SCFA) are produced as a result of fermentation of carbohydrates and are used by the host. Phenolic metabolites produced by protein fermentation may have harmful effects on the host. These metabolites can be detoxified by the liver and the intestines. Additionally, the gut microbiota synthesizes a number of molecules, including vitamin B components and vitamin K. Certain substances may have a direct impact on human nutrition by way of intestinal absorption. The host is unlikely to receive vitamin B12 directly from the gut microbiota. The absorption of vitamin B12 is regulated by physiology, which calls for complex absorption in the terminal ileum, transfer to intrinsic factor in the small intestine, and binding to R factor in the stomach.

The human gut microbiota was found to have three enterotypes, and an analysis of metabolic pathways produced some intriguing findings. Since the microbes of enterotype 1 were enriched for genes corresponding to saccharolytic enzymes, galactosidases, hexosaminidases, proteases, and enzymes in the glycolysis and pentose phosphate pathways, it was hypothesized that they obtained their energy primarily from the fermentation of proteins and carbohydrates. Enterotypes 2 and 3 were thought to primarily obtain their energy from the breakdown of mucin, though the latter likely also possessed the capacity to ferment carbohydrates due to the presence of a considerable number of Bacteroides species. Enzymes involved in the biosynthesis of biotin, riboflavin, pantothenate, and ascorbate were found to be enriched in enterotype 1, whereas thiamine and folate were found to be enriched in enterotype 2. Age-related increases in starch degradation enzymes are consistent with shifting dietary habits. ATPase complexes were found to be two marker modules that correlated significantly with the host body mass index, supporting a connection between the gut microbiota and the energy nutrition state of the host.

Table 9.1. Energy Sources Available for Bacterial Fermentation in the Human Colon

Substrate	Components	Structure	Amount Consumed (g Per Day)
Carbohydrates	**Resistant Starch (RS)**	**RS**—polymer of α1,4 linked glucose residues	10–40
	Non-starch polysaccharides (e.g., cellulose, xylan, pectin, inulin)	**Cellulose**—homopolymer of β1,4 linked glucose residues **Xylan**—polymer of β1,4 linked xylose residues with arabinose **Pectin**—complex polymer of α1,4 linked D-galacturonic acid or rhamnogalacturonan backbone with side-chain sugars of xylose, galactose, and arabinose	10–30
		Inulin—polymer of β 2,1 D-fructose residues with a terminal α1,2 D-glucose (DP > 10)	3–11
	Oligosaccharides (e.g., raffinose, stachyose, fructo-, xylo- and galacto-oligosaccharides)	**FOS**—polymer of β 2,1 D-fructose residues with a terminal α1,2 D-glucose (DP < 10)	2–10
	Unabsorbed sugars (e.g., lactose, sugar alcohols)	**Lactose**—dimer of β D-galactose (1,4) D-glucose	2–12
Proteins	**Unabsorbed dietary residues**	Mix of amino acids (meat protein should provide all required essential amino acids)	2–10
	Endogenous secretions (e.g., pancreatic enzymes and bile, mucus)	Mucins are high-molecular-weight glycoproteins consisting of a protein backbone, rich in serine and threonine, surrounded by O- and N-linked oligosaccharide side chains terminated by sialic acids or sulfate groups	2–8
Other	**Bacterial fermentation products** (cross-feeding)	Mainly formate, acetate, lactate, and succinate	

Source: Duncan SH, Conti E, Ricci L, Walker AW. Links between diet, intestinal anaerobes, microbial metabolites and health. Biomedicines. 2023; 11(5):1338. https://doi.org/10.3390/biomedicines11051338.

9.5.2. Colonic Fermentation and Production of SCFA

10–20% of the carbohydrates that are consumed through diet are not easily broken down in the small intestine. These non-digestible dietary carbohydrates (NDC) include non-starch polysaccharides (NSPs) and some types of starch that are resistant to amylase digestion (resistant starch [RS]). The NSP contains materials like cellulose that are not fermented by colonic bacteria as well as materials like pectin, which are substrates for the metabolism of colonic bacteria. Dietary carbohydrates that are not digested reach the colon, where fermentable NSP and RS are converted by colonic bacteria into lactate, SCFA, and gases like CO_2, H_2, and methane. For colonic fermentation, RS—which is mostly derived from cereals but can also be found in raw bananas and potatoes—is an essential substrate. While a considerable amount of type 2 RS (i.e., naturally occurring in the food source), the cooking and eating techniques may increase the food's RS content. As a result, cooked and cooled rice or potatoes may have a higher RS content than raw food. Between 10 and 20% of the starch consumed daily may be RS, depending on these factors. Research conducted both in vivo and in vitro has demonstrated that colonic bacteria quickly ferment starch to SCFA. The three main SCFAs that are obtained from the colon during carbohydrate fermentation are butyrate, propionate, and acetate. The primary energy source for colonic epithelial cells is butyrate.

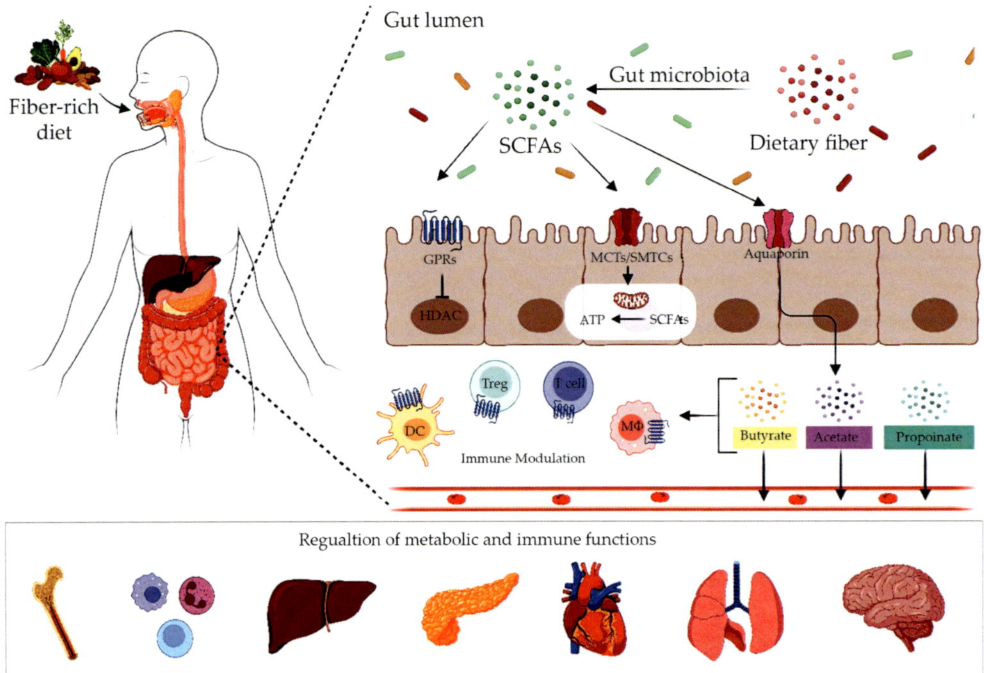

Figure 9.4. *SFCAs and gut microbes: SCFAs; short-chain fatty acids, GPRs; G protein-coupled receptors, MCTs; Monocarboxylate transporters, SMTCs; Sodium-coupled monocarboxylate transporter; DC, dendritic cell, Treg; T regulatory cell, Mϕ; Macrophage.*

Source: Al-Qadami GH, Secombe KR, Subramaniam CB, Wardill HR, Bowen JM. Gut microbiota-derived short-chain fatty acids: impact on cancer treatment response and toxicities. Microorganisms. 2022; 10(10):2048. https://doi.org/10.3390/microorganisms10102048.

In addition to facilitating epithelial cell differentiation, which has anticancer effects, SCFAs also promote tight junction integrity in the colon, accelerate epithelial repair in response to injury, and increase the rate of epithelial cell proliferation. Propionate and acetate enter the portal circulation and undergo liver metabolism. When non-digestible carbohydrates are taken orally, a portion of the acetate produced in the colon by bacterial fermentation is detected in the peripheral circulation as an increase in acetate levels in the blood. Adipose tissue is among the other tissues where this is metabolized. The majority of propionate's metabolism occurs in the liver, where it also lowers blood sugar and serum cholesterol. When all of these SCFA are present, the small intestine's "lost" energy is preserved. Approximately 2 kcal of energy is recovered per gram of starch through fermentation to SCFA, as opposed to 4 kcal per gram if the starch were fully hydrolyzed to glucose. Consequently, the food industry uses RS as a low-calorie alternative since its energy absorption is less effective than that of digestible starch. Nevertheless, in underprivileged communities with weakened diets where RS makes up a large portion of the dietary starch, the capacity to store energy from ingested RS is likely of major nutritional importance (Figure 9.4).

Many different enzymes are needed for the fermentation of unabsorbed carbohydrates, and these enzymes are produced by a variety of gut microbes. The main fermenters of carbohydrates are now identified. Because they have adapted to live there, the majority of colonic microbial communities are able to use complex carbohydrates. For example, it has been demonstrated that lactobacilli originating from the human gut possess the required machinery to utilize complex carbohydrates, an ability absent in lactobacilli strains originating from dairy products. Bacteroides species have genes for a wide range of enzymes involved in the utilization of carbohydrates, such as glycoside hydrolases, glycosyl transferases, polysaccharide lyases, and carbohydrate esterases, according to an analysis of the genetic potential of gut microbiota. In situations where dietary NDCs are scarce, bacteria may prefer to break down host carbohydrates, such as mucus proteins, in addition to dietary NDCs.

Clostridium leptum, *Ruminococcus bromii*, and *Faecalibacterium prausnitzii* are the members of Clostridium cluster IV, while Clostridium XIV (*C. Cobboides*, *E. rectale*, *Roseburia* species, and *Butyrivibrio fibrisolvens*) are regarded as highly significant bacteria that ferment carbohydrates. They are especially good at fermenting starch and producing butyrate. High amylose starch (type 3 RS) has been reported to be very well hydrolyzed by Bifidobacterium strains.

Novel metabolic pathways found in bifidobacteria make use of host glycoproteins and oligosaccharides found in human milk. While *Bifidobacterium adolescentis* and *Bifidobacterium longum* both produce acetate from glucose, the former is also capable of producing acetate from fructose thanks to an ATP-binding cassette-type carbohydrate transporter. Studies in an *in vitro* human colon model suggested that *R. bromii* and related species were the primary starch degraders in most cases, but metabolic cross-feeding of *Prevotella* species, *B. adolescentis*, and *E. rectale* occurred resulting in fermentation to acetate, butyrate, and propionate. The fact that members of *Clostridium* cluster XIVa convert lactate produced by multiple microbial species from carbohydrate to butyrate and members of Clostridium cluster IX convert lactate to propionate further highlights the requirement for a consortium of bacteria to complete these processes.

9.5.3. The Gut Microbiota and Obesity

Human association studies conducted around the globe have confirmed that obese people have different gut microbiomes than lean people, but the specific microbial communities involved have varied. *F. prausnitzii* was increased in the fecal microbiota of obese children in southern India that used real-time polymerase chain reaction to quantitate specific bacterial groups. Conversely, a higher concentration of fecal SCFA and an enrichment of Bacteroides and Archaea in the fecal microbiota were observed in obese adults from central India. In France, studies on obese adults revealed lower levels of Bacteroidetes and higher levels of Lactobacillus. Conversely, when compared to their healthy counterparts, obese preschoolers in Sweden had lower levels of *Desulfovibrio* and *Akkermanseae* and higher levels of *Enterobacteriaceae*.

Many attempts have been undertaken to clarify the causal relationship between gut microbiota and obesity. When twin pairs with similar body mass indices were examined, it was discovered that a large number of microbial genes were shared, which may indicate the existence of a core microbiome. Reduced microbial diversity, changes in genes involved in metabolic pathways, and differences in the microbiota at the phylum level (with significantly fewer Bacteroidetes and Actinobacteria found in obese twins without significant changes in the phylum Firmicutes) were all associated with obesity. *Gammaproteobacteria* increased and Firmicutes decreased in obese patients undergoing gastric bypass surgery.

There are multiple possible mechanisms that could account for the relationship between gut microbiota and nutrition (Figure 9.5). Numerous microbial communities within the phylum Firmicutes are significant fermenters of carbohydrates and may aid in the recovery of energy from dietary carbohydrates that are not absorbed. Obese people had higher levels of fecal SCFA, which is the colon's fermentation of unabsorbed carbohydrates. Increased food-based energy recovery efficiency could be a factor in weight gain. In lean volunteers, increasing the daily calorie load from 2400 to 3400 kcal led to alterations in the gut microbiota and a rise in the fractional energy absorbed from the diet. These researchers determined that an increase in energy absorption equal to 150 kcal/day was linked to a 20% increase in Firmicutes and a corresponding decrease in Bacteroidetes. Of interest, the abundant fecal microbial communities *Bacteroides* and *F. prausnitzii* were reduced, and Enterobacteriaceae increased in frail elderly individuals. Restriction of dietary carbohydrate intake in obese adults resulted in reduced abundance in stool of several carbohydrate-fermenting Firmicutes including *E. rectale*.

Microbial fermentation products influence energy metabolism and salvage through multiple neuroendocrine mechanisms, in addition to directly supplying energy in the form of SCFA. Peptide YY (PYY) and glucagon-like peptide (GLP) are released when SCFA binds to and activates G protein-coupled receptors Gpr41 (FFAR3) and Gpr43 (FFAR2) on colonic epithelial cells and enteroendocrine cells. Gpr41-deficient individuals were obese, had low energy expenditure, and had less PYY expression—which typically inhibits gut motility—which was linked to an increase in intestinal transit rate and a decrease in energy harvesting. Gpr41 is also present in other tissues, such as sympathetic ganglia and pancreatic β-cells. These are bound by the SCFA acetate and propionate, which then suppress insulin release and heighten sympathetic activity. Other researchers' studies indicate that the first two SCFA-induced gut hormones and decreased food intake, while butyrate, propionate, and acetate all protected against diet-induced obesity and insulin resistance.

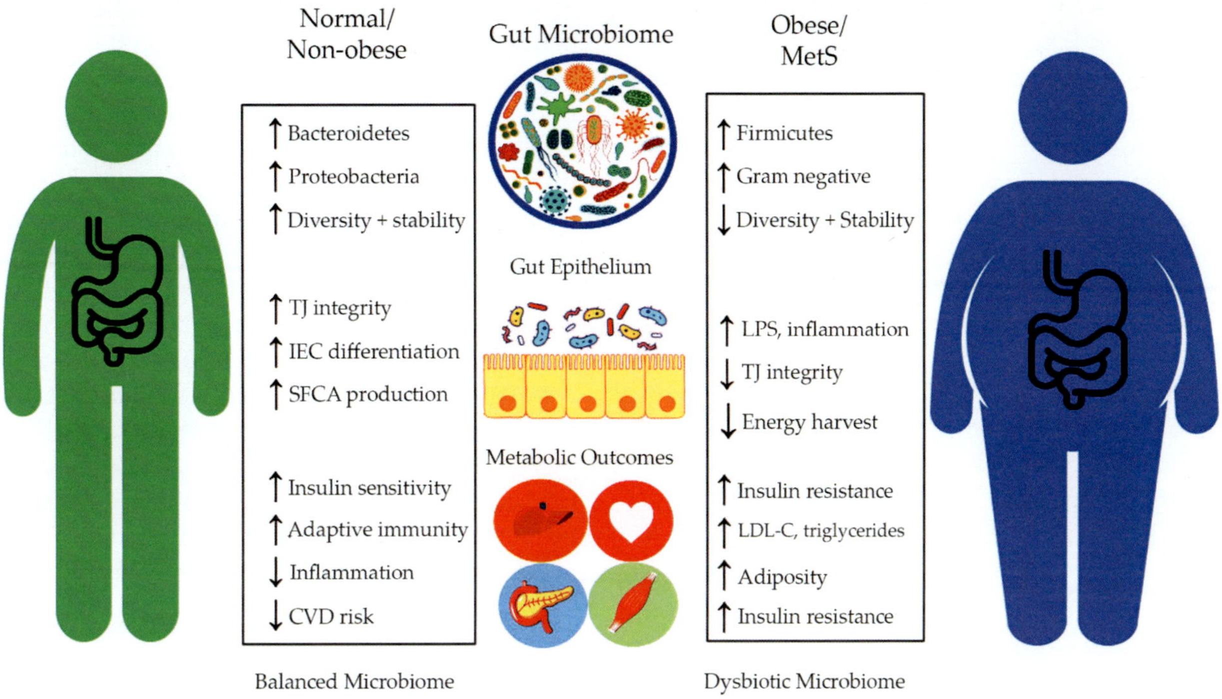

Figure 9.5. *Putative pathways that link the gut microbiota to obesity.*

Source: Green M, Arora K, Prakash S. Microbial medicine: Prebiotic and probiotic functional foods to target obesity and metabolic syndrome. International Journal of Molecular Sciences. 2020; 21(8):2890. https://doi.org/10.3390/ijms21082890.

An additional potential connection between peripheral fat accumulation and gut microbiota could be the existence of a mild systemic inflammatory state brought on by specific gut microbial communities. It has been demonstrated that obesity induced in otherwise normal animals by feeding them a high-fat diet is linked to elevated intestinal permeability and lipopolysaccharide plasma levels. It was hypothesized that the high-fat diet would induce toll-like receptor 4 (TLR4), which would cause obesity in these animals. Other consequences and associations of obesity, such as non-alcoholic fatty liver disease (NAFLD), may also result from a systemic inflammatory state.

9.5.4. Gut Microbiota and Energy Malnutrition

Gut mucosal inflammation may be linked to a lean body mass index in and of itself. In patients with overt inflammatory bowel disease, this is clinically evident. However, in subclinical gut mucosal inflammatory states like tropical enteropathy, which is characterized by a lymphoplasmacytic inflammatory cell infiltration of the gut's lamina propria, a lean body habitus may also be observed. SCFAs, especially butyrate, work through nuclear factor kappa B signaling to decrease the production of inflammatory cytokines and intestinal inflammation. In animal models of overt colitis, manipulation of the gut microbiota (by administering specific microbial communities) reduces gut inflammation and increases body weight. The relationship between gut microbiota and malnutrition has only recently been studied, and it is unclear whether changes in the gut microbiome cause or are a result of malnutrition. Research on Bangladeshi children suffering from marasmus—a type of malnutrition marked by energy deprivation—showed that the diversity of gut microbial species was lower in these children, with Proteobacteria accounting for 46% and Bacteroidetes for 18%, respectively, while Proteobacteria (including pathogenic bacterial genera) accounted for 56% and 44%, respectively, in healthy children. Recent research has also focused on kwashiorkor, a condition in which children are malnourished in protein but not in energy. Three years of the lives of 317 pairs of Malawian twins were studied for the gut microbiota. Of these twin pairs, 7% had both twins develop kwashiorkor, and 43% had one twin develop the condition. Research on the gut microbiome metabolic capacity in kwashiorkor children revealed that when high-protein dietary supplements were fed, the capacity temporarily matured and then reverted to abnormal when the supplementation was stopped. Most intriguingly, it was discovered that feeding a Malawian diet to the kwashiorkor young and transferring their gut microbiota into gnotobiotic caused the animals to significantly lose weight and experience abnormalities in their metabolism of carbohydrates and amino acids. Therefore, it would seem that the gut microbiota plays a part in the development of malnutrition as well.

9.5.5. Gut Microbiota and Mineral Absorption

There are several other correlations between human nutrition and gut microbiota. Accordingly, research on people with iron deficiency anemia reveals that the gut microbiota of those people is comparatively lacking in lactobacilli. It is unclear if iron deficiency causes the decline in lactobacilli or if the decrease in lactobacilli is the result of iron deficiency. Due to their significant iron growth requirement, lactobacilli may be less common in the intestines of people who are iron deficient. However, in the right colon, bacteria that ferment carbohydrates produce SCFA and lower the luminal pH, which encourages the absorption of divalent cations through transporters in the cecum. It is now known that the enterocyte transporters involved in iron transport are also expressed in the cecum and right colon, despite the duodenum being the primary site of iron absorption. In animal models, readily fermented carbohydrates encourage the growth of bacteria that produce propionic acid, thereby promoting colonic absorption of iron. The conversion of lactate to propionate in fermentation systems is facilitated by lactobacilli, which offers a logical explanation for the causal relationship between the decline in lactobacilli and iron-deficiency anemia.

9.5.6. Gut Microbiota and Glucose Metabolism

The development of type 2 diabetes has been linked to changes in the gut microbiota. It has been shown that there are modifications that result in impaired insulin signaling. These include decreased phosphorylation of the insulin receptor, insulin receptor substrate (IRS), and Akt, as well as increased inhibitory serine phosphorylation of IRS-1. The metabolic syndrome that resulted from TLR2 knockout was linked to a significant rise in Firmicutes and a slight increase in *Bacteroides*. An increase in the abundance of *E. rectale-C. coccoides* belonging to the phylum Firmicutes has been noted in women with metabolic syndrome, where this population correlated with metabolic dysfunction. Male recipients with metabolic syndrome received intestinal infusions of microbiota from lean donors (or the patient's own microbiota as a control) in an intriguing randomized trial. Insulin sensitivity (rate of glucose disappearance) increased significantly in recipients receiving microbiota from lean donors six weeks after the infusions. This was linked to a rise in the number of bacteria in the feces that produce butyrate. It is yet unknown, though, whether the gut microbiota plays a significant part in the onset of diabetes and by what mechanisms.

9.5.7. Gut Microbiota and Lipid Metabolism

By producing bile salt hydrolases, some gut microbiota, especially lactobacilli, are able to hydrolyze bile salts. The diversion of cholesterol to bile acid synthesis disrupts the enterohepatic cycle of bile salt reabsorption, increasing the loss of bile salt in the stools and causing a secondary decrease in serum cholesterol. This is one of the two mechanisms that connect dyslipidemia and the gut microbiota; the other is the inhibition of 3-Hydroxy-3-Methyl Glutaryl-Coenzyme A synthase activity in the liver by propionic acid, which is produced by gut bacteria and reduces cholesterol synthesis.

9.5.8. Gut Microbiota and Protein Metabolism

In a healthy individual, the majority of protein that enters the colon and is subject to microbial metabolism is likely derived from the host, with a small amount coming from unabsorbed dietary protein. Branching-chain amino acids and various phenolic and other metabolites that could be harmful to the host are produced during protein fermentation. The liver and intestinal wall do the majority of the detoxification for these. Since microbial metabolites of protein are primarily responsible for hepatic encephalopathy, protein metabolism in the colon becomes important in the presence of liver disease. This can be mitigated by giving fermentable carbohydrates, like lactulose, which change the fermentation profile to metabolites that do not affect cognition. According to recent research, liver disease patients' gut microbiome composition may have an impact on their cognitive function. When cirrhosis patients with hepatic encephalopathy were compared to those without encephalopathy, a higher concentration of Veillonellaceae was discovered. Increases in *Alcaligenaceae* and *Porphyromonadaceae*, or a change to pathogenic microbiota in the gut, have been linked to cognitive deficits. When rifaximin was given to cirrhotics with mild hepatic encephalopathy, the microbiota's composition remained largely unchanged, but there were increases in serum saturated and unsaturated fatty acids and a shift in the metabolic networks of the gut microbiome from pathogenic to beneficial profiles. While it is unlikely that the gut microbiota is primarily responsible for the metabolic disturbances associated with hepatic dysfunction, research on this topic will undoubtedly concentrate in the near future.

9.6. Microbiome-Based Therapeutics

Gaining knowledge about the metabolic capacities of gut microbiota in every part of the body could be the key to unlocking the secrets of health and illness-related processes. Novel approaches to the prevention and treatment of extraintestinal inflammatory diseases, such as IBD, may be made possible by the latest insights into GM modulation mechanisms. Pre-, pro-, and post-biotics or synbiotics included in diets increased saccharolytic fermentation and decreased proteolytic fermentation simultaneously. Significant advancements have been made thus far in the field of microbial analysis tools and therapeutic strategies, including the use of fecal microbiota transplantation (FMT) and dietary intervention with microbes (Figure 9.6). Probiotics are live microorganisms that, when taken in sufficient quantities, provide health benefits to the body. Despite the consistent definition for 17 years, public understanding of probiotics is still evolving.

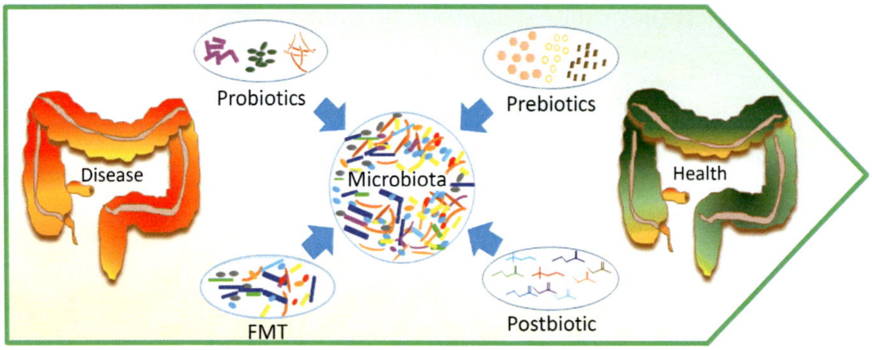

Figure 9.6. *Gut microbiota modulation. Beneficial effect on the intestinal environment through microbial composition modification, by using probiotic, prebiotic, and postbiotic administration and fecal microbiota transplantation (FMT). All these approaches can be optimized by patient-tailored treatments for the better management of the individual's physiology and pathology.*

Source: Vernocchi P, Del Chierico F, Putignani L. Gut microbiota metabolism and interaction with food components. International Journal of Molecular Sciences. 2020; 21(10):3688. https://doi.org/10.3390/ijms21103688.

Scientists often categorize probiotics based on the targeted system or potential illness they are meant to address. Some probiotic products are designed for specific diseases, rather than general health benefits, making it important to understand how probiotics work and their effects on the body to effectively treat a range of human illnesses. Probiotics are known for their antimicrobial effects, ability to improve mucosal barrier integrity, and their role in modulating the immune system.

Although other microorganisms, like the yeast *Saccharomyces*, are now also widely used, *Bifidobacterium* and *Lactobacillus* strains make up the majority of the widely commercialized probiotics. Different probiotic strains, however, do not have the same potency, and the complex gut microbial ecosystem and host immune response interactions mediate their effects. Researchers may uncover the intricate relationship between microbiota and host through targeted or untargeted metagenomics techniques and anticipated pathways, paving the way for the creation of probiotics for the coming generation. In human clinical trials, the use of recombinant LAB, which expresses advantageous molecules to promote the suppression of the inflammatory systemic immune response, has produced some encouraging results.

Conversely, in pediatric GI and respiratory infections, dietary treatment with cow's milk fermented with *Lactobacillus paracasei* CBA L74 (FM-CBAL74) has been linked to high abundance of predicted genes involved in butyrate synthesis. These days, live recombinant vectors can be produced using genetically modified lactic acid bacteria, such as *Lactococcus lactis* and some species of Lactobacilli, to advance the development of novel nontoxic mucosal vaccines. The goal of personalized probiotic therapy is to improve metabolic disorders, asthma, arthritis, and cancer by modifying the host's genetic makeup.

As previously mentioned, a number of plant polysaccharide complexes found in food are insoluble or lack hydrolytic enzymes encoded in human DNA, making them undigestible by human enzymes. These food substrates are referred to as prebiotics. Prebiotics are defined as dietary supplements and are resistant starch, β-glucans, inulin, pectin, and other GOS and FOS, and are taken to increase the level of beneficial bacteria (i.e., Bifidobacteria and LAB). After bacterial metabolism, prebiotics are substances that specifically affect the makeup or function of GM, thereby benefiting the host. They can, however, be broken down by certain bacteria that function as probiotics, and polysaccharide ingestion is crucial to their development.

Moreover, the safety and possible side effects of using probiotics to treat various pediatric illnesses have not been examined in clinical practice guidelines. Thus, more research is required to determine whether probiotic administration is appropriate for producing noticeable benefits in healthy adults. Prebiotics may have a promising therapeutic role in treating metabolic syndrome or inflammatory bowel syndrome (IBS), according to omics-based analyzes. However, more research is needed to fully understand the mode of action of prebiotics and how they affect various microbiome ecosystems. However, the response to dietary supplements varies between individuals, which can be partly explained by the makeup of the microbiome.

Furthermore, a more comprehensive dietary strategy known as "personalized nutrition" (PN) makes use of bioinformatic tools and a large set of metadata specific to a population, including a rich dataset of microbiome features. This enables personalized dietary interventions that have the potential to alter the microbiome by influencing metabolic homeostasis. Several factors may impact genetic modification (GM), with diet potentially playing a crucial role. Not only is it appealing to modify the composition and activity of genetically modified organisms through customized dietary interventions, but it also serves as a catalyst for further investigation into disease prevention and wellness maintenance.

Precision lifestyle medicine is made possible by developments in the fields of precision nutrition and human genome sequencing. This allows for the classification of various nutrient metabolisms among subgroups (e.g., lifestyle, cultural preferences, ethnicity, health status, and clinical variables) as well as inter-individual variation in responses to dietary interventions. To determine the extent to which the spread of the Western diet and lifestyle has impacted our microbial symbionts and how this has affected human health, a number of studies have focused on the co-evolution of humans and their GM counterparts. Individualized approaches to suggest optimal nutrition are being combined, but additional research is required to enhance the understanding of PN obtained from microbiome studies. Using synbiotics, which combine prebiotics and probiotics in beneficial ways, is an additional option for managing genetically modified organisms.

Prior research has indicated that synbiotics, rather than probiotics or prebiotics alone, may have a significant impact on the modulation of GM metabolic activity.

It has also been reported that synbiotic administration can improve (i) metabolic status (total cholesterol, low-density lipoprotein cholesterol (LDL-c), high-density lipoprotein cholesterol (HDL-c), triglycerides, etc.), and (ii) serum level of liver function enzymes and inflammatory biomarkers by changing the composition and/or function of the GM.

"Postbiotics" are the non-viable bacterial byproducts or metabolic byproducts obtained from probiotics. Functional products obtained from fermentation are known as postbiotics. These include teichoic acid, peptidoglycan-derived muropeptides, extracellular polysaccharides (EPS), microbial fractions, hydrogen peroxide, hydrogen peroxide, ethanol, diacetyl, acetaldehydes, and SCFAs, which may be utilized in conjunction with nutritional components to support health. These metabolic products can be used in place of antibiotics because they have a variety of inhibitory qualities against pathogenic microorganisms.

Fermented infant formulas (FIFs) and paraprobiotics are two common types of postbiotics. Paraprobiotics, also referred to as "ghost probiotics," are non-viable or inactivated probiotics that, according to the general definition, "give benefits to the host when administered in sufficient amounts." Infant formulas known as FIFs—which frequently lack live bacteria—are fermented by lactic acid-producing or other bacteria. Because of our growing understanding of the mechanisms underlying microbiota–host metabolism, the use of postbiotic molecules has emerged as a potential treatment option for a variety of inflammatory diseases. In fact, these molecules mimic the health benefits and therapeutic effects of probiotics without requiring the administration of live microorganisms to a host that has a weakened immune system.

FMT, in which a patient receives a healthy donor microbiome to correct the patient's own disease-associated microbiome, is a potentially effective microbiome intervention.

The patient will receive a fecal suspension infusion from a healthy donor rather than specific strains of bacteria as part of the probiotic-based approach to GM modulation by FMT. This treatment is currently being tested in various clinical procedures for treating a variety of pathological conditions, ranging from metabolic and neoplastic disorders to autoimmune disorders, in both adult and pediatric patients. It is also approved for the treatment of recurrent *Clostridium difficile* infections (rCDI) in adults. However, there are risks associated with transplanting an entire microbial community. When a pathogen/pathobiont is introduced into a new host with a different genetic, immunological, metabolic, and nutritional environment, it can have unfavorable effects on the transplanted microbiome and lead to incomplete long-term stabilization of an extraneous microbial configuration. To maximize the effectiveness of this method and expand the use of FMT as a clinical treatment outside of rCDI, more research is required. Clinical trials are required to standardize the registration of adverse events, patient registrations, and experimental techniques for the identification of metabolites and metagenomes linked to various disease treatments through FMT. For this reason, international agreements and/or recommendations are required for donor screening against a variety of illnesses. It has recently been proposed that the microbial diversity and composition of the donor determine the success of FMT, leading to the hypothesis of the existence of FMT super-donors and highlighting the significance of donor screening. The identification and description of super-donor gut microbes will contribute to our understanding of the bacterial causes of disease and enable the development of future therapies that are more precisely targeted.

9.7. The Latest Technical Development in the Microbiome Field

9.7.1. The Rise of Machine Learning in Gut Microbiota Analyzes

In today's world, artificial intelligence (AI) is becoming essential. AI can assist in interpreting patterns in the real world, from cars to mobile phones (smart phones). This is also true in the medical field, and particularly in the field of gut microbiome research. The gut microbiome species interact with both the host and one another, but these relationships are frequently non-linear. The majority of machine learning techniques enable the capture of these non-linear patterns. There is always a trade-off between the model's complexity (e.g., complexity and performance) the quantity of samples as well as the number of variables, trees, or layers. The number of subjects in studies involving gut microbiome interventions ranges from two to four digits. Furthermore, the model's performance is highly dependent on the target phenotype. Microbiome studies typically have a relatively small number of samples when it comes to machine learning or AI concepts. Decision-tree-based models, such as XGBoost, gradient boosting, and extreme random decision trees, are frequently used for these kinds of studies where only a small number of subjects are included. This is because these models are known to perform well when dealing with many variables relative to the number of subjects. While research questions vary amongst studies, the kind of data generated by these approaches can be applied generally, i.e., which characteristics or biomarkers are used to identify the target of interest. These machine-learning models identify more distinct, but uncultivated, species and sequences as features of interest in conjunction with the application of improved sequencing techniques.

Decision trees, for instance, have the ability to identify biomarkers based on feature importance that seem to be risk factors for the development of colorectal carcinoma. These include *Fusobacterium nucleatum*, *parvimonas* spp., and *Solobacterium moorei*, species that were also suggested to be important in earlier colon cancer studies. In contrast to what might be expected, it has been demonstrated that patients with carcinomas exhibit greater bacterial alpha diversity in comparison to healthy individuals. They may also contain a comparatively high number of species that are orally derived, which could account for the increased diversity of the gut microbiome. Similarly, a decision-tree-based machine learning technique could be used to identify T2D South Asian and African Surinamese participants. Novel T2D biomarkers may be found using machine learning. In this instance, bacterial strains linked to the butyrate-producing species *Anaerostipes hadrus* were linked to health. *Anaerostipes hadrus* has been found to have a strong association with Bacteroides enterotypes, despite being a producer of butyrate, a characteristic that is frequently, though not always, associated with health. Nonetheless, the majority of Surinamese residents in Amsterdam, particularly those with South Asian ancestry, belong to the *Bacteroides* enterotype. There is a great deal of variation within this enterotype, and *Anaerostipes hadrus* is probably a good indicator of health because it is considered to be at the top of the food pyramid for metabolic products and produces butyrate as an end product, which is a sign of a sufficient fermentative capacity. Furthermore, a multivariate analysis of the use of metformin by both ethnic groups shows that there is a strong correlation between the drug and Escherichia/shigella, which is known to be associated with the Bacteroides 2 enterotype, suggesting that metformin use may have a mediating or confounding effect on the development of the gut microbiome profile associated with the enterotype. Interestingly, when comparing the two ethnic groups, a confounding effect that may be driven by ethnicity is visible correlations in South Asian Surinamese with metformin use were stronger for a variety of species, including *Faecalibacterium* spp., *Blautia* spp., and *Anaerostipes*. Moreover, only South Asian Surinamese with type 2 diabetes who took metformin exhibited significantly reduced alpha diversity when compared to those without the condition. It is noteworthy that the alpha diversity of African Surinamese people is higher than that of Asian Surinamese people, since the latter frequently lack species related to these groups and the families *Christensenellaceae* and *Methanobrevibacter*. Pathway analyzes have shown that ethnicity and medication use have similar effects, with significant negative associations found in the isoleucine and lysine pathways and a slight positive association found in the pathways for the production of menaquinone and demethylmenaquinol. This suggests that, despite the fact that machine learning models can provide novel targets and insights, it is still difficult to relate these discoveries to functionality or causality because of a number of possible confounding factors. To enhance comprehension of the consequences revealed by the exposed targets acquired by these intricate non-linear machine learning models, one can utilize or investigate cross-sectional processes spanning numerous data domains (e.g., the metabolomic, clinical, epigenome, or microbiome) (Figure 9.7).

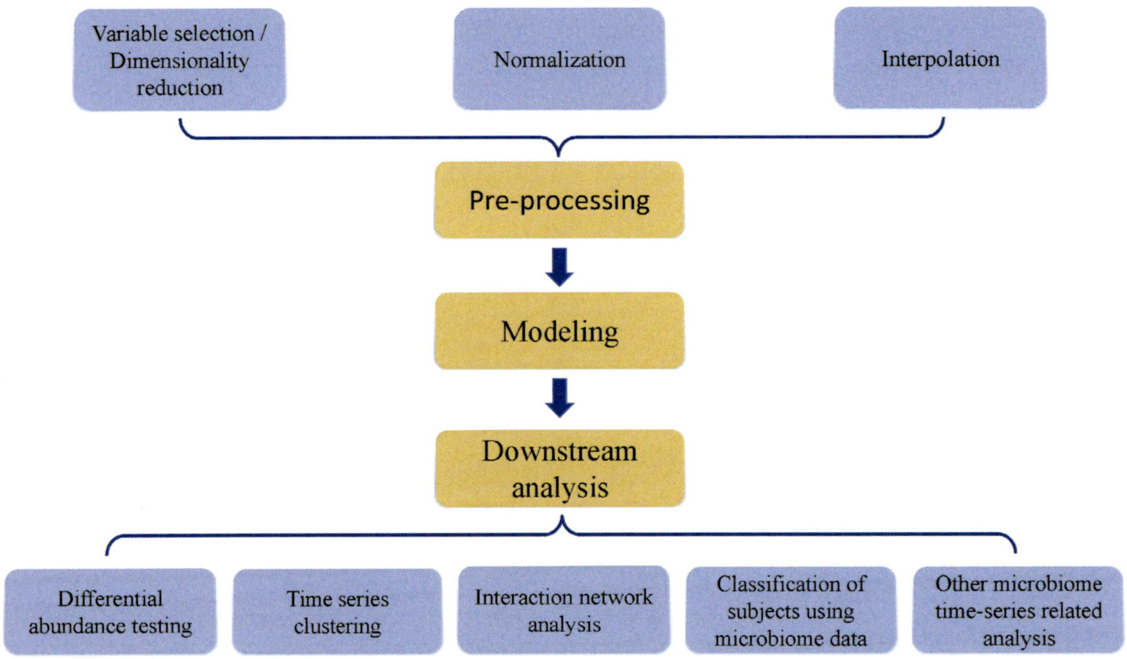

Figure 9.7. *Overview of the most commonly used methodologies to examine microbiome data and the corresponding information accordingly.*

Source: Lyu R, Qu Y, Divaris K, Wu D. Methodological considerations in longitudinal analyzes of microbiome data: A comprehensive review. Genes. 2024; 15(1):51. https://doi.org/10.3390/genes15010051.

9.7.2. Multi-Omics

The use of multi-omics techniques is growing to comprehend the relationships and operation of microbiome biomarkers in relation to a target phenotype (e.g., illness or the result of a treatment), in addition to other data kinds like clinical, metabolomic, and epigenomic data. The main components of these multi-omics analyzes are multivariate regression models, either alone or in conjunction with separately trained machine learning models. Using a combination of conventional statistics, clustering techniques, and rigid regression models, microbiome and metabolomic profiles were generated that demonstrated a strong impact of FMT on both bacterial diversity and insulin sensitivity. A small number of species, including *Lactobacillus salivarius*, *Butyrivibrio*, *Clostridium symbiosum*, and *Eubacterium* spp., were identified as producing butyrate and lactate. that differentiate autologous recipients (feces from the self) from allogeneic (feces from a donor). Additionally, responders in the allogeneic group exhibited an increase in *Akkermansia*, a condition that is frequently linked to health. This suggested that changes in DNA methylation in plasma blood mononuclear cells and certain plasma metabolite levels could be linked to changes in the gut microbiota, particularly elevated levels of *Prevotella* following an allogeneic FMT. Only a small percentage of allogeneic FMT recipients showed an increase in *Prevotella*, as the majority of FMT donors also did not exhibit significant *Prevotella* levels.

Combining various data sources is still difficult, though, because some states—like illness or health—are frequently reflected in several data domains. One may think about using a manifold approach to integrate the knowledge from the various domains, but this method might not be directly applicable to the transfer of knowledge to a single target domain. To take this issue into account, a strategy based on manifold mixing in conjunction with stacked regularization was created. The method combined all of the different data types into a single meta-model by first creating a mixed manifold of the various data modalities. More direct effects across various data domains, and consequently across various system components or systems, can be revealed by incorporating a meta-model. A follow-up study demonstrated how stacked regularization models, in conjunction with additional data sources like plasma metabolomics, clinical, nutrition, and fecal microbiome data, can produce excellent model performance and identify biomarkers linked to the effects of the intervention under investigation. It is evident that mediators, including genetics, diet, and sex, in the modality significantly helped in the interpretability of the data, and even suggested possible gut-axial linkage associations across various domains, even though several cofounders were controlled for in these studies. Many species of Bifidobacterium have been demonstrated to have a close relationship with blood levels of glutamate, lactic, and succinic acid; of particular note is the relationship between intestinal GABA levels and *Veillonella*, which is linked to brain diseases.

9.7.3. Behind Microbiome Machine Learning Analysis

In addition to current models, the application of machine learning in the microbiological field is expanding along with new techniques to uncover particularly novel species. During the development of these novel techniques, considerable emphasis has been placed on improving the interpretability of the model's decision-making. Decision trees employ feature-importance-based techniques to identify the characteristics or variables that are connected to a model's ability to successfully discriminate between two or more groups. While decision tree feature importance offers insights into the model's development process, it only offers a veiled explanation of the model's reasoning behind a particular decision. This problem has been addressed by a number of methods, such as pairwise permutated importance, local interpretable model-agnostic explanations (LIME), and permutated importance, which can be applied to other machine learning and deep learning models. These methods give direct information about the effects of the variables and evaluate how each one affects the overall model. These models, which are based on non-linear decision trees, are more intricate than conventional linear regression models. In comparison to deep neural networks, they are not as complex, and relationships and information that are pertinent to biology may go unnoticed. Inspired by the imaging world, where neural networks are becoming the gold standard for segmentation and classification purposes for various imaging types (e.g., CT, MRI, and PET), including additional artificially generated data might improve the development of such deep neural networks for microbial-based predictive purposes since a massive amount of data is required. Generative adversarial networks, or GANs, are developed in the imaging domain to produce artificial images from real data that typically contain more noise. GANs have been embraced in a variety of domains, including biomedical research, because of their exceptional performance. When compared to actual gut microbe data, the properties of the gut microbiome—such as sparsity, diversities, and taxa-taxa correlations—remained intact after the application of Microbiome Generative Adversarial Networks (MB-GANs).

While significant progress has been made in identifying new cultured and uncultured species over the years, there is still a lack of developed methodologies to comprehend the non-linear relationships between the species and features sourced from other data domains. These relationships have historically been highlighted within species and between other areas primarily through the use of traditional statistical techniques like correlations, linear regression, and univariate tests. Making certain connections between what the machine learning model has observed and phenotype becomes easier and/or more critical when linear relationships and patterns are examined and compared with similar studies. Since the results of linear analyzes are compared and reflected with the non-linear biomarkers, one could question, from a technical and biological standpoint, whether these standard approaches are able to accurately represent the outputs of machine learning. Determining causal relationships frequently requires laboratory research using models like cell cultures. However, from a practical standpoint, it is often impossible to decipher all of these intricate relationships among the (many) pertinent features through laboratory investigations. However, more biologically grounded methods are becoming available and are being applied in the field of microbiomes to analyze pathways. These methods include the analysis of metabolic pathways utilizing energy generation and composition-based models, as well as kinetic/ordinary differential equation (ODE) models.

9.7.4. Microbiome Viability and Origin

Assuming that the species found through sequencing are strains that were alive at the time of sampling, many analyzes have been conducted. The ability to sequence a specific microbial strain found in a sample with such high microbial biomass as feces led many people to conclude that this assumption is accurate. This is probably true for extremely abundant strains, but it's not always evident for many strains that are of intermediate abundance. It is now possible to determine the degree of viability in terms of active duplication thanks to recent technological developments. A single peak and a single trough lead are present in the read coverage for different microbial genomes, and these leads subsequently correspond to the replication source of the bacteria. A quantitative way to evaluate a species' viability or rate of growth is to find the ratio between its peak and trough. While this approach has potential, it is currently challenging to apply in microbiome studies for all species because all strains present in a sample must have complete reference genomes, and each strain's sequencing coverage must be sufficiently high. Gao and Li developed a multisampling method called the dynamic estimator of microbial communities (DEMIC) based on contigs and coverage values to estimate the growth rates of species that are still unknown or not fully sequenced. This method uses the relative distance from the origin of replication to determine growth rates. Reliable performance was achieved over the course of the study for various sample sizes and assemblies. Though these technological developments are very promising, it should be noted that they are limited to strain-level analysis at the species level.

Strain-tracking techniques have shown links between the microbiomes of different body sites, such as the gut and oral microbiomes, regarding the origin of species themselves. Single-nucleotide variants (SNV), from which a transmission score was derived, were the basis for associations or correlations. More convincing proof of the strain engraftment of the microbiome from the oral area into the gut is being obtained through new techniques. These techniques combine probabilistic or non-probabilistic shotgun-read metagenomics sequencing of SNV. Previous research has demonstrated that probabilistic methods offer superior sensitivity and precision. The field is still developing quickly, and in the next years, even more effective approaches should be accessible. Although strain tracking is still in its early stages, studies focused on FMT and gut microbiome intervention studies have already shown promise.

9.7.5. Sequencing Limitations and Future Directions

In the field of microbiomes, 16S sequencing remains one of the most widely used sequencing methods. Within the 16S ribosomal gene, one or combinations of multiple so-called variable regions (e.g., v1 and v3) are sequenced and subsequently analyzed with various pipelines and reference libraries to ascertain the relative abundances of microbial groups. If raw reads are processed through the same pipelines, studies using the same variable regions can be somewhat compared. However, batch effects can still occur due to variations in the DNA isolation protocol, primer selection, or operator differences. Therefore, the only comparisons that are usually possible are qualitative ones. Over time, shotgun sequencing studies have gained popularity because of their many benefits, including the fact that they are not dependent on primer selection or a particular variable region. However, batch effects still affect comparisons between studies because of variations in the pre-sequencing processing steps. Furthermore, because fractions do not equal the absolute bacterial abundances, it is difficult to compare samples in the same way even though relative abundance describes abundances within a single sample. Using a 2D method that takes into account the relative abundance of microbial groups as well as the absolute microbial load is one way to address this problem. This can be done by counting the number of cells in each sample or by adding a positive control of a known quantity before performing DNA isolation. Apart from the expense, one current drawback of shotgun sequencing is that its data analysis pipelines still rely on reference libraries, whereas the most recent 16S data analysis pipelines produce Amplicon Sequencing Variants (ASVs) without the need for a reference library. The speed at which sequencing technologies are developing is remarkable, especially when it comes to Nanopore sequencing. Because samples are sequenced individually rather than in batches, it can sequence the entire 16S gene at high sequencing depth and accuracy, enabling species-level identification. Its utility was previously limited due to high error rates, but it is now a viable alternative to 16S and shotgun sequencing. Additionally, it has the advantage of speed and may even be useful for clinical diagnostics at a relatively low cost.

A Closer Look

Acquisition in Human Infants

For the gastrointestinal tract to function properly and for an adult's health, gut flora must be established. Within a year or two of birth, humans develop an adult-like gut flora because microbiota are transferred from parent to child and from food, water, and other environmental sources. The conventional understanding of a typical fetus's digestive system is that it is sterile, however, in recent years, this understanding has been questioned. There are now several lines of evidence that point to the possibility of bacteria in the intrauterine environment. Research on humans has demonstrated that the fetus may experience microbial colonization; one study found Lactobacillus and Bifidobacterium species in placental biopsies.

The baby's stomach is quickly colonized by bacteria from the mother and the surroundings after birth. Although the precise sources of bacteria are unknown, they may come from the birth canal, other people (parents, siblings, hospital staff), food, breastmilk, and the baby's surroundings in general. Research indicates that babies delivered vaginally inherit most of their gut bacteria from their mother, whereas babies delivered by cesarean section had more bacteria linked to hospital environments. These findings highlight the significant differences in the microbiomes of babies delivered vaginally and babies delivered by cesarean section. The gut flora's composition is typically simple during the first year of life, but it varies greatly over time and amongst people. Researchers think that because the first colonizers lower the oxygen concentration in the gut, obligately anaerobic bacteria like *Bacteroidota*, *Actinomycetota*, and *Bacillota* can establish and flourish. The initial bacterial population is typically facultative anaerobic organisms. Breast milk contains prebiotic components that promote healthy bacterial growth, and it may also contain bifidobacterial growth factors, which contribute to the dominance of bifidobacteria in breastfed babies. Higher concentrations of immunoglobulin A (IgA) found in breast milk also aid in the tolerance and control of the developing child's immune system. Infants fed formula, on the other hand, have a more varied microbiota, with higher concentrations of *Bacteroides*, Clostridium, Bifidobacteria, *Enterobact*eriaceae, and enterococci.

Antibiotics, formula feeding, and Cesarean section may change the makeup of the gut microbiome. Antibiotic-treated children have less varied and stable floral communities. Cesarean sections have been demonstrated to disrupt the transmission of bacteria from mother to child, which affects the offspring's general health by increasing the risk of conditions like type 1 diabetes, asthma, and celiac disease. This provides more proof of the significance of a balanced gut microbiome. Many approaches to microbiome restoration are being investigated; these usually include giving the baby exposure to the mother's vaginal secretions and using oral probiotics.

Summary

- The gut microbiota is mainly composed of strict anaerobes, which outnumber the facultative anaerobes— organisms able to grow both aerobically and anaerobically— and the aerobes by up to 100-fold.
- The microbial composition of the gut microbiota varies across the digestive tract. In the stomach and small intestine, relatively few species of bacteria are generally present.
- Microbial colonization of the human gut begins at birth. The infant's intestines are believed to be sterile or contain a very low level of microbes at birth, but the GIT is quickly colonized during and after delivery.
- The gut flora community plays a direct role in defending against pathogens by fully colonizing the space, making use of all available nutrients, and by secreting compounds known as cytokines that kill or inhibit unwelcome organisms that would compete for nutrients with it.
- In humans, a gut flora similar to an adult's is formed within one to two years of birth. As the gut flora gets established, the lining of the intestines – the intestinal epithelium and the intestinal mucosal barrier that it secretes – develop as well, in a way that is tolerant to, and even supportive of, commensalistic microorganisms to a certain extent and also provides a barrier to pathogenic ones.
- Without gut flora, the human body would be unable to utilize some of the undigested carbohydrates it consumes, because some types of gut flora have enzymes that human cells lack for breaking down certain polysaccharides.
- The gut–brain axis is the biochemical signaling that takes place between the gastrointestinal tract and the central nervous system. That term has been expanded to include the role of the gut flora in the interplay; the term "microbiome--brain axis" is sometimes used to describe paradigms explicitly including the gut flora.
- Dysbiosis (also called dysbacteriosis) is characterized by a disruption to the microbiome resulting in an imbalance in the microbiota, changes in their functional composition and metabolic activities, or a shift in their local distribution.
- The GI tract is home to vast microbial communities including bacteria, fungi, archaea, and viruses. The microbe population is more sparse in the upper gut (stomach, duodenum, and jejunum) with approximately 10^3 bacteria per mL of aspirate, where there are approximately 10^{7}-10^{12} bacteria per mL of aspirate in the lower gut (ileum and proximal colon).
- The gut microbiota provides its host with essential health benefits primarily by maintaining healthy gut homeostasis.
- Any disruption of the body's microbiota can lead to dysbiosis. Dysbiosis in the gut happens when the bacteria in the gastrointestinal tract become unbalanced.
- The microbiota composition is subject to shaping by host and environmental selective pressures. To protect from injury and maintain homeostasis, the GI tract limits exposure of the host immune system to the microbiota by recruitment of a multifactorial and

dynamic intestinal barrier.

- Owing to its large genomic content and metabolic complement, the gut microbiota provides a range of beneficial properties to the host. Some of the most important roles of these microbes are to help to maintain the integrity of the mucosal barrier, to provide nutrients such as vitamins or to protect against pathogens.
- Probiotics are defined as live microorganisms that, when administered in adequate amounts, confer a health benefit to the host.
- Artificial intelligence (AI) is becoming indispensable in today's world. From cars to mobile (smart) phones, AI can help interpret patterns in the real world and the same is true in the medical world, and, more specifically, in the gut microbiome field.
- Multi-omics approaches are increasingly being implemented to understand the associations and functionality of how microbiome biomarkers are linked to a target phenotype (e.g., disease or the outcome of an intervention), as well as with other data types, such as clinical, metabolomic, and epigenomic data.

References

1. Arumugam, M., et al. (2011). Enterotypes of the human gut microbiome. *Nature, 473*(7346), 174–180.
2. Brestoff, J. R., & Artis, D. (2013). Commensal bacteria at the interface of host metabolism and the immune system. *Nature Immunology, 14*, 676–684.
3. Canny, G. O., & McCormick, B. A. (2008). Bacteria in the intestine, helpful residents or enemies from within. *Infection and Immunity, 76*(8), 3360–3373.
4. Clarke, G., Stilling, R. M., Kennedy, P. J., Stanton, C., Cryan, J. F., & Dinan, T. G. (2014). Gut microbiota: The neglected endocrine organ. *Molecular Endocrinology, 28*, 1221–1238.
5. De Preter, V., Hamer, H. M., Windey, K., & Verbeke, K. (2011). The impact of pre- and/or probiotics on human colonic metabolism: Does it affect human health? *Molecular Nutrition & Food Research, 55*(1), 46–57.
6. Delzenne, N. M., & Williams, C. M. (2002). Prebiotics and lipid metabolism. *Current Opinion in Lipidology, 13*, 61–67.
7. den Besten, G., et al. (2013). The role of short-chain fatty acids in the interplay between diet, gut microbiota, and host energy metabolism. *Journal of Lipid Research, 54*(9), 2325–2340.
8. Fasano, A. (2012). Zonulin, regulation of tight junctions, and autoimmune diseases. Ann N Y Acad Sci. 2012 Jul; 1258(1): 25–33.
9. Hills RD Jr, Pontefract BA, Mishcon HR, Black CA, Sutton SC, Theberge CR. Gut Microbiome: Profound Implications for Diet and Disease. Nutrients. 2019 Jul 16;11(7):1613.
10. Hinnebusch, B. F., Meng, S., Wu, J. T., Archer, S. Y., & Hodin, R. A. (2002). The effects of short-chain fatty acids on human colon cancer cell phenotype are associated with histone hyperacetylation. *Journal of Nutrition, 132*, 1012–1017.
11. Hooper, L. V., Littman, D. R., & Macpherson, A. J. (2012). Interactions between the microbiota and the immune system. *Science, 336*, 1268–1273.

12. Hsiao, E. Y., et al. (2013). Microbiota modulate behavioral and physiological abnormalities associated with neurodevelopmental disorders. *Cell, 155*, 1451–1463.

13. Jandhyala, S. M. (2015). Role of the normal gut microbiota. *World Journal of Gastroenterology, 21*(29), 8787–8803.

14. Lan, A., Lagadic-Gossmann, D., Lemaire, C., Brenner, C., & Jan, G. (2007). Acidic extracellular pH shifts colorectal cancer cell death from apoptosis to necrosis upon exposure to propionate and acetate, major end-products of the human probiotic propionibacteria. *Apoptosis, 12*, 573–591.

15. Leech B, McIntyre E, Steel A, Sibbritt D. Risk factors associated with intestinal permeability in an adult population: A systematic review. Int J Clin Pract. 2019 Oct;73(10):e13385.

16. Maranduba, C. M. da C., De Castro, S. B. R., Souza, G. T. de, Rossato, C., Da Guia, F. C., Valente, M. A. S., Macedo, G. C. (2015). Intestinal microbiota as modulators of the immune system and neuroimmune system: Impact on the host health and homeostasis. *Journal of Immunology Research, 2015*, 931574.

17. Martinez, K. B., Leone, V., & Chang, E. B. (2017). Microbial metabolites in health and disease: Navigating the unknown in search of function. *Journal of Biological Chemistry, 292*, 8553–8559.

18. Maurice, C. F., Haiser, H. J., & Turnbaugh, P. J. (2013). Xenobiotics shape the physiology and gene expression of the active human gut microbiome. *Cell, 152*, 39–50.

19. Morowitz, M. J., Carlisle, E., & Alverdy, J. C. (2011). Contributions of intestinal bacteria to nutrition and metabolism in the critically ill. *Surgical Clinics of North America, 91*(4), 771–785.

20. Mu Q, Kirby J, Reilly CM, Luo XM. Leaky Gut As a Danger Signal for Autoimmune Diseases. Front Immunol. 2017 May 23;8:598.

21. Nicholson, J. K., et al. (2012). Host-gut microbiota metabolic interactions. *Science, 336*, 1262–1267.

22. Portune KJ, Benítez-Páez A, Del Pulgar EM, Cerrudo V, Sanz Y. Gut microbiota, diet, and obesity-related disorders-The good, the bad, and the future challenges. Mol Nutr Food Res. 2017 Jan;61(1).

23. Prakash, S., Rodes, L., Coussa-Charley, M., Tomaro-Duchesneau, C., & Coussa-Charley, R. (2011). Gut microbiota: Next frontier in understanding human health and development of biotherapeutics. *Biologics: Targets and Therapy, 5*, 71–86.

24. Quinn, R. A., et al. (2014). Biogeochemical forces shape the composition and physiology of polymicrobial communities in the cystic fibrosis lung. *mBio, 5*, e00956–13.

25. Sharon, G., et al. (2014). Specialized metabolites from the microbiome in health and disease. *Cell Metabolism, 20*, 719–730.

26. Sheflin, A. M., Melby, C. L., Carbonero, F., & Weir, T. L. (2017). Linking dietary patterns with gut microbial composition and function. *Gut Microbes, 8*, 113–129.

27. Soret, R., Chevalier, J., De Coppet, P., Poupeau, G., Derkinderen, P., Segain, J. P., & Neunlist, M. (2010). Short-chain fatty acids regulate the enteric neurons and control gastrointestinal motility in rats. *Gastroenterology, 138*, 1772–1782.

28. Sung, J., Kim, S., Cabatbat, J. J. T., Jang, S., Jin, Y.-S., Jung, G. Y., Chia, N., & Kim, P. J. (2017). Global metabolic interaction network of the human gut microbiota for context-specific community-scale analysis. *Nature Communications, 8*, 15393.

29. Tremaroli, V., & Bäckhed, F. (2012). Functional interactions between the gut microbiota and host metabolism. *Nature, 489*, 242–249.

30. Visconti, A., Le Roy, C. I., Rosa, F., Rossi, N., Martin, T. C., Mohney, R. P., Li, W., de Rinaldis, E., Bell, J. T., Venter, J. C., & et al. (2019). Interplay between the human gut microbiome and host metabolism. *Nature Communications, 10*, 4505.

31. Wu, G. D., Chen, J., Hoffmann, C., Bittinger, K., Chen, Y. Y., Keilbaugh, S. A., Bewtra, M., Knights, D., Walters, W. A., Knight, R., Sinha, R., Gilroy, E., Gupta, K., Baldassano, R., Nessel, L., Li, H., Bushman, F. D., & Lewis, J. D. (2011). Linking long-term dietary patterns with gut microbial enterotypes. *Science, 334*(6052), 105–108.

32. Yadav, M., Verma, M. K., & Chauhan, N. S. (2018). A review of metabolic potential of human gut microbiome in human nutrition. *Archives of Microbiology, 200*, 203–217.

Chapter 10

DISEASES OF THE DIGESTIVE SYSTEM

Contents

Introduction

The gastrointestinal tract (GI), liver, pancreas, and gallbladder comprise the digestive system, which aids in the body's food digestion. The process of digestion is critical for the breakdown of food into the nutrients your body needs for growth, repair, and energy. A wide spectrum of illnesses, from mild to severe, fall under the category of digestive disorders. Gastroesophageal reflux disease, hiatal hernias, lactose intolerance, cancer, and irritable bowel syndrome are common digestive disorders. Digestion disorders are most commonly characterized by bleeding, bloating, constipation, diarrhea, heartburn, pain, nausea, and vomiting. Gaining a precise diagnosis of digestive disorders requires both a physical examination and a comprehensive medical history. For patients suffering from digestive disorders, more thorough diagnostic evaluations involving endoscopic procedures, laboratory testing, and imaging may be necessary.

Orientation and Directional Terms

Term	Definition	Illustration
Gastroesophageal Reflux Disease (GERD)	Heartburn happens, but if it occurs regularly, you may need to be evaluated for GERD. A medical provider can often diagnose GERD based on a description of symptoms alone, but if the problem has been ongoing for some time, additional diagnostic testing may be necessary to evaluate if the disease has caused damage to the esophagus.	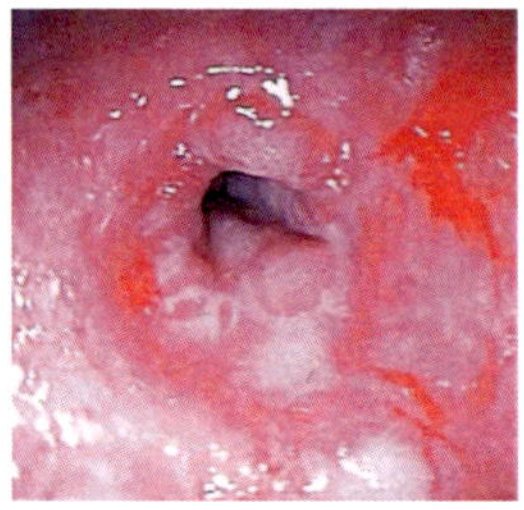
Helicobacter pylori	*Helicobacter pylori*, previously known as Campylobacter pylori, is a gram-negative, flagellated, helical bacterium. Mutants can have a rod or curved rod shape, and these are less effective.	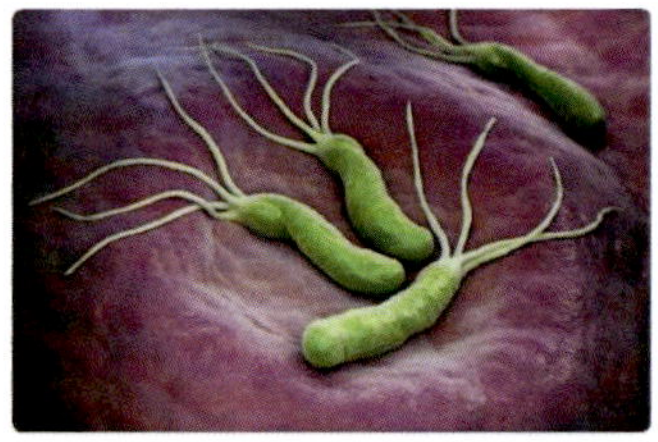
Gastroparesis	Gastroparesis is a paralysis of your stomach muscles. It's often caused by nerve damage, most commonly from diabetes.	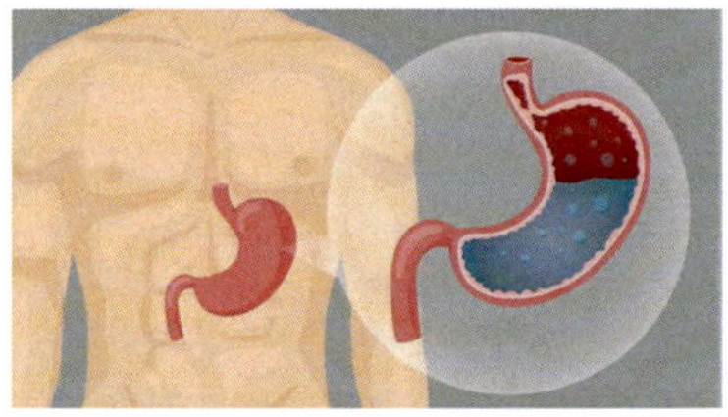
Pancreatitis	Pancreatitis is a painful inflammation in your pancreas, an organ in the middle of your abdomen. It can be chronic or acute.	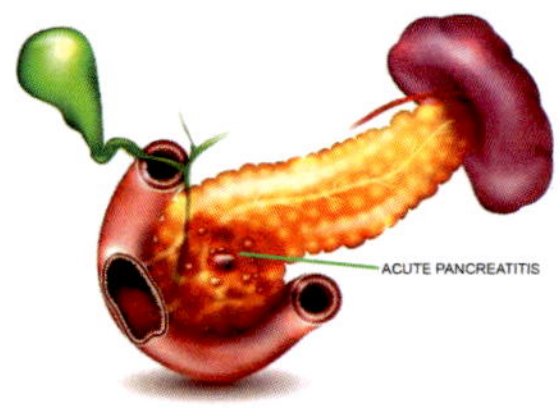
Liver Cirrhosis	Cirrhosis is a condition in which your liver is scarred and permanently damaged. Scar tissue replaces healthy liver tissue and prevents your liver from working normally. As cirrhosis gets worse, your liver begins to fail.	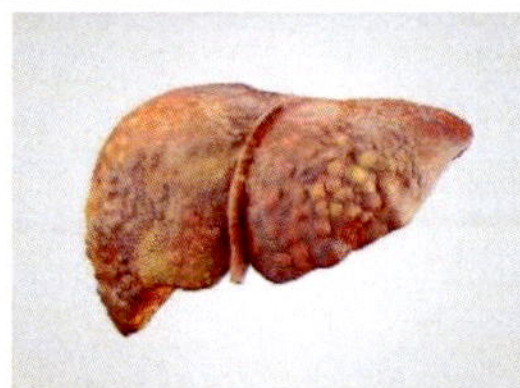
Crohn's Disease	Crohn's disease is a type of inflammatory bowel disease (IBD) that causes your digestive tract to become swollen and irritated.	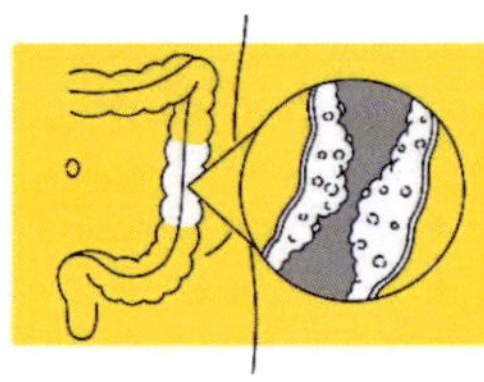

10.1. Disorders in Esophagus

The esophagus, which is the tube that transports food from your mouth to your stomach, is impacted by esophageal disorders. The most typical kind is GERD. Heartburn and difficulty swallowing are symptoms of disorders such as GERD, achalasia, and Barrett's esophagus, which also raise the risk of esophageal cancer. Medication can be helpful, as can dietary and lifestyle modifications.

10.1.1. GERD

Acid reflux from the stomach constantly running back into the esophagus, the tube that connects your mouth and stomach, is known as gastroesophageal reflux disease (GERD). The lining of your esophagus may become irritated by this backwash, or acid reflux. Periodically, a lot of people experience acid reflux. GERD can develop, though, if acid reflux occurs frequently over an extended period of time. With medication and lifestyle modifications, the majority of people can control their GERD discomfort. Even though it's rare, some people may require surgery to relieve their symptoms.

10.1.1.1. Symptoms

The following are typical GERD signs and symptoms.

- Heartburn is a burning feeling in your chest that usually occurs after eating and may be worse at night or while you're lying down.
- Regurgitating food or sour liquids, or backwashing.
- Upper abdominal or chest pain
- Trouble swallowing (dysphagia)
- Sensation of a lump in your throat
- If you have nighttime acid reflux, you might also experience:
- An ongoing cough
- Vocal cord inflammation (laryngitis).
- New or worsening asthma

When to See a Doctor. If you experience arm, jaw, or chest pain, or shortness of breath, get medical attention right away. These could be heart attack warning signs and symptoms.

Schedule a visit with your physician in the event that:

- Suffer from frequent or severe GERD symptoms
- Utilize over-the-counter heartburn remedies more than twice a week

10.1.1.2. Causes

Frequent stomach acid reflux or reflux of nonacidic content is the cause of GERD. The lower esophageal sphincter, a circular band of muscle that surrounds the bottom of your esophagus, relaxes during swallowing to let food and liquids pass into your stomach. The sphincter then shuts once more.

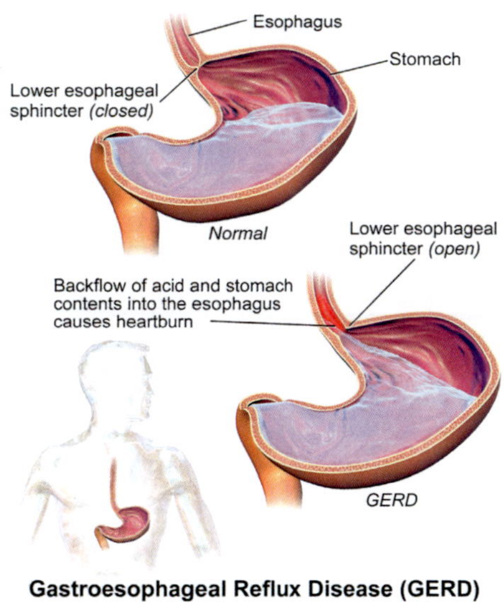

Figure 10.1. *A comparison of a healthy condition to GERD.*

Source: By BruceBlaus – Own work, CC BY-SA 4.0, https://commons.wikimedia.org/w/index.php?curid=44923646.

Stomach acid can return to your esophagus if the sphincter weakens or fails to relax as it should. The lining of your esophagus becomes irritated by this continuous backwash of acid, which frequently results in inflammation (Figure 10.1).

10.1.1.3. Risk Factors for GERD

Over 15 million adults in America, including many pregnant women, experience heartburn every day, and over 60 million adults experience it at least once a month. Unbeknownst to medical professionals, GERD in infants and children is more common than previously believed. Recurrent episodes of vomiting may result from it. In addition, it may result in coughing and other respiratory issues. Hiatal hernias are thought by some medical professionals to weaken the LES and increase the risk of reflux disease. When the upper portion of your stomach pushes through a tiny hole in your diaphragm and into your chest, it is called a hiatal hernia (diaphragmatic hiatus). The muscle that divides the chest and abdomen is called the diaphragm. According to recent research, the diaphragm's opening aids in supporting the lower portion of the esophagus.

Heartburn or reflux is rare in many patients with hiatal hernias. However, a hiatal hernia may make it easier for stomach contents to reflux into the esophagus. A hiatal hernia can result from sudden physical exertion, vomiting, coughing, or straining that increases pressure in the abdomen. Many fifty and older adults in otherwise good health have a small one. Hiatal hernias can affect people of any age, but they typically affect those in their middle years. Most of the time, hiatal hernias heal on their own. However, it might be required if there is a risk that the hernia could become strangulated or twisted in a way that would cut off the blood supply. If you have one and severe GERD or esophagitis (esophageal inflammation), you might also need to treat it. Your physician might operate to reduce the size of the hernia or avoid strangulation. There are numerous other factors that can increase your risk of developing GERD that include:

- Being overweight or obese
- Pregnancy
- Delayed stomach emptying (gastroparesis).
- Disorders of the connective tissue, like lupus, scleroderma, and rheumatoid arthritis.
- If you already have acid reflux, certain dietary and lifestyle choices may exacerbate it:
- Smoking
- Some foods and beverages, such as chocolate, fried or fatty foods, coffee, and alcohol.
- Large meals
- Eating too soon before bed
- Certain medications, including aspirin

10.1.1.4. GERD Symptoms

Acid reflux disease, also known as heartburn, is the most typical GERD symptom. Usually, it feels like a searing pain in your chest that travels up to your neck and throat from behind your breastbone. A lot of people report feeling as though food is returning to their mouths, leaving behind an acidic or bitter taste. Heartburn can cause pressure, burning, or pain that lasts for up to two hours. Usually, it gets worse after eating. Additionally, bending over or lying down can cause heartburn. Many people find that standing up straight or taking an antacid that removes acid from the esophagus helps them feel better.

There are distinctions between the pain of heartburn and that of heart disease or a heart attack, which is sometimes the case. While resting may lessen heart disease pain, exercise may exacerbate it. Physical activity has a lower correlation with heartburn pain. You can't tell the difference, though, so if you experience any chest pain, get medical attention straight away. Other than pain, you might experience:

- Nausea
- Bad breath
- Trouble breathing
- A hard time swallowing
- Vomiting
- Wearing a way of tooth enamel
- A lump in your throat
- You might also have the following if you experience acid reflux at night.
- A lingering cough
- Laryngitis
- Asthma that comes on suddenly or gets worse
- Sleep problems

10.1.1.5. GERD Treatment and Home Remedies

The goal of GERD treatment is to reduce reflux or the harm that refluxed materials cause to the lining of the esophagus. To treat your symptoms, your doctor might suggest over-the-counter or prescription drugs.

- Antacids: These medications can help prevent heartburn by neutralizing stomach and esophageal acid. A lot of people discover that over-the-counter antacids offer fleeting or incomplete relief. For certain people, combining an antacid with a foaming agent is helpful. Scientists believe that these substances create a foam layer over the stomach to prevent acid reflux. However, prolonged antacid use can cause a buildup of magnesium in the body, altered calcium metabolism (a change in how the body breaks down and uses calcium), and diarrhea. For those with kidney disease, an excess of magnesium can be dangerous. See your doctor if you require antacids for a period longer than two weeks.
- H2 blockers: In cases of persistent reflux and heartburn, the physician might suggest drugs that lower stomach acid. Among these medications are H2 blockers, which assist in preventing the stomach's production of acid. Cimetidine (Tagamet), famotidine (Pepcid), and nizatidine are examples of H2 blockers.
- Proton pump inhibitors (PPIs): These medications, also called acid pumps, inhibit a protein required for the production of stomach acid. PPIs consist of pantoprazole (Protonix), rabeprazole (Aciphex), omeprazole (Prilosec), lansoprazole (Prevacid), esomeprazole (Nexium), and dexlansoprazole (Dexilant).
- Prokinetics: In certain instances, these medications can assist in speeding up the emptying of your stomach to reduce the amount of remaining acid. They may also alleviate symptoms such as bloating, nausea, and vomiting. However, they do come with potential harmful side effects. Not everyone is able to tolerate these medications and those who can should only use them for a short period. Examples of prokinetics are domperidone and metoclopramide (Clopra, Maxolon, Metozolv, Reglan).

10.1.1.6. Diet and Lifestyle Changes

Doctors advise you to modify your lifestyle in a few ways to help reduce your GERD symptoms.

- **Avoid Foods and Beverage Triggers:** Foods like chocolate, peppermint, fatty foods, caffeine, and alcoholic beverages should be avoided as they can relax the LES. Citrus fruits and juices, tomato products, and pepper are among the foods and drinks that should be avoided if they cause symptoms due to their potential to irritate a damaged esophageal lining.
- **Eat Smaller Servings:** Reducing the size of meals may also aid in symptom management. Additionally, eating meals two to three hours before going to bed allows your stomach to partially empty and reduce acid production.
- **Eat Slowly:** Take your time at every meal.
- Chew your food thoroughly: If you put down your fork after a bite, it might help you remember to do this. Only pick it back up after you've fully chewed and swallowed that bite.
- **Stop Smoking:** Smoking cigarettes weakens the LES. It's critical to give up smoking to lessen GERD symptoms.
- **Elevate Your Head:** Gravity can reduce the amount that refluxes into your esophagus when you sleep on a specially made wedge or raise the head of your bed on 6-inch blocks. Avoid using pillows as self-support. That only makes the stomach feel more compressed.
- **Stay at a Healthy Weight:** Symptoms are frequently made worse by obesity. When they lose weight, many overweight people experience relief.
- **Wear loose clothes:** Wearing clothing that clings to your waist puts strain on your lower esophagus and belly.
- **Acupuncture:** Acupuncture treatment prevented reflux in the test group more effectively than proton pump inhibitors, with longer-lasting effects.

10.1.1.7. Severe GERD Diagnosis

You might require testing to get a more accurate diagnosis if you have severe, chronic reflux disease or if treatment doesn't improve your symptoms. To do this, your doctor might perform one or more procedures as follows:

- **Endoscopy**: Your physician will insert an endoscope—a tiny, illuminated tube with a tiny video camera on the end—into your esophagus to check for tissue irritation or inflammation (esophagitis). They might take a tiny tissue sample for additional testing (biopsy) if the results are unusual or dubious.
- **Upper GI Series:** One of your doctor's initial tests might be this one. This type of X-ray displays your stomach, duodenum, and upper portion of your small intestine. It can help rule out other conditions, like peptic ulcers, but it provides limited information about potential reflux.
- **Esophageal Manometry and Impedance Study:** This test looks

for signs of low esophageal pressure. It may also reveal abnormalities in the contraction of your esophageal muscles.

- **pH testing:** Your doctor may use this test to measure the acid levels in your esophagus if a definitive diagnosis is difficult to make. It monitors your esophageal acid production during meals, physical activity, and sleep. This is a more useful tool now that longer-term pH tracking has been done using newer methods.

10.1.1.8. Surgery for Severe GERD

You might require GERD surgery if your symptoms cannot be controlled with medicine, you have a hiatal hernia, and you require frequent high doses of PPIs. However, you ought to exhaust all alternative therapies first.

- **Fundoplication:** Your lower esophageal pressure will rise as a result of this operation. Your stomach's upper region will be wound around the LES by the doctor. To stop reflux, this tightens the muscle and increases the pressure in your lower esophagus. They will either perform open surgery or use a laparoscope, which is a device that pokes tiny holes in the abdomen.
- **Transoral Incisionless Fundoplication (TIF):** An endoscope, a tiny tube with a camera, is used in a more recent version of this procedure to wrap the stomach around the LES using plastic fasteners. It requires less incision than a typical fundoplication.
- **Stretta Procedure:** Your LES will be reshaped by your doctor using low-radiofrequency heat and a tiny tube that is inserted down your esophagus.
- **LINX Surgery:** Your esophageal-gastric junction is bandaged by your physician with magnetic titanium beads. The beads' magnetic pull keeps it just tight enough to prevent reflux but loose enough to allow food to pass through into the stomach.

10.1.1.9. GERD Complications

Sometimes GERD leads to serious complications:

- **Esophageal Ulcer:** Your esophagus is eroded by stomach acid until an open sore appears. These sores may bleed and are frequently painful. They could make swallowing difficult.
- **Esophageal Stricture:** The lower portion of your esophagus is harmed by stomach acid, which also forms scar tissue. The accumulation of scar tissue causes the esophagus to narrow, making it difficult to swallow food.
- **Barrett's Esophagus:** Acid reflux modifies the esophageal lining's cellular composition. The lining thickens and becomes crimson. This illness is associated with an increased risk of esophageal cancer.
- **Lung Problems:** Reflux can irritate and hurt your throat if it reaches the back. It can then enter the lungs through perspiration from there. You might get hoarse if this occurs. It's also possible that you

have a persistent cough and chest congestion. You run the risk of developing pneumonia, bronchitis, and asthma if your lungs become inflamed.

10.1.2. Achalasia

The esophagus, which is the tube that connects the throat and stomach, is impacted by the uncommon swallowing disorder achalasia. The esophageal muscles malfunction in achalasia sufferers, making it difficult for food to pass down toward the stomach. Simultaneously, the lower esophageal sphincter (LES), a ring of muscle at the base of the esophagus, is unable to relax and allow food to pass into the stomach. Adults with achalasia usually range in age from 30 to 60, peaking in their 40s. Men are roughly twice as likely as women to have the disorder.

10.1.2.1. Achalasia Causes

Although achalasia's causes are unknown, researchers are investigating several theories. One has to do with the deterioration of the nerve cells that lie in the space between the esophageal muscles' layers. Food can be forced into and into the stomach by the esophagus thanks to these nerve cells. A possible correlation between parasitic or viral infections and achalasia has been suggested by certain studies. Individuals diagnosed with achalasia may exhibit a higher likelihood of presenting symptoms of prior infections, including antibodies to the measles virus, human papillomavirus, and herpes simplex virus. Additionally, there is evidence that suggests achalasia could be an inflammatory autoimmune disorder, meaning the body could attack itself to cause the condition. Scientists have observed immune system activity in the nerve cells that supply strength to the esophageal muscles. Additionally, autoimmune diseases like uveitis, type I diabetes, rheumatoid arthritis, systemic lupus erythematosus, and Sjögren's syndrome are three to six times more common in patients with achalasia.

10.1.2.2. Achalasia Symptoms

Food buildup in the esophagus that prevents it from passing into the stomach can contribute to certain symptoms of achalasia. The esophagus widens and may twist as it fills up. The abnormal contractions of the esophageal muscles are linked to additional symptoms of achalasia. Achalasia symptoms usually appear during or right after meals. Among them are:

- The most common symptom of achalasia is the sensation that food or liquids are difficult to swallow and are "sticking" or getting caught in the esophagus on the way down to the stomach.
- Regurgitation or the backflow of food and liquids into the mouth following swallowing.
- Chest pain, which can be very intense and cause a person to wake up.
- Heartburn
- Coughing, especially at night
- Choking or aspirating food particles or liquids into one's airways.

One or more of the initial symptoms of achalasia, such as regurgitation and chest pain, are also linked to gastroesophageal reflux disease (GERD). The two situations are not the same, though. Too much slack in the lower esophageal sphincter allows stomach acid to pass through and cause GERD. The sphincter is overly constricted in achalasia. The symptoms of achalasia can worsen. Severe achalasia can cause severe exhaustion, weight loss, malnourishment, and chest pain. Food particles can cause pneumonia, an inflammation of the airways that can be fatal if they get into the airways as a result of coughing or choking during eating.

10.1.2.3. Types of Achalasia

There are differences in the way esophageal muscles contract in individuals with achalasia. The lower esophageal sphincter, which regulates the passage between the esophagus and the stomach, malfunctions to relax at the appropriate moment in all cases of achalasia. Three types of achalasia have been identified by medical professionals based on concurrent problems.

- Sometimes, type 1 achalasia is referred to as classic achalasia. Food descends due to gravity alone in this type of reflux because the esophageal muscles hardly contract.
- The esophagus becomes compressed in Type 2 achalasia as a result of increased pressure inside it. Compared to type I, this is the most prevalent type of achalasia and frequently results in more severe symptoms.
- Atypical contractions occur at the base of the esophagus where it joins the stomach, causing type 3 achalasia, also known as spastic achalasia. The severity of this achalasia type is the highest. The chest pain that the contractions may produce can mimic the signs of a heart attack and wake someone up from sleep.

10.1.2.4. Achalasia Diagnosis

Apart from a comprehensive physical assessment and a review of your medical background and symptoms, your physician might suggest the following tests to aid in the diagnosis of achalasia.

- Using pharyngeal and esophageal manometry, you can monitor and document variations in the pressure in your throat and esophagus while you swallow. Because manometry can identify the location and degree of muscle contractions that impair swallowing ability—or lack thereof—some believe it to be the most accurate test for achalasia.
- Upper endoscopy: This procedure uses an endoscope, a thin tube with a camera inserted through the mouth, to examine the stomach and esophagus. This test aids in identifying esophageal abnormalities such as tumors and strictures, or narrowing. Your doctor may take a biopsy or remove any abnormal tissue for additional examination during an endoscopy.
- To assess the level of acidity in the esophagus over an extended period and rule out other conditions like GERD, use wireless pH testing or 24-hour pH impedance testing.
- Barium swallow is an imaging test that produces images of the upper gastrointestinal (GI) tract using X-rays and the contrast medium barium. A significant narrowing of the esophagus, sometimes referred to as an achalasia bird beak, may be detected by this test.

10.1.2.5. Achalasia Treatment

Although there are currently no cures for achalasia, there are a number of ways to manage the condition's symptoms, including dilation, surgery, injections of botulinum toxin, and medication. The aim of treatment is to help the sphincter relax and permit food to pass into the stomach while also returning the esophageal contractions to normal.

- **Dilation of the Esophageal Sphincter:** Dilation refers to the act of widening a passageway. In a dilation procedure for achalasia, a gastroenterologist gently inflates a balloon close to the lower esophageal sphincter while the patient is sedated and an endoscope is inserted into the mouth and esophagus. By doing this, you can stretch the sphincter muscles and lower the pressure inside the esophagus, allowing food and liquids to pass through more easily. Probably the most popular method of treating achalasia is balloon dilation. Following the procedure, the majority of patients (65–80%) report a significant improvement in their ability to swallow. The relief, though, might only last temporarily, as achalasia symptoms can recur and necessitate additional care.
- **Achalasia Surgery — Esophageal Myotomy:** To keep the muscles in the esophagus, lower stomach, and esophageal sphincter from tightening, a gastroenterologist performs a myotomy. An achalasia myotomy can be executed through multiple small abdominal incisions (laparoscopic Heller myotomy) or through the mouth using an endoscope (peroral endoscopic myotomy, or POEM). Just enough muscle is disrupted by a lower esophageal sphincter myotomy to relieve the symptoms of achalasia, but not enough to result in acid reflux. Although it is not suitable for all patients, this is the most long-term treatment for achalasia.
- **Botulinum Toxin Injections:** Certain patients with achalasia have shown improvement after receiving a botulinum toxin injection into the lower esophageal sphincter. Older patients and those who are not candidates for dilation or myotomy benefit most from these treatments. The sphincter and nearby nerves are made numb by botulinum toxin injections, which causes the sphincter to relax. An endoscope is used to insert a special needle during the injections. Their limited impact lasts for approximately a year. Injections may need to be given again. Following this treatment, there have been reports of skin rashes and mild chest pain in certain patients.
- **Medications for Achalasia:** In general, achalasia cannot be effectively treated with medication. Lower esophageal sphincter temporary relaxation is possible with certain medications that contain calcium channel blockers or nitrates. But they have to be taken before every meal, and generally speaking, the negative effects outweigh the positive ones.

10.1.2.6. Living with Achalasia

Following achalasia treatment, you should work with your doctor to look into other options if your symptoms persist. Changing your eating habits, diet, or other aspects of your lifestyle may improve your quality of life.

10.1.3. Barrett's Esophagus

Barrett's esophagus is a disorder where acid reflux damages the lining of the esophagus, the flat, pink tube that connects the mouth to the stomach. As a result, the lining thickens and turns red. The lower esophageal sphincter (LES) is a vital valve that sits between the esophagus and the stomach. Gastroesophageal reflux disease (GERD) is a condition caused by acid and chemical damage to the esophagus caused by the LES failing over time. Heartburn and regurgitation are common symptoms of GERD. Barrett's esophagus is a condition where the lining of the lower esophagus changes as a result of GERD in certain individuals.

An increased risk of esophageal cancer is linked to Barrett's esophagus. Despite the low risk of esophageal cancer, it is crucial to have frequent examinations with meticulous imaging and thorough esophageal biopsies to screen for precancerous cells (dysplasia). To stop esophageal cancer, precancerous cells can be treated if they are found.

10.1.3.1. Symptoms

The most common cause of Barrett's esophagus is chronic GERD, which can manifest as any of the following symptoms:

- Frequent reflux of stomach contents and heartburn.
- Difficulty swallowing food
- Less commonly, chest pain

It's interesting to note that only about 50% of patients with Barrett's esophagus report having minimal to no symptoms of acid reflux. Therefore, you should talk to your doctor about the possibility of Barrett's esophagus in relation to your digestive health.

- **When to See a Doctor:** Consult your physician regarding your risk of Barrett's esophagus if you have experienced heartburn, regurgitation, or acid reflux for longer than five years. Get aid right away if you:
    - Feel pain in your chest, which could be a sign of a heart attack.
    - Have difficulty swallowing
    - Are throwing up blood in the form of coffee grounds or red blood.
    - Are passing black, tarry or bloody stools
    - Are unintentionally losing weight

10.1.3.2. Causes

It is unknown what specifically causes Barrett's esophagus. Although GERD is common in people with Barrett's esophagus, many also have silent reflux or no reflux symptoms at all. Barrett's esophagus is caused by stomach acid and chemicals that wash back into the esophagus, damaging tissue and altering the swallowing tube's lining whether or not GERD symptoms are present.

10.1.3.3. Risk factors

The following variables raise your risk of Barrett's esophagus:

- **Family History:** If esophageal cancer or Barrett's esophagus run in your family, your chances of developing these conditions rise.
- **Being male:** Men are far more likely to develop Barrett's esophagus.
- **Being White:** Compared to people of other races, white people are more likely to contract the illness.
- **Age**: Although it can happen at any age, adults over 50 are more likely

to have Barrett's esophagus.

- Acid reflux disease and chronic heartburn. Barrett's esophagus is more common in people with GERD that is unresponsive to proton pump inhibitor treatment or in people with GERD that needs ongoing medication.
- Current or past smoking.
- Being overweight. Your risk is further increased by abdominal body fat.

10.1.3.4. Complications

Barrett's esophagus is not a serious medical emergency. However, in a small percentage of cases, Barrett's esophagus can result in precancerous changes. Less than 1% of individuals with Barrett's esophagus go on to develop esophageal adenocarcinoma, a dangerous and potentially fatal esophageal cancer. This is a very tiny increase in risk if you have Barrett's esophagus. Regular checkups will help your doctor detect precancerous and cancerous cells early on, when the disease is easier to treat and before they can spread.

10.1.3.5. Diagnosis

The most common method for identifying Barrett's esophagus is endoscopy. Your throat is examined with an endoscope, a lit tube with a camera at the end, to look for indications of shifting esophageal tissue. Normal esophageal tissue has a glossy, pale appearance. The tissue in Barrett's esophagus has a velvety, red appearance. Your esophagus will be biopsied, or tissue removed, by your doctor. To ascertain the extent of change, the biopsied tissue can be examined.

- **Determining the Degree of Tissue Change:** The level of dysplasia in your esophageal cells is assessed by a pathologist, a medical professional who specializes in analyzing tissue in a lab. It is best to have two pathologists agree on your diagnosis because dysplasia in the esophagus can be challenging to diagnose, with at least one of them specializing in gastroenterology pathology. You could categorize your tissue as:
  - If Barrett's esophagus is present but there are no precancerous alterations in the cells, there is no dysplasia.
  - Low-grade dysplasia, in which cells exhibit minute indications of cancerous alterations.
  - Elevated dysplasia, if numerous alterations are seen in the cells. It is believed that high-grade dysplasia is the last stage before cells transform into esophageal cancer.
- **Screening for Barrett's Esophagus:** According to the American College of Gastroenterology, screening may be advised for men who have at least two additional risk factors, such as the following, and who have experienced GERD symptoms at least once a week that do not improve after taking a proton pump inhibitor medication.
  - Barrett's esophagus or esophageal cancer running in the family.
  - Being male
  - Being white
  - Being over 50
  - Being a current or past smoker
  - Having a lot of abdominal fat

Despite the fact that women are much less likely than men to have Barrett's esophagus, if they have uncontrolled reflux or other risk factors, they should get screened.

10.1.3.6. Treatment

The degree of aberrant cell growth in your esophagus and your general state of health will determine how you are treated for Barrett's esophagus.

- **No Dysplasia:** Your doctor will likely recommend:
  - Routine endoscopy to keep an eye on the esophageal cells. You will likely have a follow-up endoscopy in a year if your biopsies reveal no dysplasia, and then every three to five years if no changes take place.
  - Treatment for GERD. Changes in lifestyle and medication can reduce your symptoms. The lower esophageal sphincter, which regulates the flow of stomach acid, can be tightened or a hiatal hernia can be corrected surgically or by endoscopic procedures.
  - **Low-grade Dysplasia:** Low-grade dysplasia is thought to represent the initial stage of precancerous alterations. If low-grade dysplasia is discovered, a qualified pathologist should confirm it. Your doctor might suggest an additional endoscopy in six months for low-grade dysplasia, along with additional follow-up every six to twelve months. However, if the diagnosis is confirmed, treatment might be advised due to the risk of esophageal cancer. Among the recommended therapies are:
  - Endoscopic resection: This procedure helps identify dysplasia and cancer by removing damaged cells with the help of an endoscope.
  - Heat is applied during radiofrequency ablation to eliminate abnormal esophageal tissue. It might be advised to undergo radiofrequency ablation following endoscopic resection.
  - Cryotherapy involves applying a cold liquid or gas to abnormal cells in the esophagus using an endoscope. The cells are first allowed to thaw before being frozen once more. The aberrant cells are harmed by the freezing and thawing cycle.

After you've had three or four months of treatment to lower stomach acid, another endoscopy is done if there is noticeable esophageal inflammation at the first one.

- **High-grade Dysplasia:** Most people believe that high-grade dysplasia is a sign of esophageal cancer. Your doctor might therefore suggest radiofrequency ablation, cryotherapy, or endoscopic resection. Surgery is an additional option that entails cutting out the damaged section of your esophagus and joining the remaining section to your stomach. Following treatment, Barrett's esophagus recurrence is possible. Find out from your doctor how frequently you must return for additional testing. Your doctor may prescribe lifelong medication to lower acid and promote esophageal healing if your course of treatment involves anything other than surgery to remove abnormal esophageal tissue.

10.1.3.7. Lifestyle and Home Remedies

Controlling acid reflux is another treatment objective that can be attained by modifying one's lifestyle. You may attempt to:

- Make dietary adjustments. Reflux can be made worse by chocolate, caffeine, fatty meals, spicy foods, and peppermint.
  - Avoid alcohol, caffeinated drinks, and tobacco.
  - Reduce your weight. The risk of reflux is increased by being overweight because excess weight around the abdomen can compress the stomach and push acid up into the esophagus.
  - Elevate the head of your bed while you sleep. Elevating your head during sleep could potentially mitigate the risk of stomach acid refluxing up into the esophagus.
  - Adjust the time you eat. Eat frequently in small portions rather than in large ones, and avoid lying down for at least three hours after eating.
  - Take all medicines with plenty of water.

10.1.4. Esophageal Cancer

Cancer that develops in the esophagus, a long, hollow tube that connects your throat to your stomach, is known as esophageal cancer. The food you swallow is moved from the back of your throat to your stomach via your esophagus, where it is broken down for digestion. Usually, the cells lining the inside of the esophagus are where esophageal cancer starts. Anywhere along the esophagus is susceptible to esophageal cancer. Esophageal cancer affects men more often than women. The sixth most common cause of cancer-related deaths globally is esophageal cancer. The incidence rates in various geographical areas differ. Certain dietary practices, obesity, and tobacco and alcohol use may be linked to a higher incidence of esophageal cancer in some areas.

10.1.4.1. Symptoms

Esophageal cancer symptoms and signs include:

- Difficulty swallowing (dysphagia)
- Weight loss without trying
- Chest pain, pressure or burning
- Worsening indigestion or heartburn
- Coughing or hoarseness

Most of the time, early esophageal cancer shows no symptoms at all.

- **When to See a Doctor:** If you are concerned about any persistent signs or symptoms, schedule an appointment with your doctor. Your risk of developing esophageal cancer is increased if you have been diagnosed with Barrett's esophagus, a precancerous condition brought on by persistent acid reflux. Consult your doctor about the symptoms and indicators that could indicate that your illness is getting worse. People with Barrett's esophagus may be candidates for esophageal cancer screening. Talk to your doctor about the benefits and drawbacks of screening if you have Barrett's esophagus.

10.1.4.2. Causes

The exact cause of esophageal cancer is unknown. DNA alterations, or mutations, in esophageal cells lead to esophageal cancer. The alterations cause uncontrollably growing and dividing cells. The abnormal cells build up to form a tumor in the esophagus, which can spread to other parts of the body and invade neighboring structures.

10.1.4.3. Types of Esophageal Cancer

The type of cells involved in esophageal cancer determines the classification of the disease. The kind of esophageal cancer you have affects the available treatments. Esophageal cancer comes in various forms.

- **Adenocarcinoma**: The cells of the mucus-secreting glands in the esophagus are where adenocarcinoma starts. The lower part of the esophagus is where adenocarcinomas most frequently occur. The most prevalent type of esophageal cancer in the US is called adenocarcinoma, and it mainly affects white men.
- **Squamous Cell Carcinoma:** The thin, flat cells that border the esophageal surface are called squamous cells. Most cases of squamous cell carcinoma are found in the middle and upper regions of the esophagus. Globally, squamous cell carcinoma is the most common type of esophageal cancer.
- **Other Rare Types:** Sarcoma, lymphoma, melanoma, small cell carcinoma, and choriocarcinoma are a few uncommon types of esophageal cancer.

10.1.4.4. Risk Factors

Chronic esophageal irritation is thought to be a factor in the alterations that lead to esophageal cancer. The following are some of the factors that irritate the esophageal cells and raise your risk of esophageal cancer:

- Having gastroesophageal reflux disease (GERD)
- Smoking
- Possessing Barrett's esophageal cells, which are precancerous in nature.
- Being obese
- Drinking alcohol
- Having bile reflux
- Experiencing dysphagia due to a non-relaxing esophageal sphincter (achalasia).
- Drinking hot beverages on a regular basis.
- Not eating enough fruits and vegetables
- Undergoing radiation treatment to the chest or upper abdomen

10.1.4.5. Complications

As esophageal cancer spreads, it may result in complications like these.

- Obstruction of the esophagus. Cancer can potentially hinder the movement of food and liquid through your esophagus
- Pain. Pain can arise from advanced esophageal cancer
- Bleeding in the esophagus. Hemorrhage may result from esophageal cancer. Bleeding typically occurs gradually, but occasionally it can happen suddenly and severely

10.1.4.6. Prevention

It is possible for you to lower your risk of esophageal cancer. For example:

- **Quit Smoking:** If you smoke, discuss quitting methods with your physician. There are options for counseling and medication to assist with quitting. Don't start using tobacco if you don't already.
- If you use alcohol at all, do so in moderation. If you decide to use alcohol, use it sparingly. This translates to up to one drink for women and up to two for men per day for healthy adults.
- Consume more veggies and fruits. Increase the amount of vibrant fruits and vegetables in your diet.
- **Sustain a Healthy Weight:** See your doctor about weight loss techniques if you are obese or overweight. Aim for a weekly weight loss of one or two pounds, done slowly and steadily.

10.1.4.7. Diagnosis

Esophageal cancer is diagnosed using the following tests and procedures:

- Barium swallow investigation. You will swallow a barium-containing liquid during this study, and you will then get X-rays. Your esophagus's interior is coated with barium, which causes any changes to the tissue to show up on an X-ray.
- Examining your esophagus with a scope (endoscopy). A flexible tube called a video endoscope is passed down your throat and into your esophagus by your doctor during an endoscopy. Your doctor looks for cancer or irritated areas in your esophagus with the endoscope.
- Obtaining a tissue sample for examination (biopsy). To take a sample of suspicious tissue for a biopsy, your doctor may use an endoscope, a special scope that is inserted down your throat and into your esophagus. A lab receives the tissue sample to search for cancerous cells.
- **Determining the Extent of the Cancer:** To ascertain whether your cancer has spread to your lymph nodes or other parts of your body, your doctor might advise further testing if esophageal cancer is diagnosed.

Tests may include:

- Bronchoscopy
- Endoscopic ultrasound (EUS)
- Computerized tomography (CT)
- Positron emission tomography (PET)

Your doctor stages your cancer based on the data gathered from these procedures. Roman numerals 0 through IV represent the stages of esophageal cancer; the lowest stage signifies a small cancer that only affects the outermost layers of the esophagus. When a cancer reaches stage IV, it is thought to be advanced and to have spread to other bodily parts. As medical professionals advance in the diagnosis and treatment of cancer, the system for staging the disease keeps changing and growing more intricate. Your doctor determines the best course of treatment for you based on the stage of your cancer.

10.1.4.8. Treatment

The kind of cells causing your esophageal cancer, its stage, your general health, and your treatment preferences will all influence the treatments you receive.

- **Surgery:** Cancer removal surgery can be used either as a stand-alone treatment or in conjunction with other therapies.

Operations used to treat esophageal cancer include:

- Surgery to cut out tiny tumors. In case your esophageal cancer is localized to the outermost layers and hasn't spread, your surgeon might suggest excising the cancer along with the surrounding healthy tissue margin. An endoscope that is inserted down your throat and into your esophagus can be used for surgery.
- Esophagectomy is a surgical procedure where a portion of the esophagus is removed, typically due to cancer. During the surgery, the affected section of the esophagus, along with a portion of the upper stomach and nearby lymph nodes, is excised. The remaining parts of the esophagus and stomach are then reconnected, usually by pulling the stomach up to meet the remaining esophagus.
- Esophagogastrectomy involves removing a section of your esophagus and upper stomach. The procedure includes removing part of the esophagus, adjacent lymph nodes, and a significant portion of the stomach. The remaining stomach is then brought up and connected back to the esophagus. In some cases, a portion of the colon may be utilized to assist in connecting the two organs.

Serious side effects from esophageal cancer surgery include bleeding, infection, and leakage from the site where the stomach and remaining esophagus are reattached. Your esophagus can be removed surgically through an open procedure involving large incisions or laparoscopically, using a series of small skin incisions to insert special surgical instruments. Your surgeon's unique management strategy and the specifics of your case will determine how your surgery is carried out.

10.1.4.9. Treatments for Complications

Some possible treatments for esophageal obstruction and difficulty swallowing (dysphagia) may include:

- Relieving esophageal obstruction. A metal tube, or stent, may be inserted by a surgeon using an endoscope and specialized instruments to hold your esophagus open if your esophageal cancer has caused it to narrow. Additional choices consist of laser therapy, photodynamic therapy, chemotherapy, radiation therapy, and surgery.
- Providing nutrition. If you're having esophageal surgery or are experiencing difficulty swallowing, your doctor might suggest a feeding tube. With the use of a feeding tube, you can receive nutrition directly into your stomach or small intestine, allowing your esophagus to heal from cancer treatment.

10.1.4.10. Chemotherapy

Chemotherapy is a medication used to destroy cancer cells with chemicals. In patients with esophageal cancer, chemotherapy medications are usually administered either before (neoadjuvant) or after (adjuvant) surgery. Radiation therapy and chemotherapy can also be used in tandem. Chemotherapy may be used alone in patients with advanced cancer that has spread outside of the esophagus to help relieve the disease's symptoms. The specific chemotherapy drugs you are prescribed will determine the side effects you experience.

10.1.4.11. Radiation Therapy

High-energy beams, like protons and X-rays, are used in radiation therapy to destroy cancer cells. Usually, radiation is directed toward your cancer by a machine outside of your body (external beam radiation). Or, less frequently, radiation therapy (brachytherapy) can be applied inside your body in the vicinity of the cancer. For patients with esophageal cancer, chemotherapy is most frequently combined with radiation therapy. It is usually used either before or occasionally following surgery. Additionally, radiation therapy is used to treat complications resulting from advanced esophageal cancer, such as tumor growth that prevents food from reaching the stomach. Radiation to the esophagus can cause adverse effects such as skin reactions similar to sunburn, difficulty or agony when swallowing, and harm to neighboring organs like the heart and lungs.

10.1.4.12. Combined Chemotherapy and Radiation

The efficacy of radiation therapy and chemotherapy combined may be increased. You might only receive combined chemotherapy and radiation therapy, or you might receive combined therapy and surgery at the same time. However, the chance and intensity of side effects are increased when radiation and chemotherapy are administered together.

10.1.4.13. Targeted Drug Therapy

Treatments with targeted drugs concentrate on particular flaws in cancer cells. Targeted drug therapies can kill cancer cells by obstructing these vulnerabilities. Targeted medications are typically used in conjunction with chemotherapy to treat esophageal cancers that are advanced or resistant to other forms of treatment.

10.1.4.14. Immunotherapy

A medication called immunotherapy strengthens your body's defenses against cancer. Because cancer cells produce proteins that make it difficult for immune system cells to identify cancer cells as dangerous, your body's disease-fighting immune system may not attack cancer. Immunotherapy functions by obstructing that procedure. Immunotherapy may be used to treat esophageal cancer in cases where it has progressed, returned, or spread to other body parts.

10.2. Disorders in Stomach

An organ situated between the esophagus and the small intestine is the stomach. That is the starting point for protein digestion. Three jobs for the stomach. Swallowed food is stored there. It incorporates stomach acids into the meal. The mixture is subsequently sent to the small intestine. Most people have experienced stomach issues at some point. Heartburn and reflux are frequent issues. Certain gastrointestinal issues can be resolved with over-the-counter medications and dietary modifications, like cutting back on fattening foods or eating more slowly. Other issues like GERD or stomach ulcers need to be treated by a doctor.

10.2.1. Helicobacter Pylori

Helicobacter pylori (H. pylori) infection occurs when *Helicobacter pylori* (H. pylori) bacteria infect your stomach. Usually, this occurs in childhood. A common cause of stomach ulcers (peptic ulcers), H. pylori infection may be present in more than half the people in the world.Most people are unaware that they are

H. pylori infection because it never causes them to become ill. Your doctor will likely perform an H test on you if you exhibit symptoms and indicators of a peptic ulcer. H. pylori infection. A peptic ulcer is a sore on the stomach (gastric ulcer) or the duodenum, the first portion of the small intestine. A. Antibiotics are used to treat *Helicobacter pylori* cases.

10.2.1.1. Symptoms

Most people with *H. pylori* infection will never have any signs or symptoms. Many people don't exhibit symptoms, but why is unknown. However, some people may be born with more resistance to the harmful effects of H. pylori. When signs or symptoms do occur with *H. pylori* infection, they are typically related to gastritis or a peptic ulcer and may include:

- An ache or burning pain in your stomach (abdomen)
- Stomach pain that may be worse when your stomach is empty
- Nausea
- Loss of appetite
- Frequent burping
- Bloating
- Unintentional weight loss

When to See a Doctor. If you experience any symptoms that could indicate gastritis or a peptic ulcer, schedule a visit with your doctor. Get medical attention right away if you have:

- Severe or persistent abdominal pain that has the potential to wake you up.
- Bloody or black tarry stools
- Vomit that is bloody, black, or resembles coffee grinds.

10.2.1.2. Causes

H. pylori infection occurs when *H. pylori* bacteria infect your stomach. The most common way that the pylori bacteria spread from person to person is by direct contact with saliva, vomit, or feces. *H. pylori* may also be spread through contaminated food or water. The exact way *H. pylori* bacteria causes gastritis or a peptic ulcer in some people is still unknown.

10.2.1.3. Risk Factors

Individuals frequently receive *H. pylori* infection in the early years. Hazard variables for *H. pylori* infection are linked to certain childhood living circumstances, like:

- Living in close quarters. Living in a house with lots of other people can make you more susceptible to *H. pylori* infection.
- Living without a consistent source of pure water. Reliability in the provision of uncontaminated, flowing water mitigates the risk of H. pylori.
- Living in a nation in development. Individuals in developing nations are more likely to contract *H. pylori* infection. This could be as a result of the prevalence of filthy and cramped living arrangements in developing nations.
- Living with someone who has an *H. pylori* infection. You're more likely to have *H. pylori* infection if you live with someone who has *H. pylori* infection.

10.2.1.4. Complications

Complications associated with *H. pylori* infection include:

- Ulcers. *H. pylori* can harm the small intestine's and stomach's protective lining. This can lead to the formation of an ulcer (open sore) from stomach acid. 10% or so of those who have *H. pylori* will experience ulceration.

- Inflammation of the stomach lining. *H. pylori* infection can affect the stomach, causing irritation and swelling (gastritis).
- Stomach cancer. *H. pylori* infection is a strong risk factor for certain types of stomach cancer (Figure 10.2).

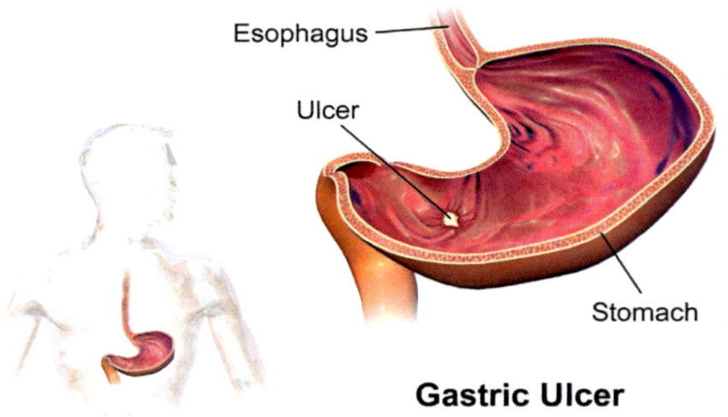

Figure 10.2. *Gastric ulcer.*

Source: By BruceBlaus – Own work, CC BY-SA 4.0, https://commons.wikimedia.org/w/index.php?curid=44923645.

10.2.1.5. Prevention

In areas of the world where *H. pylori* infection and its complications are common, healthcare providers sometimes test healthy people for *H. pylori*. Whether there is a benefit to testing for *H. pylori* infection when you have no signs or symptoms of infection is controversial among experts. If you're concerned about *H. pylori* infection or you think you may have a high risk of stomach cancer, talk to your healthcare provider. Together you can decide whether you may benefit from *H. pylori* testing.

10.2.1.6. Diagnosis

There are multiple methods and tests used to diagnose *Helicobacter pylori* (*H. pylori*) infection. Repeat testing after treatment is important to be sure *H. pylori* is gone. Testing can be performed with an upper endoscopy examination, a breath test, and a stool sample.

- Stool Tests
  - Stool antigen examination. This is the most common stool test to detect *H. pylori*. The test looks for proteins (antigens) associated with *H. pylori* infection in the stool.
  - Stool PCR examination. *H. pylori* can be found in a laboratory test known as a stool polymerase chain reaction (PCR) test. The test can also identify mutations that may be resistant to antibiotics used to treat H. pylori. However, this test costs more than a stool antigen test, and not all hospitals may have it available.
- Breath Test

You swallow a pill, liquid, or pudding containing tagged carbon molecules during a breath test, also known as a urea breath test. If you have *H. pylori* infection, carbon is released when the solution comes in contact with *H. pylori* in your stomach. The carbon is released when you exhale because your body has absorbed it. You inflate a bag to determine the amount of carbon released. The carbon molecules are found using a specialized tool. Both adults and kids over the age of six who can cooperate with the test can use this one.

- Scope Test

A scope test also referred to as an upper endoscopy exam, may be performed by a medical professional. This test might be carried out by your doctor to look into symptoms that could be brought on by illnesses like gastritis or peptic ulcers that could be related to *H. pylori*. You will be given medication to help you relax for this exam. A long, flexible tube with a tiny camera (an endoscope) attached is threaded down your throat, esophagus, stomach, and the duodenum, the first portion of your intestine, by your healthcare provider during the examination. With the use of this device, your doctor can see any issues with your upper digestive tract. Also, your physician might obtain tissue samples (biopsy). We check these samples for *H. pylori* infection.

This test is usually performed in addition to diagnosing other digestive issues because it is more invasive than a breathalyzer or stool test *H. pylori* infection. This test can be used by medical professionals to look for additional digestive disorders and to conduct additional testing. This test may also be used to pinpoint the precise antibiotic that would be most effective in treating *H. pylori* infection, particularly if the infection persisted after the first round of antibiotics was tried. This test may be repeated after treatment, depending on what is found at the first endoscopy or if symptoms continue after *H. pylori* infection treatment.

- Testing Considerations

Antibiotics have the potential to compromise test accuracy. Retesting is typically done only, if at all possible, after four weeks without taking antibiotics. Proton pump inhibitors (PPIs) and bismuth subsalicylate (Pepto-Bismol), two acid-suppressing medications, can also affect the precision of these tests. It's possible that medications known as histamine (H-2) blockers, which suppress the stomach acid, could also affect how accurate these tests are. You may need to stop taking your medications for up to two weeks before the test, depending on what kind of medication you take. You will receive detailed instructions regarding your medications from your healthcare provider. The same tests used for diagnosis can be used to tell if *H. pylori* infection is gone. If you were previously diagnosed with *H. pylori* infection, you'll generally wait at least four weeks after you complete your antibiotic treatment to repeat these tests.

10.2.1.7. Treatment

H. pylori infections are usually treated with at least two different antibiotics at once. This helps prevent the bacteria from developing a resistance to one particular antibiotic. Medications to aid in stomach healing may also be part of your treatment. These include:

- Proton pump inhibitors (PPIs). These medications prevent the stomach from producing acid. Proton pump inhibitors, or PPIs, include medications such as pantoprazole (Protonix), lansoprazole (Prevacid), esomeprazole (Nexium), and omeprazole (Prilosec).
- Bismuth subsalicylate. This medication, which is more widely marketed under the brand name Pepto-Bismol, acts by covering the ulcer and shielding it from stomach acid.
- Histamine (H-2) blockers. These drugs inhibit a chemical known as histamine, which causes the body to produce acid. One example is cimetidine (Tagamet HB). histamine (H-2) blockers are only prescribed for *H. pylori* infection if PPIs can't be used.

Repeat testing for *H. pylori* at least four weeks after your treatment is recommended. You might require additional treatment with a different combination of antibiotics if the tests reveal that the treatment was ineffective in eliminating the infection.

10.2.2. Peptic Ulcer Disease

Open sores on the inside lining of the stomach and upper part of the small intestine are called peptic ulcers. Stomach pain is the most typical symptom of a peptic ulcer.

- Peptic ulcers include:
  - stomach ulcers that are found inside the stomach.
  - ulcers on the inside of the duodenum, which is the upper part of your small intestine.

Helicobacter pylori (*H. pylori*) infection is the most frequent cause of peptic ulcers. *H. pylori* and chronic use of nonsteroidal anti-inflammatory medications (NSAIDs), such as naproxen sodium (Aleve) and ibuprofen (Advil, Motrin IB, and other brands). Spicy food and stress are not the causes of peptic ulcers. They might, however, exacerbate your symptoms.

10.2.2.1. Symptoms

- Burning stomach pain
- Feeling of fullness, bloating or belching
- Intolerance to fatty foods
- Heartburn
- Nausea

Stomach pain that burns is the most typical symptom of a peptic ulcer. Both stomach acid and an empty stomach exacerbate the pain. Eating certain foods that buffer stomach acid or taking an acid-reducing medication can often relieve the pain, but the pain may return later. The pain might be more severe at night and in between meals. Many peptic ulcer sufferers don't even exhibit any symptoms (Figure 10.3).

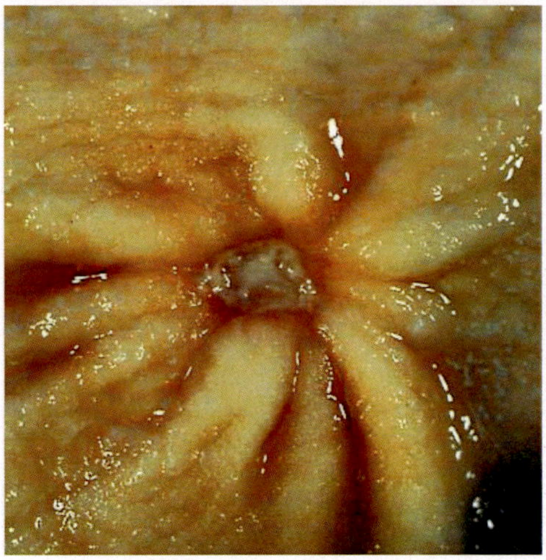

Figure 10.3. *A benign gastric ulcer (from the antrum) of a gastrectomy specimen.*

Source: By Ed Uthman, MD, public domain, https://commons.wikimedia.org/w/index.php?curid=840064.

Less frequently, severe symptoms or signs like these can indicate an ulcer.

- Vomiting or vomiting blood — which may appear red or black
- Dark blood in stools, or stools that are black or tarry
- Trouble breathing
- Feeling faint
- Nausea or vomiting
- Unexplained weight loss
- Appetite changes
- When to See a Doctor

If you experience any of the severe symptoms or signs mentioned above, consult your physician. If you take over-the-counter antacids and acid blockers for pain relief, but the pain comes back, consult your doctor as well.

10.2.2.2. Causes

Acid in the digestive system eats away at the inside surface of the stomach or small intestine, resulting in peptic ulcers. A painful, potentially bleeding open sore may be caused by the acid. A mucous layer covers your digestive tract, which typically shields it from acid. However, you run the risk of getting an ulcer if the quantity of mucus or acid decreases.

- Common causes include:
  - **A Bacterium:** The mucous layer that covers and shields the tissues lining the stomach and small intestine is home to *Helicobacter pylori* bacteria. Often, the *H. pylori* bacterium causes no problems, but it can cause inflammation of the stomach's inner layer, producing an ulcer. *H. pylori* infection can spread from person to person through intimate physical contact, like kissing. *H. pylori* can also infect people by means of food and drink.
  - **Regular Use of Certain Pain Relievers:** Aspirin and certain prescription and over-the-counter pain relievers known as nonsteroidal anti-inflammatory drugs (NSAIDs) can irritate or inflame the lining of your small intestine and stomach. These drugs include ketoprofen, naproxen sodium (Aleve, Anaprox DS), ibuprofen (Advil, Motrin IB, and others), and others. Acetaminophen (in Tylenol and other brands) is not one of them.
- **Other Medications:** The risk of developing ulcers can be significantly increased by taking certain other medications in addition to NSAIDs, including steroids, anticoagulants, low-dose aspirin, selective serotonin reuptake inhibitors (SSRIs), alendronate (Fosamax), and risedronate (Actonel).

10.2.2.3. Risk Factors

You may be more susceptible to peptic ulcers in addition to the risks associated with using NSAIDs if you:

- Smoke. Smoking may increase the risk of peptic ulcers in people who are infected with H. pylori.
- Drink alcohol. Alcohol can cause your stomach's mucous lining to become irritated and eroded, as well as increase the production of stomach acid.
- Have untreated stress.
- Eat spicy foods.

These elements do not directly cause ulcers, but they can exacerbate existing ones and make healing more challenging.

10.2.2.4. Complications

Left untreated, peptic ulcers can result in:

- **Internal Bleeding**: Bleeding can be so severe that it necessitates hospitalization or a blood transfusion, or it can be so mild that it causes anemia. Black or bloody stools or vomit are possible symptoms of severe blood loss.
- A perforation or hole in the wall of your stomach. You run the risk of developing a serious abdominal cavity infection (peritonitis) if your stomach or small intestine wall is eaten through by peptic ulcers.

- **Obstruction**: Peptic ulcers can impede food from passing through the digestive tract, making it difficult for you to feel full, causing you to throw up and lose weight due to either scarring or swelling from inflammation.
- **Gastric Cancer:** Research has indicated that individuals with *H. pylori* are more likely to develop stomach cancer.

10.2.2.5. Prevention

If you use the same techniques as suggested for treating ulcers at home, you may be able to lower your risk of developing a peptic ulcer. It could also be beneficial for:

- Protect yourself from infections. It's unclear exactly how *H. pylori* spreads, although there is some evidence that it can also be spread by food and drink or from person to person.
- You can take precautions to keep yourself safe from infections like H. pylori, by eating fully cooked food and by regularly washing your hands with soap and water.
- Use caution with pain relievers. Take precautions to lower your risk of stomach issues if you frequently use painkillers that raise your risk of peptic ulcers. Take your medication with food, for example.

Consult your physician to determine the lowest dosage that will still provide you with pain relief. Steer clear of alcohol while taking medication as the combination may make you more susceptible to stomach upset. In addition to taking an NSAID, you might also need to take an antacid, proton pump inhibitor, acid blocker, or cytoprotective agent. COX-2 inhibitors are a class of NSAIDs that may raise the risk of heart attack but may also lessen the likelihood of peptic ulcers.

10.2.2.6. Diagnosis

Your doctor may first perform a physical examination and obtain a medical history to identify an ulcer. After that, you might require diagnostic procedures like these.

- Laboratory tests for H. pylori. Your doctor may recommend tests to determine whether the bacterium *H. pylori* is present in your body. He or she might try to find *H. pylori* by means of a breath, stool, or blood test. The most accurate test is the breathalyzer.

For the breath test, you drink or eat something that contains radioactive carbon. *H. pylori* breaks down the substance in your stomach. You subsequently blow into a sealed bag. If you have an infection *H. pylori*, the radioactive carbon in your breath sample will be in the form of carbon dioxide. In the event that you take an antacid before the H. pylori, be sure to inform your physician. Because antacids can cause false-negative test results, you might need to stop taking the medication for a while, depending on the test that is used.

- **Endoscopy:** Your doctor may perform an endoscopy, or upper digestive system examination, using a scope. An endoscope is a hollow tube that your doctor inserts down your throat, into your stomach, small intestine, and esophagus during an endoscopy. Your physician uses the endoscope to check for ulcers.

If your doctor detects an ulcer, a small tissue sample (biopsy) may be removed for examination in a lab. A biopsy can also identify whether *H. pylori* is in your stomach lining. If you have recently lost weight, have bleeding symptoms, are older, or have trouble swallowing and eating, your doctor is more likely to advise an endoscopy. Even if your symptoms get better, you should still get a follow-up endoscopy to confirm that the stomach ulcer has healed if the initial one revealed one.

- Upper gastrointestinal series. This series of X-rays of your upper digestive system, sometimes known as a "barium swallow," produces images of your stomach, small intestine, and esophagus. You ingest a white liquid that contains barium before the X-ray, which coats your digestive tract and highlights any ulcers.

10.2.2.7. Treatment

The cause of peptic ulcers determines how to treat them. Typically, therapy entails eliminating the *H. pylori* bacteria, if it's present, avoiding or minimizing the use of NSAIDs, and using medicine to aid in the healing of your ulcer.

Medications can include:

- Drugs with antibiotics to eradicate H. pylori. Should *H. pylori* be discovered within your digestive system, your physician might suggest taking a mix of antibiotics to eradicate the bacterium. These might include levofloxacin, metronidazole (Flagyl), tinidazole (Tindamax), amoxicillin (Amoxil), clarithromycin (Biaxin), and tetracycline.

The antibiotics you take will depend on your location and the prevalence of antibiotic resistance at the time. You will probably require two weeks of antibiotics in addition to other medications that lower stomach acid, such as a proton pump inhibitor and maybe bismuth subsalicylate (Pepto-Bismol).

- Medications that support healing and prevent the production of acid. By preventing the parts of cells that produce acid from acting, proton pump inhibitors, or PPIs, lower stomach acid. Among these medications are omeprazole (Prilosec), lansoprazole (Prevacid), rabeprazole (Aciphex), esomeprazole (Nexium), and pantoprazole (Protonix), both prescribed and over-the-counter.

Proton pump inhibitor use over an extended period of time, especially at high doses, may raise your risk of hip, wrist, and spine fractures. Consult your physician if taking a calcium supplement could lower this risk.

- Medications that lessen the generation of acid. By lowering the quantity of stomach acid released into your digestive tract, acid blockers, also known as histamine (H-2) blockers, lessen ulcer discomfort and promote healing.

Acid blockers include the drugs famotidine (Pepcid AC), cimetidine (Tagamet HB), and nizatidine (Axid AR), which are available over-the-counter or with a prescription.

- Ants that counteract the acidity of the stomach. An antacid might be prescribed to you by your doctor. Antacids neutralize stomach acid that already exists and can relieve pain quickly. Depending on the primary ingredients, side effects may include diarrhea or constipation.
- Although they can relieve symptoms, antacids are typically not used to treat ulcers.

- Drugs that shield your stomach and small intestine's lining. Your doctor may occasionally recommend cytoprotective agents—drugs that support the preservation of the tissues lining your stomach and small intestine—to you.

Prescription drugs sucralfate (Carafate) and misoprostol (Cytotec) are among the options.

- **Follow-up after Initial Treatment:** Peptic ulcer therapy is frequently effective, resulting in ulcer healing. However, to rule out other potential causes of your symptoms, your doctor might advise endoscopy if they are severe or persist after treatment. To ensure that the ulcer has healed, your doctor might advise a follow-up endoscopy if one is found during the procedure. Consult your physician about any necessary follow-up testing following your course of treatment.
- **Ulcers that Fail to Heal:** Peptic ulcers that do not respond to treatment are referred to as refractory ulcers. There are numerous factors that can contribute to an ulcer's failure to heal, such as:
    - Not taking prescription drugs as directed.
    - The existence of antibiotic-resistant *H. pylori* strains.
    - Regular use of tobacco
    - Frequent use of medications that raise the risk of ulcers, such as NSAIDs.
    - Refractory ulcers can occur less frequently as a result of:
    - Severe excess gastric acid production, as in Zollinger-Ellison syndrome.
    - An infection other than *H. pylori*
    - Stomach cancer
    - Some illnesses, like Crohn's disease, can result in sores that resemble ulcers in the stomach and small intestine.

Refractory ulcers are typically treated with a combination of different antibiotics and the removal of any factors that may impede healing. You might need surgery if you have a serious ulcer-related complication, like severe bleeding or a perforation. However, due to the availability of numerous effective medications, surgery is no longer required as frequently as it once was.

10.2.3. Gastric Cancer

Cancer that originates in the stomach's lining cells is known as stomach (or gastric) cancer. Food is broken down in the stomach, an organ located on the left side of the upper abdomen.

A group of muscular, hollow organs connected in a long, winding tube from the mouth to the anus is called the digestive tract, of which the stomach is a component. The digestive system aids in the removal of waste from the body and breaks down nutrients from meals.

- The esophagus is the tube that carries food from the throat to the stomach.
- Food is broken down by stomach muscles that combine it with liquid and digestive juices once it reaches the stomach.
- Partially digested food travels through the small and large intestines after exiting the stomach.
- The waste from the broken down food is held in the rectum, the end

of the large intestine, until it is expelled during a bowel movement.

10.2.3.1. Symptoms

Stomach cancer symptoms and indicators could include:

- Trouble swallowing
- Belly pain
- Feeling bloated after eating
- Feeling full after eating small amounts of food
- Not experiencing hunger when you normally would
- Heartburn
- Indigestion
- Nausea
- Vomiting
- Losing weight without trying
- Feeling very tired
- Stools that look black

Early-stage stomach cancer is not always symptomatic. Indigestion and upper abdominal pain are possible symptoms when they occur. It is possible for symptoms to be hidden until the cancer has progressed. Symptoms of stomach cancer in its later stages include extreme fatigue, spontaneous weight loss, vomiting blood, and dark stools. Metastatic stomach cancer is a type of stomach cancer that has spread to other parts of the body. It manifests symptoms unique to the area it spreads to. For instance, lumps that are perceptible through the skin may develop if cancer spreads to the lymph nodes. The skin and whites of the eyes may turn yellow if the cancer spreads to the liver. The belly may fill with fluid if the cancer spreads inside the abdomen. The abdomen may appear enlarged.

- **When to See a Doctor:** Schedule a visit with your healthcare provider if you are concerned about any of the signs and symptoms listed. Similar symptoms to those of stomach cancer can be caused by several illnesses. Prior to testing for stomach cancer, your provider may do tests for those other possible causes.

10.2.3.2. Causes

The exact cause of stomach cancer is unknown. According to experts, the majority of stomach cancers begin with damage to the stomach's internal lining. Examples include eating a lot of salty foods, having chronic acid reflux, and having a stomach infection. However, not everyone who has these risk factors develops stomach cancer. Therefore, more investigation is required to determine the precise cause. The genesis of stomach cancer is caused by damage to the stomach's inner lining cells. It results in DNA alterations in the cells. The instructions that tell a cell what to do are encoded in its DNA. The alterations instruct the cells to proliferate rapidly. When healthy cells would naturally die, the cells can continue living. There are many more cells in the stomach as a result. Tumors are masses made up of cells. Healthy body tissue can be invaded and destroyed by stomach cancer cells. They may begin to protrude farther into the stomach wall. Cancer cells can split off and travel to other areas of the body over time. Metastasis is the term used to describe the spread of cancer cells to other parts of the body.

10.2.3.3. Types of Stomach Cancer

The kind of cell that gave rise to your stomach cancer determines the type of cancer you have. Types of stomach cancer include the following:

- **Adenocarcinoma:** Mucus-producing cells are the initial stage of adenocarcinoma, a stomach cancer. This kind of stomach cancer is the most prevalent one. Adenocarcinoma stomach cancers account for almost all cancers that begin in the stomach.

- **Gastrointestinal Stromal Tumors (GIST):** Special nerve cells found in the stomach wall and other digestive organs are the source of GIST. One kind of soft tissue sarcoma is called GIST.
- **Carcinoid Tumors:** Cancers that originate in the neuroendocrine cells are called carcinoid tumors. The body contains neuroendocrine cells in many different locations. They perform a portion of the tasks performed by nerve cells and hormone-producing cells. One kind of neuroendocrine tumor is a carcinoid tumor.
- **Lymphoma:** A cancer that begins in immune system cells is called lymphoma. The immune system of the body combats bacteria. When the body sends immune system cells to the stomach, lymphoma can occasionally begin there. This could occur if the body is attempting to combat an infection. Non-Hodgkin's lymphomas make up the majority of lymphomas that begin in the stomach.

10.2.3.4. Risk Factors

Stomach cancer risk factors include the following.

- Ongoing issues known as gastroesophageal reflux disease, which are caused by stomach acid backing up into the esophagus.
- A diet heavy in smoked and salty foods.
- A diet low in fruits and vegetables
- Stomach infection brought on by the *Helicobacter pylori* bacteria.
- Inflammation and swelling of the stomach's interior, also known as gastritis.
- Smoking
- Polyps are growths of noncancerous cells in the stomach.
- Family history of stomach cancer
- A family history of genetic syndromes, such as Lynch syndrome, Peutz-Jeghers syndrome, familial adenomatous polyposis, hereditary diffuse gastric cancer, and juvenile polyposis syndrome, that raise the risk of stomach cancer and other cancers.

10.2.3.5. Prevention

To lower the risk of stomach cancer, you can:

- Consume a lot of vegetables and fruits. Make an effort to consume fruits and vegetables daily. Pick an assortment of vibrant fruits and vegetables.
- Eat fewer foods that are smoked and/or salted. Limit these foods to protect your stomach.
- Stop smoking. Quit smoking if you do. Don't start if you don't already smoke. Colon cancer is one of the many cancers that smoking increases the risk of, including stomach cancer. See your doctor for assistance if you need it to stop smoking as it can be quite difficult to do so.

- Inform your healthcare provider if there is a history of stomach cancer in your family. Individuals with a significant family history of stomach cancer may be recommended for screening to detect the disease before symptoms appear.

10.2.3.6. Diagnosis

There are various tests and procedures available to diagnose and detect stomach cancer, such as:

- Looking inside the stomach. Your doctor may use a tiny camera to see inside your stomach to check for signs of cancer. We refer to this process as upper endoscopy. A tiny camera-equipped thin tube is inserted into the stomach and down the throat.
- Obtaining a tissue sample for examination. Should an apparent cancerous growth be discovered in your stomach, it may be extracted for examination. We refer to this as a biopsy. An upper endoscopy can be used to complete it. To obtain the tissue sample, special instruments are passed through the tube. For testing, the sample is sent to a lab (Figure 10.4).

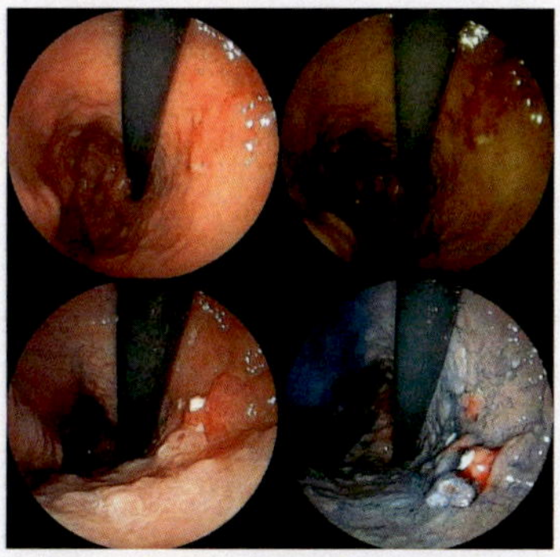

Figure 10.4. *Endoscopic images of stomach cancer in the early stage. Its histology was poorly differentiated adenocarcinoma with signet ring cells. Left above: normal, right above: FICE, left low: acetate stained, right low: AIM stained.*

- **Determining the Stage of Stomach Cancer:** If stomach cancer is diagnosed, you may undergo additional testing to determine whether the disease has spread. The cancer is assigned a stage based on this information. The stage provides information about your prognosis and the extent of your cancer to your provider. Various tests and procedures are employed to determine the stage of gastric cancer.
  - **Blood Tests:** Stomach cancer cannot be diagnosed by a blood test. Your doctor may be able to learn more about your health from blood tests. Tests to assess the health of your liver, for instance, may reveal issues brought on by stomach cancer that has spread to the liver.

A different kind of blood test searches the blood for fragments of cancer cells. A circulating tumor DNA test is what this is known as. It is only applied to patients with stomach cancer under specific circumstances. For instance, if you are unable to have a biopsy due to advanced cancer, this test may be used. Blood cell samples can provide your medical team with information that will help them plan your course of treatment.

- **Stomach Ultrasound:** An imaging test called an ultrasound creates images by using sound waves.

The images can demonstrate the extent to which stomach cancer has penetrated the stomach wall. A thin tube with a camera attached to the tip is inserted into the stomach and down the throat to take the images. An ultrasonography instrument is used to take images of the stomach.

Examining lymph nodes close to the stomach may be done with ultrasound. When removing tissue from lymph nodes with a needle, the images can be used as guidance. In a lab, the tissue is examined to check for cancerous cells.

- **Imaging Tests:** Imaging tests produce images that your healthcare team can use to search for evidence of metastases from stomach cancer. The images might depict cancer cells in adjacent lymph nodes or other body parts. CT and PET (positron emission tomography) are two possible test types.
    - **Surgery:** Surgery may be necessary to see inside the body when imaging tests are unable to provide a clear picture of your cancer. Surgery can be used to detect metastatic cancer, another name for cancer that has spread. Your physician may recommend surgery to ensure that no small cancerous tumors are present in the abdomen or liver.

In other cases, different tests might be employed. Your medical team assigns a stage to your cancer based on the results of these tests. The stomach cancer stages range from 0 to 4. The stomach's interior surface is the only area where the cancer is present at stage 0. Stomach cancer in stage 1 has spread to the stomach's inner layers. The cancer penetrates the stomach wall more deeply in stages two and three. The cancer may have moved to adjacent lymph nodes. It's possible that by stage 4, the stomach cancer has spread to neighboring organs. Cancers in stage 4 include those that have metastasized to other body parts. Metastatic cancer is the term for cancer that spreads. When stomach cancer spreads, it frequently affects the liver or lymph nodes. It may also spread to the peritoneum, the lining that surrounds the abdominal organs. After your initial treatment, your medical team may decide to move your cancer to a new stage. For stomach cancer, different staging methods can be applied following chemotherapy or surgery.

- **Understanding your Prognosis:** The stage of your cancer is used by your healthcare team to determine your prognosis. The likelihood that the cancer will be cured is known as the prognosis. The prognosis for stomach cancer is excellent when it is detected in its early stages. The likelihood of a cure decreases as the stage rises. Treatments for stomach cancer may be able to control the disease and extend your life, even in cases where there is no cure. Several factors can affect the prognosis of stomach cancer.
    - The type of cancer
    - The cancer's stage
    - Where the cancer is within the stomach
    - Your overall health
    - If surgery is used to fully remove the cancer.
    - If chemotherapy or radiation therapy proves effective in treating the cancer.

Speak with your provider if you have concerns about your prognosis. Find out how serious your cancer is.

- **Detecting Stomach Cancer before it Causes Symptoms:** In certain cases, tests are performed on individuals without symptoms to check for stomach cancer. We refer to this as screening for stomach cancer. The purpose of screening is to find stomach cancer early on when it is more curable and smaller in size. Only those who have a high risk of stomach cancer are eligible for screening tests in the United States. Should stomach cancer run in your family, you may be at a higher risk. If you have a genetic syndrome that increases the risk of stomach cancer, you may be at a higher risk. Hereditary diffuse gastric cancer, Lynch syndrome, Peutz-Jeghers syndrome, juvenile polyposis syndrome, and familial adenomatous polyposis are a few examples.

Tests for stomach cancer are used more frequently in other parts of the world where the disease is much more prevalent. The most widely used test for stomach cancer detection is upper endoscopy. X-rays are used in some nations to identify stomach cancer. One active area of cancer research is the screening for stomach cancer. Researchers are looking into blood tests and other means of identifying stomach cancer early on before symptoms appear.

10.2.3.7. Treatment

The stage and location of stomach cancer determine the available treatment options. When creating a treatment plan, your healthcare provider also takes your preferences and general health into account. Treatments for stomach cancer encompass surgery, immunotherapy, targeted therapy, chemotherapy, radiation therapy, and palliative care.

- **Surgery:** The aim of surgery for gastric cancer, also known as stomach cancer, is to remove the entire cancer. Surgery may be the initial course of treatment for small stomach cancers. If the stomach cancer invades more tissue in the stomach wall or spreads to the lymph nodes, alternative therapies may be tried first. Surgery is one method used to treat stomach cancer.
  - Removing tiny cancers from the lining of the stomach. The stomach lining can be removed to expose very tiny malignancies. A tube is inserted into the stomach and down the throat to remove the cancer. To remove the cancer, special cutting instruments are inserted through the tube. We refer to this process as an endoscopic mucosal resection. It may represent a therapeutic option for treating stomach lining stage 1 cancer.
  - Removing the stomach in part. A subtotal gastrectomy is the term for this operation. The cancerous portion of the stomach is excised, along with a portion of the surrounding healthy tissue. If the location of your stomach cancer is closest to the small intestine, then it might be a possibility.
  - The entire stomach being removed. We refer to this procedure as a total gastrectomy. The entire stomach as well as some

surrounding tissue are removed. To facilitate food passage through the digestive system, the surgeon joins the esophagus and small intestine. Cancers that affect the portion of the stomach that is closest to the esophagus can be treated with a total gastrectomy.

  - Removing lymph nodes to detect cancer. To check for cancer, the surgeon might remove some of your abdomen's lymph nodes.

- Surgery to reduce the symptoms. The symptoms of a developing cancer may be relieved by surgery to remove a portion of the stomach. If other treatments have failed and the cancer is advanced, this may be a possibility.

It is frequently possible to remove small stage 1 stomach cancers by cutting away the stomach's inner lining. However, this may not be an option if the cancer spreads to the stomach wall's muscle layer. Surgery may be required for some stage 1 cancers to remove all or part of the stomach. It is possible that surgery is not the first line of treatment for stomach cancers in stages 2 and 3. To reduce the cancer, chemotherapy and radiation therapy may be applied initially. This may facilitate a full removal of the cancer. During surgery, the stomach and/or some lymph nodes are frequently removed. Surgery may be necessary if stage 4 stomach cancer spreads beyond the stomach and into adjacent organs. Parts of the adjacent organs may also need to be removed to eradicate all of the cancer. To reduce the cancer, alternative therapies may be tried initially. If total removal of stage 4 cancer is not possible, surgery may help manage symptoms.

- **Chemotherapy:** A medication called chemotherapy employs chemicals to destroy cancer cells. Chemotherapeutic approaches include:
  - Chemotherapy is administered throughout the entire body. The most popular kind of chemotherapy uses drugs that kill cancer cells throughout your entire body. We refer to this as systemic chemotherapy. The medications can be taken as pills or administered intravenously.
  - Chemotherapy is limited to the abdominal cavity. Hyperthermic intraperitoneal chemotherapy (HIPEC) is the term used to describe this kind of chemotherapy. Following surgery, HIPEC is performed. Chemotherapy drugs are injected directly into the stomach after the stomach cancer has been removed by the surgeon. To improve their effectiveness, the medications are heated. After a predetermined period of time, the chemotherapy is drained.

For stomach cancer in stage 1, chemotherapy may not be necessary. If the cancer was completely removed during surgery and the chance of it returning is minimal, it might not be necessary. Chemotherapy is a common preoperative treatment for stage 2 and stage 3 stomach cancers. Perhaps systemic chemotherapy can help reduce the size of the cancer so that it is easier to remove. Neoadjuvant chemotherapy refers to the administration of chemotherapy prior to surgery. If there is a chance that some cancer cells were left behind after surgery, systemic chemotherapy may be used. This risk may increase if the cancer invades the stomach wall deeply or spreads to the lymph nodes. Adjuvant chemotherapy is the term for chemotherapy administered following surgery. It is possible to use chemotherapy alone or in conjunction with radiation therapy. Systemic chemotherapy may be suggested in place of surgery if that is not an option. In cases where surgery is not feasible or the cancer is too advanced, it may be used. Chemotherapy may be able to manage cancer symptoms.

For stage 4 stomach cancer, HIPEC is an experimental treatment that may be an option. It could be applied if the cancer spreads through the stomach and into adjacent organs, making complete removal of the tumor impractical. The surgeon may try to remove the majority of the cancer. Subsequently, HIVEC aids in the elimination of residual cancer cells.

- **Radiation Therapy:** High-powered energy beams are used in radiation therapy to destroy cancer cells. Protons, X-rays, and other sources may be the source of the beams. Radiation therapy involves lying on a table with a machine applying radiation to specific body points. Chemotherapy and radiation therapy are frequently administered concurrently. Doctors refer to this as "chemoradiation" at times. When treating stomach cancer in stage 1, radiation therapy may not be necessary. If the cancer was completely removed during surgery and there was little chance that it would return, it might not be necessary. When treating stage 2 and stage 3 stomach cancers, radiation therapy is occasionally used before surgery. It has the ability to reduce cancer so that removal is simpler. Neoadjuvant radiation refers to radiation administered prior to surgery. If the cancer cannot be entirely removed during surgery, radiation therapy may be used as a last resort. Adjuvant radiation is the term for radiation given after surgery. If surgery is not an option or the stomach cancer is advanced, radiation therapy may help relieve symptoms.
- **Targeted Therapy:** Medicines known as "targeted treatments" target particular chemicals found in cancer cells. Targeted therapies have the ability to kill cancer cells by preventing these substances from functioning. To determine whether targeted therapy is likely to be effective for you, your cancer cells are tested. Targeted therapy is frequently combined with systemic chemotherapy for stomach cancer. Advanced stomach cancer is usually treated with targeted therapy. This may include recurrent cancer following treatment and stomach cancer in stage 4.
- **Immunotherapy:** Immunotherapy is a medical treatment that stimulates the immune system to eradicate cancerous cells from the body. Your immune system targets bacteria and other foreign cells in your body to prevent illness. Cancer cells evade the immune system to survive. Immunotherapy aids in the immune system's ability to identify and eliminate cancerous cells. In certain cases, immunotherapy is used to treat advanced cancer. This may include recurrent cancer following

treatment or stomach cancer in stage 4.

- **Palliative Care:** A unique kind of medical care known as palliative care is designed to make you feel better when you have a life-threatening illness. Palliative care can assist in reducing pain and other symptoms if you have cancer. Palliative care is administered by a group of medical professionals. This can apply to physicians, nurses, and other professionals with specialized training. Enhancing your and your family's quality of life is their main objective. Palliative care experts collaborate with you, your loved ones, and your healthcare team to promote your well-being. They offer an additional degree of assistance during your cancer treatment. Palliative care can be provided alongside aggressive cancer treatments like radiation therapy, chemotherapy, or surgery. Palliative care may help cancer patients feel better and live longer when used in conjunction with all other appropriate treatments.

10.2.4. Stomach Motility

A class of diseases known as gastrointestinal motility disorders affect the contractions of the muscles that move food through the digestive tract, or peristalsis. The range of symptoms that may arise from this depends on the specific area of the digestive tract that is impacted. These include diarrhea, constipation, heartburn, regurgitation, and choking. Many factors can affect gastrointestinal motility.

An issue with the muscles governing peristalsis.

- A problem with the hormones or nerves that control the contraction of muscles.

One or both of these issues can arise from a variety of conditions.

10.2.4.1. Symptoms of Peristalsis Problems

Depending on the kind and site of the disturbance in motility, intestinal motility disorders can result in a variety of symptoms, such as:

- Difficulty swallowing
- Choking
- Heartburn
- Burping
- Acid reflux
- Regurgitation
- A feeling of early fullness
- Stomach pain
- Nausea
- Vomiting
- Gas
- Bloating
- Abdominal cramping
- Diarrhea
- Constipation

10.2.4.2. Types of Motility Disorders

The following six common and uncommon conditions are linked to dysfunctional gastrointestinal motility:

- **Gastroparesis:** The condition known as gastroparesis, or delayed gastric emptying, is brought on by the stomach emptying slowly. The passage of partially digested food into the small intestine is controlled by the muscles in your stomach.

Food will move too slowly when there is damage to the nerves that regulate the muscles in the stomach, which can result in nausea, burping, bloating, heartburn, indigestion, regurgitation, or vomiting.

- **Achalasia:** The lower esophageal sphincter (LES), a ring of muscle at the base of the esophagus that allows food to pass into the stomach, malfunctions in achalasia. Food doesn't travel through the esophagus as easily when you have achalasia because the LES is unable to relax during swallowing. Chest pain, regurgitation, heartburn, and trouble swallowing are among the symptoms.
- **Gastroesophageal Reflux Disease (GERD):** The inability of the LES to close completely results in the chronic digestive tract disorder known as gastroesophageal reflux disease (GERD). This makes it possible for stomach acid to reflux back into the esophagus, which can result in nausea, heartburn, chest pain, and an acidic aftertaste. Heartburn and acid reflux that happen more than twice a week could be a sign of GERD. Sometimes the symptoms are so bad they seem to be heart attack symptoms.
- **Irritable Bowel Syndrome (IBS):** As a functional digestive disorder, irritable bowel syndrome (IBS) affects how your digestive system functions but does not harm the digestive organs directly. Your digestive motility moves either too quickly or too slowly when you have IBS, which can cause mixed-type IBS (IBD-M), constipation-predominant IBS (IBS-C), or diarrhea-predominant IBS (IBS-D). Additional symptoms include cramps, nausea, bloating, gas, and pain in the stomach and rectal area.
- **Hirschsprung's Disease:** In Hirschsprung's disease, a congenital condition, the large intestine becomes blocked due to a disruption in peristalsis. The condition is more prevalent in younger boys and is frequently observed in conjunction with other congenital conditions like Down syndrome.
- **Chronic Intestinal Pseudo-Obstruction:** A rare disorder known as chronic intestinal pseudo-obstruction (CIPO) mimics the symptoms of a bowel obstruction. However, there is no obstruction of any kind when using CIPO. Peristalsis essentially just ends. The movement of food, liquid, and air through the large intestine (bowel), as well as the esophagus, stomach, small intestine, and rectum, is disturbed by nerve issues that lead to CIPO.

10.2.4.3. Causes

A rare disorder known as chronic intestinal pseudo-obstruction (CIPO) mimics the symptoms of a bowel obstruction. However, there is no obstruction of any kind when using CIPO. Peristalsis essentially just ends. The movement of food, liquid, and air through the large intestine (bowel), as well as the esophagus, stomach, small intestine, and rectum, is disturbed by nerve issues that lead to CIPO.

- **Underlying Conditions:** Diseases that either harm nerves or interfere with the production of hormones necessary for peristalsis, such as the following, are closely associated with issues with stomach motility.

- **Diabetes:** It is estimated that gastroparesis affects 20 to 50% of diabetics. The nerves that control regular peristalsis can be progressively damaged by high blood sugar levels.
- **Scleroderma:** An autoimmune condition called scleroderma tightens tissues, including those in your digestive system. GERD and CIPO are prevalent conditions in scleroderma patients.
- **Neurological Disorders:** Conditions involving the nerves that can impact stomach motility include multiple sclerosis, Parkinson's disease, and stroke.
- **Hypothyroidism:** Reduced stomach motility has been found to be closely associated with hypothyroidism (low thyroid function).

- **Genetics:** Certain gastric motility disorders, including GERD, Hirschsprung's disease, and CIP, are believed to be influenced by genes. Genetics can also play a role in autoimmune disorders linked to dysfunction in motility.
- **Medications:** Constipation can be brought on by opioid painkillers like oxycodone and hydrocodone, which slow stomach motility. Up to 81% of individuals who use opioids are estimated to experience constipation.

10.2.4.4. Treatment

Treatments for various gastric motility disorders vary. Options for treatment include surgery, medication, and dietary and lifestyle modifications.

- **Lifestyle:** Many different gastric motility disorders can be managed with a healthy diet and minor dietary adjustments. This entails consuming softer foods like the following and consuming smaller meals throughout the day to prevent overtaxing the digestive tract.
  - Ground meat, poultry, or seafood
  - Well-cooked fruits and vegetables
  - Soft pasta and rice
  - Low-fat dairy

Some people may have improved gastrointestinal motility by engaging in regular aerobic exercise. It's frequently advised to assist in treating and preventing IBS-C-related constipation. Another benefit of quitting smoking is that it lessens overall digestive tract inflammation, which can make the intestines and stomach more susceptible to food triggers.

- **Medications:** Drugs that are frequently prescribed to treat problems with stomach motility include:
  - Antacids: including GERD medications like Rolaids and Tums.
  - Antiemetics: Used to treat achalasia, gastroparesis, and nausea related to GERD.
  - Antidiarrheals: Such as Viberzi (eluxadoline) and Imodium (loperamide), which are used

  - to treat diarrhea brought on by IBS-D.
  - Botulinum toxin injections: Also referred to as Botox; used to treat gastroparesis and achalasia.
  - Calcium-channel blockers: Used to treat achalasia
  - H2 blockers: Such as the famotidine-containing Pepcid AC and Zantac 360, which are used to treat GERD.
  - Laxative and stool softeners: used to treat IBS-C-related constipation.
  - Prokinetic drugs: Such as the medications Reglan (metoclopramide) and Linzess (linaclotide), which are used to treat IBS-C and gastroparesis.
  - Proton pump inhibitors (PPIs): Such as Prilosec (omeprazole) and Nexium (esomeprazole), which are prescribed to treat gastroparesis and GERD.
- **Surgery:** If non-invasive treatments do not alleviate your symptoms, your gastroenterologist may suggest a surgery tailored to address your specific condition. Some options include:
  - **Nissen Fundoplication:** To stop acid reflux, the LES is tightened during this GERD treatment procedure.
  - **Heller Myotomy:** To treat achalasia, this procedure entails making incisions on the lower and upper esophageal sphincters to relieve persistent difficulties with swallowing.
  - **Pyloroplasty:** This procedure widens the pyloric valve, which is the valve that divides the stomach from the small intestine and is used to treat gastroparesis. This facilitates faster stomach emptying.

10.2.5. Gastroparesis

Gastroparesis is a medical condition characterized by weak stomach muscular contractions, or peristalsis, which leave food and liquid in the stomach for extended periods of time. As a result, stomach contents pass into the duodenum of the digestive tract more gradually. This may lead to poor glycemic control, insufficient nutrition, and irregular nutrient absorption. Dumping syndrome is the opposite of this, where stomach contents swiftly exit into the duodenum. Early satiety, which is the feeling of being full quickly after eating, heartburn, nausea, vomiting, and abdominal pain are among the symptoms. The most widely recognized cause is autonomic neuropathy of the vagus nerve, which innervates the stomach. One of the main causes of this nerve damage is uncontrolled diabetes mellitus; other factors include vagus nerve trauma and post-infectious diseases.

A stable isotope breath test, radioisotope gastric-emptying scan, gastric manometry, esophagogastroduodenoscopy (EGD), barium swallow X-ray, and barium beefsteak meal are some of the methods used to make the diagnosis. Malnutrition, exhaustion, loss of weight, vitamin deficiencies, intestinal blockage from bezoars, and an overgrowth of bacteria in the small intestine are among the complications. If oral intake is insufficient, the patient's nutritional status should be managed with a jejunostomy feeding tube. Otherwise, oral dietary modification should be used. Dietary changes, drugs to increase stomach emptying, drugs to lessen vomiting, and surgical techniques are all part of the treatment. Furthermore, a treatment option is gastric electrical stimulation (GES; authorized under a humanitarian device exemption). Patients with gastroparesis have a much lower overall survival rate than people in the general population. It is linked to unfavorable results.

10.2.5.1. Signs and Symptoms

Early satiety, bloating, vomiting, and epigastric pain have all been associated with gastroparesis. Eating usually makes symptoms of delayed gastric emptying worse, especially after fatty meals and indigestible solids like leafy greens and salads. As the most often reported symptom, nausea affects up to 96% of patients with gastroparesis. However, the most common symptom reported can vary depending on the etiology. The degree of symptoms is not correlated with the severity of gastric emptying dysfunction. In patients with diabetes, heartburn and inadequate glycemic control might be the only signs of delayed stomach emptying. Patients with gastroparesis may appear physically normal upon examination, or in more severe cases, there may be signs of malnutrition, dehydration, and a splashing sound.

With gastroparesis, nausea is typically postprandial, though it can also happen in the morning or last all day. Retching and the forceful evacuation of stomach contents from the stomach up to and out of the mouth are the hallmarks of vomiting. Retching may occur in certain patients but not vomiting of stomach contents.

An uncomfortable sensation of fullness in the stomach that develops after eating is called postprandial fullness. Patients may describe postprandial fullness as having food in their stomachs for a longer amount of time. After eating, satiation is the absence of hunger. It is the opposite of appetite and hunger. The loss of appetite that occurs before the absorption of nutrients during food ingestion is known as early satiety. Patients with gastroparesis may describe their early satiation as a loss of appetite or disappearance of appetite during eating. The feeling of fullness in the stomach that develops quickly after starting to eat and is not in line with the amount of food consumed is known as early satiety. Bloating is a very personal sensation of elevated abdominal pressure. It's important to distinguish between postprandial fullness and bloating without eating. It is occasionally, but not always, connected to eating. 90% of patients with gastroparesis experience abdominal pain or discomfort regularly. Patients with idiopathic gastroparesis may feel more pain in their abdomens than those with diabetic gastroparesis. Postprandial epigastric pain is thought by doctors to be the most typical sign of gastroparesis. There are numerous symptoms associated with abdominal pain. Although it can occasionally be diffuse, localized epigastric pain affects about 40% of patients. Although pain is typically categorized as postprandial, it can also happen at night and cause sleep disturbances. The degree of stomach pain has nothing to do with how well the stomach empties.

10.2.5.2. Complications

Gastroparesis can cause aspiration, bezoar formation, abnormalities in fluid and electrolyte balance, difficulty controlling blood sugar levels (which exacerbates gastric dysmotility), and inadequate nutrition intake leading to weight loss. Acute renal insufficiency and orthostatic hypotension are signs of dehydration that some patients may experience due to severe nausea and vomiting. Some individuals with severe gastroparesis experience severe weight loss and nutritional deficiencies that require access to small bowel feeding to bypass the stomach.

Gastric bezoars are also more common in people with gastroparesis. Large masses of food and foreign materials that have become lodged in the GI tract, particularly the stomach, are known as bezoars. According to a barium study, the incidence of bezoar formation in patients with gastroparesis is thought to be around 6%. Small intestinal bacterial overgrowth (SIBO) development and gastroparesis are strongly correlated. Using a glucose breath test, a study that looked at 50 patients with gastroparesis found that 60% of them had SIBO. Moreover, a longer duration of gastroparesis symptoms raises the chance of SIBO. It's thought that poor gastric acid production and gastrointestinal motility allow bacteria to grow in the small intestine. Additionally, a lot of people with gastroparesis are treated with acid-suppressive medications, which severely reduce the natural bactericidal activity of the GI tract. SIBO induces inflammation in the small intestine, which exacerbates nutritional deficiencies in gastroparesis and hinders absorption.

Patients with gastroparesis run the risk of serious nutritional abnormalities due to the incapacitating symptoms. A study involving 305 patients diagnosed with gastroparesis evaluated their nutritional status and dietary intake; the average daily caloric intake was 1168 kcal, leading to significant nutritional deficiencies. In addition, 64% of patients with gastroparesis followed a diet low in calories. Higher symptom scores also showed an inverse relationship with calorie intake. According to a different study, the length of time it took for the stomach to empty was correlated with how severe nutritional deficiencies were. Deficiencies in iron, fat-soluble vitamins, thiamine, and folate are frequently reported. A common condition among gastroparesis patients is iron deficiency. Additional problems include blood glucose swings brought on by erratic digestion times brought on by variations in the rate and volume of food entering the small intestine, a decline in quality of life as a result of the inability to keep up with work and other obligations, and extreme exhaustion as a result of calorie deficit.

10.2.5.3. Causes

Acute illnesses of any kind, certain cancer treatments, medications that impact the digestive system, and irregular eating habits can all result in transient gastroparesis. Cancer patients may experience gastroparesis as a result of chemotherapy-induced neuropathy, immunosuppression followed by GI tract viral infections, celiac block procedures, paraneoplastic neuropathy or myopathy, or graft-versus-host disease following an allogeneic bone marrow transplant.

The symptoms of gastroparesis are comparable to those of high blood pressure, slow stomach emptying brought on by some opioid, antidepressant, and allergy medications. These may exacerbate the symptoms of gastroparesis in individuals who already have it. Over half of all cases of gastroparesis have idiopathic causes, meaning they have no known cause. However, autonomic neuropathy is often the cause. About 30 to 50% of individuals with type 2 diabetes who have had the disease for a long time may experience this. Given that elevated blood glucose levels may impact chemical alterations in the nerves, diabetes mellitus has actually been identified as the most frequent cause of gastroparesis. Years of high blood sugar or inadequate glucose transport into cells damage the vagus nerve, which causes gastroparesis. Thyroid and adrenal gland issues may also be the reason.

Additionally, gastroparesis has been linked to neurological disorders like multiple system atrophy and Parkinson's disease, as well as connective tissue diseases like scleroderma and Ehlers-Danlos syndrome. It could happen as a result of a mitochondrial illness. Gastroparesis brought on by medication can be brought on by opioids and anticholinergic drugs. There are additional causes of chronic gastroparesis, including vagus nerve injury from abdominal surgery. Given that smoking damages the lining of the stomach, heavy cigarette smoking is also a possible explanation. A third of chronic cases are idiopathic gastroparesis, or gastroparesis with no known cause. It is believed that an acute viral infection triggers an autoimmune response in many of these cases. Anecdotally, the condition has been linked to the onset of gastroenteritis, mononucleosis, and other illnesses; however, no systematic study has established a link.

There is a disproportionate number of female gastroparesis patients. Women have naturally slower stomach emptying times than men-that could be one reason for this finding. Given that symptoms of gastroparesis typically worsen the week before menstruation, when progesterone levels are at their highest, a hormonal explanation has been proposed. Neither theory has received conclusive evidence.

10.2.5.4. Physiology and Mechanism

The physiology of gastric emptying (GE) provides the most insight into the symptoms of gastroparesis. Food and nutrients are stored in the stomach, where they are broken down to create chyme. After that, chyme is gradually released into the duodenum to promote optimal nutrient absorption. The stomach and small intestines' feedback mechanisms, which trigger the vagus nerve and other hormones, control the regulated rate of chyme release. Any delay in any of the gastric emptying factors results in disarray or a decrease in the frequency of antral contractions, which postpones gastric emptying.

Since the cells in the GI tract secrete nitric oxide, it is believed that gastroparesis may be caused by a loss of neuronal nitric oxide expression at the molecular level. This significant signaling molecule functions in the GI tract and in muscles all over the body. Low nitric oxide levels can impair the smooth muscle and other organs' ability to operate. The interstitial cells of Cajal (ICC), which function as a pacemaker by transducing signals from motor neurons to produce an electrical rhythm in the smooth muscle cells, are additional significant components of the stomach. Reduced nitric oxide levels are also associated with the death of ICC cells, which can eventually cause the stomach's smooth muscle and other parts of the gastrointestinal tract to stop working.

Among the pathophysiology of diabetic gastroparesis symptoms are:

- Early satiety and postprandial fullness are caused by a defective accommodation reflex, which is caused by the loss of gastric neurons that contain nitric oxide synthase (NOS).
- Delayed gastric emptying causes nausea and vomiting because of impaired electromechanical activity in the myenteric plexus.
- Epigastric pain may be caused by sensory neuropathy in the gastric wall.
- Tymparadyarrhythmia, or abnormal pacemaker activity, can produce a toxic signal that travels to the central nervous system and causes nausea and vomiting.

10.2.5.5. Diagnosis

Patients experiencing bloating, nausea, vomiting, or abdominal pain, especially after eating, are suspected of having gastroparesis. Patients should be evaluated for gastroparesis after an upper endoscopy has been conducted to rule out gastric outlet obstruction or peptic ulcer disease as the cause of their symptoms. The most reliable test for diagnosing gastroparesis at the moment is gastric emptying scintigraphy (GES), though there are other options as well.

Griffith et al. initially defined gastroparesis in 1966, and it has since evolved into the accepted diagnostic method for the condition. Within 10 minutes of this test, the patient has a low-fat, standardized meal that is bound by radiotracer after fasting for the entire night. An extended period of ingestion could change the outcome. The majority of hospitals use Egg Beaters egg whites with one or two slices of bread, strawberry jam, and water, or 99mTc sulfur colloid-labeled egg sandwiches. Studies in the past have labeled both the liquid and solid phases of meals; however, since liquid emptying is only delayed in the most severe stages of gastroparesis, current standard tests only label the solid phase of meals. Testing liquid emptying is useful, though, when looking for postsurgical anatomic problems or ruling out dumping syndrome in postsurgical patients. The patient is given standard imaging of the gastric area while standing after ingestion. At one, two, and four hours postprandially, the percentage of radioactivity remaining in the stomach is measured using computerized software and normalized to the baseline value. If there is more than 60% retention at 2 hours and/or more than 10% retention at 4 hours, gastric emptying is deemed to have occurred later than expected (Figure 10.5).

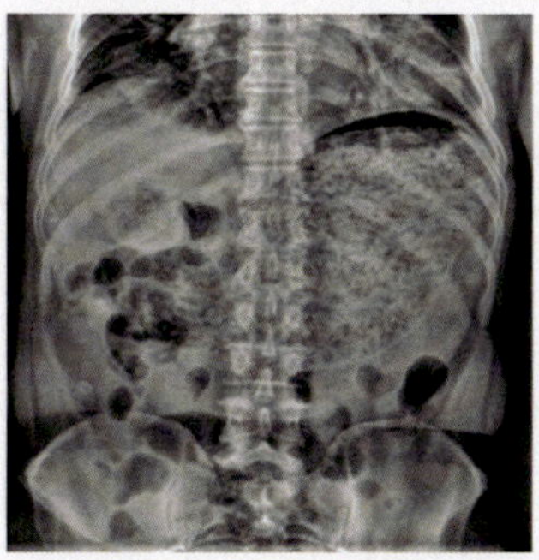

Figure 10.5. *A simple abdominal X-ray reveals a large amount of material in the stomach, suggesting severe gastric hypomotility.*

Source: By Dong Seok Lee1 and Sang Jin Lee, CC BY 3.0, https://commons.wikimedia.org/w/index.php?curid=101161694.

Using a medium-chain fatty acid substrate, such as octanoic acid, the stable isotope carbon-13 (13C) is used in the stable isotope breath test. Subsequently, the 13C-labeled substrate is affixed to either digestible food, such as muffins, or to *Spirulina plantensis*, a blue-green algae that contains 50–60% protein, 30–40% starch, and 10% fat. Meals are consumed after pre-meal breath samples are obtained after an overnight fast. 13C-octanoate is absorbed in the duodenum and becomes liquefied to form chyme following stomach emptying and feeding. After that, it travels to the liver through the portal circulation, where it is converted into 13-carbon dioxide (13CO2) and exhaled during expiration. Gastric emptying is represented by the amount of 13CO2 in an exhaled breath test because it is the rate-limiting step in the testing process. Breath samples taken after meals are taken every half an hour, and isotope-ratio mass spectrometry is used for analysis. Every 30 minutes, samples are taken for a total of 4–6 hours.

Because the stable isotope breath test involves duodenal absorption, 13C metabolism in the liver, and pulmonary exhalation of 13CO2, it is unreliable for people with small bowel diseases such as celiac disease, exocrine pancreatic insufficiency, liver disease, or lung disease. Another factor that may affect CO2 excretion is physical activity. The wireless motility capsule (WMC) has been approved by the US Food and Drug Administration to assess colonic transit time and gastric emptying in patients suspected of having slow transit constipation. The capsule measures 26.8 mm in length and 11.7 mm in width. It has three temperature, pH, and pressure sensors inside. After being consumed, the WMC measures all three variables continuously as it passes through the digestive system. Real-time, wireless data is then sent to a receiver that the patient wears around their waist to complete the study. When a pH increase of more than three units indicates that the capsule has reached the duodenum, it is said that the gastric emptying time is delayed if it lasts five hours or more. The small bowel transit time, which is measured from the point at which the pH rises by more than three units to the point at which it falls by more than one unit and is maintained for at least thirty minutes, is typically two to six hours. The capsule's journey to the cecum is indicated by this drop. The colon transit period is measured from the moment the WMC enters the cecum until it is expelled from the body, which is indicated by a sudden drop in temperature or loss of signal. The colon transit period is normally 59 hours or less. On the day of testing, patients have a set meal that includes a nutrient bar and 50 cc of water. Patients are required to fast for six hours after eating. They are required to record specific events in a diary and press the EVENT button throughout the study. After that, the receiver is collected and the data is downloaded for analysis.

Additionally, recent research has demonstrated that pressure measurements can be used to distinguish diabetic gastroparesis from other conditions. Diabetic gastroparesis is characterized by lower contraction volumes and motility indices in comparison to healthy individuals. Another benefit of employing WMC in the diagnosis of gastroparesis is the capacity to assess extragastric motility with a single test. This is helpful since gastrointestinal symptoms do not always correspond well with the gastrointestinal segment that is affected, and extragastric impaired motility affects over 40% of patients with suspected gastroparesis. In addition to measuring gastric emptying, evaluating the rest of the gastrointestinal tract can reveal information about motility in different gut segments, which can alter treatment and alleviate symptoms. Antroduodenal manometry entails inserting a manometry catheter or transducer with pressure sensors into the pyloric channel either endoscopically or under radiographic fluoroscopy to assess gastric and duodenal contractions. The pressure of antral, pyloric, and duodenal contraction waves is measured during fasting and postprandial states, typically over a period of 5–8 hours in a stationary setting or 24 hours in an ambulatory setting to evaluate duodenal motor function. This test can identify decreased antral motility in gastroparesis and help differentiate between myopathic (such as scleroderma or amyloidosis) and neuropathic (such as diabetes mellitus) causes of reduced motility. Patients with myopathic conditions exhibit decreased frequency and amplitude of migrating motor complexes, while those with neuropathic causes have normal amplitude but impaired coordination of these complexes. Antroduodenal manometry is a specialized and invasive test that requires expertise for accurate interpretation. It is technically challenging, as the catheter may shift from the pylorus during feeding and stomach dilation, and further research is needed for validation and wider availability.

While magnetic resonance imaging (MRI) and transabdominal ultrasonography (USSON) have been suggested as noninvasive diagnostic methods for gastroparesis, their application is currently limited to research. Two-dimensional ultrasonography can measure changes in the antral area to provide information about gastric emptying; the antral area returns to its preprandial baseline when complete gastric emptying has occurred. Tumor volume and meal distribution can both be determined using three-dimensional ultrasonography. Additionally, it has been suggested to use duplex sonography to assess both the liquid contents and transpyloric flow. Ultrasound seems like a safe and appealing technique, but because it requires a lot of expertise and doesn't work well on obese patients, it isn't used much in clinical settings. An additional useful tool is

MRI, which measures gastric accommodation and emptying every 15 minutes using transaxial abdominal images. Additionally, it provides information on gastric emptying and secretions by differentiating between gastric meal and air. It is expensive and requires specialized equipment, though, and its use is restricted to research alone because it is not standardized amongst centers outside of research.

10.2.5.6. Treatment

Dietary changes, drugs to increase stomach emptying, drugs to lessen vomiting, and surgical techniques are all part of the treatment. Low-fiber diets and, occasionally, restrictions on fat or solids are part of dietary treatment. It has been beneficial to eat smaller meals two to three hours apart. Eating foods like rice or beef that contribute to the specific issues, like abdominal pain or constipation, can help prevent symptoms. The dopamine D2 receptor antagonist metoclopramide improves gastric emptying by strengthening the GI tract's contractility and resting tone. Furthermore, vomiting and nausea are inhibited by the dopamine antagonist action of the central nervous system. Similarly, gastroparesis is treated with dopamine receptor antagonist domperidone. Although erythromycin is known to help with stomach emptying, its benefits are only fleeting because of tachyphylaxis and disappear after a few weeks of regular use. In cases of diabetic gastroparesis, some practitioners stimulate the gastrointestinal tract with sildenafil citrate, which increases blood flow to the genital area in men. When traditional treatment for gastroparesis is ineffective, the antidepressant mirtazapine has shown promise in treating the condition. This is because of its appetite-stimulating and antiemetic qualities. Mirtazapine and the well-known anti-emetic ondansetron both function on the same 5-HT3 serotonin receptor. A motilin agonist called caminal is used to treat gastroparesis.

Implantable gastric stimulation is a potential treatment option in certain situations where medication-resistant chronic nausea and vomiting occur. To lessen the symptoms, a medical device that applies neurostimulation to the lower stomach muscles is implanted. This is only applied in cases that are refractory and have not responded to medical management (usually after a minimum of two years of treatment). Another treatment option for medically refractory gastroparesis is a pyloromyotomy, which involves severing the circular pylorus muscle to widen the stomach outlet. This can be performed endoscopically (referred to as G-POEM) or laparoscopically. In some cases, treating gastroparesis in obese patients with a vertical sleeve gastrectomy—which involves removing all or part of the affected stomach—has even been shown to be effective in curing the condition. The small sample size of the earlier research has led to the recommendation for more investigation. Patients with postinfectious gastroparesis often experience symptoms for three weeks to six months before receiving a proper diagnosis and starting treatment.

10.3. Disorders in Pancreas

A gland located in front of the spine and behind the stomach is called the pancreas. It generates hormones that aid in blood sugar regulation and juices that aid in the breakdown of food. Numerous health issues can arise from pancreatic issues. These consist of:

- When digestive enzymes begin to break down the pancreas itself, it results in pancreatitis or inflammation of the pancreas.
- Pancreatic cancer
- In addition to clogging pancreatic tubes, thick, sticky mucus can also cause cystic fibrosis, a genetic disorder.

Diabetes is also caused in part by the pancreas. Because of an immune system attack, the pancreatic beta cells in people with type 1 diabetes are unable to produce insulin. The pancreas can no longer secrete enough insulin in response to meals if you have type 2 diabetes.

10.3.1. Pancreatitis

Inflammation of the pancreas is called pancreatitis. Immune system activity known as inflammation can result in pain, swelling, and modifications to the function of tissues or organs. Tucked behind the stomach is a long, flat gland called the pancreas. The pancreas controls blood sugar levels and aids in food digestion. Acute pancreatitis is a possible diagnosis. This indicates that it often manifests quickly and disappears quickly. Chronic pancreatitis is an enduring ailment. Over time, the pancreas damage may worsen. Acute pancreatitis might get better by itself. Severe diseases can have life-threatening consequences and need to be treated in a hospital.

10.3.1.1. Symptoms

Pancreatitis symptoms can vary. Symptoms of acute pancreatitis can include:

- Pain in the upper belly.
- Radiating pain from upper abdomen to back.
- Tenderness when touching the belly.
- Fever.
- Rapid pulse.
- Upset stomach.
- Vomiting.

Chronic pancreatitis signs and symptoms include:

- Pain in the upper belly.
- Belly pain that feels worse after eating.
- Losing weight without trying.
- Oily, smelly stools.

Some patients with chronic pancreatitis don't experience symptoms until after the condition worsens.

- **When to See a Doctor:** In the event that your stomach pain is sudden or persistent, schedule a visit with your physician. If your pain is so bad that you are unable to sit still, get medical attention right away and find a more comfortable position.

10.3.1.2. Causes

The pancreas performs two main functions. It creates insulin, which aids in the body's utilization and control of sugars. Additionally, the pancreas secretes digestive juices known as enzymes to aid in digestion. Enzyme copies that have been disabled are produced and stored by the pancreas. The enzymes are activated and begin to break down proteins in the small intestine after the pancreas delivers them there. The pancreatic enzymes may begin to function like digestive juices if they are activated prematurely. The action may cause irritation, harm, or even cell death. This issue then triggers immune system reactions that result in swelling and other things that impact the pancreas's functionality.

Acute pancreatitis can result from a number of conditions, such as:

- Gallstone-induced bile duct obstruction.
- Heavy alcohol use.
- Certain medicines.
- High triglyceride levels in the blood.
- High calcium levels in the blood.
- Pancreas cancer.
- Injuries from trauma or surgery.

- Chronic pancreatitis can result from the following conditions:
- Damage from repeated acute pancreatitis.
- Heavy alcohol use.
- Inherited genes linked to pancreatitis.
- High triglyceride levels in the blood.
- High calcium levels in the blood.

There are situations when pancreatitis has no known cause. We call this pancreatitis that is idiopathic.

10.3.1.3. Risk Factors

The following are some factors that raise your risk of pancreatitis:

- Excessive alcohol use. According to research, the risk of pancreatitis rises with four or five drinks per day.
- Cigarette smoking. Smokers have an average three-fold increased risk of developing chronic pancreatitis when compared to nonsmokers. Giving up smoking can lower the risk.
- Obesity. Pancreatitis is more common in people with a body mass index of 30 or higher.
- Diabetes. The risk of pancreatitis is higher in those with diabetes.
- Family history of pancreatitis. Chronic pancreatitis has been related to several genes. Elevated risk is associated with a family history of the condition, particularly when paired with additional risk factors.

10.3.1.4. Complications

Serious side effects from pancreatitis can include:

- **Kidney Failure:** Waste products may not be removed from the blood by the kidneys as a result of acute pancreatitis. Dialysis, or artificial filtering, may be required for either a short-term or long-term course of treatment.
- **Breathing Problems:** The functioning of the lungs can be altered by acute pancreatitis, which can lead to dangerously low blood oxygen levels.
- **Infection:** Acute pancreatitis may increase the susceptibility of the pancreas to infections. Serious pancreatic infections necessitate extensive care, including surgery or other treatments to remove infected tissue.
- **Pseudocyst:** Pancreatitis, both acute and chronic, may result in the accumulation of fluid and debris within the pancreas, forming a pseudocyst. A ruptured large pseudocyst can lead to serious complications such as internal bleeding and infection.
- **Malnutrition:** The pancreas may not generate enough digestive enzymes in cases of acute or chronic pancreatitis. Weight loss, diarrhea, and malnutrition may result from this.
- **Diabetes:** When insulin-producing cells are harmed by chronic pancreatitis, diabetes may result.
- **Pancreatic Cancer:** Pancreatic cancer is a risk factor for chronic inflammation of the pancreas.

10.3.1.5. Diagnosis

In addition to performing a general physical examination and asking you questions about your symptoms and medical history, your healthcare provider will also feel for any pain or tenderness in your abdomen.

The following are some tests and procedures that could be employed.

- Blood tests can provide information about the health of the pancreas, immune system, and other related organs.
- Pancreatitis or gallstones in the gallbladder can be seen on ultrasound images.
- The degree of inflammation and gallstones can be seen on a computerized tomography (CT) scan.
- Use magnetic resonance imaging (MRI) to check for abnormalities in the pancreas, bile ducts, and gallbladder tissues or structures.
- An ultrasound instrument on a tiny tube inserted through the mouth and into the digestive system is called an endoscopic ultrasound machine. It can reveal bile or pancreatic duct blockages, cancer, gallstones, and inflammation.
- Stool tests can measure fat levels, which may indicate that your digestive system isn't properly absorbing nutrients.

Depending on your symptoms and any other conditions you may have, your doctor might suggest additional tests.

10.3.1.6. Treatment

Pancreatitis cannot be cured with a particular medication. To manage symptoms and complications, treatment starts with a hospital stay. These consist of:

- **Analgesics:** Pain from pancreatitis can be excruciating. You will receive medication from your medical team to help manage your pain.
- **Fluids Given Intravenously (IV):** To keep you hydrated, fluids will be given to you through a vein in your arm.
- **Nutrition:** When you are able to eat again without experiencing any pain or vomiting, you will. A feeding tube is used in certain situations.
- Other treatments are used to address underlying causes once the symptoms and complications are under control. These could consist of:
- Procedures to open bile ducts. To find and remove a gallstone, a procedure known as endoscopic retrograde cholangiopancreatography (ERCP) is performed. Through the mouth and digestive tract, a long tube equipped with a camera is fed to the bile duct. This tube is also used to deliver small instruments to the location to clear the bile duct and remove the stone. Although ERCP may cause acute pancreatitis on its own, studies on risk factors have improved results.
- **Gallbladder Surgery:** Surgery to remove the gallbladder may be suggested if pancreatitis was brought on by gallstones. We refer to this procedure as a cholecystectomy.
- **Pancreas Procedures:** It is possible to remove diseased tissue or drain fluid from the pancreas using

procedures involving an endoscopic camera and tools.

- **Treatment for Alcohol Dependence:** An alcohol addiction treatment program is advised if pancreatitis was brought on by excessive alcohol consumption. Drinking alcohol continuously makes pancreatitis worse and can have major consequences.
- **Changes in Medicines:** Your healthcare provider will collaborate with you to identify alternative treatments if a medication is the likely cause of acute pancreatitis.

10.3.1.6. Additional Treatments for Chronic Pancreatitis

Additional therapies for chronic pancreatitis could include:

- **Pain Management:** Severe, chronic pain is a common symptom of chronic pancreatitis. Your healthcare provider will look for causes or complications of pain-causing chronic pancreatitis in addition to prescribing medication. Procedures to enhance pancreatic drainage or injections to obstruct nerve signals from the pancreas to the brain are examples of possible treatments. They might suggest that you see a pain specialist.
- **Enzymes to Improve Digestion:** You may use pancreatic enzyme supplements if diarrhea or weight loss are symptoms of chronic pancreatitis. These enzyme supplements, when taken with each meal, assist your body in utilizing and breaking down the nutrients in food.
- **Changes to Your Diet:** A dietitian can assist you in creating nutrient-dense, low-fat meals. Your doctor may recommend one to you.

10.3.1.8. Lifestyle and Home Remedies

Following your hospital discharge, you can continue your pancreatitis recovery by doing the following:

- **Stop Drinking Alcohol:** It is best to abstain from alcohol while recovering from pancreatitis, even if it was not the likely cause. If drinking was the expected cause, give it up. Seek assistance from your doctor if you are unable to quit drinking alcohol on your own. Your physician can recommend nearby programs to assist you in quitting drinking.
- **Stop Smoking:** Give up smoking if you do. See your doctor for assistance if you are unable to stop on your own. You can stop smoking with the aid of medication and counseling.
- **Choose a Low-Fat Diet:** Pick a diet that is low in fat and high in whole grains, lean protein, and fresh produce.
- **Drink More Fluids:** Drink more water throughout the day as pancreatitis can lead to dehydration. Having a glass or bottle of water on hand could be beneficial.

10.3.1.9. Alternative Medicine

While alternative therapies cannot cure pancreatitis, they may help manage the pain associated with chronic pancreatitis. These consist of:

- Meditation
- Relaxation exercises
- Yoga
- Acupuncture

10.3.2. Pancreatic Cancer

One kind of cancer that starts as an increase in pancreatic cells is called pancreatic cancer. The lower portion of the stomach is followed by the pancreas. It produces hormones that aid in blood sugar regulation and enzymes that aid in food digestion. Pancreatic ductal adenocarcinoma is the most prevalent kind of pancreatic cancer. This kind starts in the cells that encircle the pancreatic ducts that transport digestive enzymes. Rarely is pancreatic cancer discovered in its early stages, when there is the best chance of a cure.

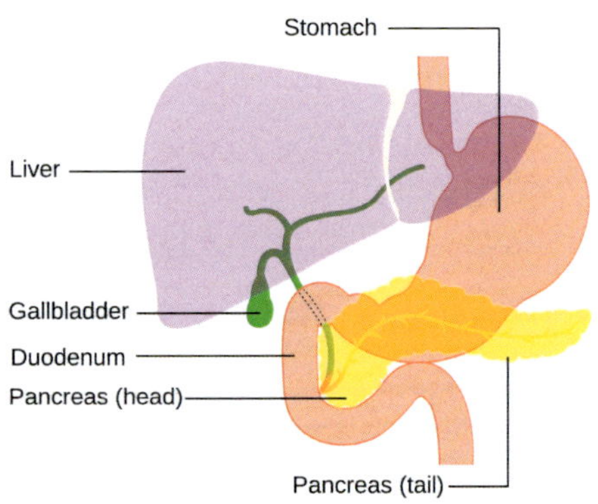

Figure 10.6. *Diagram showing the position of the pancreas.*

Source: By Cancer Research UK – original email from CRUK, CC BY-SA 4.0, https://commons.wikimedia.org/w/index.php?curid=34334263.

This is due to the fact that symptoms frequently appear only after the disease has spread to other organs. When developing your treatment plan, your healthcare team takes into account the severity of your pancreatic cancer. Radiation therapy, chemotherapy, surgery, or a combination of these may be used as treatment options (Figure 10.6).

10.3.2.1. Symptoms

Symptoms of pancreatic cancer frequently appear later in the disease's progression. Signs and symptoms of pancreatic cancer can include the following when they occur.

- Back or sides accompanied by stomach pain.
- Loss of appetite.
- Weight loss.
- Jaundice is the term for a yellowing of the skin and the whites of the eyes.
- Light-colored or floating stools.
- Dark-colored urine.
- Itching.
- Diabetes that is newly diagnosed or that is becoming more difficult to manage.
- Arm or leg pain and swelling that could be brought on by a blood clot.
- Tiredness or weakness.
- **When to See a Doctor:** If you are concerned about any symptoms, schedule a visit with a medical professional.

10.3.2.2. Causes

The cause of pancreatic cancer is unknown. Physicians have identified a few risk factors that may increase this particular cancer's likelihood. Smoking and a family history of pancreatic cancer are two of these.

- **Understanding the Pancreas:** The pancreas resembles a pear lying on its side and is roughly 6 inches (15 centimeters) long. Hormones, including insulin, are released. These hormones aid the body's digestion of the sugar that is present in food. To aid in food digestion and nutrient absorption, the pancreas also produces digestive juices.

- **How Pancreatic Cancer Forms:** When DNA alterations occur in pancreatic cells, pancreatic cancer results. The instructions that tell a cell what to do are encoded in its DNA. The instructions in healthy cells direct the cells to divide and grow at a predetermined pace. The cells have a finite lifespan. Different instructions are given by the changes in cancer cells. The alterations instruct the cancer cells to proliferate rapidly. When healthy cells die, cancer cells can survive. As a result, there are excessively many cells. The cancer cells may aggregate into a mass known as a tumor. The tumor has the potential to spread and engulf healthy bodily tissue. Cancer cells can split off and travel to other areas of the body over time. The cells lining the pancreatic ducts are where the majority of pancreatic cancer starts. We refer to this kind of cancer as pancreatic exocrine cancer or pancreatic ductal adenocarcinoma. Less frequently, pancreatic neuroendocrine or hormone-producing cells can develop cancer. Pancreatic endocrine cancer or pancreatic neuroendocrine tumors are the names given to these cancer forms.

10.3.2.3. Risk Factors

Pancreatic cancer risk factors include the following:

- Smoking.
- Type 2 diabetes.
- Pancreatitis is the term for persistent pancreatic inflammation.
- A family history of DNA alterations linked to an increased risk of cancer. The BRCA2 gene mutation, Lynch syndrome, and familial atypical multiple mole melanoma (FAMMM) syndrome are a few of these.
- Family history of pancreatic cancer.
- Obesity.
- Older age. Pancreatic cancer patients are typically older than 65.
- Drinking a lot of alcohol.

10.3.2.4. Complications

Complications from pancreatic cancer can include: as it advances.

- **Weight Loss:** Due to the fact that pancreatic cancer consumes more energy from the body, patients may experience weight loss. Eating may be difficult if cancer treatments are causing nausea and vomiting or if the cancer is pressing on the stomach. The pancreas sometimes produces insufficient digestive juices, which causes the body to have difficulties absorbing nutrients from food.
- **Jaundice:** Jaundice can result from pancreatic cancer that obstructs the bile duct in the liver. Yellowing of the skin and the whites of the eyes are symptoms. Pale stools and dark urine are two signs of jaundice. Jaundice frequently happens without abdominal pain.

A stent, which is a tube made of plastic or metal, can be inserted into the bile duct to clear obstructions. The bile duct is kept open in part by the stent. Endoscopic retrograde cholangiopancreatography, or ERCP, is the technique used to do this. An endoscopic procedure involves the insertion of a long tube, known as an endoscope, down the throat by a medical professional. The tube enters the upper portion of the small intestine after passing through the stomach. The physician inserts a dye via a tiny tube that passes through the endoscope into the pancreatic and bile ducts. On imaging tests, the dye makes the ducts more visible. Using those images, the medical professional can precisely position a stent inside the duct to help keep it open.

- Pain a developing tumor may put pressure on your abdomen's nerves, potentially resulting in excruciating pain. Painkillers may make you feel more at ease. Chemotherapy and radiation therapy are two examples of treatments that may help slow the growth of tumors and reduce pain.

If medication isn't working, a physician may recommend a celiac plexus block. Alcohol is injected via a needle into the stomach pain-regulating nerves during this procedure. Alcohol inhibits the brain from receiving pain signals from the nerves.

- Bowel blockage. Pancreatic cancer has the potential to invade or press against the duodenum, which is the first segment of the small intestine. This may stop food that has been broken down from moving from the stomach into the intestines.

A medical professional may recommend the placement of a stent, or tube, to hold the small intestine open. Occasionally, having surgery to implant a feeding tube may be beneficial. Alternatively, where the cancer isn't causing a blockage, surgery can be used to attach the stomach to a lower portion of the intestines.

10.3.2.5. Prevention

- **Screening for People with a High Risk of Pancreatic Cancer:** Tests are used in screening to look for pancreatic cancer indicators in individuals without symptoms. If you are at a very high risk of developing pancreatic cancer, it may be a possibility. If there is a significant family history of pancreatic cancer or if you have an inherited DNA mutation that raises the risk of cancer, your risk may be elevated. Imaging tests like MRIs and ultrasounds may be used in the screening process for pancreatic cancer. Typically, these exams are conducted again each year.

Finding pancreatic cancer early on, when it is small and most likely to be cured, is the aim of screening. It's unclear at this time whether screening can reduce the chance of dying from pancreatic cancer because research is still being done. It is not risk-free to screen. This includes the possibility of discovering something that needs surgery but ultimately proves not to be cancer. Discuss with your medical team the advantages and disadvantages of pancreatic cancer screening. You and your partner can determine if screening is appropriate for you (Figure 10.7).

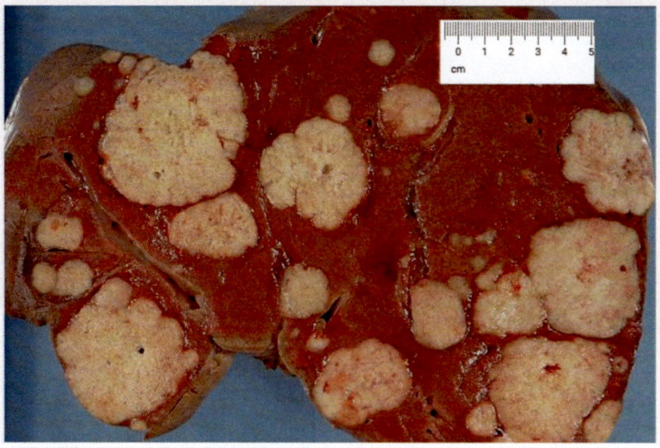

Figure 10.7. *Cross-section of a human liver, at autopsy, showing many large pale tumor deposits, that are secondary tumors derived from pancreatic cancer.*

Source: By Haymanj – Self-photographed, Public Domain, https://commons.wikimedia.org/w/index.php?curid=3662694.

- **Genetic Testing for Cancer Risk:** Talk to a healthcare provider if there is a history of pancreatic cancer in your family. Your physician can examine your family medical history and assist you in determining whether genetic testing is appropriate for you. Genetic testing can identify hereditary changes in DNA that raise the risk of cancer and run in families. You may be referred to a genetic counselor or another medical professional with training in genetics if you are interested in genetic testing.
- **Ways to Lower Risk:** Your chance of developing pancreatic cancer may be lower if you:
    - **Stop Smoking:** If you smoke, discuss quitting with a member of your healthcare team. These could consist of medications, counseling services, and nicotine replacement treatment.
    - **Maintain a Healthy Weight:** Strive to stay at your current weight if it is healthy. Aim for a gradual, consistent weight loss of one to two pounds (0.35 to one kilogram) per week if you need to lose weight. Work out most days of the week to aid in weight loss. Increase your exercise regimen gradually. Select a diet that is high in fruits, vegetables, and whole grains, but in smaller serving sizes.

10.3.2.6. Diagnosis

The following tests are used to identify pancreatic cancer:

- Imaging tests. Imaging tests produce images of the internal organs. Imaging tests such as ultrasounds, CTs, MRIs, and occasionally positron emission tomography (PET) scans are used to diagnose pancreatic cancer.
- A scope with ultrasound. The test known as endoscopic ultrasound, or EUS, creates images of the digestive tract as well as surrounding organs and tissues. The endoscope, a long, thin tube equipped with a camera, is used in EUS. The endoscope enters the stomach after passing down the throat. Sound waves are used by an ultrasound device on the endoscope to produce images of surrounding tissues. It can be applied to the creation of pancreatic images.
- Removing a sample of tissue to be examined. Taking a tiny sample of tissue for laboratory testing is

known as a biopsy. Most frequently, the sample is obtained during EUS by a medical professional. To extract tissue from the pancreas during an endoscopic procedure, specific instruments are inserted through the endoscope. It happens less frequently, but a needle inserted through the skin and into the pancreas can extract a sample of tissue. We refer to this as aspiration with fine needles.

The sample is sent to a lab to be tested for cancer. Certain DNA alterations found in cancer cells can be revealed by additional, specialized testing. The findings support the development of your treatment plan by your medical team.

- **Blood Tests:** Tumor markers are proteins produced by pancreatic cancer cells that may be detected by blood tests. The CA19–9 tumor marker test is used to detect pancreatic cancer. To monitor the cancer's response to treatment, doctors frequently repeat this test both during and after it has been started. Not all pancreatic cancers produce excess CA19–9, so not all patients benefit from this test.
- **Genetic Testing:** Discuss genetic testing with your medical team if you receive a pancreatic cancer diagnosis. A sample of blood or saliva is used in genetic testing to check for inherited DNA alterations that raise the risk of cancer. The results of genetic testing may influence how you are treated. The findings may also indicate whether there is a possible family history of pancreatic cancer.
- **Staging:** Your healthcare team investigates the cancer's extent after confirming the diagnosis of pancreatic cancer. This is referred to as the cancer's stage. The stage of your cancer is used by your healthcare team to determine a treatment plan and determine your prognosis. Pancreatic cancer stages are denoted by the numbers 0 through 4. The pancreas is the only organ affected by cancer in its lowest stages. The stage rises as the cancer spreads. Stage 4: The cancer has progressed to other bodily regions.

10.3.2.7. Treatment

The location and stage of pancreatic cancer determine the course of treatment. Your medical team also takes your preferences and general health into account. When treating pancreatic cancer, the majority of patients prioritize eliminating the cancer as much as possible. If that isn't feasible, the emphasis might be on enhancing life quality and preventing the cancer from spreading or becoming worse. Treatments for pancreatic cancer may involve radiation, chemotherapy, surgery, or a mix of these. These treatments are unlikely to be helpful when the cancer has spread. To keep you as comfortable as possible for as long as possible, the goal of treatment is to relieve symptoms.

- **Surgery:** Though not everyone has the option, surgery is a viable treatment for pancreatic cancer. Cancer that hasn't spread to other organs may be treated with it. In the event that the cancer becomes large or invades adjacent blood vessels, surgery might not be feasible. In these cases, alternative therapies, like chemotherapy, may be used as the first line of treatment. Surgery may occasionally be performed following these other therapies.

Operations used to treat pancreatic cancer include:

- Surgery to treat pancreatic head cancers. Pancreaticoduodenectomy, another name for the Whipple procedure, is an operation that removes the pancreatic head. The bile duct and the first segment of the small intestine must also be removed. An area of the stomach and adjacent lymph nodes may occasionally be removed by the surgeon. To facilitate the passage of food through the digestive system, the remaining organs are reunited.
- Surgery to treat pancreatic cancer and other body cancers. Distal pancreatectomy is the surgical term for the removal of the pancreatic body and tail. The surgeon may also need to remove the spleen during this procedure.
- Surgical excision of the entire pancreas. We refer to this as a total pancreatectomy. Following surgery, you will be on medication for the remainder of your life to replace the hormones and enzymes produced by the pancreas.
- Surgery for blood vessel-related cancers nearby. If pancreatic cancer spreads to surrounding blood vessels, a more involved procedure may be required. Parts of the blood vessels may need to be removed and rebuilt during the procedure. Surgeons skilled in performing these blood vessel operations safely are hard to come by in American medical facilities.

Bleeding and infection are risks associated with each of these operations. If the stomach has problems emptying after surgery, a condition known as delayed gastric emptying, some patients experience nausea and vomiting. After any of these procedures, a lengthy recovery is to be expected. After a few days in the hospital, you'll recuperate at home for a few weeks. According to research, pancreatic cancer surgery performed by highly skilled surgeons at facilities that perform a high volume of these procedures typically results in fewer complications. Find out about the hospital's and your surgeon's experience performing pancreatic cancer surgeries. You should seek a second opinion if you are unsure.

- **Chemotherapy:** Chemotherapy kills cancer cells with potent medications. Chemotherapy medications may be taken alone or in combination. While some chemotherapy medications are taken as pills, the majority are administered intravenously. When surgery is not an option, chemotherapy may be used as a first line of treatment. Radiation therapy and chemotherapy may also be administered concurrently. This combination of therapies can occasionally reduce the cancer to a size that allows for surgery. Treatment for this kind of pancreatic cancer is provided by specialty hospitals with a long history of treating patients with the disease. Chemotherapy is frequently used to eradicate any cancer cells that may have persisted after surgery. Chemotherapy can assist in controlling cancer that has progressed and spread to other body parts. Chemotherapy may be able to reduce pain and other symptoms.

- **Radiation Therapy:** Strong energy beams are used in radiation therapy to destroy cancer cells. Protons, X-rays, and other sources are possible sources of such energy. Radiation therapy involves lying on a table with a machine encircling you. The device targets specific areas of your body with radiation. Radiation therapy can be applied before or following surgery. It frequently follows chemotherapy. Chemotherapy and radiation can be combined as well. Chemotherapy and radiation therapy may be the first line of treatment when surgery is not an option. By reducing the cancer, this combination of treatments may enable surgery. Radiation therapy can help reduce symptoms like pain when the cancer spreads to other body parts.
- **Immunotherapy:** Immunotherapy is a medical treatment that stimulates the immune system to eliminate cancerous cells from the body. The immune system targets bacteria and other foreign cells in the body to prevent illness. Cancer cells evade the immune system to survive. Immunotherapy aids in the immune system's ability to identify and eliminate cancerous cells. If your pancreatic cancer has certain DNA alterations that increase the likelihood that the cancer will respond to these treatments, immunotherapy may be an option for you.
- **Clinical Trials:** Studies of novel treatments are called clinical trials. The opportunity to test the newest therapies is offered by these studies. The possibility of adverse effects is unknown. Find out from your medical practitioner if you could qualify for a clinical trial.
- **Palliative Care:** Palliative care is a unique form of medical care that promotes comfort for patients facing life-threatening illnesses. Palliative care can assist in reducing pain and other symptoms if you have cancer. A group of medical specialists provides palliative care. Physicians, nurses, and other professionals with specialized training may be a part of the team. Enhancing your and your family's quality of life is the team's main objective. Palliative care experts collaborate with you, your loved ones, and your healthcare team to promote your well-being. They offer an additional degree of assistance during your cancer treatment. Palliative care can be provided alongside aggressive cancer treatments like radiation therapy, chemotherapy, or surgery. Palliative care may help cancer patients feel better and live longer when combined with all other recommended treatments.

10.3.2.8. Alternative Medicine

The symptoms brought on by cancer or cancer treatments may be alleviated by certain integrative medicines and alternative therapies.

- **Treatments to Help You Cope with Distress:** Cancer patients frequently experience distress.

Distress can manifest as anxiety, fear, rage, or melancholy. Feelings like these could make it difficult for you to fall asleep. You may consider your cancer constantly. Talk to a member of your healthcare team about how you are feeling. Experts can assist you in organizing your emotions. They can assist you in coping mechanisms. Sometimes, medications can be helpful. Alternative therapies and integrative medicine may also be able to assist you in managing your emotions. Some instances are as follows:

- Art therapy.
- Exercise.
- Meditation.
- Music therapy.
- Relaxation exercises.
- Spirituality.

If any of these treatment options sound appealing to you, discuss your preferences with a member of your healthcare team.

10.3.2.9. Coping and Support

Receiving a diagnosis of a life-threatening illness can be overwhelming. The following tips may provide some relief:

- Learn about your cancer. Gain enough knowledge about your cancer to enable you to make decisions regarding your treatment. Find out the specifics of your cancer and your available treatment options by speaking with a member of your medical team. Inquire about reliable resources for additional details.
- Create a network of support. Request that your loved ones create a network of support for you. After receiving your diagnosis, they might not know what to do. They might feel more at ease and be relieved of some of your simple tasks if you help them. Consider the tasks you would like assistance with, like preparing meals or scheduling appointments.
- Look for a conversation partner. Even though they are usually your greatest allies, friends and family may occasionally find it difficult to accept your diagnosis. Speaking with a pastoral or religious counselor, a medical social worker, or a counselor might be beneficial. Seek a referral from a member of your medical team.
- Make connections with other cancer survivors. Speaking with other cancer survivors could provide you with comfort.
- Hospice care offers loved ones and those nearing the end of their lives consolation and support. It enables loved ones to be cared for and comforted at home or in a hospice setting by family and friends with the assistance of nurses, social workers, and trained volunteers. In addition, hospice care provides social, emotional, and spiritual support to patients and their loved ones.

10.3.3. Cystic Fibrosis

The genetic (inherited) disease known as cystic fibrosis (CF) results in the accumulation of thick, sticky mucus in your pancreas and lungs, among other organs. The mucus that lines your lungs, nose, and other body cavities is watery and slick if you do not have cystic fibrosis (CF). Thick mucus clogs the airways and makes breathing difficult if you have CF. Additionally, mucus clogs the pancreatic ducts, making it difficult to digest food. It's possible that CF babies and kids won't be able to get enough nutrients from their diet. In addition to affecting your liver, sinuses, intestines, and sex organs, cystic fibrosis (CF) is progressive, meaning that it gets worse over time. Additionally, there is a disease known as "atypical cystic fibrosis." It differs from classic CF in that it may only affect one organ and is a milder form. The fact that it typically manifests much later in life is another "atypical" aspect of it. "Typical" or "classic" CF typically manifests in a child during the early years of life.

10.3.3.1. Causes

Fibrosis is inherited. Individuals with CF receive one defective gene from each parent. Because two different gene variants are required to have CF, the condition is referred to as recessive. (Gene mutation is an older term for gene variant. You can have cystic fibrosis without your parents having the disease. In actuality, CF is not a family history in many of them. The person who carries the variant gene is known as a carrier if there is no history of cystic fibrosis in your family. About 1 in 31 people in the U.S. is a carrier who is free of CF symptoms.

10.3.3.2. Symptoms

- **Classic Cystic Fibrosis:** Classic CF in children manifests as the following symptoms:
  - Inability to thrive, defined as the inability to gain weight in spite of a healthy appetite and adequate caloric intake.
  - Loose or oily stools.
  - Trouble breathing.
  - Recurrent wheezing.
  - Recurring lung infections (chronic bronchitis or pneumonia).
  - Recurrent sinus infections.
  - A nagging cough.
  - Slow growth.
- **Atypical Cystic Fibrosis:** By the time they receive atypical cystic fibrosis diagnosis, some individuals may already be adults. These are a few examples of respiratory symptoms and signs.
  - Chronic sinusitis.
  - Breathing issues that could be related to chronic obstructive pulmonary disease (COPD) or asthma.
  - Nasal polyps.
  - Frequent bouts of pneumonia.
  - Other indications and manifestations of atypical CF could be:
  - Dehydration or heat stroke can result in abnormal electrolyte levels.
  - Fertility problems.
  - Diarrhea.
  - Pancreatitis.
  - Unintended weight loss.

10.3.3.3. Diagnosis

The majority of CF diagnoses occur in childhood. Several tests and a comprehensive assessment are used by doctors to diagnose cystic fibrosis (CF). They include:

- **Newborn Screening:** During a heel prick, your healthcare provider collects a small amount of blood from your newborn while they are in the hospital and places it on a Guthrie card for screening. This test checks for various conditions, including CF. All states in the U.S.

mandate newborn screening at birth and again a few weeks later.

- **Sweat Test:** Sweat test results show that CF patients have higher levels of chloride in their bodies than non-CF individuals. To induce sweating, your healthcare provider will first apply a substance known as pilocarpine to your skin and then mildly stimulate your sweat glands with electricity. After that, your provider gathers the perspiration in a plastic coil, on gauze, or on a piece of filter paper. Sweat tests are available for people of all ages. It doesn't hurt and doesn't require a needle. For CF, this test is the most conclusive.
- **Genetic Tests:** The genes that cause cystic fibrosis are tested in blood samples.
- **Chest X-rays:** A chest X-ray is one of the tests your healthcare provider will order to support or confirm a diagnosis of cystic fibrosis (CF), but it is not the only test required. Additional testing is required.
- **Sinus X-rays:** Sinus X-rays, like chest X-rays, can verify cystic fibrosis (CF) in patients exhibiting specific symptoms. Sinus X-rays are used in conjunction with other types of testing.
- **Lung Function Tests:** A tool known as a respirometer is used in the most popular lung function test. You inhale fully and then force the breath into the spirometer's mouthpiece.
- **Sputum culture:** A sample of your sputum, or spittle, is taken by your healthcare provider, who will test it for bacteria. Pseudomonas is one of the bacteria that is most frequently found in CF patients.
- **Nasal Potential Difference (NPD):** This test measures the electrical activity in your nose by using a voltmeter, electrodes positioned in two locations within your nostrils, and one placed outside of your nose. It detects the electricity produced by the movement of ions in solution through the nasal tissue. Three various solutions are used in the test.
- **Intestinal Current Measurement (ICM):** For this test, a rectal tissue biopsy is required. Chloride secreted from the tissue is then measured.

The sweat test results for chloride levels may be normal in individuals with atypical cystic fibrosis. Certain individuals with atypical CF might have been born prior to the widespread use of testing. In cases where the diagnosis is dubious, your physician might request NPD and ICM testing.

10.3.3.4. Treatment

Your medical team will likely consist of numerous caregivers as well as a cystic fibrosis specialist. Cystic fibrosis cannot be cured, but your team will assist you in managing the condition. Keeping your airways clear is the main goal of management. If necessary, your physician will also write a prescription for medication.

- **Keeping Airways Clear:** If you have cystic fibrosis, there are several ways that you can help maintain clear airways:
  - You can pick up unique techniques for breathing and coughing.
  - You can use therapy vests that

use vibrations to break up mucus, or you can use devices that fit into your mouth.

- Chest physical therapy, commonly referred to as postural drainage and percussion to release mucus, is something you can learn. This technique involves adopting specific positions to allow your lungs to empty. To assist in releasing the mucus, another person claps their hand on your back, chest, or both. You could do this while coughing.

• **Medications for Cystic Fibrosis:** These medications, which your doctor may recommend, won't treat CF but may be helpful in some circumstances. They include:
  - Antibiotics to either prevent or treat lung infections.
  - Breathed bronchodilators, which open and relax your airways to facilitate breathing.
  - Inhaled medication to thin mucus and facilitate its removal.
  - Drugs that are anti-inflammatory, including steroids and non-steroidal anti-inflammatories.
  - Medications to treat people with specific gene variants who have cystic fibrosis.
  - Digestive enzymes from the pancreas help with digestion.
  - Constipation relief products with a soft texture.

• **Surgeries for Cystic Fibrosis:** Surgery might be required if you have cystic fibrosis or one of its side effects. These might include:
  - Surgery on your nose or sinuses.
  - bowel surgery to clear obstructions.
  - Surgery related to transplants, such as liver or double lung transplants.

10.3.3.5. Complications

The following are some of the CF complications.

• Adult CF patients may experience issues with their reproductive system, digestion, and breathing.

• People with cystic fibrosis (CF) often have thick mucus, which can harbor bacteria and cause further infections.

• Individuals with cystic fibrosis (CF) are more susceptible to the bone-thinning diseases osteopenia and osteoporosis, as well as diabetes.

• Males with cystic fibrosis (CF) require the assistance of alternative reproductive technologies to become fathers. Pregnancy problems and a decline in fertility are two potential effects of cystic fibrosis (CF) in women.

10.3.3.6. Prevention

Since cystic fibrosis is a hereditary disorder, it cannot be prevented. Consider consulting a genetic counselor before deciding to start a family if you or your partner have any family history.

10.4. Disorders in Liver and Biliary System

The liver performs a wide range of diverse functions that include hepatic blood flow, protein, carbohydrate, and fat metabolism, drug and toxin excretion and detoxification, and bile formation and elimination. As a result, there are many different clinical and laboratory abnormalities linked to liver failure.

10.4.1. Liver Cirrhosis

Severe liver scarring is known as cirrhosis. Numerous types of liver diseases and disorders, including hepatitis and chronic alcoholism, can contribute to this dangerous condition. Your liver attempts to heal itself every time it sustains damage, whether from excessive alcohol use or another factor like an infection. In the process, tissue scarring develops.

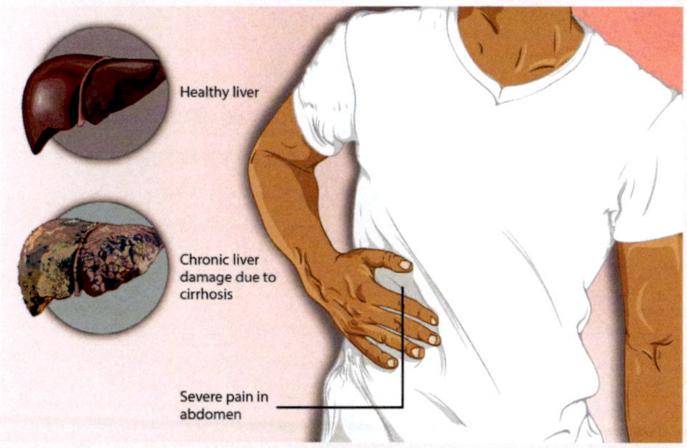

Figure 10.8. *Person with cirrhosis and associated pain in the right upper region of the abdomen.*

Source: CC BY-SA 4.0, https://commons.wikimedia.org/w/index.php?curid=82880195.

An increasing amount of scar tissue forms as cirrhosis worsens, which complicates the liver's ability to function. Advanced cirrhosis poses a serious risk to life. In most cases, cirrhosis-related liver damage is irreversible. However, additional harm can be prevented if liver cirrhosis is identified early and the underlying cause is addressed. Rarely, it might be the opposite (Figure 10.8).

10.4.1.1. Symptoms

Many times, cirrhosis is asymptomatic until significant liver damage occurs. In the event that symptoms do manifest, they could be:

- Fatigue.
- Easily bleeding or bruising.
- Loss of appetite.
- Nausea.
- Swelling in the legs, feet or ankles, called edema.
- Weight loss.
- Itchy skin.
- Jaundice is a yellow discoloration of the skin and eyes.
- A build-up of fluid in the abdomen known as ascites.
- Spiderlike bloedvate in die vel.
- Redness in the palms of the hands.
- Pale nails, particularly on the thumb and middle finger.
- Fingers that have been clubbed together spread out and rounder than normal.
- Women's loss of or inability to get their periods is unrelated to menopause.
- Male gynecomastia, which is characterized by breast enlargement, testicular shrinkage, or loss of sex drive.
- Confusion, drowsiness or slurred speech.
- **When to See a Doctor:** If you experience any of the above symptoms, schedule a visit with your physician.

10.4.1.2. Causes

Numerous illnesses and ailments have the potential to harm the liver and cause cirrhosis.

Some of the causes include:

- Long-term alcohol abuse.
- Ongoing viral hepatitis (hepatitis B, C and D).
- Fat builds up in the liver in a condition known as nonalcoholic fatty liver disease.
- A disorder called hemochromatosis leads to an accumulation of iron in the body.
- An illness of the liver brought on by the immune system is called autoimmune hepatitis.
- Bile duct destruction brought on by primary biliary cholangitis.
- Primary sclerosing cholangitis causes the bile ducts to harden and scar.
- Wilson's disease is a disorder where the liver accumulates copper.
- Cystic fibrosis.
- Alpha-1 antitrypsin deficiency.
- Biliary atresia, or poorly formed bile ducts, is a medical condition.
- Genetic diseases related to the metabolism of sugar, such as glycogen storage disease and galactosemia.
- Alagille syndrome, a genetic digestive disorder.
- Infection, like brucellosis or syphilis.
- Drugs, such as isoniazid or methotrexate.

10.4.1.3. Risk Factors

- Excessive alcohol consumption. Cirrhosis is associated with an increased risk of alcohol consumption.
- Having a weight problem. Obesity raises your risk of nonalcoholic fatty liver disease and nonalcoholic steatohepatitis, two disorders that can cause cirrhosis.
- Possessing hepatitis virus. Although cirrhosis is one of the main causes of liver disease worldwide, not everyone with chronic hepatitis will go on to develop it.

10.4.1.4. Complications

Complications of cirrhosis can include:

- Elevated blood pressure in the liver-supplying veins. Portal hypertension is the name given to this illness. The normal flow of blood through the liver is slowed by cirrhosis. The vein that supplies blood to the liver becomes more pressurized as a result.
- Swelling in the abdomen and legs. Ascites, or an accumulation of fluid in the abdomen, and edema, or swelling in the legs, are two possible outcomes of elevated portal vein pressure. When the liver is unable to produce enough albumin or other blood proteins, edema and ascites may also occur.
- **Growth of the Spleen:** White blood cells and platelets may become trapped in the spleen as a result of portal hypertension. Splenomegaly is the term for the swelling of the spleen caused by this. The initial

indication of cirrhosis may be a decrease in white blood cells and platelets in the blood.

- **Bleeding:** Blood can be diverted into smaller veins as a result of portal hypertension. These smaller veins may rupture due to the increased pressure, resulting in severe bleeding. Vascular enlargements in the stomach or esophagus known as varices can also be brought on by portal hypertension. Additionally, these varices may cause potentially fatal bleeding. Another factor that may contribute to ongoing bleeding is the liver's inability to produce enough clotting factors.
- **Infections:** It may be difficult for your body to fight infections if you have cirrhosis. Bacterial peritonitis is a dangerous infection that can result from ascites.
- **Malnutrition:** Your body may have a harder time processing nutrients if you have cirrhosis, which could result in weakness and weight loss.
- A buildup of toxins in the brain. Toxins cannot be eliminated from the blood as well by a liver damaged by cirrhosis as it can be by a healthy liver. Subsequently, these poisons may accumulate in the brain, leading to cognitive impairment and disorientation. Hepatic encephalopathy is the term for this. Hepatic encephalopathy can eventually lead to a coma or loss of consciousness.
- **Jaundice:** When your sick liver is unable to sufficiently eliminate the waste product called bilirubin from your blood, jaundice develops. Urine turns darker and the skin and whites of the eyes turn yellow due to jaundice.
- **Bone Disease:** Some cirrhosis patients experience a loss of bone mass and an increased risk of fractures.
- Increased risk of liver cancer. Cirrhosis predisposes a significant number of liver cancer patients.
- **Acute-on-Chronic Cirrhosis:** Some people eventually develop multiple organ failure. Scientists now think that some cirrhosis patients experience this complication. They're not entirely sure what causes it, though.

10.4.1.5. Prevention

By caring for your liver, you can reduce your risk of developing cirrhosis:

- Avoid consuming alcohol if you have cirrhosis or any other liver disease.
- Eat a healthy diet. Make fruit and vegetable-rich diet choices. Make sure to choose lean protein sources and whole grains. Reduce the quantity of fried and fatty foods you consume.
- Maintain a healthy weight. Overindulgence in fat can harm your liver. If you are obese or overweight, discuss a weight-loss plan with your healthcare provider.
- Reduce your risk of hepatitis. Hepatitis B and C can be contracted through unprotected sex and the sharing of needles. Inquire with your doctor about hepatitis immunizations.

Consult your healthcare provider about ways to lower your risk of liver cirrhosis if you're worried about it.

10.4.1.6. Diagnosis

Most people with early-stage liver cirrhosis do not exhibit any symptoms. Cirrhosis is frequently initially discovered during a standard blood test or examination. A combination of laboratory and imaging tests is typically performed to help confirm a diagnosis.

- **Tests:** To check your liver, your doctor may order one or more tests, such as:
  - **Laboratory Tests**: Blood tests may be prescribed by your physician to look for indicators of liver disease, such as elevated bilirubin levels or specific enzyme levels. Creatinine levels in your blood are measured to assess kidney function. They would take your blood pressure. You will undergo a hepatitis virus screening. The ability of your blood to clot is also assessed using your international normalized ratio (INR).

Your doctor may be able to determine the underlying cause of your cirrhosis based on your medical history and the results of any blood tests. Blood tests can also be used to determine the severity of your cirrhosis.

- **Imaging Tests:** It may be necessary to recommend certain imaging tests, such as magnetic resonance elastography (MRE) or transient imaging. These non-invasive imaging techniques search for liver stiffness or hardening. There may also be other imaging tests performed, including CT, MRI, and ultrasound.
- **Biopsy:** A biopsy, or sample of tissue, is not always required to make a diagnosis. However, your doctor might use it to determine the extent of liver damage and its cause.

Your doctor may advise routine testing if you have cirrhosis to monitor any progression of the liver disease or for any indications of potential complications, such as liver cancer and esophageal varices. There are more and more noninvasive tests available to track liver disease.

10.4.1.7. Treatment

The cause and degree of your liver damage will determine how you are treated for cirrhosis. Treatment aims to prevent or treat cirrhosis symptoms and complications, as well as slow the growth of scar tissue in the liver. If you have serious liver damage, you might have to stay in a hospital.

- **Treatment for the Underlying Cause of Cirrhosis:** Treating the underlying cause of early cirrhosis may enable liver damage to be minimized. Among the choices are:
  - **Treatment for Alcoholism:** Those who have cirrhosis brought on by heavy alcohol consumption ought to make an effort to cut back. If you find it difficult to give up alcohol, your doctor might suggest an alcohol addiction treatment program. It's critical to give up alcohol if you have cirrhosis because even small amounts can be harmful to your liver.

- **Weight Loss:** If nonalcoholic fatty liver disease-related cirrhosis patients reduce their body weight and manage their blood sugar, they may experience improved health.
- **Medicines to Control Hepatitis:** Medications that target hepatitis B or C viruses specifically may prevent additional harm to liver cells.
- Medications to manage cirrhosis symptoms and other underlying causes. Certain types of liver cirrhosis may progress more slowly under medication. For instance, medication may greatly slow the progression of primary biliary cholangitis to cirrhosis in patients with early diagnosis.

Alternative medications are available to alleviate specific symptoms like itching, fatigue, and pain. In cases of malnutrition related to cirrhosis, nutritional supplements may be recommended. Additionally, supplements can aid in the prevention of osteoporosis by promoting stronger bones.

- **Treatment for Complications of Cirrhosis:** Your healthcare provider will address any complications associated with cirrhosis, focusing on treatment:
    - **A Buildup of Fluid in Your Body:** Ascites and swelling may be controlled with a low-sodium diet and medications that stop the body from accumulating fluid. Severe fluid accumulation might necessitate surgery to release pressure or procedures to drain the fluid.
    - **Portal Hypertension:** Certain blood pressure medications can prevent severe bleeding by regulating portal hypertension, or elevated blood pressure in the veins supplying the liver. An upper endoscopy will be performed regularly by your physician to check for any enlarged, potentially bleeding veins in the stomach or esophagus. Varices are the name for these veins.

You will probably require medication to reduce the risk of bleeding if you develop varices. A process called band ligation may be necessary if you exhibit symptoms that indicate the varices are bleeding or are likely to bleed. A band ligation can halt the bleeding or lessen the chance that it will continue. In extreme circumstances, a transjugular intrahepatic portosystemic shunt—a tiny tube inserted into your vein to lower liver blood pressure—might be necessary.

- **Infections:** Antibiotics or other treatments for infections might be administered to you. It's also likely that your doctor will advise getting vaccinated against hepatitis, pneumonia, and influenza.
- **Increased Liver Cancer Risk:** Your physician will probably advise routine blood work and ultrasound examinations to check for liver cancer symptoms.
- **Hepatic Encephalopathy:** You might be given medication to help lessen the accumulation of toxins in your bloodstream brought on by impaired liver function.

- **Liver Transplant Surgery:** When liver function is lost due to advanced cirrhosis, liver transplantation might be the only available treatment. The process of replacing your liver with a healthy liver from a deceased donor or with a portion of a liver from a living donor is known as a liver transplant. One of the most frequent causes of liver transplantation is cirrhosis. Several tests are performed on liver transplant candidates to see if they are healthy enough to recover well from surgery.

Because of the possibility that they will resume their harmful drinking after receiving a liver transplant, people with alcoholic cirrhosis have historically not been considered candidates for the procedure. However, recent research indicates that the post-transplant survival rates of carefully chosen individuals with severe alcoholic cirrhosis are comparable to those of liver transplant recipients with other liver diseases.

In the event that you have alcoholic cirrhosis, you would have to:

- Look for a program that supports individuals with alcoholic cirrhosis.
- Fulfill the prerequisites of the course. These would include adhering to the transplant center's specific guidelines and making a lifetime commitment to alcohol abstinence.
- **Potential Future Treatments:** Efforts to broaden the current cirrhosis treatment regimen have not yielded much success thus far. There are numerous possible treatment approaches for cirrhosis due to its diverse range of etiology and complications. If initiated at an early stage, a combination of new medications, lifestyle modifications, and increased screening may improve outcomes for individuals with liver damage. Therapeutics that specifically target liver cells are being developed by researchers in an effort to slow or even reverse the fibrosis that causes cirrhosis. But no targeted treatment is quite ready yet.

10.4.1.8. Lifestyle and Home Remedies

If you have cirrhosis, take precautions to prevent further liver damage:

- **Don't Drink Alcohol:** Don't drink alcohol, regardless of whether chronic alcohol use or another illness led to your cirrhosis. Alcohol consumption may exacerbate liver damage.
- **Eat a Low-sodium Diet:** Your body may retain more fluids as a result of eating too much salt, which can exacerbate leg and abdomen swelling. Instead of using salt to season your food, use herbs. Select prepared foods with minimal sodium content.
- **Eat a Healthy Diet:** Malnutrition is a possibility in the cirrhosis patients. Eat a balanced diet that includes a range of fruits and vegetables to help combat this.

Select lean protein sources like fish, poultry, or legumes. Steer clear of raw seafood.

- **Protect Yourself from Infections:** It is more difficult to fight off infections if you have cirrhosis. Keep yourself safe by avoiding sick people and washing your hands often. Obtain vaccinations against pneumonia, influenza, and hepatitis A and B.
- **Use Over-the-Counter Medicines Carefully:** It is more difficult for your liver to process medications if you have cirrhosis. Because of this, consult your doctor before taking any medications, even over-the-counter ones. Avoid taking ibuprofen and aspirin (Advil, Motrin IB, etc.). Your doctor might advise against taking acetaminophen (Tylenol, among others) or only using small amounts of it to relieve pain if you have liver damage.

10.4.2. Jaundice

Blood contains bilirubin, a yellow-orange pigment that is left over after red blood cells die. Bilirubin is eliminated from the bloodstream by the liver and ends up in your stool. Hyperbilirubinemia is a build-up that occurs when your liver is overworked or when your system contains too much. This results in jaundice, a yellowing of the skin and the whites of the eyes. Newborns frequently contract it. Jaundice, or icterus, affects about 60% of newborns in the first few days of life. Although it's less common, adults can also contract it. See a physician as soon as possible if you suspect jaundice. It might indicate a problem with the liver, blood, or gallbladder.

10.4.2.1. Types of Jaundice

Based on where bilirubin accumulates in your body, there are four primary types of jaundice. You can find out which type you have with a blood test.

- **Prehepatic:** Prestigepatic jaundice is the term for bilirubin accumulation that occurs before blood reaching the liver. This indicates that your liver is unable to handle the excess bilirubin produced by the breakdown of red blood cells.
- **Hepatic:** Hepatic jaundice is the term for when your liver is unable to properly process bilirubin.
- **Posthepatic:** After bilirubin passes through the liver and accumulates because your body cannot remove it fast enough, it causes posthepatic jaundice.
- **Obstructive Jaundice:** This is a condition where a narrowed or blocked pancreatic duct prevents bile from draining into your intestines. Given the high mortality rate associated with this type of jaundice, early detection and treatment are crucial. (Table 10.1).

Table 10.1. Potential Causes of Jaundice, Divided into Pre-hepatic, Hepatocellular, and Post-hepatic

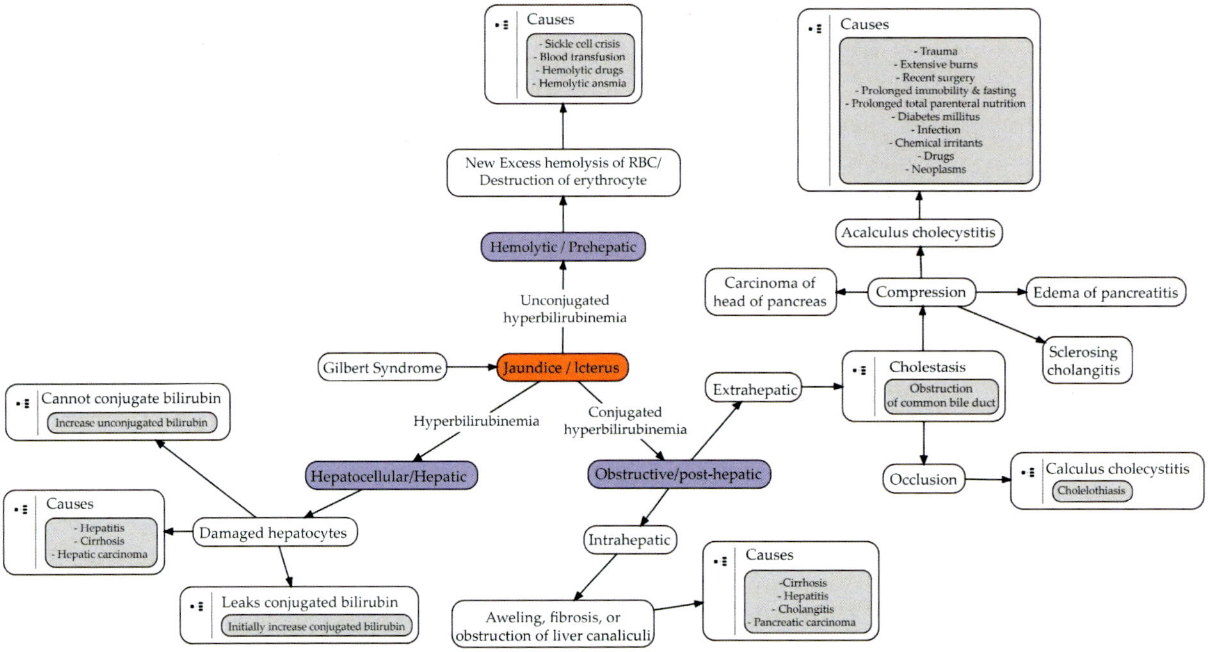

Source: GFDL, https://commons.wikimedia.org/w/index.php?curid=92928475.

10.4.2.2. Symptoms

There could be no symptoms of jaundice. Depending on how quickly the condition is deteriorating, you may experience different signs. The most well-known signs are jaundice eyes, also known as scleral icterus, and yellowing of the skin. However, there are still more to be aware of, such as:

- Fever
- Stomach pain
- Chills
- Dark urine
- Tar- or clay-colored stools
- Flu-like symptoms
- Itchy skin
- Weight loss
- Feeling unusually irritated
- Confusion
- Abnormal drowsiness

- Bruising or bleeding easily
- Bloody vomit
- **How long Does Jaundice Last in Adults?:** The cause of your jaundice and the course of treatment you need will determine how long it lasts. If jaundice is brought on by a medication, it will go away once you stop taking it. Treatment options include medication if hepatitis is the underlying cause. Surgery might be necessary if there are gallstones or a blocked bile duct (Figure 10.9).

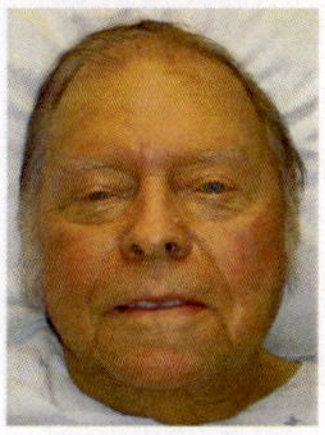

Figure 10.9. *Jaundice of the skin caused by pancreatic cancer.*

Source: By James Heilman, MD – Own work, CC BY 3.0, https://commons.wikimedia.org/w/index.php?curid=9389660.

10.4.2.3. Causes

Although it is uncommon, there are numerous causes of jaundice in adults. These include:

- **Hepatitis:** Inflammation of the liver can be brought on by viruses, autoimmune diseases, drug or alcohol abuse, or chemical exposure. It could be acute, meaning it goes away quickly, or chronic, meaning it lasts for at least six months. Jaundice can arise from chronic inflammation causing harm to the liver.
- **Alcohol-Related Liver Disease:** Over an extended period of time (eight to ten years), heavy drinking can cause significant liver damage. Particularly damaging to the liver are alcoholic hepatitis and alcoholic cirrhosis.
- **Other Liver Diseases:** Hepatitis, genetic disorders that run in the family, and autoimmune diseases can also result in cirrhosis. Nonalcoholic fatty liver disease can be brought on by a serious illness called nonalcoholic steatohepatitis. This type of liver disease causes inflammation and fat accumulation in the liver, which over time deteriorates the liver.
- **Blocked Bile Ducts:** These are tiny tubes that travel from your liver and gallbladder to your small intestine to transport a substance known as bile. You may experience jaundice if the tubes are obstructed by gallstones, cancer, inflammation, or uncommon liver diseases.
- **Pancreatic Cancer:** For men, this is the tenth most common cancer, and for women, it is the ninth. Jaundice may result from bile duct obstruction.
- **Certain Medicines:** Liver disease has been associated with drugs such as steroids, birth control pills, penicillin, and acetaminophen.
- **Blood Clots:** Your body may reabsorb a large hematoma (blot clot) under the skin, which can raise your bilirubin levels.
- **Hemolytic Anemias:** Sometimes the bloodstream's removal of destroyed blood cells occurs too quickly, which raises bilirubin levels.

10.4.2.4. Diagnosing Jaundice

Your medical history and symptoms will be questioned by your physician. After that, they'll examine you physically to check for liver swelling. Your doctor will probably order blood tests to measure cholesterol and bilirubin levels as well as a complete blood count (CBC) to gather more information. Your bilirubin level will be elevated if you are experiencing jaundice. To determine the cause and severity of your jaundice, your doctor may prescribe additional tests, such as the following.

- A blood test called a hepatitis panel determines whether you currently have or have ever had hepatitis. It tests for the three types of hepatitis: A, B, and C. You either don't have hepatitis or you had it in the past but your body has recovered if there are no hepatitis antibodies in your blood.
- Tests to measure the liver's enzyme levels and assess its overall health. Elevations or decreases in enzyme levels may indicate a condition affecting the liver or bile ducts.
- Imaging tests include CT, ultrasound, and magnetic resonance cholangiopancreatography (MRI), which looks for clogged ducts in the vicinity of the gallbladder.
- A liver biopsy to determine whether your liver is diseased or damaged. A tiny portion of your liver is taken out during the test via an abdominal incision, a vein in your neck, or a needle inserted into your abdomen.
- Prothrombin time is a metric used to determine how long blood plasma takes to clot. After drawing your blood, it will be tested in a lab to determine whether it clots more quickly or more slowly than is typical (between 10 and 13 seconds). Should it clot excessively slowly, it could indicate liver issues.

10.4.2.5. Treatment

Jaundice in adults is typically left untreated. However, your physician will address the underlying cause of it. Jaundice caused by acute viral hepatitis will go away on its own as your liver recovers. Your doctor might advise surgery to open the bile duct if it is the cause of the problem. Your doctor may recommend cholestyramine for oral use if your skin is itching. This drug is intended to flush your body of bile acids, which cause itching.

- **Phototherapy for Jaundice:** In phototherapy, bilirubin is broken down and released from the body through the use of fluorescent white or blue-spectrum light. While phototherapy is used to treat jaundice in newborns, it has not been demonstrated to be useful in treating jaundice in adults.

10.4.2.6. Preventing Jaundice

If you have hepatitis or consume excessive amounts of alcohol, you may be more susceptible to jaundice. Additionally, it is more prevalent in middle-aged individuals.

By altering your lifestyle, you can lower your risk of jaundice.

- Steer clear of herbal supplements unless your doctor directs you to do so, as they may be toxic to the liver.
- Stop smoking
- Minimize or give up alcohol completely (the CDC suggests one drink for women and two for men each day).

- Avoid using intravenous medications (drugs that enter your veins).
- Take no more prescription medication than is recommended for you.
- Obtain all advised vaccinations before international travel.
- Use safe sex practices
- Maintain a healthy weight
- Maintain a healthy cholesterol range.

Jaundice in adults is uncommon, in contrast to that in newborns. It usually goes away on its own, but if there's a medical condition causing it, your doctor might suggest treatment. See your doctor straight away if you experience any of the following symptoms of jaundice: yellowish skin or eyes, flu-like symptoms, dark urine, or stomach pain.

10.4.3. Liver Cancer

Cancer that starts in the cells of your liver is known as liver cancer. Located in the upper right section of your abdomen, beneath your diaphragm and above your stomach, is your liver, an organ the size of a football. The liver can develop into several types of cancer. Hepatocellular carcinoma is the most prevalent kind of liver cancer, and it starts in the primary hepatocyte form of liver cells. Hepatoblastoma and intrahepatic cholangiocarcinoma are two less common forms of liver cancer. Compared to cancer that starts in the liver cells, cancer that spreads to the liver occurs more frequently. Metastatic cancer, as opposed to liver cancer, is the term for cancer that starts in another part of the body, such as the colon, lung, or breast, and then spreads to the liver. This kind of cancer is called after the organ in which it first appeared; for example, cancer that starts in the colon and spreads to the liver is called metastatic colon cancer.

10.4.3.1. Classification

There are numerous subtypes of liver cancer, the most prevalent of which are listed below. Liver cancer can originate from the liver parenchyma as well as other liver structures like the bile duct, blood vessels, and immune cells (Figure 10.10).

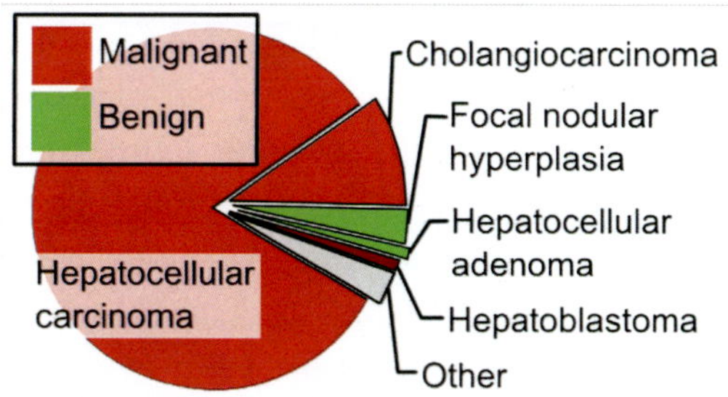

Figure 10.10. *Liver tumor types by relative incidence in adults in the United States (liver cancers in dark red color).*

Source: By Mikael Häggström, M.D. Author info- reusing images- Conflicts of interest: None Mikael Häggström, M.D. – Own work, CC0, https://commons.wikimedia.org/w/index.php?curid=87423292 hepatocellular carcinoma.

Around 75% of all primary liver cancers are hepatocellular carcinoma (HCC), the most common type of liver cancer. Hepatocytes, or malignant liver cells, give rise to HCC, a type of cancer. Globally, hepatocellular carcinoma (HCC) is ranked third in terms of cancer-related deaths. When it comes to the diagnosis of HCC, it is advised that individuals with risk factors (such as cirrhosis, known chronic liver disease, etc., ought to undergo screening ultrasonography. Patients should then have an MRI or CT scan with triple-phase contrast-enhanced if the ultrasound reveals a focal area larger than 1 centimeter in size. The Liver Imaging Reporting and Data System (LI-RADS) can then be used to diagnose HCC radiologically. A variant form of HCC exists as well, which combines elements of cholangiocarcinoma and HCC.

- **Intrahepatic Cholangiocarcinoma:** Cholangiocarcinoma and cholangiocellular cystadenocarcinoma, cancers of the bile duct, make up about 6% of primary liver cancers. An epithelial cancer of the intra-hepatic biliary tree branches is known as intrahepatic cholangiocarcinoma (CCA). The second most common cause of primary liver cancer is intrahepatic CCA. It is more common in men and typically affects people in their 60s to 70s. The following are risk factors for the development of intrahepatic CCA: exposure to trotrast and dioxins, cirrhosis, *Opisthorchus viverrini* infection, clonorchis sinensis infection, choledochal cysts, sclerosing cholangitis, and previous biliary tree procedures. Until the cancer has advanced, it usually exhibits no symptoms. Abdominal pain, fatigue, weight loss, and night sweats are some of the symptoms. Intrahepatic CCA has the potential to elevate the liver markers CA19–9, CA-125, and carcinoembryonic antigen (CEA).
- **Angiosarcoma and Hemangiosarcoma**: These are the third most common primary liver cancers, accounting for 0–1–2% of all primary liver cancers, despite being uncommon and aggressive. Hemangiosarcoma and angiosarcoma of the liver originate from the endothelium layer of blood vessels. These tumors grow quickly and spread easily, which leads to poor outcomes. Although they are difficult to diagnose, they are usually suspected based on CT or MRI scans that display focal lesions with varying signal intensities (these tumors exhibit extensive bleeding or hemorrhaging and ensuing tissue death, or necrosis). The final diagnosis is obtained through a biopsy combined with a histopathological assessment. Although the etiology is frequently unknown (idiopathic accounting for 75% of cases), exposure to chemicals like vinyl chloride, arsenic, trotrast (e.g., exposure at work). Another risk factor is radiation. These tumors are more common in males in adulthood, but more common in females in children.

The prognosis is poor even with surgery; the majority of patients do not survive for more than six months following diagnosis. Three percent of people survive for more than two years.

- **Hepatoblastoma:** Hepatoblastoma is a different kind of cancer that arises from liver cells; it is primarily caused by immature liver cells. Approximately 1 percent of all cancers in children and 79% of all primary liver cancers in people under the age of 15 are caused by this rare malignant tumor, which mostly affects children. In the right lobe, hepatoblastomas typically form.
- **Metastasis to Liver:** Many cancers that are discovered in the liver are actually metastases—cancers from other parts of the body that have traveled to the liver. Since the liver is close to many of these metabolically active, blood-rich

organs near blood vessels and lymph nodes (such as pancreatic cancer, stomach cancer, colon cancer, and carcinoid tumors, mostly of the appendix), but also from breast cancer, ovarian cancer, lung cancer, renal cancer, and prostate cancer, the gastrointestinal tract is frequently the site of origin.

- **Children:** A protocol has been developed by the Children's Oncology Group (COG) to aid in the diagnosis and treatment of liver tumors in children.

10.4.3.2. Symptoms

In the early stages of primary liver cancer, the majority of people don't exhibit any symptoms or indicators. When symptoms do materialize, they could include the following.

- Losing weight without trying
- Loss of appetite
- Upper abdominal pain
- Nausea and vomiting
- General weakness and fatigue
- Abdominal swelling
- Jaundice is the yellow discoloration of the whites of your eyes and skin.
- White, chalky stools
- **When to See a Doctor:** Schedule a visit with your physician if you notice any warning signs or symptoms that concern you.

10.4.3.3. Causes

When liver cells experience DNA alterations, or mutations, liver cancer results. The material that gives instructions for all of your body's chemical reactions is called DNA, and it is found in cells. These instructions change as a result of DNA mutations. One outcome could be the start of uncontrollably growing cells that eventually develop into a tumor, which is a mass of malignant cells. Certain cases of liver cancer, like those resulting from persistent hepatitis infections, have a known cause. However, liver cancer can also occur in healthy individuals for whom there is no known cause.

10.4.3.4. Risk Factors

The following are some factors that raise the risk of primary liver cancer.

- **Chronic HBV or HCV Infection:** Liver cancer risk is increased by persistent infection with either the hepatitis B virus (HBV) or the hepatitis C virus (HCV).
- **Cirrhosis:** The formation of scar tissue in your liver as a result of this progressive and irreversible condition raises your risk of developing liver cancer.
- Certain inherited liver diseases. Hemochromatosis and Wilson's disease are two liver conditions that can raise the risk of liver cancer.
- **Diabetes:** Compared to people without diabetes, those who have this blood sugar disorder are more likely to develop liver cancer.
- Nonalcoholic fatty liver disease. Liver cancer risk is increased by a buildup of fat in the liver.
- **Exposure to Aflatoxins:** Poisons known as aflatoxins are synthesized when molds develop on improperly stored crops. Aflatoxin contamination can occur in crops like grains and nuts, and the contaminated crops can then find their way into foods.

- **Excessive Alcohol Consumption:** Over many years, drinking more alcohol than is moderately recommended can cause irreversible liver damage and raise your risk of developing liver cancer.

10.4.3.5. Prevention

- **Reduce your Risk of Cirrhosis:** Liver cancer risk is increased by cirrhosis, which causes scarring of the liver. You have a lower chance of developing cirrhosis if you:
  - If you use alcohol at all, do so in moderation. If you decide to use alcohol, don't overindulge. This translates to women having no more than one drink per day. This translates to men having no more than two drinks per day.
  - Maintain a healthy weight. If you are currently at a healthy weight, make an effort to stay there by eating well and getting exercise most days of the week. Lower your daily calorie intake and up your exercise regimen if you need to shed some weight. Aim for a gradual weight loss of one or two pounds (0.05 to 1 kg) per week.
- **Get Vaccinated against Hepatitis B:** Getting vaccinated against hepatitis B can lower your risk of contracting the disease. Nearly everyone can receive the vaccination, including young children, the elderly, and people with weakened immune systems.
- **Take Measures to Prevent Hepatitis C:** Hepatitis C has no known vaccine, but you can lower your risk of contracting the illness.
  - Any sexual partner's health status should be known. Unless you are positive that your partner is free of HBV, HCV, or any other sexually transmitted infection, avoid having unprotected sex. Use a condom each and every time you engage in sexual activity with someone you don't know well.
  - Avoid using intravenous (IV) drugs, but if you must, make sure the needle is clean. Reducing your injection of illicit drugs can lower your risk of HIV. If you are unable to do so, however, please ensure that any needle you use is sterile and that you do not share it. Contaminated drug paraphernalia is frequently the source of an infection with hepatitis C. Use the needle-exchange services in your area, and think about getting drug treatment.
  - Make sure to choose reputable and hygienic shops when considering a piercing or tattoo. Improperly sterilized needles can potentially transmit hepatitis C. Before getting any work done, research shops in your vicinity and inquire about their safety protocols. If the staff at a particular shop is uncooperative or dismissive of your concerns, consider looking elsewhere as this may not be the best place for you.

- **Seek Treatment for Hepatitis B or C Infection:** Both hepatitis B and hepatitis C infections have treatments available. Treatment can lower the risk of liver cancer, according to research.
- **Ask your Doctor about Liver Cancer Screening:** It is not usually advised to screen for liver cancer in the general population as there is no evidence that doing so lowers the risk of dying from the disease. Individuals who have any of the following conditions, which raise the risk of liver cancer, may want to think about getting screened.
  - Hepatitis B infection
  - Hepatitis C infection
  - Liver cirrhosis

Examine the benefits and drawbacks of screening with your physician. Based on your risk, you can determine together if screening is appropriate for you. Every six months, screening usually consists of an abdominal ultrasound examination and a blood test.

10.4.3.5. Diagnosis

A number of tests and procedures are used to diagnose liver cancer.

- **Blood Tests:** Abnormal liver function may be revealed by blood tests.
- **Imaging Tests:** Your physician might advise imaging studies like an MRI, CT scan, or ultrasound.
- Removing a liver tissue sample to conduct tests. To establish a conclusive diagnosis of liver cancer, it may occasionally be required to remove a portion of liver tissue for laboratory examination.

A liver biopsy involves your doctor taking a sample of tissue from your liver by inserting a thin needle through your skin. To find cancer cells in the tissue, medical professionals examine it under a microscope in the lab. There is a chance of bleeding, bruises, and infection after a liver biopsy.

- **Determining the Extent of the Liver Cancer:** After diagnosing liver cancer, your doctor will determine the stage of the cancer to understand its extent. Staging tests such as CTs, MRIs, and bone scans help identify the size, location, and spread of the cancer. There are multiple methods for staging liver cancer, including Roman numerals I through IV and letters A through D. Your doctor will use the cancer's stage to decide the best treatment options and predict your prognosis.

10.4.3.6. Treatment

The course of treatment for primary liver cancer is determined by the disease's severity (stage), age, general health, and personal preferences.

- **Surgery:** The following procedures are used to treat liver cancer:
  - Surgery to get rid of the growth. In some cases, if your tumor is small and your liver function is good, your doctor might advise an operation to remove the liver cancer and a small amount of healthy liver tissue that surrounds it.
  - The location of the cancer within the liver, the health of your liver overall, and the function of your liver will all determine whether this is a viable option for you.

- Liver transplant surgery. Your damaged liver is removed during liver transplant surgery, and a healthy liver from a donor is used in its place. Of those with early-stage liver cancer, only a small number can undergo liver transplant surgery.

- **Localized Treatments:** Treatments for liver cancer that are applied directly to the cancer cells or the region around them are referred to as localized treatments. Options for localized liver cancer treatment include:
  - Heating cancer cells. Electric current is used in radiofrequency ablation to heat and kill cancer cells. The doctor makes tiny incisions in your abdomen and inserts one or more thin needles into them using an imaging test, like an ultrasound, as a guide. The cancer cells are destroyed by the electric current that heats the needles once they arrive at the tumor. Lasers or microwaves could be used in additional methods to heat the cancer cells.
  - Freezing cancer cells. Extreme cold is used in cryoablation to kill cancer cells. Your doctor will apply a liquid nitrogen-filled instrument called a cryoprobe directly to liver tumors during the procedure. The cryoprobe is guided by ultrasound images, which are also used to track the freezing process of the cells.
  - Injecting alcohol into the tumor. Pure alcohol is injected directly into tumors using an alcohol injection technique, either through the skin or during surgery. Alcohol kills the cancerous cells.
  - Administering chemotherapy medications intrahepaticly. One kind of chemotherapy treatment called "chemoembolization" delivers potent anti-cancer medications straight to the liver.
  - implantation of radioactive beads within the liver. Radiation-delivering tiny spheres can be inserted right into the liver to target the tumor with radiation.
- **Radiation Therapy:** X-rays and protons are two powerful energy sources that are used in this treatment to shrink tumors and kill cancer cells. Physicians carefully guide the energy toward the liver, protecting the surrounding healthy tissue in the process. If other treatments aren't working or haven't helped, radiation therapy may be an option. Radiation treatment may be able to manage the symptoms of advanced liver cancer. You lie on a table while a machine precisely targets a specific location on your body with energy beams during an external beam radiation therapy treatment. Stereotactic body radiotherapy is a specialized form of radiation therapy that involves simultaneously focusing multiple radiation beams at one specific point on your body.
- **Targeted Drug Therapy:**

Treatments with targeted drugs concentrate on particular defects found in cancer cells. Targeted drug therapies can kill cancer cells by preventing these abnormalities. There are numerous targeted medications available to treat advanced liver cancer. Certain targeted treatments are only effective in patients whose cancer cells possess specific genetic mutations. A laboratory may test your cancer cells to determine whether these medications could be beneficial to you.

- **Immunotherapy:** Immunotherapy fights cancer by boosting your immune system. The immune system that fights disease may not be able to combat your cancer because cancer cells produce proteins that cause the immune system cells to become blind. Immunotherapy functions by obstructing that procedure. Patients with advanced liver cancer are typically the only ones who receive immunotherapy treatments.
- **Chemotherapy***:* Drugs are used in chemotherapy to kill rapidly proliferating cells, including cancer cells. Chemotherapy can be taken as pills, via a vein in your arm, or a combination of both. In certain cases, chemotherapy is utilized to treat advanced liver cancer.
- **Supportive (Palliative) Care:** Palliative care refers to a specialty of medicine that aims to relieve pain and other signs and symptoms associated with a terminal illness. Palliative care specialists are a valuable resource for you, your family, and your other medical professionals. They offer an additional level of support to enhance your ongoing care. Palliative care can be utilized in conjunction with more intensive medical procedures like radiation therapy, chemotherapy, or surgery. Palliative care may help cancer patients feel better and live longer when used in conjunction with all other appropriate treatments. A group of medical professionals, nurses, and other experts in their fields offer palliative care. The goal of palliative care teams is to enhance the lives of cancer patients and their loved ones. This type of care is provided in addition to any other or curative treatments you might be receiving.

10.4.3.7. Alternative Medicine

Those with advanced liver cancer may find that alternative therapies help manage their pain. Your physician will use both medication and treatment to try to manage your pain. However, occasionally, your pain might not go away or you might wish to avoid the negative effects of painkillers.

Consult your physician about any complementary therapies that might help you manage your pain, like:

- Acupressure
- Acupuncture
- Hypnosis
- Massage
- Relaxation techniques

10.4.3.8. Coping and Support

It can be devastating to find out you have a life-threatening illness. Every individual deals with a liver cancer diagnosis in a different way. While there are no simple solutions for those suffering from liver cancer, the following advice might be helpful:

- To make decisions about your care, make sure you know enough about liver cancer. Find out everything you can from your doctor about your liver cancer, including its stage, available treatments, and, if you'd like, the prognosis. Making decisions about your course of treatment may become easier as you gain more knowledge about liver cancer.
- Maintain close relationships with family and friends. You'll be able to cope with your liver cancer if you maintain your close relationships. The practical support you'll need, like helping with housework if you're in the hospital, can be given by friends and family. Additionally, they can offer emotional support if you're feeling overtaken by cancer.
- Look for a conversation partner. Look for a sympathetic ear with whom you can share your aspirations and worries. This could be a relative or friend. Support from a clergy member, medical social worker, counselor, or cancer survivor group may also be beneficial.
- Find out from your physician about local support groups. Alternatively, consult your phone book, the library, or a cancer advocacy group like the American Cancer Society or the National Cancer Institute.
- Plan ahead for unforeseen circumstances. When you have a disease like cancer that puts your life in danger, you have to mentally prepare for the worst-case scenario. Some people find it easier to accept a life-threatening illness when they have a strong sense of faith or a connection to something bigger than themselves.

If you would like assistance planning for end-of-life care, talk to your doctor about living wills and advance directives.

10.5. Disorders in the Small Intestine

A portion of the digestive tract is the small intestine, sometimes known as the small bowel. The longest organ in the digestive system, it joins the stomach and the large intestine. Numerous illnesses can impact the small intestine and cause problems with digestion. These conditions can cause pain, bloating, constipation, and diarrhea as symptoms. Vitamins and minerals are absorbed by the small intestine during the transit of food during digestion. Small intestine issues can lead to discomfort as well as nutritional issues, which can have an impact on the body as a whole. Irritable bowel syndrome (IBS), small intestinal bacterial overgrowth (SIBO), celiac disease, and Crohn's disease are among the illnesses and ailments that can affect the small intestine.

10.5.1. Conditions That Affect the Small Intestine

Food travels down the esophagus, or food tube, into the stomach, and subsequently into the small intestine after being chewed and swallowed. It passes through the ileum, jejunum, and duodenum, the three sections of the small intestine. Food is moved along by the muscles in the small bowel walls as it breaks down and absorbs vitamins and minerals. The small intestine can experience several issues that impair its ability to properly digest food.

10.5.1.1. Crohn's Disease

One type of inflammatory bowel disease (IBD) is Crohn's disease. Both the small intestine and the remainder of the digestive tract may be impacted. It results in inflammation of the stomach wall lining. Ulcers may result from this. Difficulties with the digestive tract can also include pain, constipation, diarrhea, and poor food digestion. Symptoms of Crohn's disease can include:

- Diarrhea
- Blood in the stool
- Abdominal pain
- Reduced appetite
- Weight loss

In addition to the gastrointestinal tract, issues may also arise with the mouth, skin, eyes, and joints. Additionally, you might have full-body symptoms like exhaustion and fever.

10.5.1.2. Celiac Disease

An autoimmune condition is celiac disease. An autoimmune disease occurs when your body is attacked by your immune system by mistake. The small intestine is affected by celiac disease. Villi, which resemble tiny fingers, cover the lining of the small bowel. Nutrition is taken up by the villi from food. White blood cells attack the villi when a person with celiac disease consumes gluten, wearing them down. As a result, the small intestine is less able to absorb nutrients such as vitamins and minerals. While some people may not have any symptoms at all, those who do may have the following symptoms.

- Nausea and vomiting
- Chronic diarrhea or constipation
- Gas and bloating
- Abdominal pain
- Greasy stools that smell bad
- Lactose intolerance
- Weight loss

Additionally, especially in adults, there may be symptoms in other areas of the body such as joint pain, exhaustion, anemia (low concentration of healthy red blood cells), or other issues.

10.5.1.3. Irritable Bowel Syndrome

The intestines may be impacted by the prevalent illness known as IBS. It may result in:

- Constipation or diarrhea
- Abdominal pain
- Gas and bloating

The symptoms may be severe enough to make it difficult to go about daily activities like socializing and attending work or school.

- **Obstruction:** An obstruction or blockage in the small intestine indicates that food is being prevented from passing through. This may occur as a consequence of another illness, like Crohn's disease. Inflammation can result in scar tissue that thickens the intestinal walls or clogs the bowel. Food can become lodged in the small intestine if there is a disease known as a motility disorder that makes food move too slowly.

The following are signs of obstruction:

- Severe cramping or pain in the abdomen.
- Constipation
- Vomiting
- Swelling or fullness in the abdomen.

- Having the urge to vomit but being unable to do so.

A colon blockage may require emergency care. In a hospital, medication and fluids may be used to treat blockages. In severe situations, surgery might be required.

10.5.1.4. Small Intestine Bacterial Overgrowth (SIBO)

Microorganisms, or gut flora, are typically found in the large and small intestines and are vital to their health. It is possible for the bacteria to grow out of control. This may result in symptoms like these.

- Gas and bloating
- Constipation or diarrhea
- Weight loss

Weakness and exhaustion are among the symptoms that the illness can also produce outside of the digestive tract. It can be challenging to identify and treat SIBO. It could be linked to additional illnesses like diabetes, autoimmune diseases, or IBS.

10.5.2. Diagnosis

The symptoms may appear unrelated to digestion when small intestine issues first arise. In certain instances, getting to the core of the issue may require some time and a skilled diagnostician.

Tests that could be performed to identify issues with the small intestine include the following ones.

- **Barium Swallow and Small Bowel Follow-Through:** This test involves taking X-rays of the stomach, small intestine, and esophagus after consuming a barium contrast solution.
- **Blood Tests:** Blood tests can identify issues like anemia or vitamin deficiencies, but they cannot be used to establish a diagnosis.
- **Colonoscopy:** A colonoscopy can be used to rule out other digestive disorders, but it is primarily used to detect issues with the colon, or large intestine, as opposed to the small intestine.
- **Computed Tomography (CT) Scan:** This kind of X-ray captures fine-grained pictures of the abdominal organs.
- **Magnetic Resonance Imaging (MRI):** This test scans the abdomen with a powerful magnet to produce images.
- **Endoscopy:** The mouth, esophagus, stomach, and first segment of the small intestine are all reached by a tiny tube that has a light and camera attached to its end. It may be necessary to remove a biopsy, or a sample of tissue or fluid, for testing.
- **Breath Testing:** A breath test can identify small intestinal bacterial overgrowth or rule it out. Stool tests: Stool samples may be sent to a laboratory for analysis, which may involve a bacterial culture, to rule out issues such as infections.
- **Ultrasound:** In this test, the organs and structures in the abdomen are visible thanks to sound waves.

10.5.3. Treatment

Depending on what's causing the small bowel conditions, different treatments will be used. However, lifestyle modifications like improved diet and nutrition, lowered stress levels, or seeing a mental health professional could be a part of the treatment. Eliminating gluten is the treatment for celiac disease. Although there may be treatments for symptoms other than those related to the digestive system, there are currently no medications available to treat the condition. Treatment for Crohn's disease involves both medication and lifestyle modifications. There may be times when surgery is required, such as when the bowel narrows. Along with dietary changes and medication, lifestyle modifications are also required for the treatment of IBS. To manage their symptoms, people with IBS may also try to pinpoint the environmental cues that make them worse. Antibiotics can be used to treat SIBO to stop the bacteria's growth. Getting any related conditions under control and receiving nutritional support could be additional treatments.

A flexible tube is inserted through the nose and down into the stomach to treat bowel blockages in hospitals. This procedure is known as decompression. Surgery to remove the clogged portion of the small intestine may be required in certain situations. Small intestine illnesses and disorders are frequent. These comprise irritable bowel syndrome, small intestinal bacterial overgrowth, Crohn's disease, and celiac disease. These could result in gastrointestinal symptoms like nausea, vomiting, diarrhea, constipation, bloating, or abdominal pain. They could also result in anemia or vitamin shortages. These conditions may require several imaging tests and time to diagnose. Treatment may entail dietary and lifestyle modifications, particularly. Surgery and medication may also be used to treat the symptoms and indicators of certain conditions.

10.6. Disorders in the Colon

Numerous illnesses may impede the colon's ability to function normally. These illnesses can cause a range of symptoms, such as bleeding, infection, and perforation. They are typically categorized as benign (non-cancerous) or malignant (cancerous). Among them are a few:

- Colorectal cancer
- Colonic polyps – extra tissue that may develop into cancer is growing in the colon.
- Ulcerative colitis – stomach and colon ulcers.
- Diverticulitis – Inflammation or infection of the colon's pouches.
- Irritable bowel syndrome -a painful ailment that manifests as cramps in the abdomen and other symptoms.

Doctors may remove a portion of the colon as part of their treatment for the illness. Since the average person has 3–5 feet of colon and 8–10 feet of small bowel, removing a portion of the colon usually has no effect on the colon's ability to function normally. Depending on the illness and degree of severity, there are wide variations in treatment for colonic diseases. The course of treatment may include medication, food, and occasionally, surgery.

10.6.1. Colorectal Cancer

A growth of cells called colon cancer starts in the colon, a section of the large intestine. The first and longest segment of the large intestine is called the colon. The last segment of the digestive system is the large intestine. Food is broken down by the digestive system and used by the body. Colon cancer can strike anyone at any age, but it usually strikes older adults. Usually, it starts out as tiny cell clusters inside the colon called polyps. Although polyps don't usually cause cancer, some of them have the potential to do so in the future. Polyps frequently show no symptoms. Doctors advise routine screening tests to check for colon polyps because of this. Polyp detection and removal aids in the prevention of colon cancer. Should colon cancer arise, numerous therapies can aid in its management. Among the treatments are radiation therapy, surgery, and medications like immunotherapy, chemotherapy, and targeted therapy. Colorectal cancer is another name for colon cancer. Rectal cancer, which starts in the rectum, and colon cancer are combined under this term.

10.6.1.1. Symptoms

Many patients with colon cancer initially show no symptoms. Depending on the size and location of the cancer in the large intestine, symptoms may vary when they start.

Colon cancer symptoms can include:

- A shift in digestive patterns, such as increased frequency of diarrhea or constipation.
- Bleeding in the rectum or blood in the stool.
- Ongoing discomfort in the belly area, such as cramps, gas or pain.
- A sensation that, during a bowel movement, the bowel does not empty completely.
- Weakness or tiredness.
- Losing weight without trying.
- **When to See a Doctor:** Make an appointment with a healthcare provider if you observe persistent symptoms that cause you concern.

10.6.1.2. Causes

What causes the majority of colon cancers is unknown to doctors.

When DNA alterations occur in colon cells, colon cancer results. The instructions that tell a cell what to do are encoded in its DNA. The alterations instruct the cells to proliferate rapidly. When healthy cells naturally die as part of their lifecycle, the modifications allow the cells to live on. This results in an excess of cells. The cells may aggregate into a mass known as a tumor. Healthful bodily tissue can be invaded and destroyed by the cells. The cells may eventually separate and disperse to different areas of the body. Metastatic cancer is the term for cancer that spreads.

10.6.1.3. Risk Factors

There are several factors that could raise one's risk of colon cancer.

- **Older Age:** Any age can develop colon cancer. However, the majority of colon cancer patients are over 50. The proportion of colon cancer cases in individuals under 50 has been rising. Physicians cannot explain why.
- **Black Race:** Compared to people of other races, black Americans are more likely to develop colon cancer.
- A personal history of polyps or colorectal cancer. The risk of colon cancer is increased by prior colon cancer or colon polyps.
- **Inflammatory bowel diseases**. Inflammatory bowel diseases, which are conditions that cause swelling and pain in the intestines, can raise the risk of colon cancer. Crohn's disease and ulcerative colitis are two of these ailments.
- Inherited conditions that raise the risk of colon cancer. Certain genetic mutations that raise the risk of colon cancer are inherited. The two most prevalent hereditary syndromes that raise the risk of colon cancer are Lynch syndrome and familial adenomatous polyposis.

- **Family history of colon cancer**. The risk of colon cancer is increased if one's blood relative has the disease. The risk is higher if there are multiple family members with colon or rectal cancer.
- **High-fat, low-fiber diet**. A typical Western diet may be associated with rectal and colon cancer. This kind of diet is usually heavy in calories and fat and low in fiber. The results of this research have been inconsistent. Consuming large amounts of red and processed meat has been linked in some studies to an increased risk of colon cancer.
- Not doing regular exercise. Colon cancer is more common in those who do not exercise. Engaging in regular exercise may help reduce the risk.
- **Diabetes:** Colon cancer risk is higher in those with diabetes or insulin resistance.
- **Obesity:** Obesity raises the risk of colon cancer in people. Additionally, obesity raises the chance of dying from colon cancer.
- **Smoking**. Smokers may be at a higher risk of developing colon cancer.
- **Drinking Alcohol:** Overindulgence in alcohol consumption may raise the risk of colon cancer.
- **Cancer treatment with radiation**. The risk of colon cancer is increased by radiation therapy used to treat prior cancers that target the abdomen.

10.6.1.4. Prevention

- **Screening for Colon Cancer:** Physicians advise those with a typical risk of colon cancer to start screening for the disease at about 45 years of age. However, those who are at a higher risk ought to consider beginning screening earlier. Individuals who have a family history of colon cancer are at a higher risk. A variety of tests are employed in the screening process for colon cancer. Discuss your choices with your medical team.
- **Lifestyle Changes to Reduce the Risk of Colon Cancer:** Modest lifestyle adjustments can lower the risk of colon cancer. To reduce the likelihood of colon cancer:
    - Consume a range of whole grains, fruits, and vegetables. Vitamins, minerals, fiber, and antioxidants found in fruits, vegetables, and whole grains may help prevent cancer. To ensure you receive a range of vitamins and nutrients, choose a variety of fruits and vegetables.
    - If you use alcohol at all, do so in moderation. If you decide to consume alcohol, try to keep your intake to no more than one drink for women and two for men per day.
    - Stop smoking. Consult your medical team about quitting strategies.
    - On most days of the week, work out. Make an effort to work out for at least 30 minutes every day. If you

haven't exercised, begin slowly and increase to 30 minutes over time. Additionally, consult a medical professional before beginning an exercise regimen.

- Sustain a healthy weight. If your weight is within a healthy range, try to keep it there by eating well and exercising every day. Ask your medical team about healthy ways to reach your weight loss goals if you need to lose weight. Reduce your calorie intake and increase your physical activity to gradually lose weight.

- **Colon Cancer Prevention for People with a High Risk:** Certain medications may lower the chance of colon cancer or polyps. For example, there is evidence that regular use of aspirin or aspirin-like medications reduces the risk of polyps and colon cancer. However, it's unclear how much and for how long would be required to lower the risk of colon cancer. Daily aspirin use carries certain risks, such as bleeding in the digestive tract and ulcers. These choices are typically limited to those who have a high risk of developing colon cancer. For those with an average risk of colon cancer, these medications are not recommended due to a lack of evidence. Consult your medical team about your risk factors if you have a higher than average chance of developing colon cancer to determine whether taking preventive medication is safe for you.

10.6.1.5. Diagnosis

These are some of the tests and procedures used to diagnose colon cancer.

- **Examining the Colon's Interior with a Scope:** A long, thin, flexible tube that is connected to a monitor and video camera allows a colonoscopy to view the entire colon and rectum. A surgeon may insert surgical instruments through the tube to remove polyps and obtain tissue samples.
- **Taking a Tissue Sample Out for Analysis:** The process of taking a tissue sample for laboratory analysis is called a biopsy. The tissue sample for colon cancer is frequently taken during a colonoscopy. Occasionally, surgery is required to obtain the tissue sample. Tests conducted in the lab can determine the growth rate and cancerous nature of the cells. Additional testing may reveal more details about the cancerous cells. Your medical team makes a treatment plan and determines your prognosis based on the findings.
- **Blood Tests:** Colon cancer cannot be diagnosed by blood testing. However, blood tests can provide information about general health, including the function of the liver and kidneys. One way to check for low red blood cell counts is through a blood test. This finding could suggest that bleeding is being caused by colon cancer.

Carcinoembryonic antigen, or CEA, is a protein that is occasionally produced by colon cancers. The level of CEA can be monitored over time via blood tests. The outcome may indicate whether or not the cancer is responding to therapy. CEA blood tests may identify the recurrence of the cancer following treatment.

- **Colon Cancer Stages:** It may be necessary to do additional tests to determine the cancer's extent after a colon cancer diagnosis. This is known as the stage of cancer. When developing a treatment plan, the medical team takes the cancer's stage into account. Imaging scans of the chest, pelvis, and abdomen may be part of the staging tests. Imaging tests image the human body. They display the colon cancer's location and size. The stage of the cancer is frequently unknown to doctors until after colon cancer surgery. The range of colon cancer stages is 0 to 4. The lowest numbers indicate that all of the cancer is contained within the colon's lining. Stage 4 indicates that the cancer has progressed and has spread to different parts of the body. Metastatic cancer is the term for cancer that spreads.

10.6.1.6. Treatment

Surgery is typically required as part of colon cancer treatment to remove the cancer. Your medical team may suggest additional therapies like chemotherapy and radiation therapy. The location and stage of the cancer will determine your treatment options. When developing a treatment plan, your healthcare team also takes your preferences and general health into account.

- **Surgery for Early-stage Colon Cancer:** A very small colon cancer may be treated with a minimally invasive surgical technique like:
  - A polypectomy—the removal of polyps obtained during a colonoscopy. If the cancer is contained inside a polyp, eliminating the polyp might eradicate the cancer entirely.
  - Endoscopic removal of the mucosa. Larger polyps can be removed with this technique during a colonoscopy. The polyp and a tiny portion of the colon's lining are removed with the aid of special instruments.
  - Laparoscopic surgery is a type of minimally invasive surgery. Polyps that are too big to remove with a colonoscopy can be removed with this kind of surgery. During this process, a surgeon makes multiple tiny incisions in the abdominal wall to carry out the surgery. Through the incisions, instruments with cameras attached display the colon on a video monitor. Additionally, the surgeon might remove samples from the lymph nodes surrounding the cancer.
- **Surgery for More Advanced Colon Cancer:** A surgeon may advise the following if the cancer has spread into or through the colon:
  - Partial colectomy. Partial colectomy is the surgical term for removing a portion of the colon. The colon's cancerous portion is removed by the surgeon during this procedure. Additionally, the surgeon removes tissue from both sides of the cancer. Reconnecting the colon's or rectalhealthy sections is frequently possible. Laparoscopic surgery is a

minimally invasive method that is frequently used to perform this procedure.

- Surgery to open a channel for the body's waste to exit. After a colectomy, it is occasionally impossible to rejoin the healthy sections of the colon or rectum. A section of the remaining intestine is used by the surgeon to make an incision in the abdominal wall. The stool can be expelled from the body through this procedure, known as an ostomy, by emptying it into a bag that fits over the opening.
- Occasionally, an ostomy is placed for a brief period to allow the colon or rectum to heal from surgery. Then it's the opposite. In certain cases, the ostomy is permanent and cannot be reversed.
- Lymph node removal. During colon cancer surgery, nearby lymph nodes are typically removed and examined for cancer.

- **Surgery for Advanced Cancer:** In cases where surgical removal of the cancer is not feasible, a surgeon may opt to treat the symptoms instead of curing the cancer. Colon blockages can be removed during this procedure, which can also relieve pain and bleeding symptoms. In some cases, a healthy person's cancer has only spread to their liver or lungs. To remove the cancer, one option is surgery or other localized treatments. Chemotherapy may be applied either before or following this kind of surgery. This strategy offers a long-term chance of cancer-free living.
- **Chemotherapy:** Chemotherapy kills cancer cells with potent medications. If the colon cancer is large or has spread to the lymph nodes, chemotherapy is typically administered following surgery. Chemotherapy can eradicate cancerous cells that may remain following surgery. This lessens the possibility that the cancer will return. Before surgery, chemotherapy may also be used to reduce a large cancer so that it is easier to remove. Chemotherapy can also be used to treat colon cancer symptoms that have spread to other parts of the body or that cannot be removed surgically. It is occasionally combined with radiation treatment.
- **Radiation Therapy:** Strong energy beams are used in radiation therapy to destroy cancer cells. Protons, X-rays, and other sources are possible sources of the energy. Before surgery, radiation therapy can help a large cancer shrink so that it is easier to remove. Radiation therapy may be used to treat symptoms like pain when surgery is not an option. Some patients receive chemotherapy and radiation therapy concurrently.
- **Targeted Therapy:** Medications that target specific chemicals in cancer cells are used in targeted therapy. Targeted therapies can kill cancer cells by preventing these substances from functioning. Chemotherapy is typically given in addition to targeted therapy. Patients with

metastatic colon cancer are usually treated with targeted therapy.

- **Immunotherapy:** Immunotherapy is a medical treatment that stimulates the immune system to eliminate cancerous cells from the body. The immune system targets bacteria and other foreign cells in the body to prevent illness. Cancer cells evade the immune system to survive. Immunotherapy aids in the immune system's ability to identify and eliminate cancerous cells. Usually, immunotherapy is only used in cases of advanced colon cancer.
- **Palliative Care:** Palliative care is a specialized medical field that addresses the management of pain and other symptoms associated with life-threatening illnesses. Palliative care is provided by a group of medical specialists. Physicians, nurses, and other professionals with specialized training may be a part of the team. Enhancing the lives of those suffering from severe illnesses and their families is their main objective. Palliative care is an additional safety net for patients receiving cancer treatment. Palliative care can help cancer patients feel better and live longer when combined with all other appropriate treatments.

10.6.1.7. Coping and Support

Dealing with a cancer diagnosis can be challenging. People eventually develop coping mechanisms of their own. Until you figure out what suits you, you could attempt:

- Understand your cancer well enough to decide on a course of treatment. Find out from your medical team the kind and stage of your cancer, the side effects of your treatments, and your available options. You'll be able to participate more in decisions about your care the more informed you are. Request recommendations for additional information sources from your healthcare team, such as reliable websites.
- Keep friends and family close. Having the people you love around you can make dealing with cancer easier. If you're in the hospital, friends and family can assist you with taking care of things. Additionally, they can support you if you feel like you can't take any more.
- Find someone to talk with. Find someone who is willing to listen to you discuss your hopes and fears. This could be a relative or friend. It may also be beneficial to speak with a clergy member, medical social worker, counselor, or cancer support group.

Find out from your medical team about local support groups or get in touch with a cancer organization.

10.6.2. Colonic Polyps

A polyp is a tiny, superfluous tissue growth that frequently forms on the colon, or large intestine, lining. About 25% of men and women 45 years of age and older have colon and rectal polyps. Not every polyp will develop into cancer, and it could take a long time for a polyp to do so.

Colon and rectal polyps can occur in anybody, but they are more common in those who have the following risk factors.

- Age 45 years and older
- Colon cancer or polyps running in the family.
- A rare hereditary gene that increases the risk of polyp development in individuals.
- An inflammatory bowel condition, such as Crohn's disease or ulcerative colitis.
- High-fat, low-fiber diet
- Tobacco and alcohol use
- Little or no exercise
- Obesity

10.6.2.1. Two Types of Polyp Shapes

Polyps can grow in two different forms: sessile, or flat, and pedunculated, or having a stalk. Sessile polyps are more common than previously believed and more difficult to find during a colonoscopy. They rest level against the mucous membrane, which is the colon's lining. Pedunculated polyps are tissue growths that resemble mushrooms and adhere to the mucous membrane of the colon with a long, thin stalk.

10.6.2.2. Five Types of Polyps

Most polyps won't develop into malignancies. Some polyps have a higher chance of developing into cancer. Colonoscopy-assisted polyp removal lowers the chance of colon cancer later on. These are the most typical forms of rectal and colon polyps.

- **Adenomatous (Tubular Adenoma):** Adenomatous polyps are the most prevalent type of colon polyp, accounting for about 70% of all polyps. This kind of polyp is examined for cancer when it is discovered. Nearly all malignant polyps started off as adenomatous, but only a tiny percentage developed into cancer. Thankfully, it usually takes years for these polyps to develop into colon cancer. Regular screening will enable the removal of them before that occurs.
- **Hyperplastic:** Hyperplastic polyps are a common type of serrated polyp that is small in size and has a very low risk of developing into cancer. When found in the colon, these polyps are usually removed and tested to confirm that they are not cancerous.
- **Sessile Serrated:** Serrated polyps can have varying outcomes depending on their size and where they are located in the colon. Small serrated polyps found in the lower colon, also called hyperplastic polyps, usually do not turn cancerous. On the other hand, larger serrated polyps, often flat and hard to spot, located in the upper colon, are precancerous.
- **Inflammatory:** The majority of cases of inflammatory polyps are seen in patients with inflammatory bowel disease (IBD). Since these polyps are not actual polyps but rather form as a response to ongoing inflammation in the colon, they are also referred to as pseudopolyps. Most of the time, inflammatory polyps are benign and do not have the potential to turn into colon cancer.
- **Villous Adenoma (Tubulovillous Adenoma):** The percentage of villous or tubulovillous adenomas found during colon cancer screening is about 15%. The likelihood of this kind of polyp developing into cancer

is high. Since they are frequently sessile, removal is more challenging. While larger villous adenoma polyps may require surgery for full removal, smaller polyps may be removed during a colonoscopy. During a colonoscopy, polyps can be safely removed to stop them from developing into cancer. Large polyps might need multiple treatments, and in certain cases, surgery might be necessary to completely remove them. Consult your doctor about the appropriate test types and frequencies if you are at a higher risk of colon polyps.

10.6.2.3. Complex Polyps

Complex polyps, also known as "defiant polyps" in medical literature, are polyps that have one or more of the following characteristics: they are larger than 2 centimeters, they are in an unfavorable location or are too sessile to be removed with simpler methods, or they are just polyps that your doctor feels they cannot safely remove during a colonoscopy.

10.6.2.4. Symptoms

The majority of colon polyp patients do not exhibit any symptoms. It's possible that you won't be aware of the presence of a polyp until your doctor examines your colon.

On the other hand, some colon polyp patients might have:

- **Change in Bowel Habits:** If diarrhea or constipation persists for more than a week, it could indicate the existence of a larger colon polyp or cancer. Changes in bowel habits, however, can also be brought on by many other conditions.
- **Change in Stool Color:** Blood may appear in your stool as black particles or as red streaks. A color shift can also be brought on by specific meals, medications, or dietary supplements.
- **Iron Deficiency Anemia:** Polyp bleeding can occur gradually over time and not show up as blood in your stool. Iron deficiency anemia, which can cause fatigue and dyspnea, can be brought on by prolonged bleeding.
- **Pain:** Your bowel may become partially blocked by a large colon polyp, causing cramping pain in your abdomen.
- **Rectal Bleeding:** This may indicate the presence of colon polyps, cancer, or other disorders like hemorrhoids or small tears in the anus.
- **When to See a Doctor:** Consult your physician if you encounter:
  - Abdominal pain
  - Blood in your stool
  - a more than week-long shift in your bowel habits.

Regular polyp detection screening is recommended if:

- You're age 50 or older.
- You have a family history of colon cancer, among other risk factors. Some people who are at high risk ought to start routine screening well before they turn 50.

10.6.2.5. Causes

A healthy cell divides and grows predictably. Certain gene mutations can lead to cells proliferating even in the absence of a need for new cells. Polyps may develop in the colon and rectum as a result of these cells' ongoing growth. Anywhere in the large intestine can host polyp growth. Polyps fall into two primary categories: nonneoplastic and neoplastic. Most nonneoplastic polyps do not progress to cancer. Adenomas and serrated varieties are examples of neoplastic polyps. If given enough time to grow, adenomas have the highest chance of developing into cancer. The location and size of serrated polyps can determine whether or not they develop into cancer. The larger the polyp, the higher the risk of cancer in neoplastic polyps.

10.6.2.6. Risk Factors

Cancer and colon polyps may be brought on by the following factors.

- **Age:** Colon polyps typically affect those 50 years of age or older.
- **Suffering from inflammatory bowel diseases:** Although the polyps themselves do not pose a serious threat, having ulcerative colitis or Crohn's disease of the colon increases your overall risk of colon cancer.
- **Family History:** If you have a parent, sibling, or child with them, you have an increased risk of colon polyps or cancer. Your risk increases if a large number of your family members have them. This connection isn't inherited by some people.
- **Smoking and Excess Alcohol Use:** According to studies, individuals who consume three or more alcoholic beverages daily are more likely to develop colon polyps. It also seems that drinking alcohol and smoking together raise the risk.
- **Obesity, Lack of Exercise and Fat Intake:** If you don't exercise often, have a poor diet, and are overweight, your risk increases.
- **Race:** The risk of colon cancer is higher in Black Americans.

10.6.2.7. Hereditary Polyp Disorders

Colon polyps are rare genetic abnormalities inherited by individuals. You have a far higher chance of colon cancer if you carry one of these genes. The growth or spread of these cancers can be stopped with the aid of screening and early detection.

Colon polyps can result from the following inherited disorders.

- Hereditary nonpolyposis colorectal cancer, or Lynch syndrome. Colon polyps are rare in Lynch syndrome patients, but when they do occur, they can spread quickly and turn malignant. The most prevalent type of hereditary colon cancer is called Lynch syndrome, which is also linked to tumors in other abdominal regions.
- Familial adenomatous polyposis (FAP) is an uncommon disorder that starts in adolescence and results in the development of hundreds or even thousands of polyps in the lining of your colon. Your chance of getting colon cancer is almost 100% if the polyps are left untreated, and it usually happens before the age of 40. Your risk of FAP can be ascertained with the aid of genetic testing.
- Gardner syndrome is a kind of FAP that results in the growth of polyps in your small intestine and colon. Noncancerous tumors can also grow

in the skin, bones, and abdomen, among other areas of the body.

- MUTYH-associated polyposis (MAP) is a disorder brought on by mutations in the MYH gene that resembles FAP. Individuals with MAP frequently experience early-stage colon cancer and multiple adenomatous polyps. One way to find out if you have MAP is through genetic testing.
- Peutz-Jeghers syndrome: a disorder that typically starts with freckles appearing on the lips, gums, and feet, among other parts of the body. The intestines then begin to develop noncancerous polyps. Colon cancer is more common in those with this condition because these polyps have the potential to develop into cancer.
- Many serrated adenomatous polyps in the upper section of the colon are a symptom of serrated polyposis syndrome. These polyps could develop into cancer. They must be observed and perhaps taken out.

10.6.2.8. Complications

Certain polyps in the colon have the potential to develop into cancer. The likelihood of polyps developing into cancer decreases with the earlier they are removed.

10.6.2.9. Prevention

Regular screenings can significantly lower your risk of colon polyps and colorectal cancer. Other helpful lifestyle adjustments include:

- Adopt healthy habits. Eat a diet rich in fruits, vegetables, and whole grains while cutting back on fat. Reduce your alcohol intake and give up smoking. Continue to be physically active and keep your weight in check.
- Speak with your doctor about vitamin D and calcium. Research indicates that consuming more calcium may help stop colon adenomas from growing back. However, it's unclear if calcium offers any defense against colon cancer. According to other research, vitamin D may offer protection against colorectal cancer.
- If your risk is high, think about your options. Think about receiving genetic counseling if colon polyps run in your family. If you have been identified as having a genetic disorder that results in colon polyps, you will require routine colonoscopies beginning in your early adult years.

10.6.2.10. Diagnosis

Finding polyps before they turn malignant is made possible in large part by screening tests. In its early stages, when there is a good chance of recovery, these tests can also aid in the detection of colorectal cancer.

Screening methods include:

- **Colonoscopy:** a procedure in which your colon is examined by inserting a tiny tube into your rectum that contains a light and a camera. If polyps are discovered, your doctor may remove them right away or take tissue samples to be sent to a lab for examination.
- A test called a virtual colonoscopy looks at your colon using a CT scan. The same bowel preparations needed for a colonoscopy also apply

to virtual colonoscopies. You'll need to repeat the bowel preparation for a colonoscopy if a polyp is discovered during the scan to have it examined and removed.

- **Flexible sigmoidoscopy:** This uses a small tube with a light and camera, just like a colonoscopy, but it only looks at the sigmoid, or the last third of your colon. This screening test does not detect the majority of the colon, so certain polyps and cancers might go undetected.
- **Stool-Based Tests:** These tests look for blood in the stool or analyze the DNA in your stool to look for signs of cancer or colon polyps. A colonoscopy will be required shortly if the results of your stool test are positive.

10.6.2.11. Treatment

Most likely, your doctor will remove every polyp that is found during a bowel examination. The following are the removal options:

- **Polypectomy:** Polyps can be removed when they are smaller and in the early stages by inserting a tube into the rectum and cutting out the cancer.
- **Minimally Invasive Surgery:** Surgical removal is typically required for polyps that are too big or that cannot be safely removed during screening. This is typically accomplished by surgically removing the cancerous portion of the colon from the abdomen using a device known as a laparoscope.
- **Total Proctocolectomy:** Should you suffer from an uncommon hereditary condition like FAP, you might require surgery to remove your colon and rectum. This procedure can keep you from getting a potentially fatal cancer.
- Colostrum polyps can range in the likelihood of developing into cancer. Your polyp tissue will be examined under a microscope by a medical professional who specializes in tissue sample analysis to ascertain whether it is potentially cancerous.
- **Follow-up Care:** You have a higher chance of developing colon cancer if you have ever had an adenomatous or serrated polyp. The size, quantity, and features of the adenomatous polyps that were removed determine the degree of risk.

Polyps will require follow-up screenings. Most likely, your doctor will advise a colonoscopy:

  - If you had a single or a couple of small adenomas, in five to 10 years.
  - If you had three or four adenomas, in three to five years.
  - If you had five to ten adenomas, adenomas bigger than ten millimeters, or specific kinds of adenomas within three years.
  - If you had several adenomas, a large adenoma, or an adenoma that needed to be cut out, within six months.

- **Preparing for Your Colonoscopy:** It is imperative that you completely cleanse your colon prior to a colonoscopy. You'll probably require another colonoscopy sooner rather than later to ensure that all polyps are discovered if stool accumulates in the colon and obscures your doctor's view of the colon wall. A well-prepared colon should show up as clear liquid after bowel movements. They could have a hint of yellow or green color, depending on what liquids were consumed during preparation. Before starting your colonoscopy, you should let your provider know if you have any problems with the colon preparation or feel that you have not been completely cleaned out. Certain individuals require extra measures prior to undergoing a colonoscopy.

10.6.3. Ulcerative Colitis

An inflammatory bowel disease (IBD) called ulcerative colitis makes your digestive tract inflamed and produces ulcers or sores. The rectum and the innermost lining of your large intestine, commonly referred to as the colon, are affected by ulcerative colitis. For the majority of people, symptoms typically appear gradually as opposed to abruptly. In addition to being exhausting, ulcerative colitis occasionally results in potentially fatal complications. Although there is currently no known cure, several novel treatments can significantly lessen the disease's symptoms and induce long-term remission.

10.6.3.1. Symptoms

The location and degree of inflammation affect the symptoms of ulcerative colitis. Symptoms and indicators could be:

- Diarrhea, often with blood or pus
- A small amount of blood passing with stool is known as rectal bleeding.
- Abdominal pain and cramping
- Rectal pain
- Urgency to defecate
- Inability to defecate despite urgency
- Weight loss
- Fatigue
- Fever
- In children, failure to grow

The majority of ulcerative colitis patients experience mild to moderate symptoms. Some people experience prolonged periods of relief from ulcerative colitis. The course of the condition can vary. We refer to this as remission.

10.6.3.2. Types

Medical professionals frequently categorize ulcerative colitis based on where it occurs. Each type's symptoms frequently overlap. Ulcerative colitis comes in various forms.

- **Ulcerative Proctitis:** Only the region known as the rectum, which is closest to the anus, is inflamed. Perhaps the only indication of the illness is rectal bleeding.
- **Proctosigmoiditis:** The lower end of the colon, the rectum and sigmoid colon, are affected by inflammation. Bloody diarrhea, pain and cramping in the abdomen, and an inability to pass gas despite the strong desire to do so are some of the symptoms. We refer to this as tenesmus.
- **Left-Sided Colitis:** From the rectum, inflammation spreads to the sigmoid and lower sections of the colon. The symptoms include urgency to urinate, cramping and pain in the left side of the abdomen, and bloody diarrhea.

- **Pancolitis:** This kind frequently affects the entire colon and results in severe episodes of bloody diarrhea, exhaustion, and noticeable weight loss.
- **When to See a Doctor:** Consult your physician if your bowel habits consistently alter or if you exhibit any of the following symptoms or indicators.
  - Abdominal pain
  - Blood in your stool
  - Persistent diarrhea that is unresponsive to over-the-counter drugs.
  - Diarrhea that causes you to wake up.
  - A fever that doesn't go away after a day or two.

While ulcerative colitis is generally not life-threatening, it is a serious illness. Life-threatening complications are possible in certain cases of ulcerative colitis.

10.6.3.3. Causes

We still don't know the precise cause of ulcerative colitis. Stress and food were previously suspected. Researchers now understand that while these factors may exacerbate ulcerative colitis, they do not cause it. An immune system malfunction is one potential reason. An aberrant immune response triggers your immune system to target the cells in your digestive tract in addition to the virus or bacteria that is causing the invasion. The fact that ulcerative colitis is more common in those who have family members with the condition suggests that heredity may also be a factor. The majority of ulcerative colitis sufferers, nevertheless, do not have this family history.

10.6.3.4. Risk Factors

Males and women are affected by ulcerative colitis in roughly equal amounts. Among the risk factors are:

- **Age:** Although it can happen at any age, ulcerative colitis typically starts before the age of thirty. Some people can have the illness after the age of 60.
- **Race or Ethnicity:** Any race can contract the disease, but white people are at the highest risk. Your risk increases further if you are an Ashkenazi Jew.
- **Family History:** If you have a close relative who has the disease, like a parent, sibling, or child, your risk increases.

10.6.3.5. Complications

The following are potential ulcerative colitis side effects.

- Severe bleeding
- Severe dehydration
- A toxic megacolon, also known as a colon that is expanding quickly.
- A perforated colon, which is a hole in the colon.
- Higher risk of thrombosis in arteries and veins.
- Irritation of the eyes, joints, and skin.
- A higher chance of colon cancer.
- Bone loss, also called osteoporosis

10.6.3.6. Diagnosis

To definitively diagnose ulcerative colitis, endoscopic procedures combined with tissue biopsy are the only method available. Tests of different kinds can assist in ruling out consequences or other inflammatory bowel diseases, like Crohn's disease. You might undergo one or more of the following examinations and procedures to help confirm an ulcerative colitis diagnosis:

- Lab Tests
    - **Blood Tests:** Blood tests may be recommended by your healthcare provider to screen for infection or inflammation, or to check for anemia, a condition in which the body lacks enough red blood cells to supply enough oxygen to the tissues.
    - **Stool Studies:** Certain proteins or white blood cells in your stool may be an indication of ulcerative colitis. A stool sample can also be used to rule out other conditions, such as infections brought on by viruses, bacteria, or parasites.
- Endoscopic Procedures
    - **Colonoscopy:** During this examination, a thin, flexible, lighted tube with a camera on the end can be used to view your entire colon by your provider. Samples of tissue are removed during the process for examination in a lab. We call this a tissue biopsy. A tissue sample is required for diagnosis.
    - **Flexible Sigmoidoscopy:** Your doctor will examine the rectum and sigmoid colon—the lower end of your colon—using a thin, flexible, lighted tube. A partial colonoscopy may not be the best option if your colon is extremely inflammatory.
- Imaging Procedures
    - **X-ray:** Your doctor might perform a routine abdominal X-ray if your symptoms are severe to rule out potentially dangerous complications like a megacolon or a perforated colon.
    - **CT Scan:** If a complication from ulcerative colitis is suspected, a CT scan of your abdomen or pelvis may be conducted. Additionally, a CT scan can show how much of the colon is inflamed.
    - CT enterography and MR enterography are noninvasive tests that may be recommended to rule out inflammation in the small intestine. These tests are more effective at detecting bowel inflammation than traditional imaging tests. MR enterography is a radiation-free option.

10.6.3.7. Treatment

Treatment for ulcerative colitis typically consists of either medication therapy or surgery. Treatment for ulcerative colitis may involve using a variety of drug types. The kind you take will be determined by how serious your illness is. Some people may not benefit from the same medications that work well for others. It might take some time to locate a medicine that works for you. Additionally, you must consider the advantages and disadvantages of any course of treatment because certain drugs have harmful side effects.

- **Anti-inflammatory Medications:** For the majority of patients with ulcerative colitis, anti-inflammatory drugs are a suitable initial course of treatment. These consist of:
    - **5-aminosalicylates:** Sulfasalazine (Azulfidine), mesalamine (Delzicol, Rowasa, and other brands), balsalazide (Colazal), and olsalazine (Dipentum) are a few examples of this kind of drug. Depending on the area of your colon that is affected, the medication you take and how you take it (by mouth, as an enema, or as a suppository) will vary.
    - **Corticosteroids:** These drugs—budesonide and prednisone, among others—are usually saved for moderate-to-severe ulcerative colitis that is resistant to other forms of therapy. The immune system is suppressed by corticosteroids. They are rarely used for an extended period of time because of the side effects.
    - **Immune System Suppressors:** These drugs also lessen inflammation, but they accomplish this by stifling the immune system reaction that initiates inflammation. Some people respond better to a combination of these drugs than to any one of them by itself.

Immunosuppressant medications include:

- Mercaptopurine (Purinethol, Purixan) and azathioprine (Azasan, Imuran). These immunosuppressants are frequently used to treat inflammatory bowel disease. They are frequently taken in conjunction with drugs referred to as biologics. When taking them, you must closely monitor your healthcare provider and get regular blood work done to check for potential side effects, such as effects on the pancreas and liver.
- Cyclosporine (Sandimmune, Neoral, and Gengraf). Usually, this drug is saved for those who haven't responded well to previous ones. Cyclosporine should not be used long-term due to the possibility of major side effects.
- "Small molecule" medicationsOrally administered medications, commonly referred to as small molecules, have recently become accessible for the treatment of IBD. These consist of ozanimod (Zeposia), upadacitinib (Rinvoq), and tofacitinib (Xeljanz). When alternative therapies prove ineffective, these medications might be useful. The principal adverse effects are an elevated risk of blood clots and shingles infection.

The U.S. Food and Drug Administration (FDA) has warned against using tofacitinib because early research indicates that using this drug may increase the risk of cancer and major heart problems. If you are taking tofacitinib for ulcerative colitis, consult your doctor before stopping the medication.

- **Biologics:** These treatments focus on immune system-produced proteins. The following categories of biologics are used to treat ulcerative colitis:
    - **Infliximab (Remicade), Adalimumab (Humira) and Golimumab (Simponi):**

These drugs, known as tumor necrosis factor (TNF) inhibitors, function by preventing your immune system from producing a certain protein. These are for patients with severe ulcerative colitis who are not responsive to other treatments or who are unable to tolerate them. Another name for TNF inhibitors is a biologic.

- **Vedolizumab (Entyvio):** For those with ulcerative colitis who are unable to respond to or tolerate other treatments, this medication is approved for use. It functions by preventing proliferating cells from accessing the site of inflammation.
- **Ustekinumab (Stelara):** For those with ulcerative colitis who are unable to respond to or tolerate other treatments, this medication is approved for use. It functions by obstructing an alternative inflammatory protein.

- **Other Medications:** To treat certain ulcerative colitis symptoms, you might require additional medication. Before taking any over-the-counter medication, always consult your doctor. Your physician might suggest any one or all of the following.
  - **Anti-diarrheal Medications:** Imodium A-D, or loperamide, may work well for severe diarrhea. Do not take anti-diarrheal medications if you have ulcerative colitis without first consulting your healthcare provider. These drugs may make an enlarged colon (toxic megacolon) more likely.
  - **Pain relievers:** Your doctor might suggest acetaminophen (Tylenol, etc.) for mild pain, but not ibuprofen (Advil, Motrin IB, etc.), naproxen sodium (Aleve), or diclofenac sodium, as these medications can exacerbate symptoms and worsen the condition.
  - **Antispasmodics:** Antispasmodic medications are occasionally prescribed by medical professionals to treat cramps.
  - **Iron Supplements:** You might be prescribed iron supplements if you have chronic intestinal bleeding, which can lead to iron deficiency anemia.
- **Surgery:** A protocolectomy, which removes your entire colon and rectum, is a surgical procedure that can treat ulcerative colitis. This usually entails a surgical procedure known as ileoanal anastomosis (J-pouch) surgery. With this process, wearing a bag to collect stool is no longer necessary. Your surgeon uses the end of your small intestine to create a pouch. After that, the pouch is fastened directly to your anus, enabling you to discharge waste normally. It might take two or three steps to finish this surgery. Sometimes it is not possible to use a pouch. Rather, doctors make an ileal stoma, a permanent incision in your abdomen, through which stool is passed and collected in a bag that is attached.

- **Cancer Surveillance:** Due to your higher risk, you will require more frequent screenings for colon cancer. The recommended timetable will vary depending on where and how long you have had your illness. Proctitis, another name for rectum inflammation, does not put a person at higher risk of developing colon cancer. You will need a surveillance colonoscopy every one to two years if your disease extends beyond your rectum. If the majority of the colon is affected, this can start as soon as eight years after the initial diagnosis or, if the colon's left side is the only part affected, 15 years after the diagnosis.

10.6.3.8. Lifestyle and Home Remedies

When you have ulcerative colitis, you could occasionally feel powerless. However, making dietary and lifestyle adjustments may help manage your symptoms and increase the interval between flare-ups. There is insufficient proof to conclude that inflammatory bowel disease is genuinely brought on by food. However, some foods and drinks may make your symptoms worse, particularly if you're having a flare-up. Maintaining a food journal can help you stay on top of your eating habits and emotional state. Try cutting out certain foods if you find that they are making your symptoms worse.

The following general dietary recommendations could aid in the management of your condition:

- **Limit Dairy Products:** Many people with inflammatory bowel disease find that cutting back or giving up dairy products helps with symptoms like gas, diarrhea, and abdominal pain. You might not be able to digest the lactose (milk sugar) found in dairy products because you are lactose intolerant. Utilizing an enzyme supplement like Lactaid could also be beneficial.
- **Eat Small Meals:** Eating five or six small meals a day instead of two or three larger ones might make you feel better.
- **Drink Plenty of Liquids:** Aim to consume a lot of liquids each day. The best is water. Carbonated drinks often result in gas, while alcohol and caffeine stimulate the intestines and can exacerbate diarrhea.
- **Talk to a dietitian:** Speak with a qualified dietitian if you start to lose weight or if your diet has become extremely restrictive.
- **Stress:** While stress does not directly cause inflammatory bowel disease, it can exacerbate symptoms and possibly lead to flare-ups.

To help control stress, try:

- **Exercise:** Exercise, even modest exercise, can help relieve depression, lower stress levels, and improve bowel movements. Consult your healthcare provider about the best exercise regimen for you.
- **Biofeedback:** With the aid of a feedback machine, this stress-reduction method lowers heart rate and eases tense muscles. The intention is to assist you in achieving a relaxed state so that managing stress won't be as difficult.
- **Regular Relaxation and Breathing Exercises:** Breathing and relaxation techniques are good ways to deal

with stress. Yoga and meditation classes are available, or you can practice at home with books, CDs, or DVDs.

10.6.3.9. Alternative Medicine

Complementary and alternative medicine has been used by many patients with digestive disorders. Few well-conducted studies, nevertheless, have demonstrated the efficacy and safety of complementary and alternative medicine. There is some evidence, albeit weak, that taking probiotics in addition to other medications may be beneficial, though this has not been scientifically proven.

10.6.4. Diverticulitis

Diverticula are tiny, protruding pouches that can develop in the stomach lining. The lower portion of the large intestine is where they are most frequently found (colon). Diverticula are common and rarely cause issues, especially after the age of forty. Diverticulosis is the term for diverticula presence. Diverticulitis is the term for the condition that results from inflammation and, in some cases, infection of one or more of the pouches. Severe abdominal pain, fever, nausea, and a noticeable alteration in bowel habits are all possible symptoms of diverticulitis. Antibiotics, dietary modifications, and rest are all effective treatments for mild diverticulitis. Surgery might be necessary for diverticulitis that is severe or recurrent.

10.6.4.1. Symptoms

The signs and symptoms of diverticulitis include:

- Pain that may last for several days and be continuous. The pain typically occurs on the lower left side of the abdomen. On the other hand, the right side of the abdomen can occasionally hurt more, particularly in those who identify as Asian.
- Nausea and vomiting.
- Fever.
- Abdominal tenderness.
- Constipation or, less commonly, diarrhea.
- **When to See a Doctor:** If you experience persistent, unexplained stomach pain, see a doctor. This is especially important if you also have a fever, constipation, or diarrhea.

10.6.4.2. Causes

Diverticula typically form when your colon's naturally weak spots buckle under pressure. As a result, marble-sized pouches poke through the wall of the colon. When diverticula rupture, inflammation and occasionally infection follow, leading to diverticulitis.

10.6.4.3. Risk Factors

There are several things that can make you more likely to get diverticulitis:

- **Aging:** Diverticulitis is more common as people age.
- **Obesity:** Your risk of diverticulitis increases if you are significantly overweight.
- **Smoking:** Diverticulitis is a condition that smokers are more likely to get than nonsmokers.
- **Lack of Exercise:** Vigorous exercise seems to reduce the risk of diverticulitis.
- **A Diet High in Animal Fat and Low in Fiber**: It appears that a low-fiber diet plus a high animal fat intake increases risk, though it's unclear how low fiber works on its own.

- **Certain Medications:** Diverticulitis is linked to several medications, including steroids, opioids, and nonsteroidal anti-inflammatory drugs like naproxen sodium (Aleve) and ibuprofen (Advil, Motrin IB, and others).

10.6.4.4. Complications

Complications from acute diverticulitis can occur in about 25% of cases and can include:

- An abscess is the result of pus building up in the pouch.
- A bowel obstruction brought on by scarring.
- A fistula, or abnormal passageway, connecting the bowel and other organs or between sections of the bowel.
- If the inflamed or infected pouch bursts and spills intestinal contents into your abdominal cavity, you may develop peritonitis. As a medical emergency, peritonitis needs to be treated right away.

10.6.4.5. Prevention

To help prevent diverticulitis:

- **Exercise Regularly:** Exercise lowers colon pressure and encourages regular bowel movements. On most days, try to get in at least 30 minutes of exercise.
- **Eat More Fiber:** Diverticulitis risk is reduced by eating a diet high in fiber. Fresh fruits and vegetables, whole grains, and other foods high in fiber help soften waste and speed up its passage through your colon. There is no link between eating nuts and seeds and getting diverticulitis.
- **Drink Plenty of Fluids:** Fiber increases the amount of soft, bulky waste in your colon by absorbing water. However, fiber can cause constipation if you don't drink enough water to replace what is absorbed.
- **Avoid Smoking:** Diverticulitis is linked to a higher risk of smoking.

10.6.4.6. Diagnosis

Usually, an acute attack is used to diagnose diverticulitis. Since pain in the abdomen can be a sign of several issues, your doctor must rule out other possible reasons for your symptoms. During the initial physical examination, your doctor will feel for any tenderness in your abdomen. To rule out pelvic disease, women typically undergo a pelvic examination as well. The following tests are probably going to be performed after that:

- Tests on the blood and urine to look for infection symptoms.
- A pregnancy test to rule out pregnancy as the reason for stomach pain in women who are fertile.
- A test for liver enzymes to rule out liver-related causes of pain in the abdomen.
- A stool test to exclude infection in individuals experiencing diarrhea.
- A CT scan, which can confirm a diverticulitis diagnosis and show inflamed or infected pouches. Additionally, CT can help determine how severe diverticulitis is and direct treatment.

10.6.4.7. Treatment

The severity of your symptoms and signs will determine how you are treated.

- Uncomplicated Diverticulitis
  - You might receive care at home if your symptoms are not too severe. Your physician may advise you to:
  - Antibiotics to treat infection, though new guidelines suggest they might not be necessary in very mild cases.
  - A few days of only drinking liquids as your colon heals. You can progressively include more solid food in your diet as your symptoms get better.

For the most part, this treatment works for patients with simple diverticulitis.

- **Complicated Diverticulitis:** You will most likely need to be admitted to the hospital if you have a severe attack or other health issues. Typically, treatment entails:
  - Intravenous antibiotics
  - The insertion of a tube to drain any abscess that may have developed in the abdomen.
  - Surgery

To treat diverticulitis, you probably need surgery if:

- A bowel abscess, fistula, obstruction, or puncture (perforation) in the bowel wall are examples of complications.
- You have experienced episodes of simple diverticulitis on several occasions.
- Your immune system is compromised.
- There are two main types of surgery:
- Primary bowel resection. Your intestine is surgically divided into healthy and diseased segments, and the healthy segments are then rejoined (anastomosis). You can now have regular bowel movements as a result. Your options for surgery are open or minimally invasive (laparoscopic), depending on the degree of inflammation.
- Bowel resection with colostomy. The surgeon will perform a colostomy if your inflammation is too great for your colon and rectum to be rejoined. The healthy portion of your colon is attached to an opening (stoma) in your abdominal wall. Trash enters a bag through the opening. The bowel can be reconnected and the colostomy reversed once the inflammation has subsided.
- **Follow-up Care:** Six weeks after you recover from diverticulitis, your doctor might advise a colonoscopy, particularly if you haven't had one in the past year. It doesn't seem that diverticular disease and colon or rectal cancer are related. However, a colonoscopy, which carries some risk when performed during an episode of diverticulitis, can rule out colon cancer as the reason for your symptoms. Your doctor might advise surgery following a successful course of treatment to shield you from diverticulitis in the future. Surgery is a personal choice that is frequently determined by the frequency of attacks and the presence or absence of complications.

10.6.4.8. Alternative Medicine

Certain experts speculate that a deficiency of beneficial bacteria in the colon may be the cause of diverticulitis. Probiotics, which are meals or supplements containing good bacteria, are occasionally recommended as a diverticulitis preventive measure. However, there isn't any scientific proof for that advice.

A Closer Look

Research in Irritable Bowel Syndrome

It has been discovered that the diversity and quantity of Bacteroidetes microbiota are reduced in individuals with IBS. Based on initial research, fecal microbiota transplantation appears to be a very effective treatment for irritable bowel syndrome (IBS), with a "cure" rate of between 36 and 60% and remission of core symptoms lasting for nine to nineteen months after the procedure. Probiotic bacterial strain treatment has proven to be successful, but not all microbial strains have the same beneficial effects, and in some cases, negative side effects have been reported.

The usefulness of mesalazine (5-aminosalicylic acid) in the treatment of IBS is becoming more and more evident. Mesalazine is an anti-inflammatory medication that has been shown to dramatically lower immune-mediated inflammation in the intestines of IBS patients. This improvement in intestinal inflammation leads to a better sense of overall wellness and a reduction in IBS symptoms. Additionally, mesalazine therapy has been shown to aid in the normalization of the gut flora, which is frequently aberrant in IBS patients. It's possible that mesalazine's therapeutic advantages stem from enhanced epithelial barrier performance. It is not possible to advise treatment based on abnormally elevated IgG antibodies.

Intestinal physiology and visceral sensitivity have been found to differ in IBS. When comparing IBS to controls, there was no mucosal barrier reinforcement in response to oral 5-HTP. Those with IBS/IBD are less likely than those with upper functional gastrointestinal disease and healthy populations to be HLA DQ2/8 positive. Research on the effectiveness of mast cell-directed therapies for irritable bowel syndrome is still ongoing.

Summary

- Esophageal disorders affect your esophagus, the tube that carries food from your mouth to your stomach. The most common type is GERD. Disorders like GERD, achalasia and Barrett's esophagus cause heartburn or swallowing problems and increase your risk for esophageal cancer.
- Your stomach is an organ between your esophagus and small intestine. It is where the digestion of protein begins. The stomach has three tasks. It stores swallowed food. It mixes the food with stomach acids. Then it sends the mixture onto the small intestine.
- The pancreas is a gland behind your stomach and in front of your spine. It produces juices that help break down food and hormones that help control blood sugar levels. Problems with the pancreas can lead to many health problems.
- Pancreatitis is inflammation of the pancreas. Inflammation is an immune system activity that can cause swelling, pain, and changes in how an organ or tissues work. The pancreas is a long, flat gland that's tucked behind the stomach.
- The liver has many diverse functions related to hepatic blood flow; protein, carbohydrate, and fat metabolism; detoxification and excretion of drugs and toxins; and formation and elimination of bile.
- The small intestine, also called the small bowel, is part of the digestive tract. This organ connects the stomach and the large intestine and is the longest part of the digestive system. Many conditions can interfere with digestion and affect the small intestine. Pain, bloating, constipation, and diarrhea may occur as symptoms of these disorders.
- Several diseases can interfere with the normal functioning of the colon. These diseases can have various effects and are traditionally classified as benign (non-cancerous) or malignant (cancerous) and can cause various symptoms including bleeding, infection, and perforation.
- Colon cancer is a growth of cells that begins in a part of the large intestine called the colon.

References

1. Achkasov, E., Pugaev, A., Zabelin, M., & Posudnevskiy, V. (2019). Acute pancreatitis: clinic, diagnosis, treatment. INFRA-M Academic Publishing LLC. http://dx.doi.org/10.12737/995531.
2. Andresen, V., Banerji, V., Hall, G., Lass, A., & Emmanuel, A. V. (2018). The patient burden of opioid-induced constipation: New insights from a large, multinational survey in five European countries. *United European Gastroenterology Journal, 6*(8), 1254–1266. doi:10.1177/2050640618786145.
3. Asnacios, A., Fartoux, L., Romano, O., et al. (2008). Gemcitabine plus oxaliplatin (GEMOX) combined with cetuximab in patients with progressive advanced stage hepatocellular carcinoma: Results of a multicenter phase 2 study. *Cancer, 112*, 2733–2739.
4. Brandi, G., de Rosa, F., Agostini, V., et al. (2013). Metronomic capecitabine in advanced hepatocellular carcinoma patients: a phase II study. *Oncologist, 18*(12), 1256–1257. doi:10.1634/theoncologist.2013-0327.

5. Bruix, J., & Sherman, M. (2005). Management of hepatocellular carcinoma. *Hepatology, 42*, 1208–1230.

6. Bruix, J., Tak, W. Y., Gasbarrini, A., et al. (2013). Regorafenib as second-line therapy for intermediate or advanced hepatocellular carcinoma: multicentre, open-label, phase II safety study. *European Journal of Cancer, 49*(16), 3412–3419. doi:10.1016/j.ejca.2013.05.002.

7. Camilleri, M. (2021). Gastrointestinal motility orders in neurologic disease. *Journal of Clinical Investigation*, 2021 Feb 15;131(4):e143771, doi:10.1172/JCI143771.

8. El-Serag, H. B. (2011). Hepatocellular carcinoma. *New England Journal of Medicine, 365*, 1118–1127.

9. Enck, P., Aziz, Q., Barbara, G., et al. (2016). Irritable bowel syndrome. *Nature Reviews Disease Primers, 2*, 16014. doi:10.1038/nrdp.2016.14.

10. Fikree, A. (2019). Scleroderma and other connective tissue disorders. *Medicine, 47*(7), 460–465. doi: 10.1016/j.mpmed.2019.04.012.

11. Fong, Y., Dupey, D. E., Feng, M., & Abou-Alfa, G. (2015). Cancer of the liver. In V. T. DeVita, T. S. Lawrence, & S. A. Rosenberg (Eds.), *DeVita, Hellman, and Rosenberg's Cancer: Principles and Practice of Oncology* (10th ed., pp. 696–714). Lippincott Williams & Wilkins.

12. Forner, A., Llovet, J. M., & Bruix, J. (2012). Hepatocellular carcinoma. *The Lancet, 379*, 1245–1255.

13. Gisser, J. M., & Gariepy, C. E. (2017). Genetics of motility disorders: Gastroesophageal reflux, triple A syndrome, Hirschsprung disease, and chronic intestinal pseudo-obstruction. In *Pediatric Neurogastroenterology*. doi:10.1007/978-3-319-43268-7_18.

14. Graf, H., Jüngst, C., Straub, G., et al. (2008). Chemoembolization combined with pravastatin improves survival in patients with hepatocellular carcinoma. *Digestion, 78*, 34–38.

15. Grammatikopoulos, T. (2018). *The Pancreas*. Oxford University Press. http://dx.doi.org/10.1093/med/9780198759928.003.0050.

16. Hassan, M. M., Spitz, M. R., Thomas, M. B., et al. (2008). Effect of different types of smoking and synergism with hepatitis C virus on risk of hepatocellular carcinoma in American men and women: Case-control study. *International Journal of Cancer, 123*, 1883–1891.

17. Heo, J., Reid, T., Ruo, L., et al. (2013). Randomized dose-finding clinical trial of oncolytic immunotherapeutic vaccinia JX-594 in liver cancer. *Nature Medicine, 19*(3), 329–336. doi:10.1038/nm.3089.

18. Hoshida, Y., Villanueva, A., Kobayashi, M., et al. (2008). Gene expression in fixed tissues and outcome in hepatocellular carcinoma. *New England Journal of Medicine, 359*, 1995–2004.

19. Howlader, N., Noone, A. M., Krapcho, M., et al. (Eds.). (2012). SEER Cancer Statistics Review, 1975-2009 (Vintage 2009 Populations). National Cancer Institute. Retrieved from: http://seer.cancer.gov/csr/1975_2009_pops09/ (accessed on 23 May 2024).

20. Ishizuka, M., Kubota, K., Shimoda, M., Kita, J., Kato, M., Park, K. H., & Shiraki, T. (2012). Effect of menatetrenone, a vitamin k2 analog, on recurrence of hepatocellular carcinoma after surgical resection: a prospective randomized controlled trial. *Anticancer Research, 32*(12), 5415–5420.

21. Jemal, A., Bray, F., Center, M. M., et al. (2011). Global cancer statistics. *CA: A Cancer Journal for Clinicians, 61*, 69–90.

22. Jeon, H. H., Kim, J. H., Youn, Y. H., Park, H., & Conklin, J. L. (2017). Clinical characteristics of patients with untreated achalasia. *Journal of Neurogastroenterology and Motility, 23*(3), 378–384. doi:10.5056/jnm16177.

23. Mayerle J, Stier A, Lerch MM, Heidecke CD. Chronische Pankreatitis. Diagnostik und Therapie [Chronic pancreatitis. Diagnosis and treatment]. Chirurg. 2004 Jul;75(7):731-47; quiz 748.

24. Kim, Y. S., Song, B. K., Oh, J. S., & Woo, S. S. (2014). Aerobic exercise improves gastrointestinal motility in psychiatric inpatients. *World Journal of Gastroenterology, 20*(30), 10577–10584. doi:10.3748/wjg.v20.i30.10577.

25. Krishnasamy, S., & Abell, T. L. (2018). Diabetic gastroparesis: Principles and current trends in management. *Diabetes Therapy, 9*(Suppl 1), 1–42. doi:10.1007/s13300-018-0454-9.

26. Lee, P.J., Papachristou, G.I. Management of Severe Acute Pancreatitis. Curr Treat Options Gastro 18, 670–681 (2020).

27. Lencioni, R., & Crocetti, L. (2012). Local-regional treatment of hepatocellular carcinoma. *Radiology, 262*, 43–58.

28. Lencioni, R., Chen, X. P., Dagher, L., & Venook, A. P. (2010). Treatment of intermediate/advanced hepatocellular carcinoma in the clinic: How can outcomes be improved? *The Oncologist, 15*(suppl 4), 42–52.

29. Lewandowski, R. J., Geschwind, J. F., Liapi, E., & Salem, R. (2011). Transcatheter intraarterial therapies: Rationale and overview. *Radiology, 259*, 641–657.

30. Llovet, J. M., Ricci, S., Mazzaferro, V., et al. (2008). Sorafenib in advanced hepatocellular carcinoma. *New England Journal of Medicine, 359*, 378–390.

31. Maheshwari, S., Sarraj, A., Kramer, J., & El-Serag, H. B. (2007). Oral contraception and the risk of hepatocellular carcinoma. *Journal of Hepatology, 47*, 506–513.

32. M.W. Büchler; W. Uhl; P. Malfertheiner; M.G. Sarr, (2004), Diseases of the Pancreas: Acute Pancreatitis, Chronic Pancreatitis, Neoplasms of the Pancreas, S.Karger AG, DOI: https://doi.org/10.1159/isbn.978-3-318-01001-5.

33. Marrero, J. A., Fontana, R. J., Fu, S., et al. (2005). Alcohol, tobacco and obesity are synergistic risk factors for hepatocellular carcinoma. *Journal of Hepatology, 42*, 218–224.

34. Miyake, Y., Kobashi, H., & Yamamoto, K. (2009). Meta-analysis: The effect of interferon on development of hepatocellular carcinoma in patients with chronic hepatitis B virus infection. *Journal of Gastroenterology, 44*, 470–475.

35. Narayanan M, Reddy KM, Marsicano E. Peptic Ulcer Disease and Helicobacter pylori infection. Mo Med. 2018 May-Jun;115(3):219-224.

36. Patil, A. D. (2014). Link between hypothyroidism and small intestinal bacterial overgrowth. *Indian Journal of Endocrinology and Metabolism, 18*, 307–309. doi:10.4103/2230-8210.131155.

37. Schlosser, B., Stein, A., Neuhaus, R., et al. (2012). Liver transplant from a donor with occult HEV infection induced chronic hepatitis and cirrhosis in the recipient. *Journal of Hepatology, 56*(2), 500–502.

38. Tilghman, J. M., Ling, A. Y., Turner, T. N., et al. (2019). Molecular genetic anatomy and risk profile of Hirschsprung's disease. *New England Journal of Medicine, 380*(15), 1421–1432. doi:10.1056/NEJMoa1706594.

39. Tytgat GN., Van der Hulst RW. (1996) Helicobacter pylori and peptic ulcer disease. Scand J Gastroenterol Suppl. 1996;220:10-8.

INDEX

F

G

H

I

U

V

X

Z

FSC
www.fsc.org
MIX
Papier | Fördert gute Waldnutzung
FSC® C083411

Kolibri 360 GmbH
Ferdinand-Jühlke-Straße 7
99095 Erfurt, Deutschland
produktsicherheit@kolibri360.de